PREVENTION OF
ISCHEMIC HEART DISEASE
Principles and Practice

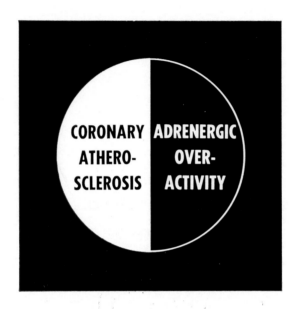

Behold the moon up there.
Half black it seems to be,
And yet it's round and fair.
Thus are we oft inclined
To scoff in our mind
At what the eyes don't see.

Matthias Claudius
(1740-1815)

PREVENTION OF
ISCHEMIC HEART DISEASE

Principles and Practice

Compiled and Edited by

WILHELM RAAB, M.D.

Emeritus Professor of Experimental Medicine
University of Vermont, College of Medicine
Burlington, Vermont

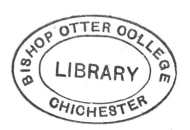
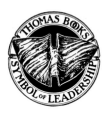

THOMAS BOOKS
SYMBOL OF LEADERSHIP

CHARLES C THOMAS • **PUBLISHER**
Springfield • Illinois • U.S.A.

Published and Distributed Throughout the World by
CHARLES C THOMAS • PUBLISHER
BANNERSTONE HOUSE
301-327 East Lawrence Avenue, Springfield, Illinois, U.S.A.

NATCHEZ PLANTATION HOUSE
735 North Atlantic Boulevard, Fort Lauderdale, Florida, U.S.A.

© *1966, by* CHARLES C THOMAS • PUBLISHER

Library of Congress Catalog Card Number: 66-16818

With THOMAS BOOKS *careful attention is given to all details of
manufacturing and design. It is the Publisher's desire to present books
that are satisfactory as to their physical qualities and artistic possibilities
and appropriate for their particular use.* THOMAS BOOKS *will be true
to those laws of quality that assure a good name and good will.*

LIST OF CONTRIBUTORS

Jiřina Adamírová, M.P.E., Assistant, School of Mathematics and Physics, Institute of Sports Medicine, Chair of Physical Education, Charles University, Prague, Czechoslovakia.

Claude C. Allard, Ph.D., Chief, Department of Biochemistry and Epidemiology, Institute of Cardiology of Montreal, Montreal, Canada.

Jan Badal, M.D., Docent, Director, Harvey Institute, Františkovy Lázně, Czechoslovakia.

Eörs Bajusz, M.D., Ph.D., Assistant Professor, Department of Pathology, University of Montreal, Montreal, Canada; Research Associate, Division of Experimental Medicine, University of Vermont, Burlington, Vermont, USA.

Peter Beckmann, M.D., Medical Director, Reconditioning Center Ohlstadt of the Unterfranken Regional Insurance Organization, German Federal Republic.

Samuel Bellet, M.D., Professor of Clinical Cardiology, Director, Division of Cardiology, Philadelphia General Hospital, University of Pennsylvania, Philadelphia, Pennsylvania, USA.

David Berkson, M.D., Staff Member, Division of Adult Health and Aging, Chicago Board of Health, Chicago, Illinois, USA.

Maria Blohmke, M.D., Institute for Social and Work Medicine, University of Heidelberg, Heidelberg, German Federal Republic.

Edward N. Brandt, M.D., Ph.D., Assistant Professor of Medical Biomathematics, Biostatistical Unit and Medical Research Computer Center, Department of Preventive Medicine and Public Health, University of Oklahoma Medical Center, Oklahoma City, Oklahoma, USA.

Daniel Brunner, M.D., Professor, Head of Donolo Institute of Physiological Hygiene, Tel Aviv University, Jaffa, Israel.

George E. Burch, M.D., Professor, Director, Department of Medicine, Tulane University, New Orleans, Louisiana, USA.

Frances Burkey, R.N., Research Assistant, Heart Disease Control Program, Chicago Board of Health, Chicago, Illinois, USA.

Gaston Choquette, M.D., Coordinator of Research Department, Institute of Cardiology of Montreal, Montreal, Canada.

Joseph Chrástek, M.D., Assistant, Institute of Sports Medicine, Medical School, Chair of Physical Education, Charles University, Prague, Czechoslovakia.

George J. Christakis, M.D., Adjunct Assistant Professor of Clinical Nutrition, Columbia University; Director, Bureau of Nutrition, Department of Health, City of New York, New York, USA.

Donald B. Cohen, M.D., Research Internist, Heart Disease Control Program, Chicago Board of Health, Chicago, Illinois, USA.

Thomas K. Cureton, Ph.D., Professor of Physical Education; Director of Physical Fitness Laboratory, University of Illinois, Urbana, Illinois, USA.

Paul David, M.D., Director, Institute of Cardiology of Montreal, Montreal, Canada.

Thomas R. Dawber, M.D., Medical Director, Heart Disease Epidemiology Study, National Heart Institute, Framingham, Massachusettes, USA.

Nicholas P. DePasquale, M.D., Assistant Professor of Medicine, Department of Medicine, Tulane University, School of Medicine, New Orleans, Louisiana, USA.

Joseph T. Doyle, M.D., Professor, Director, Cardiovascular Health Center, Albany Medical College, Union University, Albany, New York, USA.

Mort B. Epstein, Ph.D., Research Chemist, Division of Adult Health and Aging, Chicago Board of Health, Chicago, Illinois, USA.

Zdeněk Fejfar, M.D., Chief, Division of Cardiovascular Diseases, World Health Organization, Geneva, Switzerland.

Gary D. Friedman, M.D., Medical Officer, Heart Disease Epidemiology Study, National Heart Institute, Framingham, Massachusetts, USA.

Glen E. Garrison, M.D., Medical Officer, Heart Disease Control Program, Public Health Service; Instructor in Medicine; Fellow in Cardiovascular Diseases, Duke University, Medical Center, Durham, North Carolina, USA.

Menard M. Gertler, M.D., Professor, Director of Cardiovascular Research, Institute of Physical Medicine and Rehabilitation, New York University School of Medicine, New York, USA.

Viktor Gottheiner, M.D., Director, Institute for the Rehabilitation of Cardiac Patients, Tel-Aviv, Israel.

Claude Goulet, M.D., Research Associate, Institute of Cardiology of Montreal, Montreal, Canada.

Francisco Grande, M.D., Director, Jay Phillips Research Laboratory, Mount Sinai Hospital and Laboratory of Physiological Hygiene, University of Minnesota, Minneapolis, Minnesota, USA.

George C. Griffith, M.D., D.Sc. (Hon.), Emeritus Professor of Medicine, University of Southern California, Los Angeles, California, USA.

Marshall E. Groover, Jr., M.D., Associate Professor of Medicine, Department of Medicine, University of Oklahoma, Medical Center, Oklahoma City, Oklahoma, USA.

Max J. Halhuber, M.D., Professor, Department of Medicine, University of Innsbruck, Innsbruck, Austria.

Yolanda Hall, M.S., Research Nutritionist, Heart Disease Control Program, Chicago Board of Health, Chicago, Illinois, USA.

Curtis G. Hames, M.D., Chairman, Evans County Health Department, Claxton, Georgia, USA.

James W. Hampton, M.D., Assistant Professor of Medicine, Neurocardiology Research Program of the Department of Medicine, University of Oklahoma, Medical Center, Oklahoma City, Oklahoma, USA.

Harper K. Hellems, M.D., Professor of Medicine; Director, Division of Cardiovascular Diseases, New Jersey College of Medicine, Thomas J. White Cardiopulmonary Institute and B. S. Pollak Hospital for Chest Diseases, Jersey City, New Jersey, USA.

Herman K. Hellerstein, M.D., Assistant Professor of Medicine, Western Reserve University, University Hospitals, Cleveland, Ohio, USA.

Yoshikazu Hiramoto, M.D., Research Associate, Institute for Cardiovascular Diseases, Tokyo Medical and Dental University, Medical School, Tokyo, Japan.

Ernst Jokl, M.D., Professor and Director, Physical Education Research Laboratories, University of Kentucky, Lexington, Kentucky, USA.

Aubrey R. Kagan, M.D., Medical Officer, Division of Cardiovascular Diseases, World Health Organization, Geneva, Switzerland.

William B. Kannel, M.D., Associate Director, Heart Disease Epidemiology Study, National Heart Institute, Framingham, Massachusetts, USA.

Nodar N. Kipshidze, M.D., Professor, Director, Institute of Experimental and Clinical Therapy, Ministry of Health of the Georgian Socialist Soviet Republic, Tbilisi, Soviet Union.

Hans W. Kirchhoff, M.D., Director, Medical Research Institute of the Air Force of the German Federal Republic, Fürstenfeldbruck, German Federal Republic.

Mary A. Klouda, Ph.D., Research Associate, Department of Physiology, Stritch School of Medicine, Loyola University, Chicago, Illinois, USA.

Jiři Král, Dr. Sc., Professor, Director, Institute of Sports Medicine, Medical School, Chair of Physical Education, Charles University, Prague, Czechoslovakia.

Hans Kraus, M.D., Associate Professor, Department of Physical Medicine and Rehabilitation, New York University, New York City, New York, USA.

Hans J. Krzywanek, M.D., Research Associate in Experimental Medicine, University of Vermont, College of Medicine, Burlington, Vermont, USA.

Vincenzo Lapiccirella, M.D., Lecturer in Medical Pathology, University of Florence. Director, Cardiological Laboratory, Montecatini, Italy.

Serafim P. Letunov, M.D., Professor, Director, Central Research Institute of Physical Culture, Sector for Sports Medicine, Moscow, Soviet Union.

Lennart Levi, M.D., Director, Laboratory for Clinical Stress Research, Department of Medicine and Psychiatry, Karolinska Hospital, Stockholm, Sweden.

Monte Levinson, M.D., Research Internist, Heart Disease Control Program, Chicago Board of Health, Chicago, Illinois, USA.

Howard A. Lindberg, M.D., Research Internist, Heart Disease Control Program, Chicago Board of Health, Chicago, Illinois, USA.

Thomas N. Lynn, M.D., Department of Medicine, University of Oklahoma Medical Center, Oklahoma City, Oklahoma, U.S.A.

John R. McDonough, M.D., M.P.H., Medical Officer, Heart Disease Control Program, Public Health Service; Assistant Professor of Epidemiology, University of North Carolina, School of Public Health, Chapel Hill, North Carolina, USA.,

Robert B. McGandy, M.D., Assistant Professor of Nutrition, Harvard School of Public Health, Harvard University, Boston, Massachusetts, USA.

Harald Mellerowicz, M.D., Professor, Director, Institute of Fitness, Preventive and Sports Medicine, West Berlin, Germany.

Kenneth I. Melville, M.D., Professor, Head of Department of Pharmacology, McGill University, Montreal, Canada.

Wilda A. Miller, M.P.N., Research Assistant, Division of Adult Health and Aging, Chicago Board of Health, Chicago, Illinois, USA.

Salek Minc, M.D., Department of Cardiology, Royal Perth Hospital, Perth, West Australia.

Louise Mojonnier, Ph.D., Research Nutritionist, Heart Disease Control Program, Chicago Board of Health, Chicago, Illinois, USA.

Christos B. Moschos, M.D., Senior Fellow in Medicine, Division of Cardiovascular Diseases, New Jersey College of Medicine, Thomas J. White Cardiopulmonary

Institute and B. S. Pollak Hospital for Chest Diseases, Jersey City, New Jersey, USA.

Rakhil' E. Motylyanskaya, D. Med. Sci., Central Research Institute of Physical Culture, Sector for Sports Medicine, Moscow, Soviet Union.

Aleksandr L. Myasnikov, M.D., Professor, Member of the USSR Academy of Medical Sciences; Director, Institute of Therapy of the Academy, Moscow, Soviet Union.

John Naughton, M.D., Instructor in Medicine, Department of Medicine and Neurocardiology Research Program, University of Oklahoma Medical Center, Oklahoma City, Oklahoma, USA.

Henry A. Oldewurtel, Research Associate, Division of Cardiovascular Diseases, New Jersey College of Medicine, Thomas J. White Cardiopulmonary Institute and B. S. Pollak Hospital for Chest Diseases, Jersey City, New Jersey, USA.

M. N. Pertsovsky, M.D., Therapeutic Clinic of the I. M. Sechenov Research Institute, Yalta, Soviet Union.

Wilhelm Raab, M.D., Emeritus Professor of Experimental Medicine, University of Vermont, College of Medicine, Burlington, Vermont, USA.

Walter C. Randall, Ph.D., Professor, Chairman, Department of Physiology, Stritch School of Medicine, Loyola University, Chicago, Illinois, USA.

Timothy J. Regan, M.D., Associate Professor of Medicine, New Jersey College of Medicine, Thomas J. White Cardiopulmonary Institute and B. S. Pollak Hospital for Chest Diseases, Jersey City, New Jersey, USA.

James A. Richardson, Ph.D., Professor, Department of Pharmacology and Therapeutics, Medical College of South Carolina, Charleston, South Carolina, USA.

Seymour H. Rinzler, M.D., Cardiologist-in-Charge, Diet and Heart Disease Study Project, Department of Health, New York City, New York, USA.

Ray H. Rosenman, M.D., Assistant Director, Harold Brunn Institute, Mount Zion Hospital and Medical Center, San Francisco, California, USA.

Henry I. Russek, M.D., Senior Attending Cardiologist, St. Barnabas Hospital, Bronx, New York; Consultant in Cardiovascular Diseases, US Public Health Service Hospital, Staten Island, New York, USA.

Hans Schaefer, M.D., Professor, Director of the Physiological Institute and of the Institute for Social and Work Medicine, University of Heidelberg, Heidelberg, German Federal Republic.

Gustav Schimert, M.D., Professor, Department of Medicine, University of Munich; Director, Institute for the Prevention of Circulatory Diseases, Munich, German Federal Republic.

Hans Schwalb, M.D., Research Associate, University of Munich, Research Institute for the Prevention of Circulatory Diseases, Munich, German Federal Republic.

Hans Selye, M.D., Ph.D., Sc.D., Professor, Director, Institute of Experimental Medicine and Surgery, University of Montreal, Montreal, Canada.

Takio Shimamoto, M.D., Professor, Director, Institute for Cardiovascular Diseases, Tokyo Medical and Dental University, Medical School, Tokyo, Japan.

Igor K. Shkhvatsabaya, M.D., Institute of Therapy, USSR Academy of Medical Sciences, Moscow, Soviet Union. (At present: Medical Officer, Cardiovascular Diseases, World Health Organization, Geneva, Switzerland.)

Louis H. Sigler, M.D., Consulting Cardiologist, Coney Island Hospital, Peninsula General Hospital; Attending Cardiologist, Adelphi Hospital, Brooklyn, New York, USA.

Robert J. Slater, M.D., Dean, University of Vermont, College of Medicine, Burlington, Vermont, USA.

Vojin Smodlaka, M.D., Staff Physician, Department of Physical Medicine and Rehabilitation, New York University, New York City, USA. (Formerly Assistant Professor of Sports Medicine, University of Belgrade, Yugoslavia.)

Jeremiah Stamler, M.D., Director, Division of Adult Health and Aging, Chicago City Board of Health; Assistant Professor of Medicine, Northwestern University, Chicago, Illinois, USA.

Riccardo Starcich, M.D., Professor, Institute of General Clinical Medicine and Medical Therapy, University of Parma, Parma, Italy.

Clarke Stout, M.D., Assistant Professor of Medicine, Department of Medicine, University of Oklahoma Medical Center, Oklahoma City, Oklahoma, USA.

Sarah C. Stulb, M.D., Nutritionist, Heart Disease Control Program, Public Health Service; Research Associate in Epidemiology and Nutrition, University of North Carolina School of Public Health, Chapel Hill, North Carolina, USA.

Tatuzi Suzuki, M.D., Professor, Department of Physiology, Nagasaki University, School of Medicine, Nagasaki, Japan.

Mordecai Toor, M.D., Associate Clinical Professor, Hebrew University Hadassah Medical School; Director IIIrd Medical Department, Cardiopulmonary Laboratory and Department of Cardiovascular Rehabilitation, Beilinson Hospital, Petah Tikva, Israel.

Dmitri D. Venediktov, M.D., Senior Research Associate in Cardiovascular Surgery, First Moscow Medical Institute and USSR Academy of Medical Sciences, Moscow, Soviet Union. (Adviser of the USSR Mission to the United Nations, New York, USA.)

Mendel Wassermil, M.D., Assistant Director, Department of Cardiovascular Rehabilitation, Beilinson Hospital, Petah Tikva, Israel.

John B. Wells, Jr., Ph.D., Assistant Professor of Mathematics, University of Kentucky, Lexington, Kentucky, USA.

Paul Dudley White, M.D., Emeritus Clinical Professor of Medicine, Harvard Medical School, Boston, Massachusetts, USA.

Harvey H. Whiter, B.S., Research Assistant, Department of Physical Medicine and Rehabilitation, New York University, School of Medicine, New York, USA.

Stewart Wolf, M.D., Professor, Head, Department of Medicine, Neurocardiology Research Program, University of Oklahoma, Medical Center, Oklahoma City, Oklahoma, USA.

Joseph B. Wolffe, M.D., Director, Valley Forge Medical Center and Heart Hospital, Norristown, Pennsylvania, USA.

Quentin D. Young, M.D., Staff Member, Division of Adult Health and Aging, Chicago Board of Health, Chicago, Illinois, USA.

Prevention is the greatest of all goals in man's long struggle to conquer disease, and preventive cardiology is steadily bringing us closer to that goal in an area of major health concern. *

Lyndon B. Johnson

---

*From a letter of welcome from President Lyndon B. Johnson to the First International Conference on Preventive Cardiology, University of Vermont, Burlington, Vermont, August 24–28, 1964.

INTRODUCTION

THE development of preventive medicine in the United States as a specific discipline constitutes one of the major contributions made to mass health preservation throughout the world. Numerous formerly dreaded communicable diseases have been brought under control; severe nutritional deficiencies have become a thing of the past in previously ravaged populations; industrial hazards are being systematically eliminated. Alongside with these remarkable achievements, undreamed of at the turn of the century, the triumphs of modern diagnostic and curative techniques have radically changed the picture of morbidity and mortality distribution.

In highly industrialized, prosperous nations, the former numerical prevalence of infectious epidemics was taken over by chronic ailments such as cancer and, as the most devastating of all, degenerative cardiovascular diseases, with hypoxic, so-called "coronary" or "ischemic" heart disease in the lead.

According to available statistics, ischemic heart disease claims more than 500,000 lives per year in the United States alone, with about 250,000 of these deaths being "premature" (i.e., occurring before the 65th year, the arbitrarily set age limit of "social usefulness"). Other particularly heavily afflicted countries are Canada, Great Britain, Australia, and Finland.

The reasons for the wide gap between the effective prevention of so many nondegenerative conditions, including rheumatic heart disease, on the one hand, and the near absence in Western countries of organized preventive action against uncontrolled mass mortality from ischemic heart disease on the other, are not generally appreciated.

In answer to mounting criticism which is being vented by an alarmed public against the medical profession as a whole and against responsible health authorities, it should be pointed out that they are not unaware of the gravity of the situation. In fact, the term "prevention" is being widely used in programmatic declarations and statements of policy. Beyond such merely verbal exercises, some governments (e.g., Great Britain and Italy) have implemented legislative measures against the unrestricted advertising of cigarettes whose pathogenic role in ischemic heart disease has been convincingly established. The Surgeon General of the United States attempted to introduce similar reforms in this country in the face of economic and political obstacles with limited success.

Dietary recommendations against the excessive consumption of saturated fats and cholesterol, based on epidemiologic studies over more than three decades, have been published by the American Medical Association and

by the American Heart Association. In consideration of the apparent preventive value of physical activity, the President's Council on Physical Fitness
has issued a booklet on home exercises for adults. Definite improvements
in the therapy of arterial hypertension have even contributed to a slight
decrease in the incidence of degenerative heart disease over recent years by
curbing at least one pathogenic factor.

By far the most dynamic initiative in the prevention of heart disease is
being displayed by those European countries which, following the longstanding example of the Soviet Union, have launched large-scale, empirically-
organized, preventive mass reconditioning programs under the sponsorship
of governments, insurance groups, and private industries. By constrast, no
comparable measures have yet been initiated in the most heart-disease-
ridden nations of the Western hemisphere.

This seeming paradox can be ascribed to several specific circumstances:

1. The one-sided fascination of Western clinicians and medical practitioners with the spectacular diagnostic and curative achievements of modern
medicine, as compared with plain, unglamorous health preservation.

2. The general lack of adequate interdisciplinary and intercontinental
information concerning numerous available but widely scattered, uncoor-
dinated, and unutilized data, pertinent to the multifaceted problem of the
origin and preventability of ischemic heart disease.

3. The skepticism of conservative health agencies which hesitate to take
the calculated risk of large-scale educational and administrative action unless
"all the facts are known," and whose constant emphasis on the obvious
"need for more research" cannot adequately replace the necessary thorough
familiarization with already existing but poorly integrated knowledge.

4. The fact that most of the measures which constitute the basis of active
prevention against ischemic heart disease require a certain amount of
personal effort and self-discipline and thus do not appeal to an affluent,
comfort-loving, "soft" society which prefers "pill power" to will power.

5. Possibly a subconscious feeling by some that cardiac death may not be
the worst of alternatives, even if it occurs "prematurely."

In order to overcome part of the above outlined difficulties, the *First
International Conference on Preventive Cardiology,** on which this book is largely
based, was held at the University of Vermont in August, 1964.

*The program was deliberately focused on the nonvascular, neurogenic and hormonal
mechanisms which, by interfering in myocardial oxygen and electrolyte metabolism,
determine the degree of vulnerability of the heart muscle to existing coronary atherosclerosis and which, under certain conditions, destroy myocardial tissue even in the
absence of vascular lesions.*

Unquestionably, coronary atherosclerosis represents the most common and
the most important predisposing single pathogenic factor in pluricausal
ischemic heart disease. It is primarily and directly involved in those 50 or

---

*The term "Preventive Cardiology" had been coined in 1958. (W. Raab, *Maine State Medical Jour-
nal*, January, 1958.)

more per cent of all myocardial infarctions which are caused by occlusion of the coronary lumen through thrombi or intramural hemorrhage, and as a contributory element in the vast majority of all instances of ischemic heart disease. However, until not long ago, very little attention had been paid to the logical necessity of taking both vascular oxygen supply and (autonomic nerve-dominated) myocardial oxygen consumption jointly into account as the inseparably interrelated prerequisites of myocardial metabolic health or hypoxic injury, respectively.

With the purpose in mind to counterbalance the traditional, one-sidedly vascular and mechanistic approach to the problem of ischemic heart disease, investigative materials dealing with the field of coronary atherogenesis were excluded from the Vermont Conference and from this book, with the exception of only a few particularly important contributions.

Significantly, soon after the Conference, the official summary of the policy-proposing Second National Conference on Cardiovascular Diseases (Washington, D.C., November, 1964, authored by I. H. Page) stated that "higher nervous functions have received far less attention than their importance deserves" and that such studies should be given a "new public face."

The present book is being published in compliance with that postulate. In order to comprehend its general philosophy, *the readers are urged to beware of the still widespread and misleading semantic confusion of coronary atherosclerosis as such with its pathogenic corollary, i.e., myocardial metabolic vulnerability and resulting hypoxic disease of the heart muscle.* The greater ease with which a narrow vascular tube can be visualized does not absolve from the necessity to reason simultaneously also in terms of invisible features such as neurohormones, oxygen economy, and electrolyte balance.

Many contributors to this book have replaced the purely vascular-oriented designations "coronary heart disease" or "coronary disease" by the less prejudicial "ischemic heart disease." This term is not quite adequate either in that it fails to clearly point at the crucial principle: a disproportion between two interrelated elements, namely vascular oxygen supply and myocardial oxygen consumption. However, it does come closer to reality and symbolizes a less limited view of the problem complex of hypoxic myocardial destruction and death. The designation "hypoxic heart disease" is herewith being recommended as the most descriptive one available, and will be used by the editor in his own statements and comments.

The subject matter of the book is arranged in such a fashion as to proceed, step by step, from experimental biochemical, pathophysiological, neuro-endocrinological, pathomorphological, clinical, psychological, sociological and epidemiological considerations to the fundamental rationale and practical application of preventive measures, their organization and preliminary objective results, and to the deducible academic, professional, and lay educational requirements for their large-scale effective implementation.

W. Raab, M.D.
Editor

ACKNOWLEDGMENTS

THE FIRST International Conference on Preventive Cardiology at the University of Vermont, Burlington, Vermont (August 24-28, 1964), on the proceedings of which the greater part of this book is based, was aided by financial contributions from the Vermont Heart Association, the Vermont State Department of Health with Federal matching funds, pharmaceutical industries (Burroughs Wellcome and Co., Inc., Tuckahoe, New York; CIBA Pharmaceutical Company, Summit, New Jersey; Knoll Pharmaceutical Company, Orange, New Jersey; Sandoz Pharmaceuticals, Hanover, New Jersey; Smith, Kline and French Laboratories, Philadelphia, Pennsylvania); local industries in Vermont (Thermal Wire of America, Inc., Thermo Tape Corporation; Vermont Fruit and Grocery Company, Inc.), and local residents of Burlington, Vermont.

Several European governments and private agencies facilitated the participation of some of the speakers from abroad.

Additional funds for publication of the book were received from Sandoz Pharmaceuticals, Hanover, New Jersey, and from Farbwerke Hoechst A.G., Frankfurt/Main, West Germany.

Mrs. Olga E. Raab carried out all secretarial work connected with organization of the 1964 conference and with obtaining and editing the manuscripts contained in this book.

The editor wishes to express his sincere appreciation to all those who have made the conference and the publication of the book possible.

W. R.

CONDENSED SURVEY OF CONTENTS

As explained in the introduction, this book is devoted to the problem of pluricausal vulnerability of the heart muscle and *not* to the already abundantly but still inconclusively explored problem of atherogenesis. It directs attention primarily to those long disregarded contributory neurogenic and hormonal, functional and metabolic factors which (usually, but not necessarily, in conjunction with coronary atherosclerosis) possess fundamental pathogenic significance and appear rationally amenable to systematic prevention.

SECTION I
Pathophysiological Fundamentals

The long familiar phenomenon of multiple focal necrosis formation in the heart muscle caused by exogenously administered, oxygen-wasting adrenergic catecholamines (adrenomedullary epinephrine and neurogenic norepinephrine) was investigated in depth from various points of view:

Regan discusses the connections between the epinephrine-induced gradual loss of myocardial glycogen and potassium, changes of lipid metabolism, and a decline of myocardial contractility as prenecrotic manifestations. (see Chapter 1).

Early and reversible, electronmicroscopically discernible alterations of myocardial microstructure after injection of minute doses of epinephrine are described by *Shimamoto* (see Chapter 2). Larger doses were found by *Bajusz* (see Chapter 3) to cause within minutes after injection (i.e., hours before appearance of the well-known destructive lesions) a dramatic upheaval in the subendocardial distribution of potassium, glycogen, and phosphorylase activity, in a pattern analagous to that produced by experimental myocardial anoxia.

Melville (see Chapter 4) and *Shkhvatsabaya* (see Chapter 5), by electrically and mechanically stimulating the central nervous system of cats and rabbits, elicited sympathogenic hypoxic changes of the electrocardiogram and the subsequent development of focal necroses in the subendocardium. The hearts of such animals showed an excess accumulation of catecholamines (see Chapter 5).

Aside of myocardial necroses which had been previously seen after stimulation of the cardiac sympathetic nerves (see Chapter 14, ref. 36), subendocardial hemorrhages were produced by *Klouda* (see Chapter 6) with a similar technique. They seem to be caused by an intraventricular friction effect.

Groover (see Chapter 7) who, like others (see Chapter 7, ref. 5, 7) had described emotion-induced, presumably sympathogenic, myocardial necroses in animals with intact coronary vessels (see Chapter 7, ref. 4) reports the still unexplained observation that stimulation of the cardiac vagus nerves can likewise elicit myocardial lesions.

Physical stress is ordinarily associated with a marked augmentation of myocardial oxygen demands. Massive infarctions of the heart muscle, which appeared in *Kipshidze's* (see Chapter 8) coronary atherosclerotic rabbits after exhausting (but in normal animals innocuous) exercise, demonstrate the importance of vulnerability-augmenting, not primarily vascular, functional elements in the origin of myocardial necrosis.

The integrity of the heart muscle depends on the degree of compensatory dilatability of the coronary system whenever myocardial oxygen requirements rise. This was evidenced by electrocardiographic signs of myocardial anoxia during (otherwise inert) sympathetic stimulations or catecholamine administrations when a coronary artery was mechanically prevented from dilating (see Chapter 12, ref. 7). The same principle was demonstrated by *Bellet* (see Chapter 9) in dogs with restricted coronary arteries when catecholamine-liberating, myocardial oxygen-wasting nicotine was administered.

Studies by *Levi* (see Chapter 10) revealed in man a usually marked increase of urinary catecholamine excretion under occupational tensions, emotional arousal, and sensory annoyances, whereas emotionally relaxing experiences produced the opposite effect.

According to *Richardson* (see Chapter 11) and *Starcich* (see Chapter 12), patients suffering from angina pectoris display a characteristic tendency to discharge abnormally large amounts of catecholamines into the circulation both during spontaneous attacks and under the influence of exercise (see Chapters 11, 12) or emotional excitement (see Chapter 12). Since angina patients were found oversensitive even to small doses of infused epinephrine (see Chapter 12) a causal role of exaggerated adrenomedullary and sympathetic catecholamine discharges in the anginal syndrome appears highly probable (see Chapters 11, 12). The therapeutic effectiveness of various antiadrenergic measures seems to agree with this concept (27) (see Chapter 12).

Elevated plasma catecholamine concentrations after acute myocardial infarction (see Chapters 11, 12) and in patients with congestive heart failure (see Chapter 12, ref. 54) are presumably secondary phenomena without major primarily pathogenic significance.

Transient electrocardiographic changes under emotional stress in tense, excitable persons were observed by *Sigler* (see Chapter 13), and an intensified adrenergic response of the hearts of such individuals under standard sensory and mental stresses by *Raab* (see Chapter 14).

An elevated cardiac sympathetic tone and stress response was found to be a (potentially pathogenic) characteristic also of sedentary people (see Chapter 14), in sharp contrast to the well-known augmented antiadrenergic counter-regulation of trained individuals (see Chapter 15, ref. 20). In the latter, *Jokl* (see Chapter 15) demonstrated by means of ballistocardiography an increase of the ventricular stroke force.

Schimert (see Chapter 16), by defining the "coronary reserve" as the range of vascular circulatory and oxidative metabolic conditions which jointly determine the availability of oxygen to myocardial tissue, elucidates the most fundamental pathophysiological principle of hypoxic* heart disease. He points out that maintenance of the ratio:

$$\frac{\text{Vascular } O_2 \text{ supply}}{\text{Myocardial } O_2 \text{ consumption}} = 1.0$$

is responsible for the metabolic and structural integrity of the heart muscle. The antiadrenergic effectiveness of physical training possesses cardiopro-tective value by preventing the denominator of the ratio from exceeding the numerator and from thus lowering the ratio to the hypoxic level of <1.0. Muscular training also seems to favor the development of the coronary collateral network (see Chapter 16, ref. 22).

Minc (see Chapter 17) suspects the "civilized pattern" of physical activity which demands deliberate motion without appropriate emotional drive, as a possible additional factor in autonomic nervous imbalance.

Selye's (see Chapter 18) discovery of the sensitization of the myocardium to the cardiotoxicity of stresses (i.e., of catecholamine action) (see Chapters 3, 14, ref. 32) by adrenal corticoids suggests an important accessory pathogenic role of these electrolyte-regulating hormones in myocardial destruction. This applies especially under conditions of emotional stress (see Chapter 14, ref. 21) whereas according to *Suzuki* (see Chapter 19), physical exercise is devoid of an over-secretion of corticoids.

The acquisition of a cardioprotective resistance against unaccustomed severe stresses by preceding stresses of a lesser degree (e.g., exercise, cold baths), as described by *Selye* (see Chapter 18), may be of outstanding pre-ventive importance.

Still underexplored enzymatic, immunological and other possibilities of myocardial pathogenesis and protection are enumerated by *Griffith* (see Chapter 20), together with a call for positive preventive action instead of timid procrastination until all theoretical problems are solved.

SECTION II
Epidemiologic Data

The role of the above-mentioned primarily non-vascular factors which (mostly in conjunction with coronary atherosclerosis) contribute to the

---

*Preference of the term "hypoxic" over "coronary" or "ischemic" is explained in the Introduction (p. xv).

origin of hypoxic heart disease, namely (a) emotional stress, (b) lack of exercise, and (c) the abuse of nicotine, is reflected in certain epidemiologic data concerning the incidence and prognosis of that disease.

Statistically identified criteria for so-called coronary-proneness, like those obtained by the Framingham Study (see Chapter 31, ref. 1) and by *Gertler* (see Chapter 21), are useful for screening purposes and provide clues for the planning of rational preventive measures, as far as the respective, presumably pathogenic conditions are amenable to correction (e.g., lack of exercise, smoking, emotional stress, arterial hypertension, excessive consumption of saturated fats and hypercholesterolemia).

Doyle (see Chapter 22) provides statistical evidence regarding the highly pathogenic effect of transiently catecholamine-liberating cigarette smoking. In addition, he states that cessation of smoking drastically reduces the risk of developing hypoxic heart disease.

This latter observation was confirmed by *Russek* (see Chapter 23), who suspects a participation of emotional factors in the motivation for smoking as well as for abstaining from it. He ascribes the high incidence of clinical hypoxic heart disease in connection with occupational mental stresses to combined circumstantial and personality-linked pathogenic predispositions.

Rosenman (see Chapter 24) concentrates his attention more specifically on the last-named element. A high degree of coronary (or rather myocardial hypoxia)-proneness could be ascertained by his team in persons with an ambitious, hard-driving, impatient personality pattern. These individuals were characterized by an exaggerated urinary catecholamine excretion, high serum lipid levels, and accelerated blood clotting.

The part played by severe, insolvable personal conflicts and by acute emotional stresses in causing or aggravating manifestations of myocardial hypoxia is discussed by *Wolffe* (see Chapter 25) and *Lapiccirella* (see Chapter 26).

By contrast, the absense of socioeconomic emotional tensions and pressures in an unusually carefree living community of Italian immigrants in Pennsylvania and in a primitive Somali tribe is credited by *Brandt* and co-workers (see Chapter 27) and by *Lapiccirella,* (see Chapter 26), respectively, with an observed low incidence of hypoxic heart disease in these population groups despite a high dietary consumption of fat. Urinary catecholamines in the Somalis were uniformly low (see Chapter 26).

The detrimental influence of modern urban living on the cardiac fitness of a highly civilized population was demonstrated by *Allard* (see Chapter 28) on French Canadian city employees of Montreal.

Brunner's (see Chapter 29) studies on racially, environmentally and nutritionally homogeneous members of communal settlements in Israel provide evidence of a significant cardioprotective effect of physical activity with regard to both incidence and survival chance of myocardial infarction.

Similar conclusions are drawn by *Hames* (see Chapter 30) from observations on physically inactive upper-class white inhabitants of the state of Georgia, as compared with lower-class white and Negro farmers and laborers.

Dawber (see Chapter 31) calls attention to a special feature of possible predictive value and apparently connected with lack of physical exercise, namely, a low vital breathing capacity in coronary-prone subjects.

None of the conventional tests for early cardiac risk evaluation is based on parameters derived from the heart muscle itself, and none concerns the directly pathogenic involvement of the autonomic nervous system. In an attempt to remedy this defect, *Raab* (see Chapter 14) proposes a sensitive test which measures the heart rate and isometric period of the left ventricle at rest and in response to standard sensory and mental stresses, as criteria of adrenergic neurohormonal activity and excitability.

One of the reasons for not including atherogenesis in the subject matter of this review, despite its outstanding importance as a leading contributory cause of hypoxic heart disease, was the fact that the large-scale "National Diet-Heart Study" must await completion before a final statement concerning the role of dietary fat in atherogenesis can be made. A report on the initial, so-called "feasibility" phase of that study is presented by *McGandy* (see Chapter 32).

SECTION III

Preventive Measures

In view of statistical data which strongly suggest a causal link between hypercholesterolemia and hypoxic heart disease, efforts are being made to normalize elevated serum cholesterol levels by dietary adjustments as a means of prevention.

One of the most important advances in this field was the discovery of anticholesterolemic properties of polyunsaturated fats. Up-to-date studies on predictably optimal compositions of the diet are discussed by *Grande* (see Chapter 33).

The "Anti-Coronary Club" of the New York City Health Department, under the direction of *Rinzler* (see Chapter 34) has succeeded in gradually lowering the serum cholesterol level, the general risk factor prevalence, and the actual incidence of hypoxic heart disease among its members by prolonged adherence to a "prudent" diet with an adjusted content of saturated and unsaturated fats.

Effective simultaneous correction of several predisposing factors, such as hypercholesterolemia, obesity, hypertension, smoking and lack of exercise, has been achieved in coronary-prone middle-aged men by *Stamler* (35) and co-workers in the "Coronary Prevention Evaluation Program" of the Chicago Board of Health.

Since *Kraus's* (see Chapter 36) description of physical inactivity as the background of a variety of "hypokinetic" morbid conditions, including hypoxic heart disease, the importance of muscular exercise as a cardinal feature of preventive cardiology has received steadily increasing attention. Nevertheless, its physiological essentials are widely ignored, and in the current semantic confusion, exercise is frequently misinterpreted as a means to prevent coronary atherosclerosis. Even though some still inconclusive indications of such a possibility exist (e.g., a somewhat irregular tendency toward lowering serum cholesterol) (see Chapters 14, 38, 40, 41), the most striking effects of physical training are manifested in the autonomic nervous regulation of myocardial function and metabolism (see Chapters 14, 15, 16). The oxygen-economizing influence of physical training upon the heart muscle is pointed out by *Mellerowicz* (see Chapter 37).

On the grounds of his extensive cardiological experience with the traditional practice of physical culture in the Soviet Union, which includes all age categories, *Letunov* (see Chapter 38) recommends "universal prophylactic application" of regular physical activity as "one of the foremost tasks of modern medicine."

In the United States, systematic adult training programs have been initiated within the last decade by *Cureton* (see Chapter 39), followed by *Hellerstein* (see Chapter 40), *Naughton* (see Chapter 41), and others, both for primary prevention of degenerative heart disease and for the secondary prevention of recurrences of myocardial infarctions (see Chapters 40, 41).

In these carefully graded and supervised programs, the risk of untoward cardiac accidents proved unexpectedly low and results were satisfactory in several respects: amelioration of subjective well-being; marked improvement of work capacity (see Chapters 38, 39, 40, 41); partial or complete normalization of some of the pathological electro- and ballistocardiograms obtained before training (see Chapters 38, 39, 40); lowering of serum lipid levels (see Chapters 38, 39, 41); reduction of hypertensive blood pressure values (see Chapters 38, 40, 41) and of peripheral vascular resistance; diminution of the heart rate at rest (see Chapters 38, 39, 40, 41) and of the exercise-induced cardiac acceleration (see Chapter 40), and prolongation of the left ventricular isometric period (see Chapter 38). The last-named cardiac phenomena represent clear indications of a desirably diminished sympathetic, and an augmented vagal tone (see Chapters 14, 38) in the autonomic nervous regulation of myocardial function and metabolism.

Cureton (see Chapter 39) emphasizes the superior cardiac fitness value of strenuous, rhythmic and regular endurance exercises, as contrasted with that of various inadequate mild exercise schemes and more or less useless or unnecessary gadgets.

In agreement with these principles, *Gottheiner* (see Chapter 42) has created in Israel a sports organization, chiefly for post-infarction patients, which promotes slowly upgraded group sports activities such as swimming, hiking, running, and rowing.

Angina pectoris on effort was found not to constitute a definite contraindication, and improvements of the anginal syndrome were observed also among the cardiac trainees of another calisthenics and hiking program in Israel, conducted by *Wassermil* (see Chapter 43) with beneficial results.

Special merits in the reconditioning and rehabilitation of cardiac patients and prepatients are attributed by *Smodlaka* (see Chapter 44) to the system of periodically interrupted "interval training."

The reducing influence of physical training upon the blood pressure level (see Chapters 37, 38, 40, 41) is far less impressive than its antiadrenergic effects on the heart muscle (see Chapters 38, 39, 40, 41, 44). Nevertheless, *Král* (see Chapter 45) could show that the transient post-exertion fall of the systolic blood pressure develops into a more sustained lowering of the systolic blood pressure level after periods of physical training in a rural, mountainous surrounding.

Myasnikov (see Chapter 46) and *Venediktov* (see Chapter 47) describe the complex Soviet system of cardiovascular prevention by means of diagnostic mass screening, people's "health universities," operation of dispensaries, "day and night preventoria," regional cardiology centers, organization of physical culture activities for all age groups, exercise breaks in industry, maintenance of a very large network of reconditioning centers in scenic mountainous or coastal areas, and perennial educational campaigns for the nation-wide promotion of health rules.

Similar large-scale preventive activities are being conducted by the Czechoslovakian government with modernized methods in formerly fashionable bathing resorts and in numerous rural reconditioning and recreation centers, as reported by *Badal* (see Chapter 48).

The Alpine reconditioning centers of West Germany place even more emphasis than those of Eastern Europe on individually graded, systematic physical training of pre-cardiac as well as already diseased executives, workers and employees. *Beckmann* (see Chapter 49) explains the "terrain" treatment (hiking, mountain climbing), combined with breathing exercises, relaxation periods, and the emotionally equilibrating influence of the scenic environment. Under the impact of their invigorating personal experience at these centers, the trainees are said to be optimally receptive to the simultaneous indoctrination of health rules for lifelong adherence.

Prospective statistical data regarding the influence of the cardiac reconditioning system on cardiac morbidity and mortality are at present being collected in West Germany over a five-year period. In the meantime, specially established research institutes in the USSR, West Germany, Czechoslovakia, and Austria are evaluating various functional effects produced by reconditioning periods. *Kirchhoff* (see Chapter 50) observed reductions of the heart rate and blood pressure at rest and in response to physical effort, improved electrocardiographic reactions to artificially-induced hypoxia and other favorable changes.

Similar effects, suggesting a diminution of cardiac sympathetic tone and excitability were recorded by *Blohmke* (see Chapter 51) at a reconditioning center for mine workers.

In the planning of rural reconditioning programs it is important to take altitude and climatic factors with autonomic nervous regulatory implications into account, as shown by *Halhuber* (see Chapter 52). *Pertsovsky* (see Chapter 53) presents data indicating a favorable effect of environmental and climatic influences on the electrocardiogram and ballistocardiogram of patients with hypoxic heart disease in reconditioning centers on the Black Sea coast. *Burch* (see Chapter 54) warns against the intensive stimulation of the sympathetic nervous system which is induced by a hot humid atmosphere, and points out its potential dangers, especially for patients already afflicted with overt heart disease.

SECTION IV

Educational Aspects

The success or failure of attempts to induce sophisticated population groups to a change of cherished living habits in the interest of health maintenance will depend on their own willpower and motivation, as well as on the strength of conviction and persuasiveness of their responsible advisors.

Opinions are divided as to whether or not professional and lay educational campaigns could or should be initiated on the basis of our present state of knowledge.

Kagan (see Chapter 55), representing the administrative viewpoint of the World Health Organization, wishes to see a clearer demonstration of the preventive effectiveness of reconditioning programs before advocating them on a government or community level.

Such information is definitely desirable and it is to be hoped that those countries which possess the widest and longest experience in this matter make appropriate use of their ample facilities for a precise and conclusive long-range statistical evaluation of results.

Schaefer (see Chapter 56) points out the paradox that conventional medicine, although having successfully extended the average life span, is neglecting the remaining most fatal diseases in their preclinical stage and, due to its extensive preoccupation with merely symptomatic, palliative therapy, has failed to reduce overall morbidity. He criticizes the general pattern of medical education for its outdated lack of interdisciplinary coordination, and proposes a new type of medical training with the aim to keep both teachers and students in close touch with sociological problems and with the practical requirements of early prevention of the rampant degenerative diseases.

Slater (see Chapter 57), voicing the opinion of the prevention-oriented Vermont school of thought, appears encouraged by the unprecedented integration of interdisciplinary data which evolved from the First International Conference on Preventive Cardiology. He advocates the teaching of basic and practical principles of that subject to medical students and instilling in them a philosophy of prevention-mindedness as a major and timely feature of their future professional responsibilities.

Finally, the patriarch of American cardiology and champion of self-practiced preventive endeavors against hypoxic heart disease, *Paul Dudley White* (see Chapter 58), stresses the obligation of the medical profession to "practice what they preach" (or should preach) in order to instigate cardiac health-preserving habits among their patients and pre-patients by their own personal example.

CONTENTS

SECTION I
PATHOPHYSIOLOGICAL FUNDAMENTALS

SECTION II
EPIDEMIOLOGIC DATA

SECTION IV
EDUCATIONAL ASPECTS

PREVENTION OF
ISCHEMIC HEART DISEASE

Principles and Practice

SECTION I
PATHOPHYSIOLOGICAL FUNDAMENTALS

Chapter I

METABOLIC ROLE OF CATECHOLAMINES AND THE PRODUCTION OF MYOCARDIAL NECROSIS*

TIMOTHY J. REGAN, CHRISTOS B. MOSCHOS, HENRY A. OLDEWURTEL
and HARPER K. HELLEMS

(*Jersey City, New Jersey, U.S.A.*)

IN VIEW of current interest in the critical position of catecholamines in modification of cardiac function and structure (1), the following experiments were performed in the intact dog in continuation of previous studies concerning the influence of insulin, strophantidin and glucagon on myocardial metabolism (2, 3).

METHODS

Healthy male mongrel dogs (20 to 25 kg) were anesthetized 18 hours postprandial with morphine sulfate, 3mg per kg and pentobarbital (Nembutal, 12® mg per kg) and studied without opening the chest. After insertion of an endotracheal tube, respiration was regulated with a Harvard respiratory pump. Catheters were placed in the coronary sinus and aorta for blood sampling and pressure determinations. A Sones catheter was passed to the major branches of the left coronary artery via a carotid artery for the purpose of delivering 1-epinephrine bitartrate with minimal systemic effects on metabolites, and to measure

coronary blood flow by the Kr (85) method (4). A brass cannula was passed into the left ventricle from the other carotid to record pressure and the maximum rate of pressure rise (MRPR) as an indicator of left ventricular contractility (5).

Semicontinuous recordings of left ventricular pressures and their first derivative together with lead II of the electrocardiogram were made. Blood samples were taken at 20, 10 and 5 minutes before epinephrine injection while normal saline was continuously infused into the coronary artery at a rate of 0.1 ml per minute. Samples were drawn at 1 to 5 minute intervals for 50 minutes after epinephrine to determine arterial-coronary sinus differences of glucose (6), lactate (7), pyruvate (8), free fatty acids (9), and triglyceride (10), as well as the metabolites mentioned below. Excess lactate was calculated according to the Huckabee formula: $(L_V-L_A) - (P_V-P_A) (L_A/P_A)$ where L_A, L_V and P_A, P_V are lactate and pyruvate concentrations in arterial and coronary sinus bloods, respectively (11). Duplicate determinations of oxygen and carbon dioxide were performed by the Van Slyke method, and arterial pH on

*This study was supported by grants from the American Heart Association (61 F 82 E), the Morris County Heart Association, and from the Public Health Service (H-5483 and H-06376).

5

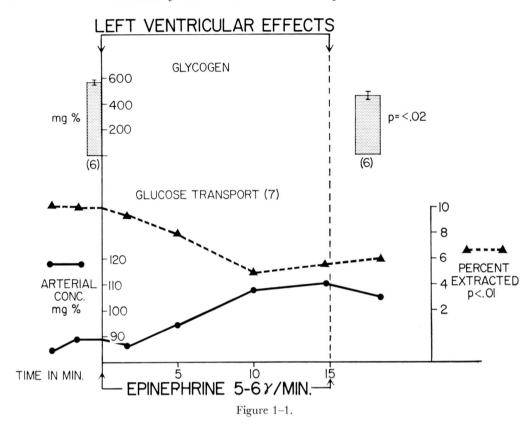

Figure 1–1.

RESULTS AND DISCUSSION

Contractility and Glycogenolytic Effects

a Beckman pH meter at 37°C. Fresh donor blood was used for replacement after each sampling. There was no apparent effect of the individual 30 ml blood replacements upon substrate extractions in the control period or, presumably in the experimental period. Continuous saline infusions in the coronary artery catheter in control animals were found to produce no change in coronary blood flow and no evidence of ischemia on the epicardial EKG taken from the same catheter.

The well-established effect of catecholamines in stimulating glycogenolysis was evidenced by a 20 per cent decrease in left ventricular glycogen content after the intracoronary infusion of 1-epinephrine for 15 minutes (Fig. 1-1). There was a simultaneous decrease in the extraction of glucose by the myocardium which was presumably mediated by the high tissue levels of hexophosphate occurring during glycogen breakdown. This regulatory mechanism is apparently not operative during the glycogenolysis induced by glucagon, since enhanced glucose uptake has been found during exposure to this hormone (3). It has been postulated that this effect on carbohydrate metabolism, mediated in large part through the activation of phosphorylase b to a, is related to the contractile response of left ventricle effected by epinephrine (12). It has been possible, however, to dissociate this biochemical pro-

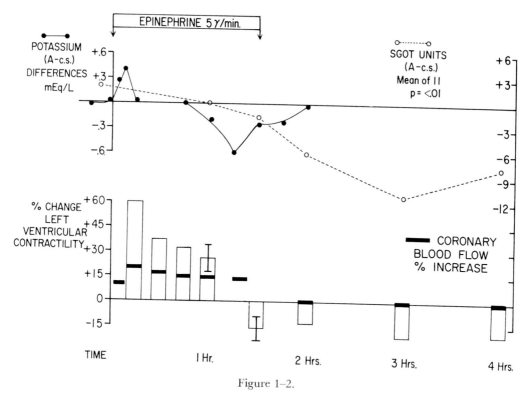

Figure 1–2.

cess from the inotropic response of left ventricle, particularly at lower dosages of the hormone, where one sees no change in glycogen or in phosphorylase activity despite the presence of a significant increase in cardiac contractility (13). Further when glycogenolysis does occur, it is more transient than the contractile response of the ventricle (14).

The inotropic response itself is certainly time dependent as observed during the sustained infusion of epinephrine over a 90-minute period into the left coronary artery (Fig. 1-2). In this situation the peak increase in the left ventricular contractility occurs at 30 to 45 minutes with an increase in the maximum rate of pressure rise (MRPR) and a decrease in end-diastolic pressure. Subsequently, there is a decline of contractility during

the infusion until at 90 minutes the state of ventricular contractility is usually below the control values, persisting through the 4 hours of observation. The stroke output response of the ventricle falls in a similar manner. In agreement with previous findings (15), the ECG (Standard II) revealed ST segment depression and increased height of T-wave during the infusion, with ST segment elevation and T-wave inversion after the infusion. Ventricular arrhythmias were seen in 60 per cent of the animals from 90 to 160 minutes.

Coronary blood flow changes appear to parallel the inotropic response and there is an increase of about 15 per cent during the peak contractility increase, which declines to a small degree throughout the infusion of epinephrine, but at no time during the 4 hours of observation is coronary flow significantly below the control value (Fig. 1-2). In addition, during the flow increment there is a rise in the coronary venous oxygen content relative to arterial so that the overall extraction of oxygen by the myocardium is reduced and the peak increase in oxygen uptake by the left ventricle is about 12 per cent at 30 minutes. The extraction of potassium and phosphate ion is significantly changed by epinephrine infusion. There is a brief 15 to 20 minute period in which there is uptake of these ions by the myocardium (16), following in about 45 minutes by a net loss of the ions from the heart. Subsequently, the enzyme glutamic oxalacetic transaminase (17) is found significantly increased in the coronary venous blood. This pattern of ion and enzyme loss from the myocardium is the same as occurs after obstruction of the left coronary artery (18).

If coronary flow is actually inadequate, the mechanism may be related to an increase in extravascular resistance associated with the increase in contractile force of heart muscle after epinephrine, which should impede coronary flow during systole. Electromagnetic measurements of phasic blood flow have actually indicated a proportionally greater increase in coronary systolic than diastolic flow after epinephrine (19, 20), so that enhanced extravascular compression does not appear to effectively interfere with coronary blood flow during the epinephrine response. The possibility remains, however, that the subendocardial layers may in special circumstances be selectively effected, as for instance when a large increase of left ventricular luminal pressures occurs in the presence of a reduced arterial perfusion pressure (21).

Since total coronary blood flow was not diminished, an increase in cardiac activity that was not met by an adequate oxygen supply increase may be invoked as a possible cause of necrosis. There was an approximately 60 per cent increase in all the measured parameters of left ventricular activity (stroke output, stroke and minute work and the first derivative of left ventricular pressure), while the coronary blood flow increment was on the order of 15 per cent. That a contractility increase may occur without an oxygen consumption increment has been observed during the positive inotropic response to strophanthidin which may sustain an equivalent increase in contractility as that observed with epinephrine in the 5 μg min experiments, without an increase in cardiac oxygen uptake. Since no effects of necrosis in the form of a contractility decline below control or a sustained period of potassium loss during the declining positive inotropic effect was observed, it appears that myocardial function may be enhanced in the absence of stimulation of oxidative metabolism, without inducing muscle damage. Further, when coronary blood flow was known to be inadequate, as during coronary artery obstruction, a compensatory increase in the extraction of oxygen would usually be expected in the presence of ischemia (18, 22). Instead, the arterial-coronary sinus difference of oxygen was reduced after epinephrine. It has also been observed on electron-micrographs that the catecholamine, isoproterenol, can produce early myocardial pathology without detectable alterations of the mitochondria, whereas during ischemia the mitochondria undergo drastic changes in a short time (23).

The experimental design of this study

enabled the production of left ventricular necrosis by epinephrine in the absence of an increase in cardiac rate or arterial pressure. The former in particular may be substantially increased during systemic administration of catecholamines, and may facilitate the necrosis of tissue. However, the current study demonstrates that it is not necessary for the production of necrosis. Prior studies have indicated a substantial rise in oxygen consumption out of proportion to the cardiac work increase (24, 25). This is not a necessary condition for the production of myocardial lesions, since without a rise in cardiac rate or arterial pressure, the coronary blood flow and myocardial oxygen consumption increase was proportionately less than the rise in cardiac contractility.

Another, perhaps separate, aspect of cardiac damage induced by catecholamines is here relevant. Virtually all animals at the 5 μg level incurred subendocardial hemorrhage notably in the mitral valve cusps, posterior papillary muscle and occasionally on the epicardial surface. A mechanical cause has been postulated on the basis of the marked squeezing of the chambers during the inotropic effect (26), despite the fact that one of these amines, norepinephrine, apparently produces no increase in intramyocardial pressure (27). Since the peak inotropic effect occurs during the initial 30 to 45 minutes of infusion and hemorrhages are generally absent in hearts taken at this time, such would seem an unlikely mechanism. Further, such changes are absent after the approximately equal inotropic response following strophanthidin (2). Since the earliest lesion during sympathetic stimulation would appear to involve the mitral valve cusps, a direct effect of this hormone on the endothelial lining of the valves and, eventually, of the endocardium may be the basis for this lesion, analogous to the right heart valvular effects of another biogenic amine, serotonin.

Myocardial Metabolism During Sustained 1-Epinephrine Infusion

The peak contractility increase was associated with the maximum rise in the myocardial respiratory quotient (Fig. 1-3), presumably a reflection of the utilization of endogenous carbohydrate during glycogenolysis. The production of excess lactate by the heart is significantly increased during this time, presumably related to the increased formation of reduced diphosphopyridine nucleotide (DPNH) during the oxidation of glyceraldyde-3-P and its subsequent interaction with the lactate-pyruvate system (28). This transient appearance of lactate occurred during the period of inotropic response to epinephrine in contrast to its production during coronary obstruction where it follows upon the onset of declining contractility (18). Since inhibition of glycogenolysis prevents the reduction of diphosphopyridine nucleotide (DPN) (28), the phenomenon of lactate production appears to be a biochemical effect of the hormone that is not closely related to the physiologic or pathophysiologic responses. In addition, the early cardiac lesions induced by isoproterenol, in contrast with epinephrine, are not associated with glycogen changes on electron microscopy (23). On the assumption that the basis for necrosis production by the different catecholamines is similar, glycogenolysis would not appear to be an essential metabolic feature for this phenomenon.

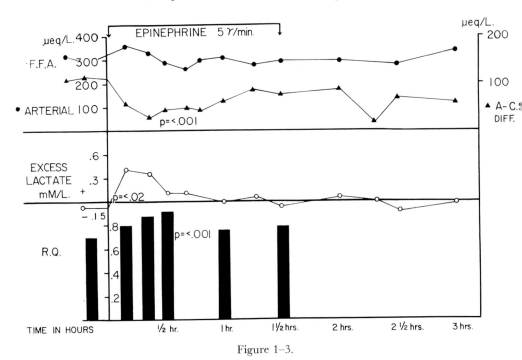

Figure 1–3.

Uptake of free fatty acid usually provides the myocardium with its major substrate in the fasted state. Unexpectedly, in view of the previous correlations of calorigenic effects of catechols with free fatty acid usage (29), the arteriovenous differences were reduced by epinephrine, which effect persisted throughout the 3 hours of observation (Fig. 1-3). Since hydrolysis of lipid in muscle could presumably release fatty acid into the coronary venous system, a series of experiments were designed to assess this possibility. Thirty microcuries of Palmitate - l-C^{14} complexed with serum was continuously infused into a systemic vein of control animals and a group receiving l-epinephrine into the left coronary artery, so that relatively constant arterial concentrations were present. A sizable arterial-coronary sinus difference of this isotope was evident in control animals, whereas the hormone

treated group exhibited significantly les extraction of the isotope (Fig. 1-4) which was not corrected by the 10 pe cent coronary flow increase, so that les C^{14} palmitate was incorporated into lef ventricular triglyceride. As a further re flection of the reduced uptake of fatt acid, there was a 60 per cent declin in the production of $C^{14}O_2$ by the hear representing a substantial lowering c fatty acid oxidation (Fig. 1-5). This phe nomenon was evident in animals receiv ing doses of l-epinephrine as low as 0. $\mu g/min$, which produced no increase c coronary blood flow or oxygen consump tion, and is in accord with decrease free-fatty acid oxidation in the bod during systemic epinephrine administra tion (30). Hence the rise in coronar sinus free-fatty acid concentrations ir duced by this hormone appears to repr sent a true decrease in uptake of th substrate. This effect of epinephrine cor

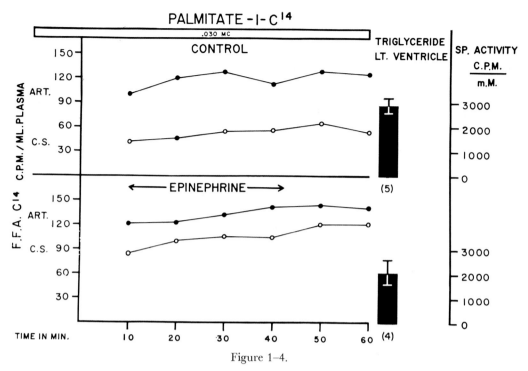

Figure 1–4.

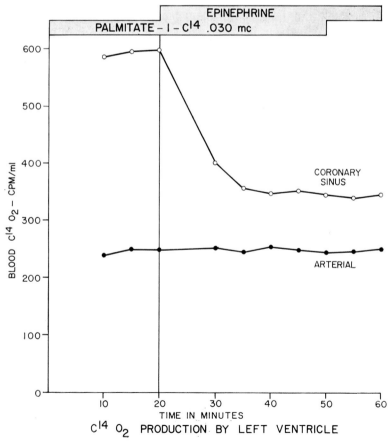

$C^{14} O_2$ PRODUCTION BY LEFT VENTRICLE

Figure 1–5.

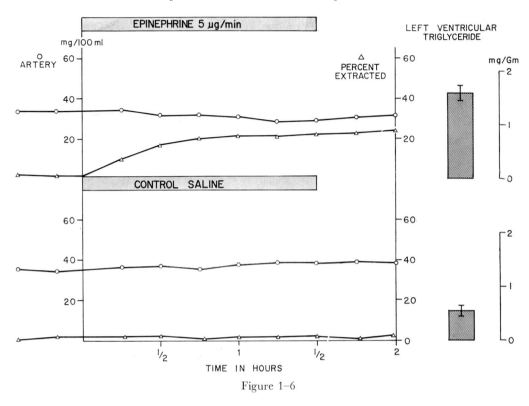

Figure 1–6

trasts with the disposition of fatty acid during ischemia where C_{14} palmitate has been found to be incorporated into tissue triglyceride to a greater extent than in controls (31).

Since the extraction of the two major substrates ordinarily utilized by the myocardium was significantly diminished it, seemed evident that another substrate must be transported to a greater extent into the cardiac cells under the condition of epinephrine stimulation. While this requirement was not met by ketone bodies, sequential sampling of arterial and coronary sinus blood for triglyceride revealed substantial uptake of this lipid persisting after the epinephrine infusion, while its arterial concentration was unaffected (Fig. 1-6). Control animals receiving intracoronary saline did not extract triglyceride significantly.

While this lipid may qualify as the major source of oxidative energy during epinephrine infusion particularly after the initial transient glycogenolysis, it is noteworthy that the accelerated transport eventuates by 2 to 3 hours in accumulation of triglyceride in left ventricular tissue (Fig. 1-6) which appears to have its counterpart in the electron microscopic findings of diffuse lipid deposition after isoproterenol (23). Since the production of glycerol phosphate from glycogenolysis probably occurs only in the early phase of epinephrine administration, the tissue triglyceride increment would not appear to be dependent upon this substrate for re-esterification of fatty acid derived from plasma triglyceride. Presumably, if the accelerated uptake is accomplished with triglyceride entering the cell intact, lipid accumulation might occur due to the following: (a) a bio-chemical barrier to the intracellular transport of this lipid to mitochondrial oxidative sites; (b) saturation of the nor-mal oxidative capability for this sub-strate, or (c) ultimate inhibition of the oxidative system by either the hormone or the accumulated lipid.

Despite the above-mentioned differ-ences, there are notable similarities in the biochemical response to ischemia and catecholamines. Interruption of coronary blood flow produces a similar transient increase in the conversion of phosphory-lase b to a, which is, at least in part, prevented by the beta-receptor inhibitor, Nethalide (32). The response to ischemia, therefore, probably involves some degree of sympathetic stimulation. Both situa-tions are associated with early accumu-lation of triglyceride (33, 34), although during ischemia this may be dependent on augmented free-fatty acid transport (31) rather than triglyceride. In addition to the ECG evidence of tissue necrosis and ventricular arrhythmias which occur in both situations, chronic cardiac aneu-rysm and congestive heart failure have been found after isoproterenol (35) and are a well-known effect of myocardial ischemia. Since definite evidence for a vascular basis of the necrosis after cate-chols is not available, many of these similarities may be explained as a com-mon response to tissue damage. Other important circumstances producing bio-chemical or histologic evidence of necrosis without definite evidence of a coronary blood flow deficit include the introduc-tion of extracorporal circulation (36), hemorrhagic schock (37), acute adminis-tration of ethanol (38), diphtheria myo-carditis (39), and depletion (40) or excess (41) of potassium ion by exogenous means. In many of these situations blood catecholamines are elevated but their precise role in the genesis of the described pathology remains to be proven.

SUMMARY

During a sustained infusion of l-epinephrine into the left coronary artery of the intact dog, the phasic nature of the metabolic as well as the hemody-namic effects of sympathetic stimulation have been observed. After an initial in-crease of left ventricular contractility, there was a progressive decline to below control levels. Biochemical evidence of myocardial necrosis appeared by 60 minutes with tissue release of K+ and PO$_4$ ions as well as the transaminase enzyme. The probability of a nonvascular basis for this lesion was discussed.

The metabolic concomitants included a transient increased rate of glycogenol-ysis, lactate production, and carbohy-drate oxidation, followed by a shift to enhanced oxidation of lipid. Plasma tri-glyceride rather than free-fatty acid be-came the major substrate transported in-to the myocardium. This latter process appeared to exceed utilization and ac-cumulation of triglyceride in the left ventricle occurred. The precise nature of this reaction as well as those naturally occurring factors which promote the pathophysiologic response of the myo-cardium to lesser degrees of sympathetic stimulation are among the issues for future resolution.

REFERENCES

1. RAAB, W.: The nonvascular metabolic myocar-dial vulnerability factor in "coronary heart dis-ease." *Amer Heart J, 66:*685, 1963.
2. REGAN, T. J., FRANK, M. J., LEHAN, P. H., and HELLEMS, H. K.: Relationship of insulin and strophanthidin to myocardial metabolism and function. *Amer J Physiol, 205:*790, 1963.

3. REGAN, T. J., LEHAN, P. H., HENNEMAN, D. H., BEHAR, A., and HELLEMS, H. K.: Myocardial metabolic and contractile response to glucagon and epinephrine. *J Lab Clin Med, 63:*638, 1964.

4. HERD, J. A., HOLLENBERG, M., THORNBURN, G. D., KOPALD, H. H., and BARGER, A. C.: Myocardial blood flow determined with Krypton-85 in unanesthetized dogs. *Amer J Physiol, 203:*122, 1963.

5. REEVES, T. J., HEFNER, L. L., JONES, W. B., COGHLAN, C., PRIETO, G., and CARROLL, J.: Hemodynamic determinants of the rate of change in pressure in the left ventricle during isometric contraction. *Amer Heart J, 60:*745, 1960.

6. NELSON, N.: A photometric adaptation of the Somogyi method for the determination of glucose. *J Biol Chem, 153:*375, 1944.

7. BARKER, S. B., and SUMMERSON, W. H.: The colorimetric determination of lactic acid in biological material. *J Biol Chem, 138:*535, 1941.

8. FRIEDMANN, T. E., and HAUGEN, G. E.: Pyruvic acid. II. The determination of Keto acids in blood and urine. *J Biol, Chem. 147:*415, 1943.

9. GORDON, R. S., JR., and CHERKES, A.: Unesterified fatty acid in human blood plasma. II. The transport function of unesterified fatty acid. *J Clin Invest, 36:*810, 1957.

10. CARLSON, L. A., and WADSTROM, L. B.: Determination of glycerides in blood serum. *Clin Chim Acta, 4:*197, 1959.

11. HUCKABEE, W. E.: Relationship of pyruvate and lactate during anaerobic metabolism. V. Coronary adequacy. *Amer J Physiol, 200:*1169, 1961.

12. ELLIS, S.: The metabolic effects of epinephrine and related amines. *Pharm Rev, 8:*485, 1956.

13. MAYER, S. E., COTTEN, M. DE V., and MORAN, N. C.: Dissociation of the augmentation of cardiac contractile force from the activation of myocardial phosphorylase by catecholamines. *J Pharmacol Exp Ther, 139:*275, 1963.

14. WILLIAMSON, J. R.: Metabolic effects of epinephrine in the isolated, perfused rat heart. *J Biol Chem, 239:*2721, 1964.

15. BARGER, A. C., HERD, J. A., and LIEBOWITZ, M. R.: Chronic catheterization of coronary artery: Induction of ECG pattern of myocardial ischemia by intracoronary epinephrine. *Proc Soc Exp Biol Med, 107:*474, 1961.

16. SARNOFF, S. J., MANSFIELD, P. B., DAGGETT, W. M.: Myocardial K+ changes resulting from inotropic agents. *Fed Proc, 23:*357, 1964.

17. KARMEN, A., WROBLEWSKI, F., and LADUE, J. S.: Transaminase activity in human blood. *J Clin Invest, 34:*126, 1955.

18. REGAN, T. J., MOSCHOS, C. B., WEISSE, A. B., and HELLEMS, H. K.: Left ventricular function and metabolism during development of coronary artery thrombosis. *Fed Proc, 23:*566, 1964.

19. GREGG, D. E., and FISHER, L. C.: Blood supply to the heart. *Handbook of Physiology Circulation* Baltimore, Williams and Wilkins Co., 1963 p. 1551.

20. CASANEGRA, P., PACIFICO, A., HELLEMS, H. K. and LEHAN, P. H.: Catecholamine action on phasic coronary flow patterns. *Clin Res, 11:*392 1963.

21. SALISBURY, P. F., CROSS, C. E., and RIEBE, P. A. Acute ischemia of inner layers of ventricular wall. *Amer Heart J, 66:*650, 1963.

22. COFFMAN, J. D., and GREGG, D. E.: Oxygen metabolism and oxygen debt repayment after myocardial ischemia. *Amer J Physiol, 201:*881 1963.

23. FERRANS, V. J., HIBBS, R. G., BLACK, W. C. and WEILBAECHER, D. G.: Isoproterenol-induced myocardial necrosis. A Histochemical and Electron Miscoscopic Study. *Amer Heart J, 68:*71 1964.

24. KATZ, L. N., WILLIAMS, F. L., LAURENT, D. BOLENE-WILLIAMS, C., and FEINBERG, H.: Effect of l-norepinephrine and 1-epinephrine on coronary flow and oxygen consumption of the intact open chest dog. *Fed Proc, 15:*106, 1956.

25. ECKSTEIN, R. W., STROUD, M., ECKEL, R., DOWLING, C. V., and PRITCHARD, W. H.: Effects on control of cardiac work upon coronary flow and O_2 consumption after sympathetic nerve stimulation. *Amer J Physiol, 163:*539, 1950.

26. KAYE, M. P., McDONALD, R. H., and RANDALL W. C.: Systolic hypertension and subendocardial hemorrhages produced by electrical stimulation of the stellate ganglion. *Circ Res, 9:*1164, 1961

27. D'SILVA, J. L., MENDEL, D., and WINTERTON M. C.: Effect of sympathomimetic amines on intramyocardial pressure in the rabbit. *Amer J Physiol, 205:*10, 1963.

28. WILLIAMSON, J. R., and CHANCE, B.: Control steps of Glycolysis in perfused rat heart. *International Congress of Biochemistry,* New York, 1964 p. 736.

29. STEINBERG, D., NESTEL, P. H., BUSKIRK, E. R. and THOMPSON, R. H.: Calorigenic effect of norepinephrine correlated with plasma free fatty acid turnover and oxidation. *J Clin Invest 43:*167, 1964.

30. HAVEL, R. J.: Transport of fatty acids in the blood: Pathways of transport and the role of catecholamines and the sympathetic nervous system. First International Pharmacy Meeting 2:43, 1964. MacMillan, New York, 1963.

31. EVANS, J. R.: Importance of fatty acid in myocardial metabolism. *Circ Res, 15:*96, Supp. 2 1964.

32. WOLLENBERGER, A., KRAUSE, E. G., and MACHO L: Thyroid state and the activity of glycogen

phosphorylade in ischemic myocardium. *Nature*, *201:*789, 1964.

33. MALING, H. M., HIGHMAN, B., and THOMPSON, E. C.: Some similar effects after large doses of catecholamines and myocardial infarction in dogs. *Amer J Cardiol, 5:*628, 1960.

34. SCHNITKA, T. K., and NACHLAS, M. M.: Histochemical alterations in ischemic heart muscle and early myocardial infarction. *Amer J Path, 42:* 507, 1963.

35. RONA, G., CHAPPEL, C. I., and KAHN, D. S.: Experimental production of chronic cardiac aneurysm and congestive heart failure in the rat. *Exp Molec Path, 2:*40, 1963.

36. COOPER, T., JELLINEK, M., WILLIAM, V. L., GANTNER, G. A., JR., and HANLON, C. R.: Biochemical studies of myocardium and blood during extracorporeal circulation in man. *Circulation, 29:*111, 1964.

37. LaFORCE, M., BLOCK, J., and REGAN, T. J.: Myocardial function during hemorrhagic shock. *Clin Res, 10:*390, 1962.

38. REGAN, T. J., MOSCHOS, C. B., and HELLEMS, H. K.: Ethanol-induced alteration of myocardial metabolism and function. *Circulation, 28:*788, 1963.

39. WITTELS, B., and BRESSLER, R.: Biochemical lesion of diphtheria toxin in the heart. *J Clin Invest, 42:*995, 1963.

40. MOLNAR, Z., LARSEN, K., and SPARGO, B.: Cardiac changes in the potassium-depleted rat. *Arch Path, 74:*339, 1962.

41. McFARLAND, J. A., THOMAS, L. B., GILBERT, J. W., and MORROW, A. G.: Myocardial necrosis following elective cardiac arrest induced with potassium citrate. *J Thorac Cardiov Surg, 40:* 200, 1960.

Chapter II

ELECTRON MICROSCOPIC OBSERVATIONS ON EDEMATOUS MYOCARDIAL RESPONSE TO EPINEPHRINE *

TAKIO SHIMAMOTO and YOSHIKAZU HIRAMOTO

(*Tokyo, Japan*)

THE pathophysiological significance of the catecholamines has been extensively investigated by Raab and others (1) and the author (2) found that the effect of high molecular weight substances in inducing myocardial necrosis is significantly enhanced by a concomitant application of epinephrine.

During the "emergency reaction" of Cannon (3) induced by a physiologically significant dose of epinephrine, the author (4) has found an edematous arterial reaction, which consists of an acute and transient enlargement of amorphous extracellular spaces of the subendothelial and medial layers of arteries, caused by an invasion of serous substances, and of a sticking of platelets and leucocytes to some parts of endothelial surfaces as its major phenomena.

In the following experiments on rabbits, a physiologically significant dose of epinephrine was administered intravenously by a single injection, and the electronmicrographic changes of the ventricular myocardium, coincident with the above mentioned arterial reaction, were observed.

*This study was supported by US Public Health Service Grant No. H-5196.

MATERIALS AND METHODS

Twenty-six albino male and female rabbits weighing 2.2 ± 10.27 kg were divided into an untreated and a treated group. All 20 animals of the treated group received 1 injection of epinephrine into the marginal ear vein in a dose of 0.1 μg per kg. For the sampling of myocardial specimens, the chest was quickly opened at 3, 5, 15, and 30 minutes and 1 hour after the injection, after the animals had been given a stunning blow on the head without anesthesia. Tissue specimens were taken from the ventricular myocardium.

In order to avoid morphological changes of the myocardium by stress or by anoxia, the sampling and immersion of the specimens into the fixative were performed within 20 seconds after cutting the skin of the chest. Two per cent osmium tetroxide, buffered with veronal acetate at pH 7.4 (0-4 °C), was used as fixative. In the fixative, the specimen was cut into cubes, measuring 1 mm or less in length and width. These cubes were left in the above mentioned fixative for 1 hour, dehydrated in graded concentrations of ethanol, and embedded in Epon 812, according to Luft (5). Thin sections, estimated to be about 400 to

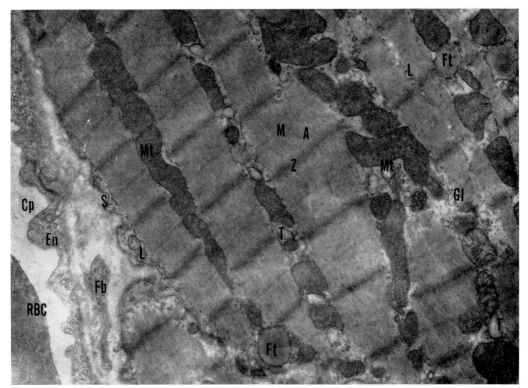

Figure 2–1. Rabbit myocardium. Control. Electron micrograph delineating the general cyto-
logic features of the heart muscle. The sarcolemma (S) is composed of an inner, dense plasma
membrane and an outer basement membrane. The myofibrils show Z, M, and A bands
(Z, M, A). The mitochondria (Mt) contain numerous cristae. No specific localization of the
mitochondria in relation to the cross striations of the myofibrils is observed. The limiting
membrane of the transverse system of the sarcoplasmic reticulum (T) is structurally quite
similar to the sarcolemma. Many small vesicles in the cytoplasm constitute the longitudinal
system of the sarcoplasmic reticulum (L). Fat droplets (Ft) are seen adjacent to mitochondria.
Fine, electron dense granules, dispersed throughout the cytoplasm, are glycogen particles (G1).
A capillary (Cp) and a fibroblast (Fb) are seen in the extracellular space. The endothelial
cell (En) of the capillary contains many pinocytotic vesicles. A red blood corpuscle (RBC)
is seen in the capillary.—X 14,500.

600 Å thick, were cut on a LKB Ultro-
tome and stained with a saturated aque-
ous solution of uranyl acetate. Using a
Hitachi HU-11A electron microscope,
the sections were observed and photographed at the direct magnification of
5,000 to 25,000.

RESULTS

The specimens sampled 1 to 3 minutes
after the intravenous injection of epinephrine, immediately after cessation of the
chronotropic and pressor response to
epinephrine, exhibited no appreciable
or only minimal changes, if compared
with specimens from untreated animals
(Fig. 2-1).

However, the specimens sampled 15
and especially 30 minutes after the injection of epinephrine, exhibited a definite change, showing a typical intracellular edema of the muscle cells as

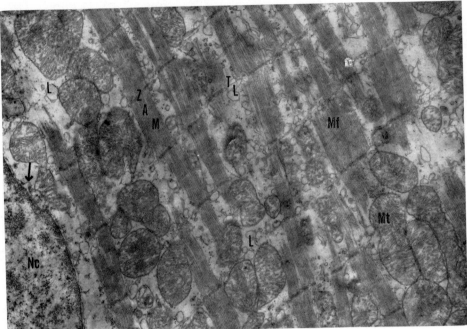

Figure 2–2. Rabbit myocardium 30 minutes after epinephrine administration. Vesicles of the longitudinal system of the sarcoplasmic reticulum (L) are markedly swollen and the cytoplasm also appears swollen with a decrease in its density and a slight increase in separation of the myofibrils. The changes mentioned above may be described as intracellular edema. The outer membrane of the nuclear envelope protrudes into the cytoplasm (*arrow*), and here fluid retention may be present in the cavity of the nuclear envelope. The number of the glycogen particles is decreased in the cytoplasm. Mitochondria (Mt) and myofibrils (Mf) are intact.—X 14,500.

described by Caulfield (6). As shown in Figures 2-2 and 2-3, the changes consist of a definite expansion of the vesicles of the longitudinal system of sarcoplasmic reticulum, an increase of the intracellular clear spaces around the mitochondria and between the myofibrils, an increase in number of fat droplets, a decrease in number of glycogen particles in the cytoplasm, and an appearance of dense bodies in the mitochondria. In some places the outer membrane of the nuclear envelope protrudes into the cytoplasm, indicating a retention of fluid in the cavity of the nuclear envelope. I bands often appear in the myofibrils.

The distribution of the "intracellular edema" seems not to be uniform, because some specimens exhibited striking changes (Fig. 2-2) whereas specimens taken from closely adjacent regions exhibited only relatively slight changes (Fig. 2-3).

In the specimens taken 1 hour after the injection of epinephrine, the "intracellular edema" was no longer seen, except for a slightly increased appearance of fat droplets inside the cytoplasm of muscle cells. Also the number of glycogen particles seemed to have been restored. In the specimens obtained 2 hours after epinephrine injection, there were almost no appreciable changes left as compared with the specimens from untreated animals.

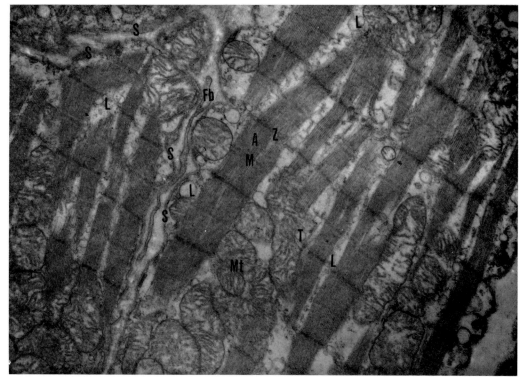

Figure 2–3. Electron micrograph showing another part of the myocardium taken from the same animal as in Figure 2–2. Intracellular edema and a decrease in the number of the glycogen particles are observed but the edematous changes are less distinct than in Figure 2–2. S: Sarcolemma. Z, M, A : Z, M, and A bands. L: longitudinal system of the sarcoplasmic reticulum. Mt: mitochondria. Fb: fibroblast.—X 14,500.

DISCUSSION

In experiments with rabbits we found that the intravenous injection of epinephrine in the dose of 0.1 μg per kg produces elevations of the blood pressure up to 10 mm Hg and a reflex reduction of the heart rate, ranging from 200 to 180 per minute. However, these changes disappeared completely within 20 to 40 seconds. Morphological changes were detected 15 to 30 minutes later. They seem to represent the morphological manifestation of metabolic effects elicited by epinephrine.

An analogous expansion of the longitudinal system and increase of the clear spaces around mitochondria and myofibrils of the cardiac muscle cells, accompanied by a definite decrease in number of glycogen particles and an alteration of mitochondria, has been observed previously in the early stages of anoxia, induced by coronary artery ligation in rabbits by Caulfield (6) and in rats by Bryant (7). The changes of cardiac muscle cells observed by us 30 minutes after a single injection of 0.1 μg per kg of epinephrine in the present experiments, exhibit principally the same characteristics, even though slighter, as those described by Caulfield (6) and Bryant (7) in anoxic heart muscles.

The longitudinal system of the sarcoplasmic reticulum is thought to be a transporting system for metabolites and ions between the extracellular spaces and the intracellular compartment. Thus, the expansion of the longitudinal system may be interpreted as being due to an influx of a large quantity of extracellular fluid into the muscle cells. Poche (8) has also described similar myocardial changes in potassium deficient rats.

The administration of epinephrine is known to exaggerate the oxygen consumption of the myocardium (1) and to dislocate potassium in the myocardial tissue aside of the well-known glycolytic effect and the release of free-fatty acids. However, the basic mechanism involved in the epinephrine-induced morphological changes of the heart muscle is still obscure.

These alterations of myocardial structure by epinephrine are as reversible as the edematous arterial reaction previously described by us (4), and the delayed appearance of the changes and their duration after epinephrine injection are likewise almost the same as those of the edematous arterial reaction. The physiological and pathophysiological significance of the early epinephrine-induced changes of the heart muscle will be the subject of further study.

SUMMARY

In 20 albino rabbits 0.1 μg per kg of epinephrine was administered in single intravenous injections. Three, 5, 15 and 30 minutes and 1 hour later, the animals were sacrificed and myocardial specimens were collected from the ventricle for electron microscopic observation. In the specimens collected 30 minutes after epinephrine injection, the heart muscle exhibited intracellular edema, accompanied by a definite expansion of the longitudinal system of sarcoplasmic reticulum, a decrease in number of glycogen particles, an increase in number of fat droplets in the cytoplasm, and the appearance of dense bodies in the mitochondria. I bands were also often observed in the myofibrils.

These changes resemble those elicited by myocardial anoxia. They were irregularly distributed and reversible. They disappeared almost completely within 1 hour after epinephrine injection.

Addendum: The authors have also performed recently a similar experiment with norepinephrine in rabbits, and it was found that norepinephrine (0.1 to 1.0 μg/kg i.v.) remained entirely without effect.

REFERENCES

1. RAAB, W.: The nonvascular myocardial vulnerability factor in "coronary heart disease." *Amer Heart J, 66:*685, 1963.
2. SHIMAMOTO, T., FUJITA, T., SHIMURA, H., YAMAZAKI, H., IWAHARA, S., and YAJIMA, G.: Myocardial infarction-like lesions and arteriosclerosis induced by high-molecular substances and prevention by magnesium salt. *Amer Heart J, 57:* 273, 1959.
3. CANNON, W. B.: *The Wisdom of the Body.* New York, W. W. Norton Co., 1939.
4. SHIMAMOTO, T., and SUNAGA, T.: Edematous arterial reaction by adrenaline and cholesterol and its prevention by MAO inhibitor observed by electron microscopic technique. *Japan Heart J, 3:*581, 1962.
5. LUFT, J. H.: Improvements in epoxy resin embedding methods. *J Biophys Biochem Cytol, 9:*409, 1961.
6. CAULFIELD, J., and KILONSKY, B.: Myocardial ischemia and early infarction. An electron microscopic study. *Amer J Path, 35:*489, 1959.
7. BRYANT, R. E., THOMAS, W. A., and O'NEAL, R. M.: An electron microscopic study of myocardial ischemia in the rat. *Circ Res, 6:*699, 1958.
8. POCHE, R.: Submikroskopische Beitrage zur Pathologie der Herzmuskelzelle bei Phosphorvergiftung, Hypertrophie, Atrophie und Kaliummangel. *Virchow Arch Path Anat, 331:*165, 1958.

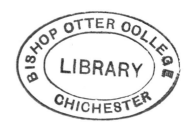

Chapter III

EARLY METABOLIC ABERRATIONS THROUGH WHICH EPINEPHRINE ELICITS MYOCARDIAL NECROSIS*

EÖRS BAJUSZ and WILHELM RAAB

(Montreal, Canada and Burlington, Vermont, U.S.A.)

Some forms of human necrotizing cardiomyopathies may be directly attributable to the reflex liberation of catecholamines which under certain circumstances exert a contributory noxious effect ou cardiac metabolism (1).

The potential danger of sympathetic (catecholamine) overactivity to the functional and structural integrity of the heart muscle may be attributed largely to the development of a discrepancy between the vascular oxygen supply (coronary blood flow) and the oxygen requirement of cardiac muscle cells.

For nearly five decades nothing definite was known concerning the precise mechanism through which catecholamines produce myocardial necrosis, except for the hypoxia-producing action of these amines in the heart muscle.

New possibilities of elucidating fundamental cardiotoxic biochemical processes were provided by recent histochemical studies on the enzyme-histogenesis of anoxic and "metabolic" (nonanoxic) myocardial lesions; the former were induced by occlusion of coronary arteries or by injection of coronary constrictor substances, the latter by dietary means and by administration of metabolic inhibitors and other cardiotoxic compounds (2, 3).

Comparative histochemical studies showed that (a) an early decline in myocardial phosphorylase activity and in the amount of the stainable, labile fraction of glycogen is a sensitive index of anoxic myocardial damage and (b) the behavior of phosphorylase and glycogen during the development of anoxic cardiac lesions is different from that seen during the development of the "metabolic" type of lesions (2-5). Differences were also established in the reaction of other enzymes (e.g., cytochrome oxidase, succinic dehydrogenase, etc.) consequently, it was suggested that certain histochemical techniques are applicable for purposes of morphologic differential diagnosis between anoxic and "metabolic" cardiomyopathies.

The present paper will demonstrate results obtained by applying these histochemical approaches to the study of cardiac damage, typically elicited by injection of epinephrine.

MATERIALS AND METHODS

In the first experimental series the effect of epinephrine upon the behavior of cardiac enzymes (phosphorylase, cyto-

*This study was aided by Research Grant HE-02169 from the National Heart Institute.

chrome oxidase, succinic dehydrogenase) and metabolites (glycogen, potassium) was studied by means of histochemical techniques. One hundred and twelve female rats of the Sprague-Dawley Farm, with a mean initial body weight of 152 g (range: 140 to 168 g) were subdivided in to two equal groups; Group 1 was treated with epinephrine; group 2 served as untreated controls.

Epinephrine was injected subcutanously, in a single dose of 450 μg/100 g of body weight, in 0.2 ml of physiologic saline, the control animals receiving only the 0.2 ml of physiologic saline. Following injection, the rats (always 4 animals at a time) were killed by decapitation at different intervals, ranging from 5 minutes to 96 hours (an equal number of epinephrine-treated animals and controls being sacrificed at the same time). Autopsies were performed 5, 10, 15 and 30 minutes, and 1, 3, 5, 8, 12, 24, 48, 72 and 96 hours after the injection. At autopsy, transventricular ablation was rapidly performed (after which cardiac contraction ceases almost instantaneously), and the remaining lower two-thirds of each ventricle was mounted on chucks, frozen with liquid air, and stored in a deep-freezing cabinet at $-70°$C. Serial sections were cut from each specimen on the same or the following day in a Pearse-Cryostat at $-20°$C; the thickness of the sections was always 10 μ.

The activity and distribution of phosphorylase was demonstrated by the method of Takeuchi et al. (6, 7) (incubation time: 120 minutes); succinic dehydrogenase by the teterazolium (MTT) technique of Pearse (8) (incubation time: 20 minutes); cytochrome oxidase with the method of Burstone (9), using a mixture of p-aminodiphenylamine and p-methoxy-p-aminodiphenylamine as substrate (incubation time: 20 minutes). Glycogen was identified by its staining characteristics with the periodic-acid-Schiff (PAS) reaction (on frozen sections following fixation with Rossman's fluid), and by its digestibility with diastase. For the histochemical localization of potassium, Poppen et al. (10) modification of the technique originally described by Macallum (11) was used, as applied to frozen sections. The sections were fixed for 10 minutes in 10 per cent acetic acid. For the purpose of routine morphologic studies, the frozen sections were post-fixed with formalin and stained with hematoxylin-phloxine-saffron (HPS).

In the second experimental series, 24 rats of the same sex and weight as those of the previous experimental series were subdivided into 3 equal groups; group 1 was treated with fluorocortisol, group 2 with epinephrine, and group 3 with fluorocortisol plus epinephrine. Fluorocortisol (9-fluorocortisol acetate) was injected in the form of a microcrystal suspension, subcutaneously, at a dose of 250 μg/100 g of body weight, always in 0.2 ml of physiologic saline, once daily, during 5 days. Epinephrine was administered also subcutaneously, in a single dose of 200 μg/100 g of body weight, on the 5th day of the experiment (i.e., 6 hours after the last injection of fluorocortisol). The animals were killed by decapitation 30 minutes later.

In a third experimental series, 7 cats of both sexes were used; 4 of them were injected with epinephrine while the remaining 3 served as controls. Epinephrine was given once, intraperitoneally, in a dose of 600 μg/kg of body weight. The animals were killed by decapitation 30 minutes later. Altogether, 10 specimens were taken from each heart; 5 from the

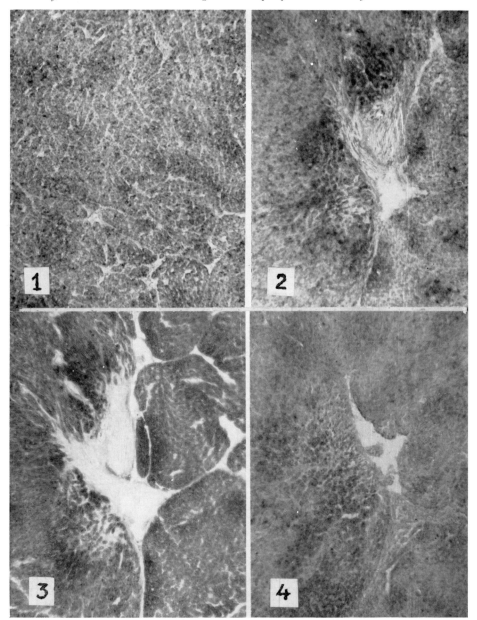

Figures 3–1 to 4. *Comparative behavior of the histochemically demonstrable potassium, glycogen and cytochrome oxidase in the heart muscle of a rat, 30 minutes following injection of epinephrine. Figure 3–1.* Distribution of potassium in a normal control heart. *Figure 3–2.* A marked depletion of myocardial potassium within some presumably affected subendocardial regions. Note that there is a zonal alteration in the distribution of potassium; fibers surrounding the depleted foci reveal markedly increased staining intensity, suggesting increased potassium content. *Figure 3–3.* The depletion of glycogen in, and its accumulation around, the affected areas always parallel the alteration in myocardial potassium content. *Figure 3–4.* At the same time, cytochrome oxidase activity is still normal, or even elevated, within those parts of the heart where potassium and glycogen are already significantly depleted. (Serial frozen sections.)

TABLE 3–I

THE EFFECT OF EPINEPHRINE ON THE POTASSIUM CONCENTRATION OF SELECTED
SUBEPICARDIAL AND SUBENDOCARDIAL REGIONS OF CAT HEARTS

Cat. No.	Treatment	Potassium Concentration in Heart Muscle (mEq/100 g dry weight)											
		Subepicardial Samples						Subendocardial Samples					
		1	2	3	4	5	Mean Values	1	2	3	4	5	Mean Values
1	None	34.6	33.7	32.8	33.9	34.1	33.8	33.8	34.5	33.5	32.1	34.8	33.7
2	None	31.3	32.7	36.8	33.0	32.9	33.3	34.9	32.6	36.0	31.0	34.6	33.8
3	None	35.2	32.5	33.6	35.4	31.6	33.6	31.7	34.8	32.6	35.1	32.1	33.2
4	Epinephrine	30.9	31.3	36.4	38.8	32.3	33.9	30.5	31.7	30.9	21.3[†]	32.1	29.3
5	Epinephrine	35.3	32.2	33.6	33.0	34.8	33.7	30.1	32.4	48.8[†]	31.9	34.7	35.5
6	Epinephrine	34.0	34.5	31.6	32.0	33.5	33.1	32.8	56.4[†]	20.6[†]	34.1	28.6[†]	34.4
7	Epinephrine	32.3	36.1	32.8	33.3	34.2	33.7	35.3	21.7[†]	34.4	26.0[†]	31.5	29.7

†Values marked are not within the range of variability normally to be expected.

subepicardial and 5 from the subendocardial areas of both ventricles. A small portion of the myocardial specimens so obtained was immediately frozen for the histochemical demonstration of potassium, while the overall concentration of potassium was measured by flame photometry in the remaining portion. The values of these determinations, as expressed in mEq/100 g dry weight for the heart (i.e., ventricular muscle) are listed in Table 3–I.

RESULTS

First Experimental Series. In the control hearts the activity of phosphorylase, succinic dehyrdogenase, and cytochrome oxidase was confined to the myocardial fibers. Within the individual muscle fibers the reactions for these enzymes were morphologically associated with the cytoplasmic structures, the nuclei remaining unstained. The intensity of enzyme activities was found to be remarkably uniform from fiber to fiber under normal conditions. The amount of the stainable labile fraction of glycogen was also remarkably constant.

Potassium appeared as a chrome-yellow precipitate, intracellular in location. This granular precipitate could be observed even more clearly under the microscope when converted to black-brown by treatment with ammonium sulfide; it was densely but evenly distributed in the cytoplasm of muscle cells and, in the longitudinally sectioned fibers, it followed the configuration of the myofibrils.

In the **hearts affected by epinephrine,** a spotty decline or even complete loss of phosphorylase activity was observed within some subendocardial regions as early as 10 to 15 minutes following the injection of the catecholamine. In addition, a depletion of the stainable glycogen reserves and a disturbance in the normal distribution of potassium were distinguishable after 10 to 15 minutes in some hearts only, but subsequently some fibers or fiber segments were seen to become completely devoid of potassium and glycogen. In some muscle fibers, bordering on the depleted foci, the amount of precipitate indicating the presence and level of potassium and glycogen respectively was increased. Such an abnormal deposition of these two substances was a more constant finding between 15 to 60 minutes after injection of epinephrine than during later stages.

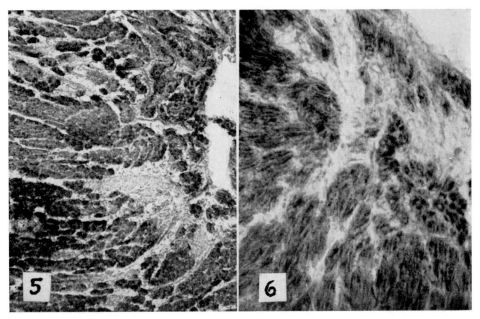

Figures 3–5 and 6. *Effect of epinephrine on distribution of potassium in the subendocardial regions of a rat heart. Figure 3–5.* Spotty subendocardial areas completely devoid of histochemically demonstrable potassium 30 minutes after administration of the amine. *Figure 3–6.* The extent of potassium loss is even more clearly demonstrated through high magnification of a section obtained from the same heart.

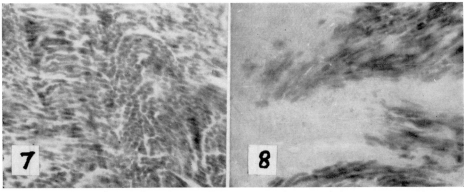

Figures 3–7 and 8. *Behavior of myocardial phosphorylase during early stages of anoxic heart damage. Figure 3–7.* Normal distribution of phosphorylase activity in the heart of a control rat. *Figure 3–8.* Disappearance of phosphorylase activity wihtin subendocardial areas 15 minutes after injection of epinephrine.

The areas depleted of potassium were always also the areas devoid of phosphorylase activity and glycogen content. The foci showing loss of phosphorylase activity—and a parallel depletion of glycogen reserves and potassium content—were spotty and mainly located in the subendocardium and apex, where necrotic lesions usually ensue. On the other hand, during such early stages of myo-

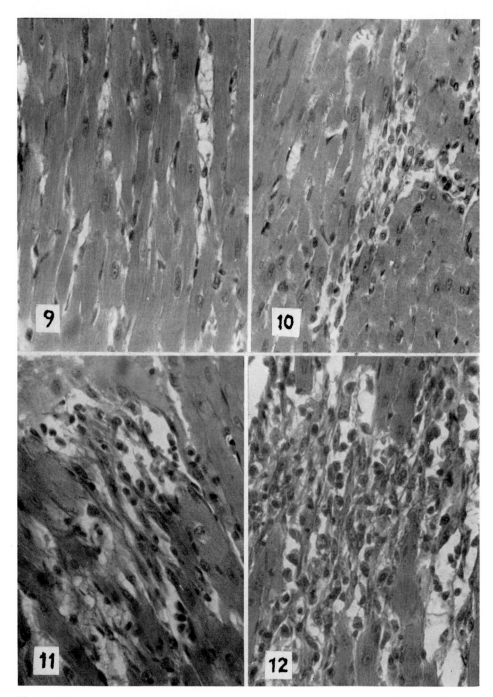

Figures 3–9 to 12. *Appearance of morphologic lesions in the heart muscle of rats following injection of epinephrine. Figure 3–9.* By using a conventional staining technique (hematoxylin-phloxine-saffron—HPS), very little damage can be demonstrated even 12 hours after the injection of the amine. Note the appearance of initial myolysis as well as swelling of a few individual muscle fibers or fiber segments. *Figure 3–10.* At 24 hours, the lesions are usually better defined, nevertheless still spotty in appearance. *Figure 3–11.* At 48 and (*Figure 3–12*) 72 hours, the morphologic lesions are fully developed as characterized by more or less confluent subendocardial areas of myolysis with inflammatory infiltration.

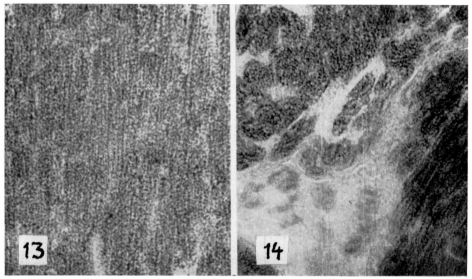

Figures 3-13 and 14. *Succinic dehydrogenase in the rat heart as influenced by epinephrine. Figure 3-13.* The activity and distribution of succinic dehydrogenase in a normal control heart. *Figure 3-14.* Partial decrease and loss of enzyme activity in myocardial fibers that are already in various stages of degeneration. Note increased succinic dehydrogenase activity in fibers surrounding the necrotic and, hence, enzymatically more or less inactive region.

cardial damage, the reactions for oxidative enzymes (succinic dehydrogenase and cytochrome oxidase) remained normal or were even somewhat elevated within the areas devoid of phosphorylase, glycogen, and potassium.

When the conventional HPS stain was used, morphologically detectable changes did not occur in the myocardium until 5 to 8 hours following treatment with epinephrine. Between 8 to 24 hours, the necrotic and myolytic foci were somewhat better defined but the HPS technique was found sufficiently informative only when dealing with lesions of at least 24 hours' duration. Only in the obviously necrotic fibers was a decrease or loss in the activity of oxidative enzymes observed.

Second Experimental Series. Neither treatment with fluorocortisol alone nor with smaller doses of epinephrine alone produced any major cardiac damage detectable by histochemical and conventional staining techniques.

On the other hand, a brief sensitization with fluorocortisol proved extremely potent in enhancing the susceptibility of the heart muscle to the potentially cardiotoxic action of subsequently injected epinephrine. This combination of agents resulted in the development of large and sometimes confluent areas, completely devoid of phosphorylase, potassium and glycogen, in 100 per cent of the hearts studied. Here again, the affected areas were mainly located within the subendocardium and the apex.

Third Experimental Series. Histochemical studies on the distribution of potassium in the heart of cats injected with epinephrine indicated that a spotty subendocardial depletion in potassium content also occurs in this species. Normally there is no significant difference in the concentration of potassium between the subendocardial and subepicardial muscle areas. By contrast, in the epinephrine-affected hearts, the subendocardial samples showed a much greater variation in the concentration of potassium than did the subepicardial muscle samples (Table 3–I).

DISCUSSION

The present studies indicate that following injection of epinephrine some histochemically clearly demonstrable alterations occur in the heart muscle long before any morphologic abnormalities can be detected by conventional staining techniques. These early (prenecrotic) histochemical alterations consist of a spotty decrease or even complete loss in the activity of phosphorylase and a parallel decline or total depletion in the stainable glycogen reserves, as well as in the concentration of the myocardial potassium. All these changes are mainly located in the subendocardium and the apex where necrotic lesions usually develop in epinephrine-affected hearts.

An alteration in the normal distribution of myocardial potassium appears to be an early prenecrotic change that precedes the development of structural abnormalities. Such zonal alterations in the distribution of potassium cannot be satisfactorily demonstrated by biochemical techniques using the whole heart as one sample, since the potassium lost from certain muscle fibers accumulates in others, especially in the cells bordering on the depleted foci. These pathologic potassium relocations disappear later during advanced stages of the development of myocardial lesions.

It is highly probable that there exists a close causal relationship between the cardiac necrotizing properties of the catecholamines and their influence on myocardial electrolyte metabolism (12-14). Potassium losses have been observed to occur following the administration of catecholamines (15-19); however, the present studies were the first to show (a) that epinephrine elicits potassium losses only from those limited focal areas of the myocardium in which it produces local hypoxia and (b) that this early spotty depletion of potassium is definitely prenecrotic in nature. The conclusion that localized hypoxia plays a primary role in the development of potassium depletion as well as in the parallel alterations in the activity of phosphorylase and in the glycogen content, was derived from observations which had shown that these histochemical alterations are identical with those seen following coronary artery occlusion (3, 5).

It is thus evident that potassium, glycogen, and phosphorylase are sensitive and early indices of the onset and extent of hypoxic damage inflicted by epinephrine on myocardial fibers. Our histochemical investigations are in agreement with earlier data (20-24) by demonstrating that potassium, glycogen and phosphorylase are intimately related to each other intracellularly.

The greatly enhanced potassium-depleting action of epinephrine after brief sensitization with a corticoid hormone may be of considerable clinical significance. Emotional, sensory, and many other stresses are accompanied by an augmented secretion of adrenocorticoid hormones, and the sensitizing action of the latter may play an important contributory role in catecholamine-induced myocardial injury (1).

SUMMARY

Studies in rats indicated that a decline or loss of histochemically demonstrable potassium occurs within some areas of the myocardium as early as 10 to 15 minutes following administration of epinephrine (i.e., long before structural changes can be demonstrated by conventional staining techniques). The foci showing loss of potassium—and a parallel depletion of glycogen reserves, as well as a decline in phosphorylase activity—were spotty and mainly located in the subendocardium and apex, where necrotic lesions usually ensue.

The reactions for oxidative enzymes (succinic dehydrogenase, cytochrome oxidase) remained normal or were even somewhat elevated within the respective areas.

Determination of the potassium concentration in hearts of epinephrine-treated cats suggested that a zonal alteration in the normal distribution of myocardial potassium is one of the earliest detectable signs of cardiac damage.

The early histochemically demonstrable alterations in the heart muscle following injection of epinephrine are identical with those seen in anoxic areas following coronary artery ligature.

A brief pretreatment with a potent corticoid hormone greatly sensitizes the subendocardial areas to the potentially cardiotoxic action of epinephrine.

The clinical significance of these findings is discussed.

REFERENCES

1. RAAB, W.: Neurogenic multifocal destruction of myocardial tissue. *Rev Canad Biol,* 22:217, 1963.
2. BAJUSZ, E., and JASMIN, G.: Comparative morphogenesis and enzyme histogenesis of some occlusive and metabolic cardiac necroses. *Rev Canad Biol,* 22:181, 1963.
3. BAJUSZ, E., and JASMIN, G.: Observations on histochemical differential diagnosis between primary and secondary cardiomyopathies. *Amer Heart J, 69:*83, 1965.
4. BAJUSZ, E., and JASMIN, G.: Histochemically demonstrable phosphorylase as an early index of anoxic myocardial damage. *Experientia, 29:* 373, 1964.
5. BAJUSZ, E., and JASMIN, G.: Histochemical studies on the myocardium following experimental interference with coronary circulation in the rat. Parts I and II. *Acta Histochem, 18:*222, 238, 1964.
6. TAKEUCHI, T., and KURIAKI, H.: Histochemical detection of phosphorylase in animal tissues. *J Histochem Cytochem, 3:*153, 1955.
7. TAKEUCHI, T., HIGASHI, K., and WATANUKI, S.: Distribution of amylophosphorylase in various tissues of human and mammalian organs. *J Histochem Cytochem, 3:*485, 1955.
8. PEARSE, A. G. E.: *Histochemistry. Theoretical and Applied.* London, Churchill Ltd., 1960.
9. BURSTONE, M. S.: Histochemical demonstration of cytochrome oxidase with new amine reagents. *J Histochem Cytochem, 8:*63, 1960.
10. POPPEN, K. J., GREEN, D. M., and WRENN, H. T.: The histochemical localization of potassium and glycogen. *J Histochem Cytochem, 1:*160, 1953.
11. MACALLUM, A. B.: On the distribution of potassium in animal and vegetable cells. *J Physiol, 32:*95, 1905.
12. SELYE, H.: *The Pluricausal Cardiopathies.* Springfield, Thomas, 1961.
13. BAJUSZ, E.: *Nutritional Aspects of Cardiovascular Diseases.* Crosby Lockwood, London, and Lippincott, Philadelphia 1965.
14. BAJUSZ, E. (Ed.): *Electrolytes and Cardiovascular Diseases: Physiology—Pathology—Therapy.* Vol. 1: *Fundamental Aspects;* Vol. 2: *Clinical Aspects.* Basel/New York, S. Karger, 1965.
15. MELVILLE, K. I., and KOROL, B.: Cardiac drug responses and potassium shifts. Studies on the interrelated effects of drugs on coronary flow, heart action and cardiac potassium movement. *Amer J Cardiol, 2:*81, 189, 1958.
16. NASMYTH, P. A.: Effect of corticosteroids on isolated mammalian heart and its response to adrenaline. *J Physiol, 139:*323, 1957.
17. ROBERTSON, W. v.B., and PEYSER, P.: Changes in water and electrolytes of cardiac muscle following epinephrine. *Amer J Physiol, 166:*277, 1951.
18. GOOTT, B., ROSENBERG, J. C., LILLEHEI, R. C., and MILLER, F. A.: The relationship of the sympatho-adrenal system to potassium flux and cardiac irritability induced by alterations in blood pH. *J Thorac Surg., 40:*625, 1960.

19. LEPESCHKIN, E., HERRLICH, H. C., and STAR-CHESKA, Y. K.: Personal communication.

20. BUCHANAN, J. M., HASTINGS, A. B., and NESBETT, F. B.: The effect of ionic environment on the synthesis of glycogen from glucose in rat liver slices. *J Biol Chem, 180:*435, 1949.

21. FENN, W. D.: The deposition of potassium and phosphate with glycogen in rat livers. *J Biol Chem, 128:*297, 1939.

22. HASTINGS, A. B., TENG, C. T., NESBETT, F. B., and SINEX, M.: Studies on carbohydrate metabolism. *J Biol Chem, 194:*69, 1952.

23. HOLLER, J. W.: Potassium deficiency occurring during treatment of diabetic acidosis. *JAMA, 131:*1186, 1946.

24. BAJUSZ, E.: Elektrolyt-Verschiebungsmechanismus im Herzmuskel und seine Bedetung für Pathogenese und Prophylaxe nekrotisierender Cardiopathien. *Arzneimittelforschung, 14:*1115, 1964.

Chapter IV

CARDIAC ISCHEMIC CHANGES INDUCED BY CENTRAL NERVOUS SYSTEM STIMULATION*

K. I. MELVILLE

(Montreal, Canada)

IN RECENT studies from this laboratory (2), it was demonstrated that centrally mediated adrenergic mechanisms can induce characteristic cardiac ischemic electrocardiographic changes. While it has long been known (3, 4) that electrical stiumlation of the brain can lead to autonomic cardiovascular disturbances, the exact role of the central nervous system in the initiation of cardiac ischemic or degenerative disease in man is still obscure.

Burdenko and Mogilnitzki (5) and Watts and Fulton (6) reported that experimental hypothalamic lesions can lead to cardiac and gastrointestinal hemorrhages. These authors and others (see review of Sheehan (7) concluded that the outflow from the posterior hypothalamus was mainly sympathetic, while that from the anterior was mainly parasympathetic. It was therefore postulated that the observed cardiac and gastrointestinal vascular changes were caused by increased sympathetic tone resulting from some kind of "autonomic imbalance," although Keller (8) concludes that these disturbances are only "indirect results of generalized physiological deteriora-

tions occasioned by the hypothalamic stimulation." The complexity of this problem has been reviewed by various workers in a recent Symposium of the American Physiological Society (9) on the central nervous system control of circulation. In addition, abundant clinical evidence (10-12) also shows that electrocardiographic abnormalities (prolongation of Q-T interval, deeply inverted and widened T waves and prominent U waves), simulating those of myocardial ischemia or infarction, can occur in patients with cerebrovascular accidents.

Following injections of the central nervous system stimulant, picrotoxin, into the lateral cerebral ventricles of rabbits, Varma, Share and Melville (13) have also shown that various types of cardiac ischemic changes (ST-T alterations) and arrhythmias ensued. It was suggested that these were mediated through central excitation of adrenergic mechanisms, probably involving catecholamines. Vogt (14) has shown that, following subcutaneous injections of picrotoxin, there is a marked decrease of catecholamines (norepinephrine and epinephrine) in the hypothalamus and midbrain. Dikshit (15) has also reported that intraventricular injections of caffeine can lead to sym-

*Aided by grants from the Canadian Heart Foundation and the Medical Research Council of Canada.

pathetic cardiovascular manifestations, presumably due to hypothalamic excitation. Marked cardiac ischemic changes (ST-T alterations) have also been described by Huq and Melville (16) following injections of pentylenetetrazol (metrazol) and caffeine into the lateral cerebral ventricle of cats. However, the exact site of action of these agents remains to be established. Evidence exists that both vagal and sympathetic pathways might be involved, and Bircher, Kanai and Wang (17) conclude that the cardiac arrhythmias induced by injections of pentylenetetrazol, picrotoxin and deslanoside in dogs were mediated mainly through vagus and to a less extent through sympathetic pathways. It is therefore clear that the role of the central nervous system in the initiation of cardiac ischemic changes requires further study.

METHODOLOGY

Full details of the procedures employed in these studies have been described in earlier papers from this Laboratory (12). Cats were used in all experiments. In most experiments ether chloralose anesthesia with succinylcholine and artificial respiration was employed. For electrical stimulation, after trephining the skull, stainless steel electrodes with bare tips of approximately 20 μ, were inserted stereotaxically into the anterior, posterior or lateral hypothalamic areas, using the Horseley-Clarke coordinate system, according to the atlases of Jasper and Ajmone-Marsan (18) and of Bleier (19). Final placements of the electrodes were verified anatomically and histologically by the method of Hess.

In the first series of experiments unipolar stimulations consisting of short (30 sec) trains of square wave pulses—100 cycles per second frequency and 1 msec duration—were repeated at 10-minute intervals. The stimulus strength ranged from 1 to 2 ma, continuously monitored on the oscilloscope and delivered through an isolation transformer. Electrocardiograms (praecordial lead V, approximately over the apical area with the animal in the left lateral position) were recorded continuously before, during, and after stimulation. Femoral arterial blood pressure was recorded concomitantly with a Statham Transducer, using a Sanborn Two-Channel recorder. The effects of the stimulation were compared (a) before and after double cervical vagotomy; (b) before and after spinal cord section at the second cervical (C2) level (in order to remove sympathetic pathways to the heart and (c) after combined C2 section and vagotomy.

In order to assess the effects of more intense and more prolonged stimulations, in a second series of similar experiments trains of stimuli (for 1 to 5 min durations) were applied in the lateral hypothalamic areas using frequencies of 100 per sec and 1 msec duration at intervals of 3 to 10 minutes. In these experiments the trains of stimulation were also repeated 20 to 40 times. For postmortem histologic examinations, the hearts were excised either immediately after the last stimulus or 12 to 20 hours later. For the prolonged experiments the animals were kept under chloralose with artificial respiration, following previous intramuscular injection of 200,000 IU of penicillin G procaine, mixed with 0.25 streptomycin sulfate. Immediately after excision all hearts were placed in formalin (10 per cent). Histologic examinations were also made of the hearts of 20 normal cats as controls.

For the experiments in which the effects

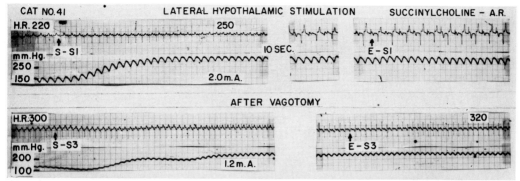

Figure 4–1. Cat No. 41. *Lateral hypothalamic stimulation.* Simultaneous electrocardiographic (lead V) and blood pressure changes recorded during and following anterior hypothalamic stimulation, before and after double cervical vagotomy. The figure shows sections of the tracings obtained during 30 sec trains of stimulation starting at arrows marked S-S and ending at arrows marked E-S. The numbers following S-S and E-S refer to the numbers of the successive trains of stimuli repeated in the experiment; an interval of 10 min elapsed between successive trains. The stimulus strength in milliamperes, as employed, is also shown. HR = heart rate per minute. (Reproduced from *Amer. J Cardiol, 12:*785, 1963.)

of intraventricular injections of drugs are considered (2, 13, and 16), the cats or rabbits were either anesthetized with chloralose or pentobarbital sodium, and the drugs (picrotoxin and pentylenetetrazol) injected into the lateral cerebral ventricle through a Collison cannula, using the method of Feldberg and Sherwood (20). Electrocardiograms (lead II) and femoral arterial blood pressure (using a Sanborn Transducer) were also simultaneously recorded at frequent intervals.

RESULTS

Cardiovascular Effects of Hypothalamic Stimulation.

Cardiovascular effects of short periods (30 sec) of stimulation were compared in 40 cats as follows: 14 with anterior, 10 with posterior, and 16 with lateral hypothalamic stimulation. In all of these experiments, both in normal and vagotomized animals, during stimulation there was always a sustained rise in blood pressure ranging from increases of 100 to 150 mm Hg (anterior), and from 175

to 200 mm Hg (posterior and lateral). These pressor responses were associated with varying degrees of electrocardiographic disturbances, which may be summarized as follows:

1. In normal nonvagotomized cats, anterior stimulation invariably induced striking S-T changes, ectopic beats and T inversion, which persisted for some time after stimulation. On the other hand, with posterior stimulation there were less marked ST-T changes and only occasional ectopic beats, but sinus bradycardia, T inversion and P-R segment depression occurred to varying degrees in different experiments. With lateral stimulation the most striking sinus tachycardia, ST-T changes and ectopic beats (multifocal, coupled) ensued. A typical example of these latter changes is shown in Figure 4–1 (upper records).

2. Following vagotomy, as can be seen from Figure 4–1 (lower records), arrhythmias (ectopic beats) were abolished, but ST-T changes still ensued with persistent T wave negativity during the post-

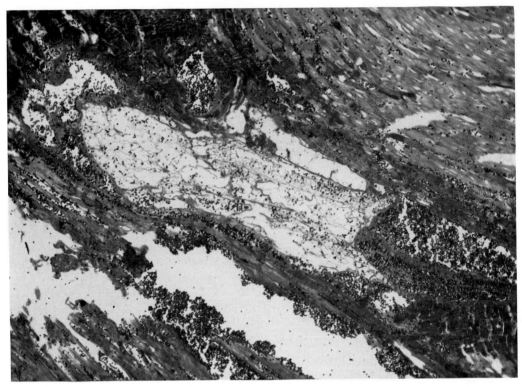

Figure 4–2. Cat No. 19. *Microphotograph of section of heart* showing general view of muscle with an area of hemorrhagic infarction in the interventricular septum. (Hematoxylin and eosin, x 100.) (Reproduced from *Amer. J Cardiol, 12:*788, 1963.)

stimulation period. Vagotomy similarly abolished the arrhythmias observed during both anterior and posterior stimulation and intensified the appearance of ischemic (ST-T) changes. The blood pressure responses were not strikingly altered by vagotomy.

3. Following spinal C2 section with the vagus nerves intact, both the pressor responses and tachycardia from stimulation of all three hypothalamic areas were abolished. However, during anterior stimulation there was rather a fall in blood pressure associated with bradycardia, suggesting stimulation of vagal pathways from this area. On the other hand, even with the most intense stimulation of the lateral hypothalamic areas

after spinal C2 section, there was no evidence of any vagal responses, suggesting that only sympathetic pathways were activated by lateral hypothalamic stimulation. The responses to posterior stimulation after spinal C2 section were more variable, and with high intensity stimulation showed some vagal responses, suggesting a mixed vagal-sympathetic response from this area. However, these vagal responses might conceivably result from current spread in this area. Beattie, Brow and Long (21) have postulated fiber pathways from the posterior hypothalamus to the thalamus, and through the reticular formation to the midbrain and medulla, without synapsing the hypothalamus. It is, therefore, concluded

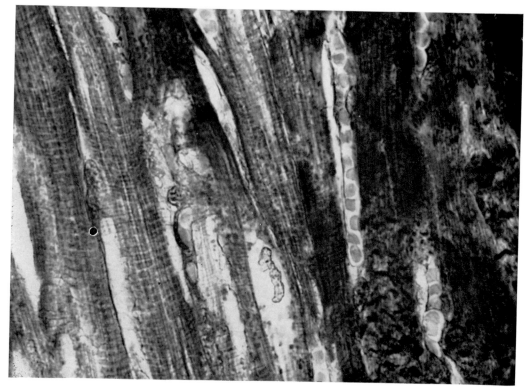

Figure 4–3. *Microphotograph of heart* under higher magnification, showing cardiac fibers at the edge of the area of infarction demonstrated in Figure 4–2. The cross striations seen in areas of normal muscle contrast with an intervening tongue of muscle fibers showing disruptions and loss of cross striations due to tissue damage. (Phosphotungstic acid, hematoxylin, x 1000.) (Reproduced from *Amer. J Cardiol, 12:*789, 1963.)

that there is no significant direct cardiac vagal connection arising either from the posterior or lateral hypothalamus.

4. Following spinal C2 section and double vagotomy, stimulation of anterior, posterior, or lateral hypothalamus induced no changes in blood pressure or electrocardiogram. It is, therefore, concluded that no hormonal or humoral (i.e., non-nervous) mechanism is involved in the above recorded changes.

Routine histological examination of the hearts of these animals showed no significant pathologic changes. In comparison with a group of 20 nonstimulated normal cat hearts similarly examined,

there were no detectable differences. In both groups, however, there were aggregates of round cells in the periadventitial tissue of small arteries in most hearts. Occasionally, small foci of interstitial myocarditis were found scattered indiscriminately throughout the myocardium, but no muscle changes were noted in relation to these foci.

These changes were rather like those described by Miller (22) as occurring spontaneously in rabbits. It is therefore concluded that under the conditions of stimulation employed in these experiments there was no postmortem evidence of myocardial damage.

In connection with the above studies it was also observed that with more prolonged repeated stimulations, of the lateral hypothalamus (15 experiments) using unilateral (9 cats) or bi-lateral (6 cats) stimulations, there was increasing evidence of cardiac ischemic changes. Thus, after 20 to 40 successive trains of such stimulations, it was observed that there was an exaggeration of the initially recorded ST-T changes, characterized by marked elevation of the S-T segment and tall peaked T waves associated with tachycardia.

After an interval of 6 hours following the last stimulation, the electrocardiogram also showed a regular sinus rhythm with plateau type S-T and distinctly inverted T waves, as well as a relative prolongation of the Q-T interval. Subsequently (after 16 to 20 hours) there was a sinus tachycardia with sagging S-T and persistent diphasic T waves, suggesting myocardial ischemic damage.

In regard to the postmortem findings in the group of 9 cats submitted to prolonged repeated unilateral stimulations, there were no abnormal pathologic changes seen, whether the hearts were excised immediately after the last stimulation or 12 hours later. However, in the group of 6 cats submitted to prolonged repeated or sustained bilateral hypothalamic stimulation, 3 animals showed definite myocardial involvement, and in 2 of these there was distinct myocardial infarction when the hearts were excised several hours after stimulation. Figures 4–2 and 3 illustrate the histopathologic changes seen in one of the animals. The heart of this animal weighed 17 g and was contracted in systole. Small irregular areas of pallor were seen in the subepicardial myocardium on gross examination. Microscopically (hematoxylin and eosin stain) an area of intense vascular congestion with associated small hemorrhages was found in the center of the interventricular muscle mass. Occasional leucocytes were seen, but the inflammatory reaction was not marked. Myocardial fibers in this area were infarcted. Their cytoplasm was brightly acidophilic and either homogeneous or in small clumps. Cross striations and nuclei were not apparent except at the borders of the lesions where the nuclei showed degenerative changes. The coronary vessels had normal appearances, and no occlusion was demonstrated.

DISCUSSION

It is clear from the above observations that brief stimulation of all three discrete hypothalamic areas studied can induce a rise in blood pressure associated with varying degrees of ischemic-like electrocardiographic changes (ST-T deviations) and arrhythmias. The data presented also show that the pressor response, tachycardia, ST-T changes, and ectopic beats resulting from stimulation of the different areas are all of sympathetic origin, since they still occurred after vagotomy and are abolished by spinal C2 section. All of these changes were also most marked during and after lateral stimulation, confirming the observations on the nonvagotomized animals that stimulation of the lateral hypothalamus leads mainly to sympathetic responses.

The above findings also indicate that only anterior hypothalamic stimulation directly activates vagal or parasympathetic effects, and the observed vagal effects arising from either posterior or lateral hypothalamic stimulation may only be due to current spread.

It is also evident from the data presented that even the most intense types of unilateral hypothalamic stimulation employed do not induce acute fatal or delayed myocardial damage. On the other hand, repeated bilateral hypothalamic stimulation intensifies both the electrocardiographic disturbances and postmortem cardiac changes. By prolonging the duration of the stimulation, profound electrocardiographic changes of an ischemic nature as well as arrhythmias and even electric alternans can occur. It is, however, curious that even the most intense degrees of stimulation employed in such experiments do not precipitate fatal ventricular fibrillation.

The electrocardiographic alterations observed in these experiments and in those concerned with the effects of intraventricular injections of picrotoxin (see above) closely resemble those previously described by Melville and Shister (23) following norepinephrine injections, and are clearly due to stimulation of the sympathetic nerves. As previously shown in rabbits, intravenous norepinephrine in doses as high as 500 to 1,000 μg induces similar characteristic anoxic ST-T changes but no ventricular fibrillation.

In conclusion, the arrhythmias described also resemble these reported in patients with cerebrovascular accidents, suggesting that hypothalamic stimulation might be involved in some of these cases. It is also postulated that sustained sympathetic cardiac stimulation of central nervous system origin can induce cardiac pathology and should be considered in any preventive regime.

SUMMARY

Stimulation of different brain areas can induce cardiac ischemic changes and arrhythmias. Increased or abnormal central nervous system excitation might, therefore, be an important factor in the genesis of human cardiac pathology.

Blood pressure and electrocardiographic changes (precordial lead V) were recorded continuously before, during, and after electrical stimulation of anterior, posterior, or lateral hypothalamic areas in cats.

Short periods of stimulation were applied repeatedly at 10-minute intervals. They induced from each area repeatable pressor responses associated with ischemia-like changes (ST-T deviations) and arrhythmias (bradycardia, tachycardia, ectopic beats). The pressor response, tachycardia and ST-T changes were all of sympathetic origin, and were abolished by spinal C2 section. These changes also appeared to be specifically mediated from the lateral hypothalamus. Parasympathetic cardiac changes (bradycardia), however, appeared to be mediated only from the anterior hypothalamus.

More intense and prolonged stimulations (repeated at 3- to 10-minute intervals 20 to 40 times) produced more marked and more persistent ischemia-like changes without ventricular fibrillation, and in some animals distinct myocardial infarction ensued.

It is concluded that sustained sympathetic cardiac stimulation of central nervous system origin can induce cardiac pathology and should be considered in any preventive regime.

REFERENCES

1. MELVILLE, K. I., BLUM, B., SHISTER, H. E., and SILVER, M. D.: Cardiac ischemic changes and arrhythmias induced by hypothalamic stimulation. *Amer J Cardiol*, *12*:781, 1963.
2. MELVILLE, K. I., and SHARE, N. N.: Cardiovascular responses following injection of picro-

toxin into the lateral cerebral ventricle. *Rev Canad Biol*, *22*:265, 1963.

3. KARPLUS, J. P., and KREIDL, A.: Gehirn und Sympathicus. I. Zwischenhirnbasis im Halssympathicus. *Arch Ges Physiol*, *129*:138, 1909.

4. KARPLUS, J. P., and KREIDL, A.: Gehirn und Sympathicus. II. Ein Sympathicus-Zentrum im Zwischenhirn. *Arch Ges Physiol*, *135*:401, 1910.

5. BURDENKO, N., and MOGILNITZKI, B. Z.: Zur Pathogenese einiger Formen des runden Magen-Darm Geschwürs. *Z Ges Neurol Psychiat*, *103*:42, 1926.

6. WATTS, J. W., and FULTON, J. F.: The effect of lesions of the hypothalamus upon the gastrointestinal tract and heart in monkeys. *Ann Surg*, *101*:363, 1935.

7. SHEEHAN, D.: The hypothalamus and gastrointestinal regulation. *Res Publ Ass Res Nerv Ment Dis*, *20*:589, 1940.

8. KELLER, A. D.: Ablation and stimulation of the hypothalamus; circulatory effects. *Physiol Rev*, *40*:116, 1960.

9. Symposium, American Physiological Society: Central nervous system control of circulation. *Physiol Rev*, *40*:1, 1960.

10. WEINBERG, S. J.: Hypothalamic dysfunction. *Calif Med*, *77*:253, 1952.

11. FENTZ, V., and GORMSEN, J.: Electrocardiographic patterns in patients with cerebrovascular accidents. *Circulation*, *25*:22, 1962.

12. HUGENHOLTZ, P. G.: Electrocardiographic abnormalities in cerebral disorders. Report of six cases and review of the literature. *Amer Heart J*, *63*:451, 1962.

13. VARMA, D. R., SHARE, N. N., and MELVILLE, K. I.: Cardiovascular responses following injection of picrotoxin into the lateral cerebral ventricle of rabbits. *Int J Neuropharmacol*, *1*:203, 1962.

14. VOGT, M.: The concentration of sympathin in different parts of the central nervous system under normal conditions and after administration of drugs. *J Physiol*, *123*:451, 1954.

15. DIKSHIT, B. B.: The production of cardiac irregularities by excitation of the hypothalamic centres. *J Physiol*, *81*:382, 1934.

16. HUQ, S., and MELVILE, K. I.: Centrally mediated cardiovascular responses induced by leptazol and caffeine. *Proc Canad Fed Biol Soc*, *6*:31, 1963.

17. BIRCHER, R. P., KANAI, T., and WANG, S. C.: Intravenous, cortical and intraventricular doseeffect relationships of pentylenetetrazol, picrotoxin, and deslanoside in dogs. *Electroenceph. Clin Neurophysiol*, *14*:256, 1962.

18. JASPER, H. H., and AJMONE-MARSAN, C.: *A Stereotaxic Atlas of the Diencephalon of the Cat.* Ottawa, Canada, Nat. Res. Council of Canada, 1960.

19. BLEIER, R.: *The Hypothalamus of the Cat.* Baltimore, Johns Hopkins Press, 1961.

20. FELDBERG, W., and SHERWOOD, S. L.: Permanent cannula for intraventricular injections. *J Physiol*, *120*:3P, 1953.

21. BEATTIE, J., BROW, G. R., and LONG, C. N. H.: Physiological and anatomical evidence for the existence of nerve tracts connecting the hypothalamus with spinal sympathetic centers. *Proc Roy Soc*, *106*:253, Series B, 1930.

22. MILLER, C. P.: Spontaneous interstitial myocarditis in rabbits. *J Exp Med*, *40*:543, 1924.

23. MELVILLE, K. I., and SHISTER, H. E.: Cardiac responses to epinephrine and norepinephrine during prolonged cholesterol and high fat feeding in rabbits. *Amer J Cardiol*, *4*:391, 1959.

Chapter V

EXPERIMENTAL PRODUCTION OF MYOCARDIAL LESIONS BY DISTURBING THE CENTRAL NERVOUS SYSTEM

(Role of Adreno-Sympathogenic Catecholamines)

IGOR K. SHKHVATSABAYA

(Moscow, USSR and Geneva, Switzerland)

DISTURBANCES of the nervous regulation of coronary circulation and myocardial metabolism are of definite importance in the pathogenesis of myocardial infarction. Many interesting observations on these problems have been made by L. A. Korejsha (1), T. M. Vihert (2), B. C. Livshiz (3), N. N. Vinogradova (4), S. S. Vail (5) and others.

Various methods of experimental production of neurogenic affections of the myocardium have been used, such as irritating and damaging various regions of the brain and spinal cord by such means as micro-electrodes; irritating extracardial nerves, and applying a glass crescent to the sella turcica (technique devised by A. D. Speransky).

As a result of each of the above-mentioned experiments, more or less conspicuous changes have been observed in coronary circulation, and structural alterations of the myocardium, although the latter were obtained only in isolated experiments and did not occur regularly.

We attempted to induce disorders of the myocardium in rabbits by disturbing the central nervous system without im-mediately affecting the coronary arteries. In trying to find an efficacious method to attain our aim, we devised a simple and reliable technique whereby we could directly affect the system of the brain ventricles.

In essence this method consists in insufflating air in the lateral ventricle of the brain of rabbits under local novocain anesthesia. The volume of air which we forced into the ventricle with the help of a thin needle did not exceed 1 cc, and the duration of the manipulation did not go beyond 5 to 10 sec. The above method differs essentially from the method of pneumoventriculography in that it does not require any partial suction of liquor prior to air insufflation and, since the air is being injected quickly under pressure, the manipulation can be repeated if necessary.

In all the animals which underwent this experiment, electrocardiograms were taken in three standard leads and in the fourth chest derivation. Pupillary reactions, as well as respiration, and in some cases arterial blood pressure, were also examined, the latter being measured on a carotid artery placed in a skin box.

The duration of our experiments varied from 4 minutes to 22 days from the moment of air insufflation, depending on how long the test animals survived. Death of the animals usually occurred after repeated insufflations, upon which a thorough morphological study of the organs was carried out, together with a detailed histological study of the heart.

RESULTS OF THE EXPERIMENTS

The response of the animals to air insufflation into the lateral ventricle of the brain consisted in motor expressions of anxiety, dilatation of the pupils, tachypnoea, reaching 120 to 160 per min., and in some cases the rhythm of respiration was disturbed. Arterial pressure at the moment of air insufflation was often decreased 10 to 90 mm Hg from the initial level, but it never fell below 60 mm.

The ECG showed various rhythmic disorders together with signs of ischemia of the myocardium. Among the most frequent disorders of rhythm were bradycardia and various forms of extrasystoles (auricular, ventricular, nodal, polytopic, single and group extrasystoles, allorhythmias, and more or less protracted periods of ectopical rhythm). In some rare cases alternation of the heart was observed. The order in which the above forms of arrhythmias appeared was as follows: first the ectopical rhythm appeared, then single and group extrasystoles, including polytopic ones, and in the end allorhythmias and alternation of the heart. Arrhythmias were accompanied by slowing of intraventricular conduction, sometimes manifested as bundle branch block (Fig. 5–1).

The main changes found in the electrocardiograms were characterized by signs of myocardial hypoxia, appearing as early as the period of rhythmic disorders. They consisted in a discordant shift of the ST interval in standard leads, in a deep depression of the ST interval in the first lead and an acute arched elevation in the third lead. The shape of the ECG resembled a monophasic curve.

The above-mentioned electrocardiographic changes were observed mainly during the first 30 minutes. Later on, from the 40th to the 60th minute, the ST interval was close to the isoelectric line, though slightly shifted, and a negative coronary T_3 appeared. The electrocardiographic changes in the third standard lead were the most durable ones and were still present several days after beginning of the experiment (Fig. 5–2).

Morphological examination of the rabbits' organs revealed distinct changes, mainly in the heart and lungs. Macroscopic investigation of the heart disclosed small hemorrhages in the epicardium mainly along the course of coronary arteries. In the lungs, areas of massive hemorrhages were observed in some cases.

Histological examination of the heart showed changes in all regions, but mainly in the septum and in the wall of the left and of the right ventricle, where these changes were far more severe and massive than elsewhere.

A marked constriction of small and large intramural arterial branches of the coronary arteries was observed, while venous sinusoids, filled with blood, were usually dilated. As a rule, hemorrhages were observed around the dilated sinusoids and in the perivascular tissue close to the contracted arterial branches. These features suggested an acute disturbance of heart vascularization.

In the myocardium we found disseminated necrobiotic areas in the form of

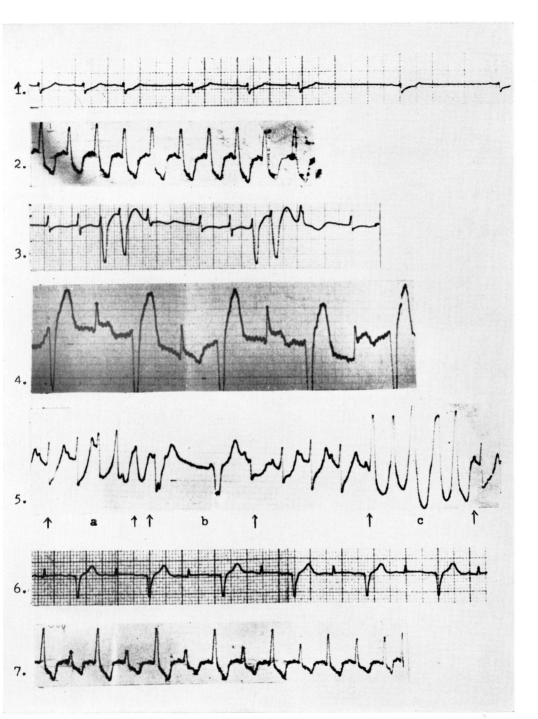

Figure 5–1. Examples of rhythm disturbances and alterations of conducting system, arising from air insufflation into the lateral ventricle of rabbit's brain: 1. Sinus bradycardia (first lead); 2. Ectopic rhythm (first lead); 3. Group ventricular extrasystoles (third lead); 4. Bigeminy (third lead); 5. Intraventricular blockade and ectopic rhythm on the background of ischemic curve; ((a) initial complexes, (b) intraventricular block, (c) ectopic rhythm); 6. Intermittent blockade (first lead); 7. Heart alternation.

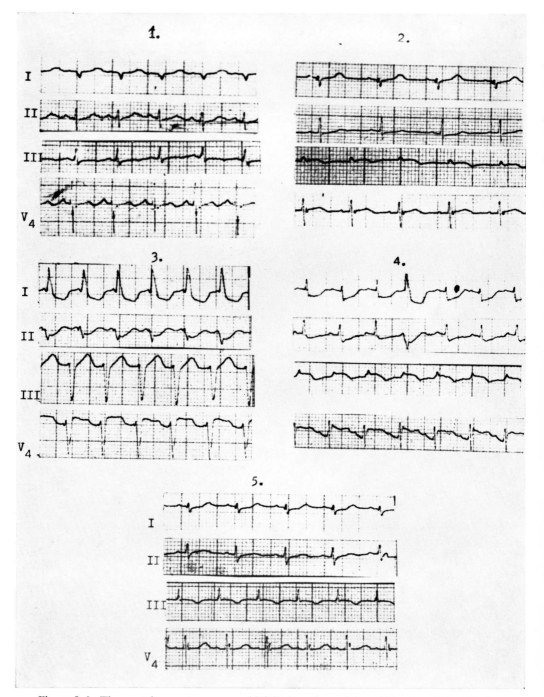

Figure 5–2. The most frequent sequence of ECG alterations of the rabbit after air insufflation into the lateral ventricle of the brain: 1. Initial ECG; 2. ECG at the moment of insufflation. Bradycardia; 3. ECG 1 min after the insufflation. Ectopic rhythm; 4. ECG 10 min after the insufflation. Markedly ischemic curve; 5. ECG after 2 days. Alterations are still present in the third standard lead.

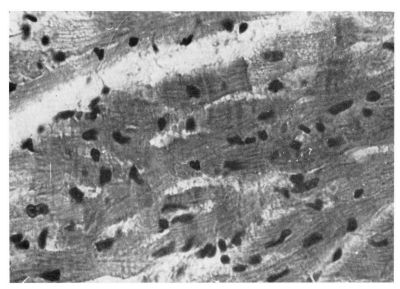

Figure 5–3. Eosinophil degeneration of muscular fibers of the myocardium. (Microphoto, 486:1.)

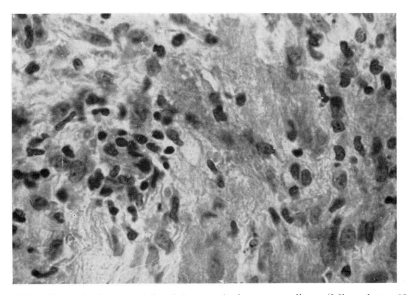

Figure 5–4. Necrotic changes of the right ventricular myocardium. (Microphoto, 486:1.)

eosinophil degeneration together with small areas of necrosis, varying in degree and volume (Figs. 5–3 and 4). Confluent areas of necrosis were also found in the right ventricle and in the septum. Most commonly they showed a subendocardial localization and in some cases they penetrated the entire thickness of the ventricular wall (Fig. 5–5). In almost all 20 rabbits (excluding 2 that died several minutes after the air insufflation), a growth of granulated tissue was observed

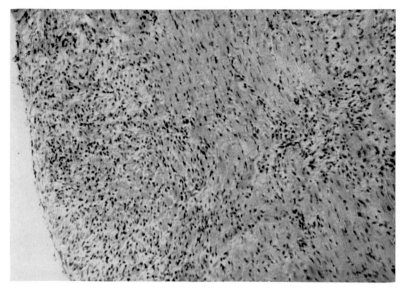

Figure 5–5. Confluent areas of necrosis and development of granulated tissue in the myo cardium of the right ventricle. The alterations have transmural character. (Microphoto, 66:1.)

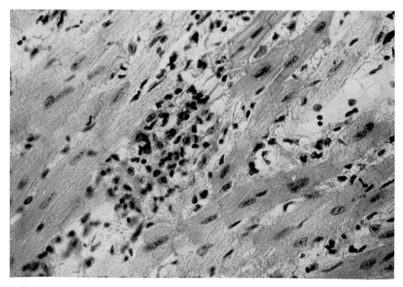

Figure 5–6. Region of granulated tissue replacing necrotized muscular fibers of the heart. (Microphoto, 258:1.)

in the affected regions (Fig. 5–6) along-side with eosinophil degeneration and myocardial necrosis. Such a combination of the earliest changes of the myocardium with those which set in later could be ascribed either to the effects of repeated insufflations, whereby the changes did not develop simultaneously, or it might be that the initial intensity of the lesions in the various regions of the myocardium was not of the same order.

Thus, the general and stereotypic character of the pathological reactions and the speed with which they appear following air insufflation into the brain ventricles prove that they are a direct consequence of the experimental disturbance of the central nervous system. Apparently, an acute, sudden and massive irritation of various regions of the brain takes place with an apparent increase of intracranial pressure. This is further evidenced by the appearance of pronounced bradycardia in the test animals.

We carried out further experiments with the purpose of studying the role played by extracardiac nerves in the origin of myocardial changes, resulting from air insufflation into a lateral ventricle.

For this purpose we used neurovegetative pharmacological agents which were administered to rabbits before the disturbance test. To induce adrenergic reactions, 0.2 mg of norepinephrine was injected intravenously to each of 6 rabbits; to block adrenergic reactions, 20 mg of hexamethonium was administered to each of 5 other rabbits. To elicit parasympathetic action, carbocholin (0.1 to 0.15 mg) was administered intramuscularly to 6 animals. Five rabbits underwent a bilateral vagotomy.

The results can be summarized as follows:

1. Air insufflation into the ventricles of the brain during parasympathetic reactions induced by carbocholin* and during blockade of sympathoadrenal effects with hexamethonium was not accompanied by ECG changes indicative

---

*Acetylcholine and carbocholin are capable of augmenting coronary flow and of reducing myocardial oxygen consumption. (KAVERINA, N. V.: *Pharmacology of Coronary Circulation*, Moscow, Medgiz, 1963. RAISKINA, M. E.: *Biochemistry of Nervous Regulation of the Heart*, Moscow, Medgiz, 1962.)

of myocardial hypoxia; no necroses in the myocardium were found under these conditions.

2. Blocking parasympathetic stimuli by severance of the vagi, as well as the adrenergic effects of administered norepinephrine, do not preclude the appearance of ECG changes or morphological lesions in the heart muscle after insufflation of air into the brain ventricle.

The above findings permit the conclusion that pathological changes in the heart are elicited by intensive activation of the sympathoadrenal system via irritation of vegetative nervous centers as a result of air insufflation into the brain ventricle.

In collaboration with Dr. V. V. Menshikov, we carried out a series of biochemical experiments to investigate the behavior of the sympathoadrenal system in connection with pathological reactions of the heart when the latter is subjected to neurogenic disturbances. In these studies we proceeded from the principle postulated by W. Raab (6, 7) concerning the role of catecholamine-induced local metabolic changes in the origin of myocardial lesions. According to Raab, the central stimulation of the sympathetic nervous system exposes the heart to an intensified, potentially hypoxiating action of epinephrine and norepinephrine, which can produce necroses in the myocardium.

In these experiments, rabbits were again subjected to air insufflation into the lateral brain ventricle and the catecholamine content in the tissue of the myocardium and adrenal glands was examined within 10 to 15 minutes after the appearance of signs of ischemia in the ECG. The animals' heads were severed, their hearts and adrenals were

TABLE 5–I

CATECHOLAMINE CONTENT OF THE TISSUE OF HEARTS AND ADRENALS
IN CONTROL AND EXPERIMENTAL RABBITS

	Control Series				Experimental Series		
		Heart	Adrenal Glands			Heart	Adrenal Glands
No. of Rabbits	Epinephrine in gamma/g	Norepinephrine in gamma/g	Epinephrine in gamma/g	No. of Rabbits	Epinephrine in gamma/g	Norepinephrine in gamma/g	Epinephrine in gamma/g
30	0.041	0.752	–	40	0.107	0.984	–
33	0.043	1.229	183.2	31	0.252	1.897	135.4
36	0.088	0.893	246.3	32	0.172	1.061	195.4
38	0.138	0.760	242.3	35	0.154	0.951	200.3
41	0.111	0.839	270.8	37	0.198	0.950	140.6
	0.084±0.036	0.894±0.192	235.65±32	45	0.158	0.986	160.3
				47	0.270	1.183	91.1
				48	0.226	1.147	90.79
				44	0.122	0.693	127.1
					0.184±0.036 220% of control level.	1.094±0.348 120.9% of control level.	142.6±57.4 60.5% of control level.

weighed, extracted and promptly ground in a 10 per cent solution of trichloracetic acid. Then the extracts were examined for their epinephrine and norepinephrine content by means of the modified fluorometric method described by V. V. Menshikov (8). These experiments were conducted on 9 male rabbits, each weighing 2.5 to 3 kg.

Five rabbits of the same sex and weight, used as controls, were submitted to conditions similar to those of the test rabbits: they underwent the same preliminary manipulations, including holes bored in their craniums above the lateral brain ventricle, without, however, insufflating air in the ventricles. The procedures which followed were the same as in the test group.

The results are presented in Table 5–I. In the experimental group the epinephrine content of the heart was 220 per cent of the control level while that of the adrenal glands was only approximately 60 per cent of the control level.

The norepinephrine content in the hearts of the experimental rabbits was also higher than in the controls; however, the difference was not found to be statistically significant.

Thus, due to centrogenic action, the epinephrine content of the adrenals appeared diminished and the epinephrine content of the myocardium greatly increased. Evidently, a gross disturbance of the central nervous system causes a massive secretion of epinephrine, the "alarm hormone," from the adrenals, which is then avidly absorbed by the heart muscle from the blood. It is probable that the centrally induced accumulation of large concentrations of epinephrine in the heart stimulates augmented oxidative metabolic processes in the myocardium and that these hypoxiating metabolic changes in the myocardium, alongside with disorders in the coronary blood flow within the heart, give rise to pathological changes of the ECG and dystrophic lesions of the myocardium.

According to widespread opinion, based on clinical and pathological observations, there are at least two mechanical factors which are very common and

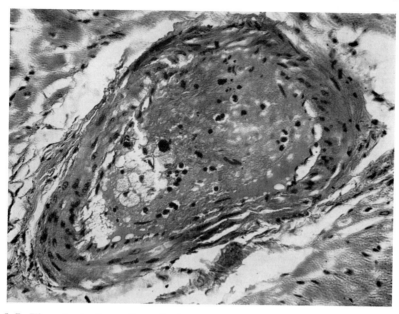

Figure 5–7. Thrombosis of a medium-sized coronary artery in cholesterol-fed rabbit subjected to air insufflation into the lateral brain ventricle. (Microphoto, 250:1.)

important for the development of myocardial infarctions. These are atherosclerosis of coronary arteries and coronary thrombosis. Both of them were absent in our above-described experiments. In order to approximate the conditions of our experiments to the clinical situation, we carried out a further series of experiments on cholesterol-fed rabbits, subjected to air insufflation into the lateral ventricle of the brain. Detailed results of these previously published experiments (9) will not be discussed here. The most important facts obtained were the following:

Apart from marked disturbances of cardiac vascularisation, capillary and venous thrombi were found (mostly of the spodogenous and hyaline type). One out of 10 rabbits showed typical thrombosis of a medium sized coronary artery (Fig. 5–7). This has never been observed in our previous experiments in rabbits without cholesterol atherosclerosis, subjected to air insufflation into the lateral ventricle of the brain (10). The arterial thrombus was characterized by proliferation of intimal cells with invasion of fibrin, leucocytes, and endothelial cells into the mass of the thrombus. This finding could be interpreted as indicating the beginning of organization of the thrombus.

In our opinion, special attention should be paid to this fact, since in plain cholesterol-induced atherosclerosis in rabbits there is no tendency to thrombus formation in the coronary arteries, in contrast to human atherosclerosis where thrombosis is frequently present (11).

So far, we can conclude that an acute disturbance of neuroregulatory mechanisms of the heart in the presence of atherosclerosis may predisope to thrombus formation in the coronary arteries of the rabbit.

Recently we investigated the changes

of blood coagulation mechanisms (blood level of fibrinogen, plasma tolerance to heparin, unbound heparin in plasma, fibrinolytic activity, thrombo-elastography) in cholesterol-fed rabbits and in normal rabbits before and after air insufflation into the lateral ventricle of the brain (the data will be published in 1965). The results of these experiments showed that this procedure caused an excessive increase of coagulation and decrease of fibrinolysis when contrasted with normal rabbits. These differences may play an important role in the mechanism of intravascular thrombus formation in cholesterol-fed rabbits subjected to acute neurogenic influences.

SUMMARY

Air insufflation into the lateral brain ventricle of the rabbit is a simple and reliable experimental method to induce disorders of the heart. These are manifested by the prompt appearance of arrhythmias and of changes of the electrocardiogram which are indicative of hypoxia of the myocardium. Ultimate results of this form of neurogenic interference are structural lesions of the myocardium including formation of focal necrosis in various regions of the heart, particularly in the ventricular subendocardium and septum.

The above described abnormalities did not appear if hexamethonium or carbocholin had been previously administered. They are accompanied by an accumulation of catecholamines in the myocardium and a decrease of epinephrine in the adrenal glands.

An acute disturbance of neuroregulatory mechanisms of the heart in the presence of cholesterol-induced coronary atherosclerosis may predispose to thrombus formation in the coronary arteries of rabbits.

REFERENCES

1. KOREJSHA, L. A.: About the relationship between cerebral cortex, subcortical ganglia and hypothalamic area in the regulation of cardiovascular system in man. *Nervous Regulation of the Cardiovascular System and Respiration*, Moscow, 1952, p. 137.
2. VIHERT, T. M.: Changes of the heart in acute disturbances of the cardiocirculatory system in patients with tumor of the brain. *Nervous Regulation of the Cardiovascular System and Respiration*, Moscow, 1952, p. 130.
3. LIVSHIZ, V. S.: Influence of irritation of subcortical area on the dog's heart. *Physiology and Pathology of Cardiocirculatory System*, Moscow, 1954, p. 35.
4. VINOGRADOVA, I. N.: Acute circulatory disturbances during the experimental irritation of hypothalamic area. *The Problems of Modern Neurosurgery*, Moscow, 1957, Vol. 2, p. 70.
5. VAIL, S. S.: *Functional Morphology of Heart Disturbance*, Moscow, Medgiz, 1960.
6. RAAB, W., and GIGEE, W.: Specific avidity of the heart muscle to absorb and store epinephrine and norepinephrine. *Circ Res*, 3:553, 1955.
7. RAAB, W.: Neurogenic multifocal destruction of myocardial tissue (pathogenic mechanism and its prevention). *Rev Canad Biol*, 22:217, 1963.
8. MENSHIKOV, V. V.: The measurement of catecholamines in urine. *Lab Delo*, 4:18, 1961.
9. SHKHVATSABAYA, I. K., and POSTNOV, Y. V.: Influence of the irritation of lateral brain ventricles on the heart in rabbits with experimental atherosclerosis. *Atherosclerosis and Thrombosis*, Meditsina, 1964, p. 49.
10. SHKHVATSABAYA, I. K.: An attempt at experimental reproduction of cardiac lesions through action on the nervous system. *Kardiologiia*, 3:18, 1961.
11. ANICHKOV, N. N.: Significance of experimental investigations for the pathogenesis of atherosclerosis. *Atherosclerosis and Coronary Insufficiency*, Medgiz, 1956, p. 3.

Chapter VI

SUBENDOCARDIAL HEMORRHAGES DURING STIMULATION OF THE SYMPATHETIC CARDIAC NERVES

MARY ANN KLOUDA and WALTER C. RANDALL

(Chicago, Illinois, U.S.A.)

SUBENDOCARDIAL hemorrhages in the heart have been described under a variety of conditions. In our laboratory they have been observed following prolonged electrical stimulation of the stellate ganglion in the dog (1) and following infusion of catecholamines. Others have noted these hemorrhages after large doses of epinephrine or norepinephrine (2–5). Similar lesions occur following severe hemorrhage (6, 7). Autopsies of persons having intracranial lesions reveal subendocardial hemorrhages (8).

One effect which these four situations — stellate stimulation, catecholamine infusion, hemorrhagic shock and intracranial lesions—have in common is an increase in the level of adrenergic activity of the heart and, consequently, an increase in the force of cardiac contraction. It has been demonstrated that electrical excitation of the stellate ganglion produces an increased force of contraction of the myocardium with a resultant smaller end-systolic volume of the ventricles (9). The increased force of contraction following infusion of catecholamines has been amply demonstrated. (10). Strain gauge measurements of cardiac contractile force during a period of rapid bleeding show a profound increase above the control level (11). Increased force of contraction is likewise a common accompaniment of intracranial lesions (8).

Since it has been demonstrated that there is a reduced end-systolic volume under stellate stimulation, it seemed plausible that under the influence of an increased force of cardiac contraction the opposing walls of the ventricle may come into contact and rub against one another. This would normally be prevented by the end-systolic volume of the ventricles. But in situations where the end-systolic volume is greatly reduced, the opposing ventricular walls could possibly meet and a subendocardial hemorrhage might be produced in this manner.

In order to test this hypothesis, an experiment was devised in which the end-systolic volume of the ventricles was prevented from reaching low levels even in the face of a great increase in force of cardiac contraction.

METHODS

Mongrel dogs under the influence of Sernylan were anesthetized with α-chloralose (85 to 90 mg/kg). The chest was opened bilaterally at the second intercostal space and the sternum was cut at this point. Bipolar stimulating electrodes were attached to both the right and the left stellate ganglion. A Grass Model S5 stimulator was used to stimulate the ganglia with pulses of 5 volts having a 5 msec duration. Frequency was varied as indicated later. The stimulation voltage was read directly from a cathode-ray oscilloscope across the stimulating electrodes. The carotid blood pressure was recorded from a Statham P23 Db transducer whose output was fed into a Grass polygraph recorder. The vagus nerves were left intact in all animals used in these experiments.

RESULTS

In 5 animals, both stellate ganglia were stimulated continuously at 3 cycles per sec for periods of 2½ to 4½ hours. The carotid blood pressure tracing showed that the heart rate increased and the systolic and diastolic pressures both increased, systolic rising more than diastolic, resulting in an increased pulse pressure. Postmortem examination of the hearts of these animals showed no grossly observable lesions in 4 of the animals. In the fifth animal, a few macroscopic subendocardial hemorrhages could be seen on the free wall of the left ventricle and an even greater number could be observed on the septal wall of the left ventricle. No lesions could be observed in the right ventricle.

In 7 animals, both stellate ganglia were stimulated continuously at 10 cycles per sec for periods of 2½ to 4 hours. The cardiac response was qualitatively the same as in the previous group of animals—an increased heart rate and increased systolic, diastolic and pulse pressures—but quantitatively the responses were much more pronounced.

On postmortem examination, 6 of the 7 hearts had grossly visible subendocardial hemorrhages on the papillary muscles and on the trabeculae carneae of the free wall of the left ventricle. Similar lesions were found on the septal wall, especially in the middle third. In 2 of these 6 hearts, subendocardial lesions were also observed in the right ventricle. In the seventh heart, there were no grossly visible lesions.

In 11 animals, both stellate ganglia were stimulated as in the previous group at 10 cycles per sec. However, in this group of animals an attempt was made to prevent the ventricles from emptying completely under the influence of stellate stimulation. A thread ligature was passed around the thoracic aorta just below the aortic arch and through a glass tube. This ligature was then tightened so as to partially occlude the aorta. In addition, the animal was infused with large volumes of saline in order to increase the vascular volume. A combination of these two procedures would presumably prevent the ventricles from completely emptying even in the face of an increased force of contraction. The cardiac response of these animals was essentially the same as in the preceding group of animals. When the hearts of these 11 animals were examined postmortem, 7 had no grossly visible subendocardial hemorrhages. The remaining 4 hearts showed lesions in both the left and right ventricles. A microscopic examination of the hearts with grossly visible lesions revealed hemorrhage, capillary congestion, focal neutrophilic infiltration, and edema. The hemorrhage involved the endocardium and adjacent myocardium to a depth of 1 mm in some sections. There was also marked hemorrhage in the mitral valve leaflets.

The hearts of all the animals used in

TABLE 6–I
NOREPINEPHRINE: μg/g TISSUE

	Control (6)	Group I (5)	Group II (7)	Group III (11)
Right atrium	1.99	2.18	0.99	1.15
Left atrium	1.42	1.37	1.16	1.43
Right ventricle	0.86	0.81	0.38	0.49
Left ventricle apex	0.69	0.69	0.30	0.53
Left ventricle base	0.75	0.73	0.36	0.59
Septum	0.71	0.73	0.35	0.44

TABLE 6–II
NOREPINEPHRINE: μg/g TISSUE IN
LEFT VENTRICLE

Group II		Group III	
Lesions	No Lesions	Lesions	No Lesions
0.38	0.26	1.10	0.30
0.55		0.23	1.16
0.11		0.73	0.26
0.00		0.31	0.94
0.61			0.37
0.42			0.40
			0.37

this study were chemically analyzed for their content of catecholamines in order to determine whether there might be a relationship between the incidence of subendocardial hemorrhages and the level of norepinephrine in the tissues. A modification of the trihydroxyindole method of analysis was used and epinephrine and norepinephrine were differentiated by reading the samples at two wave lengths in an Aminco-Bowman spectrophotofluorometer. Tissue samples of approximately 1 g each were taken from 6 areas of the heart: (a) right atrium, (b) left atrium, (c) right ventricle, (d) apex of the left ventricle, (e) base of the left ventricle, and (f) septum.

Table 6–I gives the average values for norepinephrine. Group I are the animals which were stimulated at 3 cycles per sec. Group II are the animals stimulated at 10 cycles per sec. Group III are animals which had saline infusion and aortic occlusion in addition to stimulation at 10 cycles per sec.

The cardiac norepinephrine levels of the animals in Group I were essentially the same as those of the control animals. However, in the animals in groups II and III, the cardiac norepinephrine levels (with the exception of the left atrial sample) are reduced from the control levels.

When groups II and III are broken down into those animals which had lesions and those which did not have lesions, the results shown in Table 6–II are obtained. Since the lesions were most commonly observed in the left ventricle, the average left ventricular norepinephrine level was used for comparison.

There were high norepinephrine levels and low norepinephrine levels both in the hearts which did have lesions and in the hearts which did not have lesions. In some hearts, a sample of the left ventricle from an area having a lesion was analyzed separately and compared with a sample of the same left ventricle from an area which did not have lesions. The norepinephrine level of the two samples was found to be exactly the same.

After the animals had been under constant stimulation for 2½ to 4½ hours, the stimulator was turned off and the carotid blood pressure fell to a final resting level as shown in Figure 6–1. Thus, the stimulation was still having an effect on the heart. The final systolic pressure under the effect of sympathetic stimulation was calculated as a percentage of the final resting (nonstimulated) systolic pressure. This value was then plotted against the norepinephrine level in the left ventricle at the end of the experiment in order to determine whether any correlation existed.

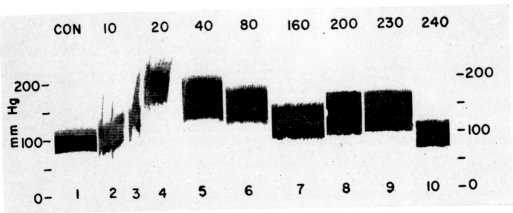

Figure 6–1. Pressure responses to stellate stimulation. Numbers at the top of the figure indicate time in minutes after control recording. Tracing at No. 1 shows the control blood pressure recording from the carotid artery. The tracing at No. 2 shows the effect of tightening the ligature around the aorta. No. 3 indicates the beginning of stimulation of both stellate ganglia. At No. 9 is shown the final blood pressure recording under stellate stimulation. No. 10 shows the final resting blood pressure recording after the stimulation has ceased.

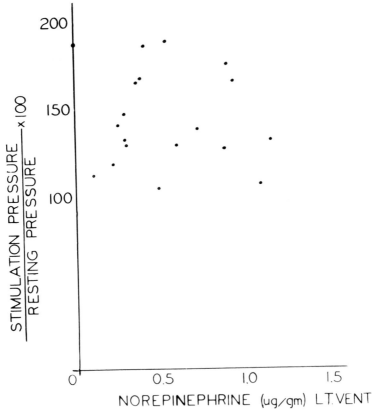

Figure 6–2. Pressure response versus norepinephrine level. The pressure response is plotted on the ordinate. Systolic pressure under stellate stimulation is plotted as a percentage of the final resting systolic pressure. On the abscissa is plotted the norepinephrine content of the left ventricle at the end of the experiment expressed as μg norepinephrine per gram of tissue.

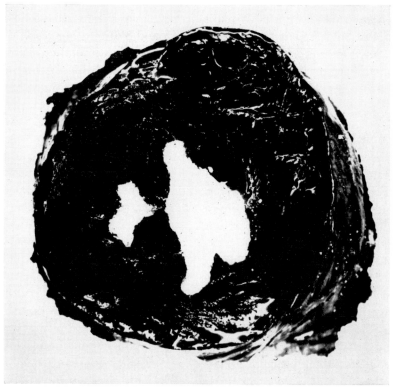

Figure 6–3. Cross section of a heart stopped in maximum systole. The left ventricle was filled with plaster of paris introduced by way of the left atrium after tying off all vessels leaving the left heart. The cross section was made near the apex of the heart so that only the left ventricle was sectioned. The right ventricle remained intact above the level of the section.

The results are shown in Figure 6–2. There was absolutely no consistent correlation between the level of norepinephrine in the left ventricle at the end of the experiment and the effect of stellate stimulation on systolic pressure at the end of the experiment.

If the development of subendocardial hemorrhages is dependent upon increased systolic emptying of the ventricles, it must also be related in some way to the maximum systolic pressure attained. Table 6–III shows a breakdown of each of the 3 groups of animals into those which had lesions and those which did not. The maximum systolic pressures attained by each animal are reported.

TABLE 6–III
MAXIMUM SYSTOLIC PRESSURE

Group I		*Group II*		*Group III*	
	No		*No*		*No*
Lesions	*Lesions*	*Lesions*	*Lesions*	*Lesions*	*Lesions*
270	140	275	235	205*	210
	130	235		220*	240
	175	210		345	260
	210	250		370	280
		250			230
		140			250
					170

*Infusion began simultaneously with stellate stimulation. Therefore, not hypervolemic at start of stimulation.

Figure 6–3 shows a cross section of a heart which has been stopped in maximum systole by calcium chloride perfusion. The anterior and posterior papillary muscles of the left ventricle are seen to be in close opposition, forming two separate chambers in the left ventricle, an inflow chamber and an outflow chamber.

DISCUSSION

It has been demonstrated that prolonged electrical stimulation of the stellate ganglion produces a systolic hypertension and that this systolic hypertension is a result of an augmented force of cardiac contraction (9, 12).

The actual apposition of the anterior and posterior papillary muscles of the left ventricle during maximum systole induced by calcium chloride injection has been demonstrated. It has also been demonstrated that prolonged stellate stimulation produces subendocardial hemorrhages in the heart (1). However, if the animal is made hypervolemic and the aorta is partially occluded, the incidence of subendocardial hemorrhages is greatly reduced. In 7 animals stimulated at 10 cycles per second (cps) in which no preventive measures were taken, 6 of the 7 animals developed subendocardial hemorrhages. However, in 11 animals which were given saline infusions and had the aorta partially occluded, only 4 animals developed the lesions. Two of these animals were used in the beginning of this series and the saline infusion was begun at the same time as the stellate stimulation. Therefore, they were not hypervolemic at the start of the stimulation. In later experiments, the infusion was begun approximately an hour before the beginning of the stellate stimulation so that the animals were hypervolemic at the start of the stimulation. The remaining 2 animals of this group which developed lesions showed systolic pressures of 345 and 370 mm Hg respectively, under sympathetic stimulation. With the development of such high pressures, it is possible that the heart may have emptied completely in spite of the hypervolemia and the aortic occlusion. It would seem, therefore, that if the ventricles can be prevented from emptying under the influence of sympathetic stimulation, the development of subendocardial hemorrhages can also be prevented.

While 6 out of 7 animals stimulated at 10 cps developed lesions, only 1 out of 5 animals stimulated at 3 cps developed lesions. The cardiac response to stimulation at 3 cycles is different from that produced by stimulation at 10 cycles (1, 13). The pressure rise under 10 cps stimulation occurs much more rapdily and reaches a greater height than that seen with 3 cps stimulation. This may account for the fact that lesions are much more prevalent with the 10 cps stimulation than with the 3 cps stimulation. In the 1 animal which did develop lesions under a 3 cps stimulation, the maximum systolic pressure attained was much greater than in the other 4 animals in this group. In general, the animals which developed lesions were the animals which attained high maximum systolic pressures. However, this does not hold true for every animal. What is actually needed is a continuous measurement of the end-systolic volume of the ventricles. It would then be possible to quantitate the degree of systolic emptying and to correlate this with the incidence of lesions.

One relationship which can be made is that there is no correlation at all, positive or negative, between the norepinephrine level in the left ventricle at the end of the experiment and the incidence of lesions. The effect of stellate stimulation on the norepinephrine level of the heart is also not consistent. The post-stimulation level may be above, below, or unchanged from the average value in control animals. Siegel has demonstrated that it is possible to show catecholamine liberation from the heart with stellate stimulation (14).

If serial biopsy samples had been taken during the course of the experiment and analyzed for norepinephrine, it might have been possible to see first an increase in tissue norepinephrine due to increased sympathetic activity (16), and then a decrease when the tissue stores become depleted (17). Since only 1 sample was taken in these experiments at the end of the stimulation, it is impossible to say what may have been happening to the norepinephrine levels during the course of the stimulation.

The fact that there was no correlation between the left ventricular norepinephrine level and the effect of stellate stimulation at the end of the experiment seems to indicate that the effectiveness of sympathetic nervous activity does not depend on the level of norepinephrine in the tissue. Obviously, other factors must be involved since it is possible to have effective sympathetic nervous activity with very low tissue levels of norepinephrine.

CONCLUSION

Subendocardial hemorrhages in the ventricles may be caused by the ventricles completely emptying themselves under sympathetic stimulation, allowing the opposing ventricular walls to meet and rub against each other.

SUMMARY

Prolonged electrical stimulation of the stellate ganglia produces systolic hypertension in dogs. The frequency of stimulation is an important factor in determining the characteristics of the hypertension. Prolonged stellate stimulation also produces subendocardial hemorrhages. The incidence of hemorrhages is higher with a 10 cps stimulation than with a 3 cps stimulation. The lesions are believed to be caused by the nearly complete emptying of the ventricles under stellate stimulation. When the ventricles are prevented from emptying completely, the lesions do not occur.

REFERENCES

1. KAYE, M., McDONALD, R., and RANDALL, W. C.: Systolic hypertension produced by electrical stimulation of the stellate ganglion. *Circ Res, 9:* 1164, 1961.
2. SZAKACS, J. E., and MEHLMAN, B.: Pathologic changes induced by l-norepinephrine: quantitative aspects. *Amer J Cardiol, 5:*619, 1960.
3. MALING, H. M., and HIGHMAN, B.: Exaggerated ventricular arrhythmias and myocardial fatty changes after large doses of norepinephrine and epinephrine in unanesthetized dogs. *Amer J Physiol, 194:*590, 1958.
4. MALING, H. M., HIGHMAN, B., and THOMPSON, E. C.: Some similar effects after large doses of catecholamines and myocardial infarction in dogs. *Amer J Cardiol, 5:*628, 1960.
5. NAHAS, G. G., BRUNSON, J. G., KING, W. M., and CAVERT, H. M.: Functional and morphologic changes in heart-lung preparations following administration of adrenal hormones. *Amer J Path, 34:*717, 1958.
6. HACKEL, D. B., and CATCHPOLE, B. N.: Pathologic and electrocardiographic effects of hemorrhagic shock in dogs treated with l-norepinephrine. *Lab Invest, 7:*358, 1958.
7. MELCHER, G. W., and WALCOTT, W. W.: Myocardial changes following shock. *Amer J Physiol, 164:*832, 1951.
8. SMITH, R. P., and TOMLINSON, B. E.: Subendocardial hemorrhages associated with intracranial lesions. *J Path Bact, 68:*327, 1954.
9. KELSO, A., and RANDALL, W. C.: Ventricular changes associated with sympathetic augmentation of cardiovascular pressure pulses. *Amer J Physiol, 196:*731, 1959.
10. MAYER, S. E., COTTEN, M. DE V., and MORAN,

N. C.: Dissociation of the augmentation of cardiac contractile force from the activation of myocardial phosphorylase by catecholamines. *J Pharmacol Exp Ther, 139:*275, 1963.

11. GREENFIELD, L., EBERT, P. A., and AUSTEN, W. G.: Effects of controlled acute hemorrhage on myocardial contractile force. *Proc. Soc Exp Biol Med, 107:*858, 1961.

12. RANDALL, W. C., and ROHSE, W.: The augmentor action of the sympathetic cardiac nerves. *Circ Res, 4:*470, 1956.

13. ROHSE, W., KAYE, M., and RANDALL, W. C.: Prolonged pressor effects of selective stimulation of the stellate ganglion. *Circ Res, 5:*144, 1959.

14. SIEGEL, J. H., GILMORE, J. P., and SARNOFF, S. J.: Myocardial extraction and production of catecholamines. *Circ Res, 9:*1336, 1961.

15. PEISS, C. N., and RANDALL, W. C.: Sympathetic control of the heart. In Cardiovascular Functions. Ed. Luisada, A. A., New York, McGraw-Hill, 1962.

16. RAAB, W., and GIGEE, W.: Specific avidity of the heart muscle to absorb and store epinephrine and norepinephrine. *Circ Res, 3:*553, 1955.

17. RAAB, W., and HUMPHREYS, R. J.: Secretory function of sympathetic neurones and sympathin formation in effector cells. *Amer J Physiol, 148:*460, 1947.

Chapter VII

NEUROGENIC MYOCARDIAL NECROSIS*

MARSHALL E. GROOVER, JR. and CLARKE STOUT

(Oklahoma City, Oklahoma, U.S.A.)

I N CLINICAL cardiology, our attention is often directed toward the neurogenic type of myocardial infarction. First, the association between emotional stress and acute myocardial infarction, and second, the absence of demonstrable coronary occlusive disease in 15 to 20 per cent of fatal cases suggests that rapid myocardial necrosis may be caused by factors other than occlusive coronary disease. This assumption is difficult to prove and indeed one is hard put to demonstrate neurogenic myocardial necrosis with the force and clarity of a well-developed coronary occlusion and its adjacent mass of necrotic tissue.

Earlier investigators have described myocardial necrosis in the absence of coronary artery disease. Josué (1) demonstrated in Paris in 1907 myocardial lesions produced by catecholamines. Many others have confirmed this phenomenon. Selye (2) described myocardial necrosis produced by various types of stress in animals previously treated with fluorohydrocortisone, and Raab (3) has shown that antiadrenergic drugs protect rats

from stress-induced myocardial necrosis. Groover et al. (4) observed abnormal electrocardiograms, myocardial scars and one fresh infarct in wild African baboons without coronary atherosclerosis, presumably caused by the emotional storm induced by trapping. Similar observations were made by Cherkovich (5) in baboons after various disturbing interferences in their living habits. Melville et al. (6) produced cardiac arrhythmias and ischemic myocardial changes by stimulation of the hypothalamus and have shown that this effect can be abolished by section of the cord at C-2, inferring that it is of sympathetic origin. Raab et al. (7) elicited myocardial necroses in 69 per cent of a series of wild rats exposed to frightening noises (tape-recorded cat-rat fight) and in 50 per cent of fluorocortisol-pretreated white rats which had been submitted to prolonged frustrating situations.

Shkhvatsabaya and Menshikov (8) found air insufflation into the brain ventricles of rabbits followed by an accumulation of catecholamines and necrosis formation in the heart muscle. Vedenyeyeva (9) has produced myocardial necroses by stimulating sympathetic nerve trunks, as well as by injecting epinephrine and norepinephrine.

On the other hand, Manning, Hall

*This work was supported in part by Public Health Service Research Grants HE-06286-04 and HE-07012-04 from the National Heart Institute, National Institutes of Health, Public Health Service, Bethesda, Maryland.

and Banting (10) very clearly demonstrated myocardial necrosis and peptic ulceration following vagus nerve stimulation in eserine-treated animals. They also demonstrated the protective effects of atropine in preventing both gastric ulceration and myocardial necrosis.

Thus we have myocardial necrosis produced by stimulation of both vagus and sympathetic nervous systems, and prevented by both atropine and antiadrenergic drugs.

If this type of neurogenic myocardial damage resembles the heart disease experienced by modern executives, for the purpose of prevention it would be desirable to classify various emotional states into adrenergic and cholinergic categories.

For an example, the situation existing at the time of myocardial infarction of one chief executive was described in a leading news magazine as one with the "terrible pressure of having many more things to do than he could possibly accomplish." There was no evidence of hostility, fear, or depression. The situation was one that could more accurately be described as one of fatigue and a sense of inability to deal with the ever increasing problems. Classification into adrenergic or cholinergic states would be extremely difficult. This suggests that cardiotoxic neurogenic activity originates in, or is mediated through, the central nervous system and reaches the myocardium by way of either one or both of the autonomic systems.

It must have been with a similar situation in mind that Manning, Hall and Banting became interested in the effects of the autonomic nervous system on the myocardium. They applied electrical stimulation to the vagus nerve, using a stimulus of sufficient intensity to give a maximum physiological response and applying it almost continuously until the animal died.

Since myocardial necrosis can be produced by such widely diverse means, we wished to determine which of these methods would more closely parallel the clinical and physiological changes seen in men in states of near rage, with slow pulse and normal blood pressure preceding the onset of myocardial infarction. We were curious to determine if electrical stimulation of nerve trunks, using a stimulus of physiological intensity, would produce myocardial necrosis.

Since the primary purpose was to find a model which could be used in the study of the role of emotional factors in myocardial infarction, a primate was selected which had some of the emotional characteristics in common with those of the modern human executive.

PROCEDURE

Preliminary dissections were done on 13 baboon cadavers to show the anatomical connections between the vagus and the sympathetic nerve trunk. A composite drawing (Fig. 7–1) shows these connections and the approximate location of nerve bundles joining the cardiac plexus from each trunk.

Eighteen female baboons (Papio anubis) weighing 10.5 to 12 kg were arranged in 6 treatment groups, designated to receive .0, .05, .1, .2, .4, and .6 mg of atropine sulphate intraperitoneally, 30 min prior to the stimulation procedure. All were healthy and had normal electrocardiograms prior to the experiment. Stimulation was applied to the unsectioned right vagus nerve in the neck, through a stainless steel electrode powered by a recently standardized Heathkit

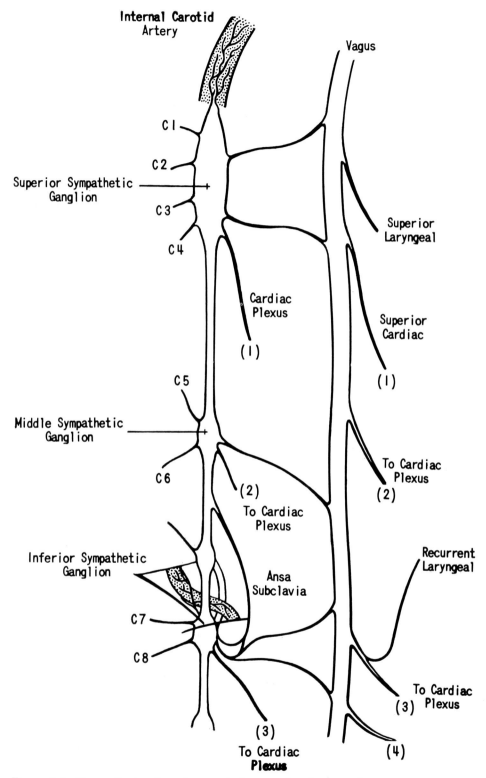

Figure 7–1. Composite drawing of anatomical connections between the vagus nerve and the sympathetic trunk, derived from the dissection of 13 baboon cadavers.

STIMULUS   RECOVERY

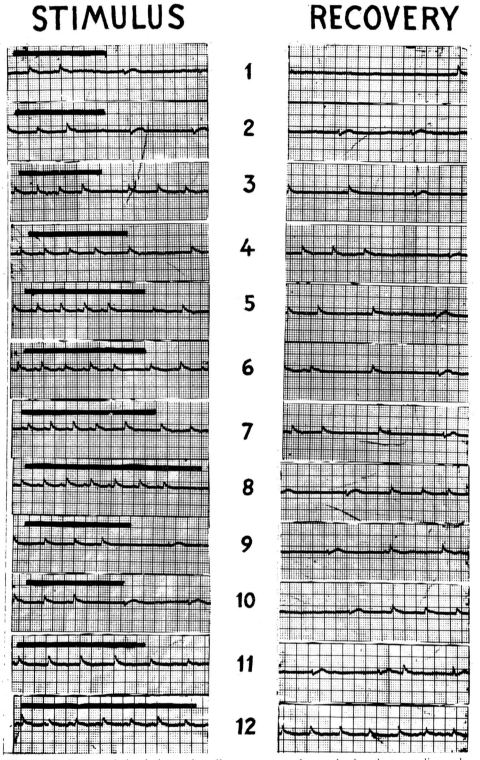

Figure 7–2, Pattern of stimulation and cardiac response on the monitoring electrocardiograph.

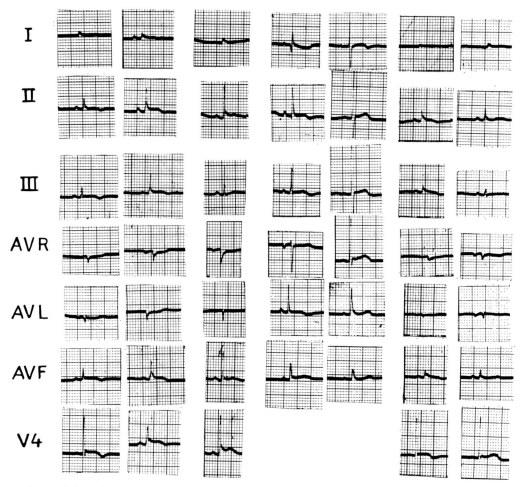

Figure 7–3. ECG tracings of 7 animals thought to be abnormal. No evidence of infarction is seen.

square wave generator. A current of .1 v at 30 cycles was used to initiate the stimulus, and the frequency gradually increased to 120 cycles per second, or until visible cardiac slowing was observed. Twelve consecutive stimulations were applied with a 1 min recovery period after each stimulation (Fig. 7–2).

Prompt cardiac slowing was obtained with the initial stimulation but the rapidity of response decreased with each successive stimulation so that little or no slowing was observed with the twelfth,

signifying vagus fatigue or perhaps injury to the conducting tissue.

After completion of the procedure, the animals were returned to holding quarters for 4 weeks, then routine ECG tracings were obtained, and they were sacrificed by exsanguination under pentobarbital anesthesia. The hearts were removed immediately, sectioned transversely, and the slices placed in a solution of blue tetrazolium at 37° for 30 min.

Seven animals had ECG tracings thought to be abnormal but the changes

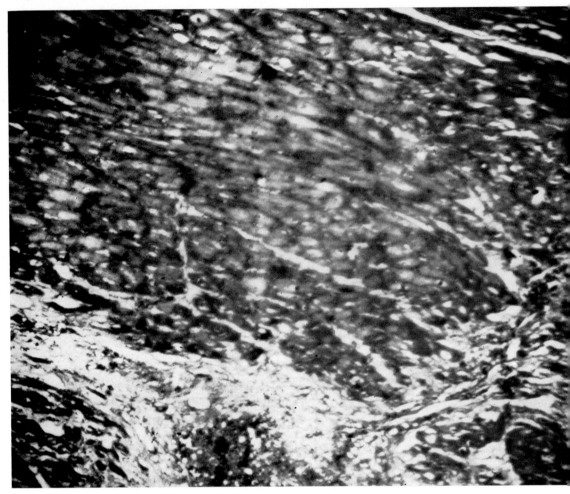

Figure 7–4. Section of H and E (Hematoxylin and Eosin) -stained tissue, taken from tetra-zolium-negative area in the septum near the anterior wall of the left ventricle.

were nonspecific and no evidence of well-developed infarction was seen (Fig. 7–3).

Blue tetrazolium stains normal dehy-drogenase-containing tissue a dark blue or black (11). Connective tissue and de-vitalized muscle are not stained, thus producing a contrast between normal myocardium and devitalized tissue. Tet-razolium negative areas were seen in the septum and adjacent ventricular wall of those animals which had received no atropine and in those which had received .05 mg.

One of the group receiving .1 mg and one of the animals receiving .2 mg showed small questionable unstained areas. Sec-tions of tissue taken from tetrazolium negative areas for histological examina-tion revealed the streaky fibrosis but not the coronary thrombi originally described by Manning, Hall and Banting (Figs. 7–4 and 5). In fact, no thrombi were seen in any of the coronary vessels even though a minimum of 20 sections were examined from each of the 8 or 9 slices. The areas of fibrosis seemed to follow the direction of muscle fibers in the septum and the direction of small arteries and nerves in the papillary muscles. The coronary arteries and epicardial surfaces were not

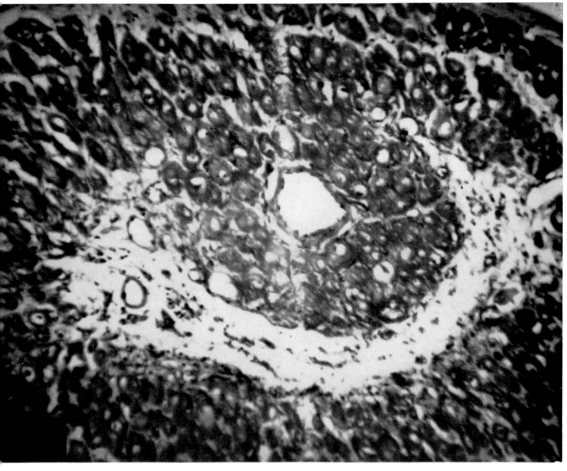

Figure 7–5. Section of H and E (Hematoxylin and Eosin) -stained tissue taken from tetra-zolium-negative area of the anterior papillary muscle.

involved and endocardial thickening was rarely seen.

The characteristic lesion was a streaky fibrosis replacing normal myocardial tissue. In the nonatropinized animals, this process was most pronounced. It was easily identified in those receiving .05 mg and in one animal receiving, 1 mg and to a lesser extent in one of the animals given .2 mg. No lesions could be detected in those receiving higher doses. Figure 7–6 is a summarizing cartoon showing the relation between atropine dosage and myocardial scarring.

It is noteworthy that one of the control animals and one of those receiving the smallest dose of atropine, .05 mg died of ventricular fibrillation during the stimulation. Even though the fibrillation was discovered immediately on the monitoring electrocardiograph and the defibrillator applied, they could not be restored to the normal rhythm and both animals died.

Autopsies disclosed no evidence of myocardial necrosis, however, microscopic areas of myocardial and subendocardial hemorrhages were noted. Subendocardial hemorrhages have been reported following electrical stimulation

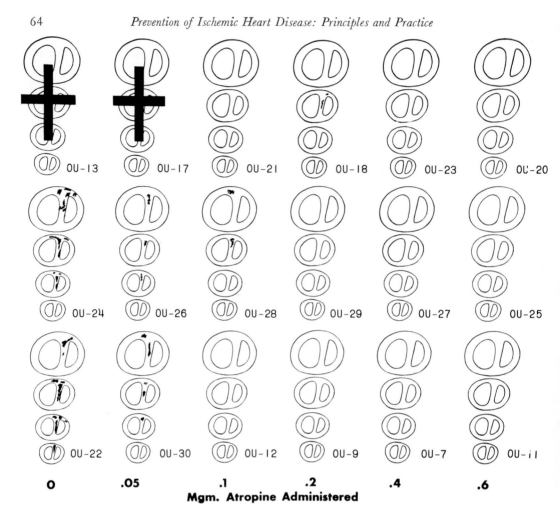

Figure 7–6. Diagrammatic representation of the location and degree of myocardial fibrosis seen with the various dosages of atropine. The two crosses represent the 2 animals which died from ventricular fibrillation.

of cardiac sympathetic trunks by Kay, McDonald and Randall (12).

DISCUSSION

The stimulus applied in the experiments was the weakest that would produce cardiac slowing. The animals were anesthetized with Sernyln*, a sensory blocking agent, which is thought to have minimal effect on cortex and basal ganglia and which was found to produce

---
*1- (1 Phenylcyclohexyl) piperidine hydrochloride manufactured by Parke, Davis and Company.

arterial hypertension in human cases. A mild elevation in blood pressure was noted in our animals. Hypotension did not occur during the stimulation procedure.

Plasma and myocardial catecholamines were not measured in these experiments and it is not possible at this time to prove that the ischemic changes were not mediated through some norepinephrine releasing mechanism. Since all lesions were confined to the anterior half of the septum and the adjacent ventricular walls, including the anterior papillary muscle, it is difficult to assign the cause of the lesion to a circulating hormone when the localized nature would suggest the distribution of some anatomical structures such as nerve ramifications. Otherwise lesions would be seen in random areas.

The protective effect of atropine in these animals and in the animals used by Manning, Hall and Banting (10), is difficult to reconcile with the findings of Josué (1), Selye (2), Raab (3), and others, unless one postulates two mechanisms for the production of myocardial necrosis. First, parasympathetic excess with an increase of acetylcholine production, augmented by eserine and inhibited by atropine, followed by a second or balancing surge of sympathetic activity as described by Gellhorn (13). In this manner, stimulation of either side will tend to increase the activity of the other. Atropine may prevent the increased vagal activity of stimulation and thus prevent the theoretically thinkable rebound sympathetic activity.

Atropine may be a much more complex drug than a simple parasympathetic blocking agent. In considering its use in these experiments one must remember that Burstein (14) has shown that atropine injected into the mesenteric vein of dogs causes the release of large amounts of heparin into the circulation. It is possible that the baboon and dog are unique in this respect. However, some of our post-myocardial infarction patients show an increase in the electrophoretic mobility of the beta lipoprotein after the oral administration of tincture of belladonna. If the beta lipoprotein mobility is an indicator of heparin activity, this would suggest that atropine not only retards acetylcholine production but by liberating heparin may reduce myocardial oxygen demand and increase the resistance of the myocardium to excess catecholamines.

On the other hand, we have found no reference in the literature to experiments proving a protective effect of heparin administration during vagus or sympathetic nerve stimulation.

SUMMARY

Myocardial lesions have been produced by electrical stimulation of the vagus nerve, using the weakest stimulus that would produce cardiac slowing for a minimal length of time. These lesions were prevented by atropine administration prior to stimulation. The mechanism involved in this phenomenon and its possible interrelation with the well-known catecholamine-induced myocardial lesions remains to be elucidated.

REFERENCES

1. Josué, O.: Hypertrophic cardiaque causée par l'adrénaline et la toxine typhique. *Compt Rend Soc Biol, 63:*285, 1907.
2. Selye, H.: *The Chemical Prevention of Cardiac Necrosis.* New York, Ronald Press Co., 1958.
3. Raab, W., Stark, E., Macmillan, W. H., and Gigee, W. R.: Sympathogenic origin and anti-adrenergic prevention of stress-induced myocardial lesions. *Amer J Cardiol, 8:*203, 1961.
4. Groover, M. E., Jr., Seljeskog, E. L., Haglin, J. J., and Hitchcock, C. R.: Myocardial infarction in the Kenya baboon without demonstrable atherosclerosis. *Angiology, 14:*409, 1963.
5. Cherkovitch, H. M.: Micronecroses in the hearts of primates resulting from experimentally induced neurosis. *Patologicheskaya fiziologiya y eksperimental'naya terapiya.* Moscow, Medgiz, 1959.
6. Melville, K. I., Blum, B., Shister, H. E., and Silver, M. D.: Cardiac ischemic change and arrhythmia induced by hypothalamic stimulation. *Amer J Cardiol, 12:*781, 1963.
7. Raab, W., Chaplin, J. P., and Bajusz, E.: Myocardial necroses produced in domesticated rats and in wild rats by sensory and emotional stresses. *Proc Exp Biol Med, 116:*665, 1964.

8. SHKHVATSABAYA, I. K., and MENSHIKOV, V. V.: The significance of the catecholamines in the pathogenesis of neurogenic lesions of the myocardium. *Kardiologiya, 2:*27, 1962.

9. VEDENYEYEVA, Z. I.: Myocardial lesions produced by sympathomimetic amines of endogenous and exogenous origin, and their analysis. *Farmakologiya y Toksikologiya, 3:*286, 1963.

10. MANNING, G. W., HALL, G. E., and BANTING, F. G.: Vagus stimulation and the production of myocardial damage. *Canad Med Ass J*, p. 215, Oct., 1937.

11. NACHLAS, M., and SHNITKA, R. K.: Macroscopic identification of early myocardial infarcts by alterations in dehydrogenase activity. *Amer J Path., 41:*279, 1963.

12. KAYE, M. P., McDONALD, R. H., and RANDALL, W. C.: Systolic hypertension and subendocardial hemorrhage produced by electrical stimulation of the stellate ganglion. *Circ Res, 9:*1164, 1961.

13. GELLHORN, E.: *Autonomic Imbalance and the Hypothalamus.* Minneapolis, Univ. of Minnesota Press, 1957, p. 137.

14. BURSTEIN, P. M.: Sur la sécrétion interne d'héparine après injection d'atropine dans la circulation hépatique. *Rev d'Hématologie, 3:*222, 1948.

Chapter VIII

ROLE OF FUNCTIONAL FACTOR IN THE PATHOGENESIS OF MYOCARDIAL INFARCTION*

NODAR N. KIPSHIDZE

(Tbilisi, U.S.S.R.)

IN THE pathogenesis of myocardial infarction primary importance is being generally ascribed to coronary atherosclerosis. N. N. Anitchkov expressed the opinion that "myocardial infarctions are practically nonexistent without atherosclerosis of the coronary arteries."

However, the exclusive role of atherosclerosis in the origin of myocardial infarction is being increasingly questioned, and a growing number of investigators attribute an at least equal pathogenic significance to functional disturbances of the coronary circulation (1–4), and/or to neurogenic and hormonal influences on myocardial oxygen and electrolyte metabolism (5–8).

It is true that according to statistical data, myocardial infarctions occur in the overwhelming majority of instances in the presence of advanced coronary atherosclerosis (9–11). However, N. N. Anitchkov et al. (12) found coronary infarctions with intact coronary arteries in 3 per cent of their autopsy material. Other cases of myocardial infarction without significant coronary arterial pathology were reported by Garshin (13), Grotel (14), Horn et al. (15), Talalayev (16) and others. Furthermore, necrotic foci of different sizes were observed in the myocardium of animals with normal coronary vessels as a result of central nervous (17, 18) and peripheral sympathetic stimulation (19) and of emotional stress (17, 20, 21), and after injection of the coronary-dilating but oxygen-wasting sympathogenic catecholamines, epinephrine and norepinephrine (22, 23).

On the other hand, despite the presence of severe, stenotic and occluding atherosclerotic lesions of individual branches or of both coronary arteries (24, 25), frequently no myocardial infarction is found; according to N. N. Anitchkov (12), in as much as 27.8 per cent of the cases. Although in a high percentage of instances myocardial infarction occurs on the basis of coronary thrombosis, no thrombi were detected in 25 to 50 per cent of several series of autopsies (26–35).

All this makes it clear that neither coronary thrombosis nor atherosclerosis per se are obligatory prerequisites for the development of myocardial infarctions and that coronary atherosclerosis must be regarded merely as an extremely important predisposing and contributory factor, but not as the exclusive pathogenic factor involved in the origin of myocardial infarction.

*Translated by W. Raab.

It appears obvious that additional functional elements must be taken into consideration to reconcile the customary vascular mechanical views concerning the pathogenesis of myocardial infarction with the above-mentioned facts.

One such functional factor is physical overstrain with resulting coronary insufficiency. This was first pointed out by F. Büchner (36). He observed disseminated necroses in the heart muscle of rabbits which, after having been made anemic, were subjected to physical strain and to an accompanying inadequacy of oxygen supply to the myocardium. This observation suggested an analogy to the exercise-induced anginal pain and to associated necrotic foci in the myocardium which are often found in the hearts of patients with coronary atherosclerosis. Raab et al. (37) have shown that galvanically-induced "exercise" of the extremities of anesthetized cats, which by itself does not cause any significant changes of the electrocardiogram, will promptly elicit the signs of severe myocardial anoxia when the normally occurring compensatory dilatation of a major coronary artery is impaired by a snugly fitting ligature. The same phenomenon occurred during stimulation of the cardiac sympathetic nerves or injection of adrenergic catecholamines (37).

A causal role of physical strain also in the formation of coronary thrombi is claimed by several investigators (38–41), but is denied by others (42).

It is believed by some that hemorrhages inside the coronary wall itself or in an atherosclerotic plaque may be provoked by the hemodynamic effects of physical or emotional stress (43–45) and that these local hemorrhages, by bulging into and obstructing the coronary arterial lumen,

give rise to secondary thrombus formation. Horn and Finkelstein (46) found intramural hemorrhages in 62.5 per cent of coronary occlusions and in only 37.5 per cent plain primary thromboses.

The following study will present evidence for the role of a functional factor, namely physical overstrain, in the development of myocardial infarction, occurring in the presence ot stenotic coronary atherosclerosis, but without thrombosis. These experiments may serve as a model for the genesis of infarctions which occur in humans with severe coronary atherosclerosis as a result of physical stress. Some instances of autoptically verified fresh infarctions were seen by us in cases of patients who, because of an earlier and already healed infarction, had spent a long time in bed and after getting up had overexerted themselves too early. Such events seem to belong in the same category.

MATERIAL AND METHODS

Our experimental rabbits (weight: 2 to 2.5 kg) were divided into 4 groups as follows:

I. (12 rabbits). Daily cholesterol-feeding during 6 months (0.3 g/kg body wieght).

II. (25 rabbits). Cholesterol-feeding as in I, plus daily physical stress (running on treadmill to exhaustion) for the same period.

III. (8 rabbits). Daily physical stress as in II, but without cholesterol-feeding.

IV. (12 rabbits). Cholesterol-feeding as in I, plus physical stress as in II and III, but the latter started only after marked coronary atherosclerosis had developed as judged by the electrocardiogram.

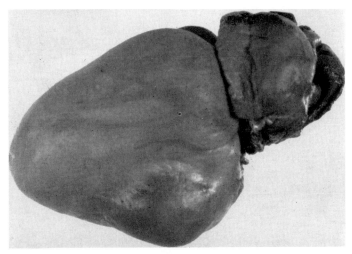

Figure 8–1.

Serum cholesterol was determined in all animals twice per month, and an electrocardiogram was recorded every tenth day. At the termination of 6 months, all surviving animals were sacrificed and the aortas and hearts were examined in the usual fashion for the presence of atherosclerotic vascular and myocardial muscular lesions.

RESULTS

In the animals of the first group (only cholesterol-feeding) the presence of stenosing atherosclerosis of the coronary arteries was ascertained. Plaques were located chiefly in the intramural branches of the left ventricle and, in part, in the subepicardial main vascular stems.

Beside the established coronary atherosclerosis within the heart muscle, particularly in the wall of the left ventricle, small focal scars of dense connective tissue were found in the vicinity of those arteries whose lumen was markedly narrowed, corresponding to the picture of disseminated microfocal cardiosclerosis.

In these instances, the electrocardiogram showed a distinctly low voltage of QRS and, in some animals, a downward dislocation of ST and depression of the T wave.

In the second group in which cholesterol-feeding and daily physical stress had been combined, some animals died within 3 to 5 months of the experiment, with signs of coronary insufficiency being recognizable in the electrocardiogram by a marked depression of the ST interval below the isoelectric line and a negative T wave. In some instances, giant T waves appeared in all leads, indicating an intense disturbance of the coronary circulation.

Within the above-mentioned time period, 11 out of 25 rabbits died. Histologic examination revealed in the hearts of all these animals extensive necroses of the left ventricle and, to a lesser extent, also of the right ventricle. In one instance, a protruding ventricular aneurysm had developed on the basis of an extensive infarct (Fig. 8–1). In 14 other animals which died spontaneously or which were killed at the end of 6 months, widespread necrotic areas were found in the left ventricular myocardium (Fig.

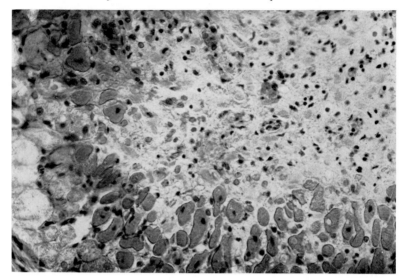

Figure 8–2.

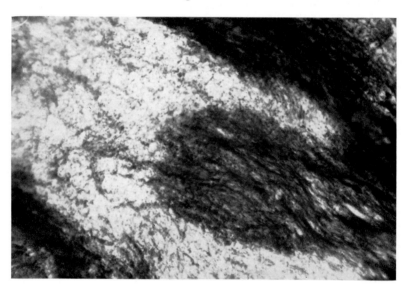

Figure 8–3.

8–2). It was possible to trace all stages of necrotization from local hemorrhages and fresh foci of proliferation to widespread tissue sclerosis (Fig. 8–3).

Larger areas of necrosis appeared more frequently in those rabbits which had displayed the highest hypercholesterolemia and the most marked atherosclerosis of the coronary arteries.

Necrotic areas were commonly distributed in the anterior and anterolateral wall of the left ventricle, less so in the posterior wall and the septum, and least frequently in the myocardium of the right ventricle (Fig. 8–4). The papillary muscles of the left ventricle were also often affected.

In the rabbits of the third group which

BACK

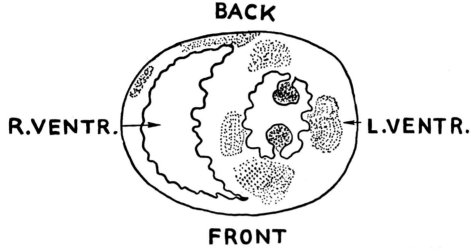

R.VENTR. ← → **L.VENTR.**

FRONT

Figure 8–4.

were stressed without cholesterol-feeding, no pathological alterations of the myocardium were seen except for a hypertrophy of the left ventricle and dilatation and congestion of some capillaries.

The rabbits of the fourth group, which were subjected to physical overstrain only after cholesterol atherosclerosis had developed, displayed rapidly progressing dyspnea, palpitations and severe hypoxic changes of the electrocardiogram. Out of these 12 animals, 8 perished within 6 to 14 days of stress. Four others survived the stress somewhat longer and died 21 to 30 days after beginning the treadmill strain.

Widespread necroses of the left ventricle were found in all rabbits of this group. Both the vicinity of arteries with atherosclerotic plaques and other areas of the myocardium exhibited numerous dystrophic foci and a great deal of scar tissue. The dystrophic areas were characterized by disintegration and extensive confluent necrosis of entire groups of myocardial fibers. Some fibers showed vacuolization. Scar formation within the heart muscle consisted, in part, of nu-

merous large regions of net-shaped connective tissue. Alongside of this loose network were scars of greater density, consisting of groups of collagenous fibers. Many myocardial fibers were separated by quantities of interstitial tissue, which contained masses of cellular elements. Among them were accumulations of lymphoid cells, histiocytes, and leucocytes with polymorphous nuclei.

The cells in the areas of infiltration frequently showed signs of disintegration. Many capillaries and veins were markedly dilated and filled with blood. In some parts, rather extensive hemorrhages were visible.

DISCUSSION

The development of multiple necrotic foci and of diffuse myocardial sclerosis in the rabbits of groups II and IV can be regarded as direct proof of the important role played by a functional factor (physical overstrain) in the origin of myocardial infarcts in the presence of stenosing coronary atherosclerosis.

A comparison of our experimental results with clinical observations concerning the occurrence of myocardial infarctions under the influence of physical stresses in patients with severe coronary atherosclerosis permits the conclusion that our experimental model of myocardial infarction is pathogenetically akin to the corresponding human pathology. Our experiments provide clear evidence of the role of physical overstrain as one factor in the pathogenesis of myocardial infarction in patients with stenotic atherosclerosis of the coronary arteries and without thrombosis.

SUMMARY

The origin of clinical myocardial infarctions cannot be explained exclusively on the basis of mechanical vascular abnormalities (coronary atherosclerosis, thrombosis). In order to prove the fundamental role of a functional vasomotor and/or metabolic factor in the development of myocardial necroses, prolonged experiments were carried out in rabbits subjected daily to an exhausting physical overstrain on a treadmill.

In otherwise untreated animals this did not elicit any significant structural lesions of the myocardium.

By contrast, widespread multiple necrotic foci and scar formation (mainly in the subendocardium) developed in all animals in which the daily physical stress was combined from the beginning with cholesterol feeding and gradual production of coronary atherosclerosis. Maximal degrees of myocardial destruction and a high mortality were observed if physical stress was imposed only after coronary atherosclerosis had fully developed.

Cholesterol-feeding alone elicited merely small disseminated focal scars.

It is concluded that, in the presence of predisposing coronary atherosclerosis, physical stress can serve as an important contributory factor in the pathogenesis of myocardial infarctions also in man, and that, in certain instances, both coronary atherosclerosis and superimposed functional overstrain of the heart are jointly responsible for the occurrence of destructive myocardial lesions.

REFERENCES

1. SMOLYANNIKOV, A. V., and APATENKO, A. K.: Pathogenesis and pathological anatomy of myocardial infarction. In: *Trudy vsyesoyuznoy konferentsu patologoanatomov,* Moscow, 1956, p. 258.
2. DAVYDOVSKY, I. V.: Discussion remark. *Op. cit.,* p. 311.
3. LAPIN, B. A.: Some peculiarities of the blood supply to the myocardium in coronary insufficiency. *Op. cit.,* p. 263.
4. MIMINOSHVILI, D. J., MEGAKYAN, G. O., and KOKAYA, G. YA.: Cortical influences on coronary circulation. *Voprosy fiziologii y patologii obyezyan,* Sukhumi, 1961.
5. MYASNIKOV, A. L.: Myocardial necroses of coronary and noncoronary genesis. *Amer J Cardiol, 13:*435, 1964.
6. SELYE, H.: The Pluricausal Cardiopathies. Springfield, Thomas, 1961.
7. RAAB, W.: Adrenergic cholinergic regulation of cardiac metabolism and function. In: *Dostizheniya Kardiologii.* Moscow, Medgiz, 1959.
8. RAYSKINA, M. E.: *Biokhimia nyervnoy regulyatsii syerdtsa.* Moscow, Medgiz, 1962.
9. McDONALD, G. E., and BENTLEY, W. B.: Acute myocardial infarction, a ten-year study. *New Eng J Med, 244:*743, 1951.
10. STRUKOV, A. I., and VINOGRADOV, C. A.: Role of coronary atherosclerosis and of functional strain of the heart in the origin of myocardial infarction. In: *Trudy XIV Vsyesoyuznogo syezda terapevtov,* Moscow, 1958, p. 296.
11. WRIGHT, J. S., MARPLE, CH. D., and BECK, D. F.: *Myocardial Infarction.* New York, Grune and Stratton, 1954.
12. ANITCHKOV, N. N., WALTER, A. V., VOLKOVA, K. G., and SINITSINA, I. A.: Morphological fundamentals of the origin of the myocardial infarct. In: *Trudy vsyesoyuznoy konferentsii patologoanatomov,* Moscow, 1956, p. 246.
13. GARSHIN, V. G.: Angiospasms in hypertensive disease. In: *Sbornik trudov, posvyashch. 35-lyetnyu*

nautchno-pedag. dyeat. N. N. Anitchkova, Leningrad, 1946, p. 44.

14. GROTEL', D. M.: *Acute Myocardial Infarction.* Leningrad Publication, 1940 ILMI, p. 219.

15. TALALAYEV, V. T.: The problem of angina pectoris vasomotorica. *Moscow Med J, 9:*112, 1928.

16. HORN, H., FIELD, L. E., DACK, S., and MASTER, A. M.: Acute coronary insufficiency: pathological and physiological aspects. *Amer Heart J, 40:*63, 1950.

17. CHERKOVICH, G. M.: Micronecroses in the heart of the monkey as a result of experimental neurosis. *Patologeecheskaya fiziologiya y eksperimental'naya terapiya.* Moscow, Medgiz, 1959.

18. SHKHVATSABAYA, I. K., and MENSHIKOV, V. V.: Significance of the catecholamines for the pathogenesis of neurogenic lesions of the myocardium. *Kardiologiya, 2:*27, 1962.

19. VEDENYEYEVA, Z. I.: Lesions of the myocardium, elicited by sympathogenic amines of endogenous or exogenous origin and their analysis. *Farmakol Toksik, 3:*286, 1962.

20. RAAB, W., CHAPLIN, J. P., and BAJUSZ, E.: Myocardial necrosis produced in domesticated rats and in wild rats by sensory and emotional stresses. *Proc Soc Exp Biol Med, 116:*665, 1964.

21. GROOVER, M. E.: Myocardial infarction without atherosclerosis in the Kenya baboon. *Circulation, 26:*645, 1962.

22. JOSUÉ, O.: Hypertrophie cardiaque causée par l'adrénaline et la toxine typhique. *Compt Rend Soc Biol, Paris, 63:*285, 1907.

23. RAAB, W.: The nonvascular metabolic myocardial vulnerability factor in "coronary heart disease." *Amer Heart J., 66:*685, 1963.

24. LEPORSKY, N. I.: Clinical observations concerning the complete occlusion of the ostia of both terminal arteries of the heart in syphilitic aortitis. *Ter Arkh, 17:*3, 1939.

25. YAROSHEVA, A. A.: Alterations of the coronary arteries of the heart in syphilitic aortitis. In: *Trudy vsyesoyuznoy konferentsii patologoanatomov,* Moscow, 1956, p. 297.

26. APPELBAUM, E., and NICOLSON, G. H.: Occlusive diseases of the coronary arteries. *Amer Heart J, 10:*662, 1935.

27. BLUMGART, H. L., SCHLESINGER, M. J., and ZOLL, P. M.: Angina pectoris, coronary failure and acute myocardial infarction. The role of coronary occlusion and collateral circulation. *JAMA, 116:* 91, 1941.

28. OBERNDORFER, L.: Pathologic anatomic findings in angina pectoris. *München Med Wschr, 72:*1495, 1925.

29. EHRLICH, J. C., and SHINOHARA, Y.: Low incidence of recent thrombotic coronary occlusion in hearts with acute myocardial infarction,

studied by serial block technique. *Circulation, 26:*710, 1962.

30. ETINGER, YA. G., and KOSTOMAROVA, M. I.: Pathology and clinic of angina pectoris of the heart in syphilitic aortitis. *Klin Med, 22:*29, 1944.

31. FRIEDBERG, C. K., and HORN, H.: Acute myocardial infarction not due to coronary artery occlusion. *JAMA, 112:*1675, 1939.

32. HAMBURGER, W. W., and SAPHIR, O.: Pulmonary embolism complicating and simulating coronary thrombosis. *Med Clin N Amer, 16:*383, 1932.

33. LIBMAN, E.: The importance of blood examinations in the recognition of thrombosis of the coronary arteries and its sequelae. *Amer Heart J, 1:*121, 1925.

34. MASTER, A. M., JAFFE, H. L., FIELD, L. E., and DONOSO, E.: Acute coronary insufficiency; its differential diagnosis and treatment. *Ann Intern Med, 45:*561, 1956.

35. MILLER, R. D., BURCHELL, H. B., and EDWARDS, J. E.: Myocardial infarction with and without coronary occlusion. *Arch Intern Med, 88:*597, 1951.

36. BÜCHNER, F.: Das morphologische Substrat der Angina pectoris im Tierexperiment. *Beitr Path Anat, 92:*311, 1933.

37. RAAB, W., VAN LITH, P., LEPESCHKIN, E., and HERRLICH, H. C.: Catecholamine-induced myocardial hypoxia in the presence of impaired coronary dilatability independent of external cardiac work. *Amer J Cardiol, 9:*455, 1962.

38. BOAS, E. P.: Angina pectoris and cardiac infarction from trauma or unusual effort. *JAMA, 112:* 1887, 1939.

39. COOKSEY, W. B.: Exertion and coronary thrombosis. *JAMA, 113:*351, 1939.

40. FITZHUGH, G., and HAMILTON, B. E.: Coronary occlusion and fatal angina pectoris. *JAMA, 100:* 475, 1933.

41. FRENCH, A. J., and DOCK, W.: Fatal coronary arteriosclerosis in young soldiers. *JAMA, 124:* 1233, 1944.

42. MASTER, A. M., DACK, S., and JAFFE, H. L.: Factors and events associated with onset of coronary artery thrombosis. *JAMA, 109:*546, 1937.

43. BOAS, E. P., and BOAS, N. F.: *Coronary Artery Disease.* Chicago, Yearbook Publisher, Inc., 1949.

44. PATERSON, J. C.: Some factors in causation of intimal hemorrhages and in precipitation of coronary thrombi. *Canad Med Ass J, 44:*114, 1941.

45. WARTMAN, W. B.: Occlusion of the coronary arteries by hemorrhage into their walls. *Amer Heart J., 15:*459, 1938.

46. HORN, H., and FINKELSTEIN, L. E.: Arteriosclerosis of the coronary arteries and the mechanism of their occlusion. *Amer Heart J, 19:*655, 1940.

Chapter IX

ADRENERGIC EFFECTS OF NICOTINE ON CORONARY BLOOD FLOW AND BLOOD LIPIDS*

SAMUEL BELLET

(*Philadelphia, Pennsylvania, U.S.A.*)

THE object of this presentation is to discuss the effect of nicotine and tobacco smoke on certain physiologic parameters, namely coronary blood flow and blood lipids. Considerable advances have been made in these fields in the past decade.

EFFECT ON CORONARY BLOOD FLOW

It has been shown that nicotine and tobacco smoke increase the coronary blood flow in the normal dog and in the human subject (1–3). This is due chiefly to the well-known effect of nicotine in releasing catecholamines (epinephrine and norepinephrine). The increase in coronary blood flow is associated with an increase in oxygen consumption and an increase in cardiac work, which can be readily accomplished in the normal heart with normal coronary arteries. Relatively few studies are available pertaining to the effect of nicotine in the presence of various types and degrees of coronary insufficiency, for example, with narrowing of the lumen of the coronary arteries or in the presence of coronary

artery disease. This point would appear to be of considerable theoretical and practical importance because many patients over the age of 45 or 50 years with varying degrees of coronary disease and/or coronary occlusion are subjected to the effects of nicotine in tobacco smoke. To meet the demand of increased cardiac work, the coronary blood flow must increase.

Experimental Procedures. The following aspects of the problem were investigated in the manner described below: (a) The effect of nicotine and tobacco smoke on the electrocardiogram of the normal dog was compared with that of dogs at various periods following coronary artery ligation, which corresponded to the acute, subacute, and healed stages of myocardial infarction, and after coronary artery narrowing produced by casein rings. (b) The effect of nicotine on the coronary blood flow was determined in a normal control group and compared with various categories of the group with myocardial infarction. (c) The effect of varying degrees of coronary artery narrowing was studied by placing casein rings around the circumflex and/or anterior descending branch of the left coronary artery. The casein swells; within a period of 2 or 3

*This work was aided by Grants #HE-9085-01 and HE-5989-01 from the National Institutes of Health, and by grants from the Tobacco Industry Research Committee and the Foundation for Cardiovascular Research.

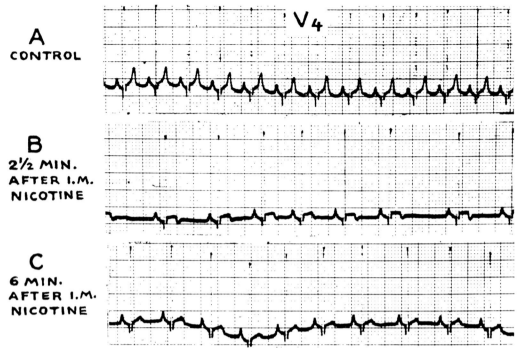

Figure 9–1. Nicotine injection in a *dog with artificial coronary insufficiency* (3 weeks after insertion of casein rings). (a) normal control tracing. (b) 2.5 min after intramuscular injection of 0.4 mg kg of nicotine. The RT segment is elevated. (c) 5.5 min after the injection. Note the upright T wave with RT no longer elevated. The T wave amplitude has not returned to normal.

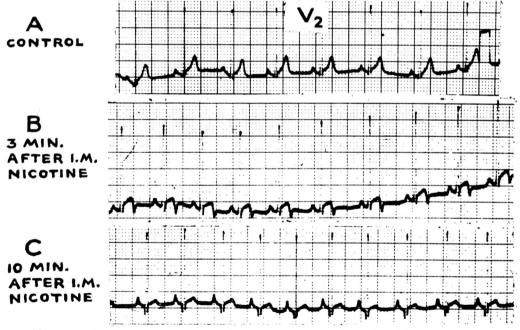

Figure 9–2. Effect of nicotine injection in a *dog prepared as in Figure 9–1*. (a) Normal control tracing (b) 3 min after intramuscular injection of 0.4 mg/kg of nicotine. The RT segment is elevated with a terminal downward dip. (c) 10 min after injection. The T wave has returned to an upright configuration.

TABLE 9–I

SUMMARY OF EXPERIMENTS SHOWING EFFECTS OF NICOTINE ON NORMAL DOGS
AND DOGS WITH MYOCARDIAL INFARCTION

| | | *Nicotine Dose Per Kilogram (Intramuscular)* | | | | | | | |
| | | 0.2 mg | | 0.4 mg | | 0.6 mg | | 0.8 mg | |
	ECG Effects	No. Exp.	Exp. In %	No. Exp.	Exp. In %	No. Exp.	Exp. In %	No. Exp.	Exp. In %
Normal dogs	Marked	0	0	0	0	0	0	2	18
	Moderate	0	0	0	0	0	0	1	9
	Slight	7	100	9	100	7	100	8	73
Infarcted dogs									
Acute (1-4 days)	Marked	13	68	11	84				
	Moderate	6	32	2	16				
	Slight	0	0	0	0				
Subacute (5–11 days)	Marked	2	33	4	33	4	66	1	100
	Moderate	2	33	3	25	1	17	0	0
	Slight	2	33	5	42	1	17	0	0
Chronic (over 18 days)	Marked	0	0	2	17	1	13	5	28
	Moderate	0	0	2	17	1	13	9	50
	Slight	2	100	8	66	5	72	4	22

weeks, the lumen is considerably narrowed and in some instances, almost obliterated (4).

Coronary blood flow was determined by directly measuring the outflow from the coronary sinus and, in some experiments, by the nitrous oxide method. Catheterization of the coronary sinus was accomplished in the intact animal with a special coronary sinus catheter (modified Morawitz cannula) inserted via the external jugular vein under fluoroscopic guidance, as previously described (4). The catheter was provided with multiple openings at the tip and an inflatable balloon for securing it in the coronary sinus. The following data were then obtained: coronary blood flow, O_2 consumption, cardiac output, cardiac work, O_2 extraction, heart rate, and blood pressure. These studies were repeated at various intervals for a period of 30 minutes after nicotene infusion. At the end of the experiment, the animals were sacrificed and carefully examined to determine the degree of coronary artery narrowing and the state of the heart muscle. In most instances, the coronary arteries were injected with Cardiographin and x rays were taken of the injected specimen.

Electrocardiographic Observations. It was found that normal unanesthetized animals were able to tolerate a fairly wide range of nicotine (0.2 to 0.8 mg/kg, intramuscularly) with the production of only slight electrocardiographic changes. Following myocardial damage produced by coronary ligation, marked electrocardiographic changes were obtained with a dose which was one-fourth of that required to produce only slight changes in the normal animal. These changes became less marked as the subacute stage was reached, and were still less evident in the chronic stage of infarction. However, the electrocardiographic changes after equivalent doses were more marked in the stage of chronic infarction than in normal controls (5). (see Table 9–I.)

Following the injection of nicotine in dogs with coronary insufficiency (con-

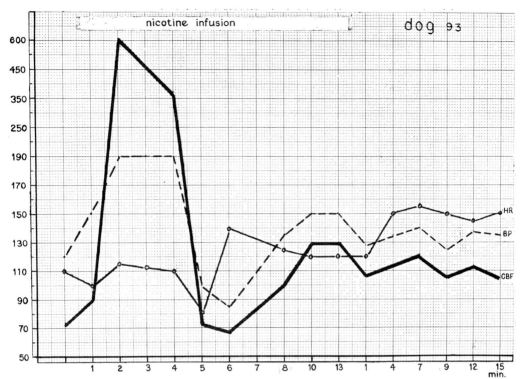

Figure 9–3. Effect of the injection of nicotine on coronary blood flow in the *normal dog*. Note the sudden increase in the coronary blood flow (CBF) between the first and fifth minute, from 70 to 600 cc/min. Following a dip down to the normal control level, the CBF is increased above the normal control value ranging between 110 and 130 cc/min, in the following 10 min. Note the increase in the heart rate (HR) and blood pressure (BP) which parallels the increase in the coronary blood flow.

striction due to casein rings) and after coronary occlusion, an elevation of the RT segments resulted (Figs. 9–1 and 2). These alterations in the ECG are believed to be due to a discrepancy between the increase in cardiac oxygen demand made by the catecholamine-liberating nicotine or the tobacco smoke and the reduced ability of coronary blood flow to increase.

Coronary Blood Flow

Normals. In 5 dogs curves similar to that shown in Figure 9–3 were obtained over periods of approximately 5 minutes. The cardiac output, work, and oxygen consumption were increased; the coro-nary a-v difference showed a decrease.

Coronary Artery Ligation. The effect of nicotine on 6 dogs, 4 to 19 days after ligation of the descending branch of the left coronary artery, is shown in Figure 9–4. The more acute and extensive the myocardial infarction, the lower and broader was the plateau of coronary flow increase. Cardiac output, work, and oxygen consumption were increased; the-coronary a-v difference was decreased.

Coronary Insufficiency Produced by Casein Rings. In the 8 dogs of this group the nicotine-induced augmentation of the coronary flow was significantly less and slower than in the controls (Fig. 9–5).

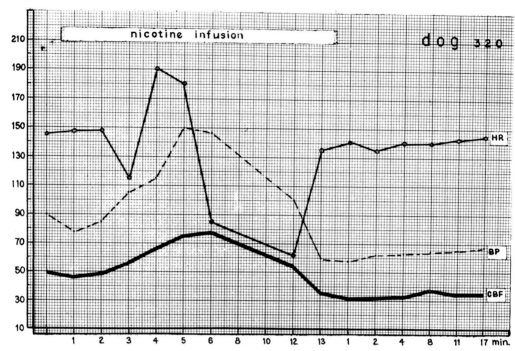

Figure 9–4. In a *dog with coronary artery ligation*, the initially low coronary blood flow (CBF) increases in a gradual manner following nicotine infusion, reaching a peak from the fifth to the eighth minute, and then gradually falling to a level below the normal control. Note the increase in the pulse rate (HR) and the blood pressure (BP) from the third to the twelfth minute.

Pathology

Coronary ligation was followed by the usual development of myocardial infarction.

Coronary insufficiency, produced by casein rings, was evident from a narrowing and, in some instances, almost complete obliteration of the coronary lumen. In this group there were no gross areas of infarction, but subendocardial necrotic foci with hemorrhages or areas of marked subendocardial fibrosis were found.

CIGARETTE SMOKING AND BLOOD LIPIDS IN HUMAN SUBJECTS

Since blood lipid variations have been generally accepted as an important factor in atherogenesis, an investigation of the effect of cigarette smoking and nicotine administration on lipid metabolism was undertaken to help clarify the relationship between smoking and coronary heart disease. The effects of nicotine in increasing the circulating catecholamines are well known.

In the present report, several phases of this investigation will be discussed: (a) the effect of cigarette smoking and nicotine on free-fatty acids (FFA) (7, 8); (b) the importance of the adrenal glands and sympathetic nervous system in the FFA response to smoking (9); (c) the effect of cigarette smoking on triglyceride tolerance following oral fat ingestion; and (d) the effect of long-term nicotine administration on serum cholesterol and triglyceride levels in dogs.

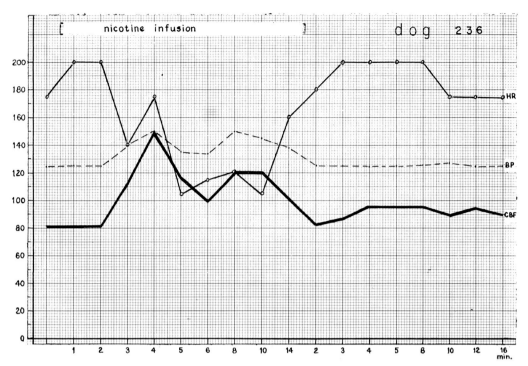

Figure 9–5. Results of nicotine infusion in a *dog with coronary insufficiency* produced by casein rings, one surrounding the anterior descending artery, and one on the circumflex branch of the left coronary artery. The relatively slight increase in coronary blood flow (CBF) reaches a peak at the fourth minute and gradually drops to the normal control level at the end of the infusion. Note the relatively high pulse rate (HR) and slight increase in blood pressure (BP).

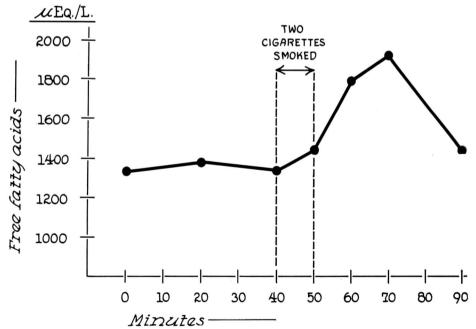

Figure 9–6. Serum FFA levels during presmoking control period and after patient smoked 2 cigarettes. Patient was a 52-year-old female with healed myocardial infarction.

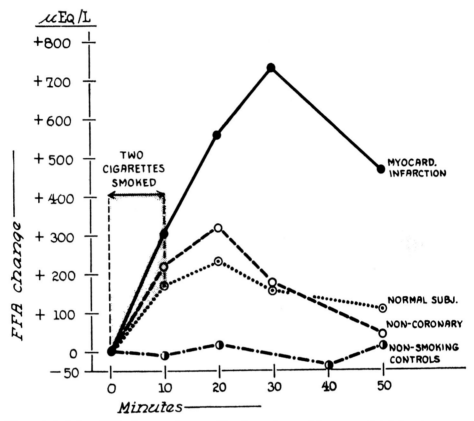

Figure 9–7. Mean FFA changes after smoking in patients with myocardial infarction, non-coronary patients, normal subjects, and nonsmoking controls. Two cigarettes were smoked during the 0 to 10 minute interval, except in nonsmoking controls.

Effect of Cigarette Smoking and Nicotine on FFA

All subjects developed a rise in serum FFA levels after smoking. Figure 9–6 shows a typical response. A mean maximal rise of 858 μEq/liter (65.6 per cent) developed in patients with myocardial infarction. Normal subjects and patients with noncoronary disorders had maximal elevations of 292 μEq liter (24.6 per cent) and 320 μEq/liter (27.2 per cent), respectively. The nonsmoking control subjects showed a mean rise of 20 μEq/liter (1.7 per cent). Figure 9–7 shows the curves of FFA changes of the three smoking groups and the nonsmoking controls.

In the dog experiments, after the intravenous administration of nicotine, the serum FFA concentration increased in 13 of 15 obersvations. The rise usually occurred at the end of 10 minutes of infusion and, in some instances, the levels further increased at the end of 20 minutes. The mean maximal elevation was 166 μEq/liter, with systemic venous blood showing the least.

Role of Adrenosympathetic System in Smoking-Induced FFA Responses

In all subjects showing a rise of the serum FFA levels there was a rise of free catecholamine excretion during smoking.

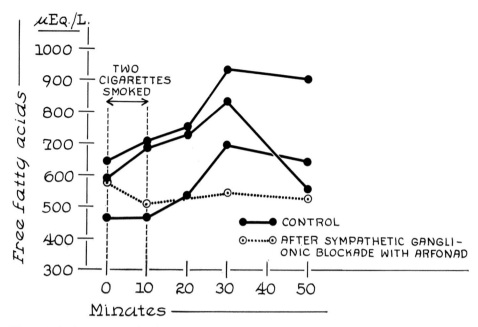

Figure 9–8. Serum FFA levels after smoking in a patient with angina pectoris before and after sympathetic ganglionic blockade with trimethaphan camphorsulfonate. Curves represent single smoking tests.

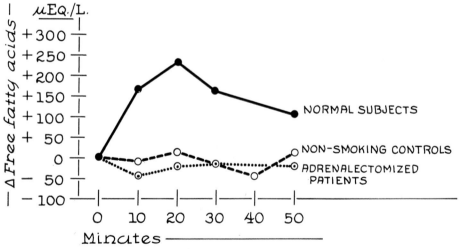

Figure 9–9. Mean FFA changes after smoking in 8 adrenalectomized patients and 10 normal subjects. Control curve represents FFA changes in 13 subjects when not smoking.

The mean increase of free catecholamines was 2.5 µg/hr (+21 per cent) and of total catecholamines 3.1 µg/hr (+16 per cent). Ganglionic blockage prevented the FFA augmentations (Fig. 9–8). Among 6 adrenalectomized subjects, FFA elevations after smoking were subnormal or absent (Fig. 9–9).

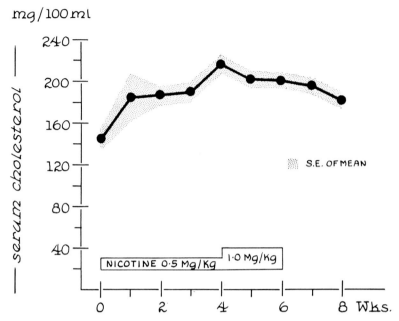

Figure 9–10. Mean cholesterol levels in dogs, given daily intramuscular injections of nicotine bitartrate in a slow absorption vehicle.

Serum Cholesterol and Triglycerides After Long-Term Nicotine Administration in Dogs

The mean serum cholesterol level increased gradually from a prenicotine value of 144 ± 11.8 mg per cent to a peak of 216 ± 15.3 mg per cent (P > 0.01) at the end of the fourth week of nicotine administration (50 per cent rise). This approximate level was maintained with nicotine until the end of the sixth week. Administration of the drug was then stopped and the cholesterol dropped to 181 ± 13.2 mg per cent (P > 0.05) after two weeks (Fig. 9–10). There was no significant change in triglyceride levels. No significant change in lipid levels occurred in the control dogs, including those receiving injections of the vehicle, but with no nicotine. There was no notable change in weight or feeding habits of dogs in the nicotine or control groups.

DISCUSSION

The effect of nicotine and tobacco smoke on dogs with coronary insufficiency showed effects which were similar to those of a stress mechanism. The findings obtained in the ECG, namely, RT segment elevations in the presence of coronary constriction, and the production of ectopic rhythms are similar to those produced in the experimental animal and in the human subject by emotional stress and/or exercise in the presence of coronary insufficiency.

Following the production of coronary insufficiency by coronary artery ligation or narrowing of the lumen of the coronary arteries, the pattern of response of the coronary blood flow was significantly different from that observed in the normal dog. The coronary blood flow showed only a slight increase as compared to the normal; this was also associated with a smaller change in cardiac output, coronary a-v difference, and oxygen consumption. The response of the coronary blood flow was similar to that observed by Foltz et al. (10), relative to the effect of anoxemia in the presence of coronary insufficiency. These studies would appear to have a bearing on the clinical problem of the effect of nicotine and tobacco smoke in the presence of coronary insufficiency.

A difference in the results, namely the observed increase in coronary blood flow in the experimental animal as contrasted to that observed in human subjects (11), is due to the fact that in the experimental animals doses far above the physiologic range were employed. Moreover, the values which were obtained in human subjects by the nitrous oxide method have their limitations in that small fluctuations in coronary blood flow are not registered by this technique.

Cigarette smoking caused a rapid, consistent and significant rise in serum FFA levels which did not appear to be related to age, sex, smoking habits, type of cigarette, or presmoking level of FFA (7). The FFA elevation after nicotine infusion in dogs indicated that the FFA effect after smoking was probably caused by nicotine and a resulting increased secretion of l-epinephrine and l-norepinephrine from the adrenal glands, extra-adrenal chromaffin tissue, and post-ganglionic sympathetic nerve endings. This is known to be followed by a rapid mobilization of FFA from adipose tissue by the released catecholamines (12, 13).

The marked rise of FFA in patients with myocardial infarction may be caused by a greater catecholamine release after nicotine stimulation. This could be due to a greater liberation of catecholamines from cardiac chromaffin tissue in ischemic hearts (14) or a greater catecholamine release from all sources in infarction patients, since these individuals have been shown to be sympathoadrenal hyper-reactors (15).

Our experiments demonstrated that (a) there was an increase in urinary catecholamine excretion during cigarette smoking; (b) sympathetic ganglionic blockade inhibited or prevented the mobilization of FFA which occurs after smoking; and (c) adrenalectomy also inhibited or prevented this mobilization. These observations permit the conclusion that, for cigarette smoking to cause an increase in serum FFA, both the adrenal glands and sympathetic nervous system must be functioning as sources of FFA-mobilizing catecholamines.

The hypercholesterolemic response in dogs to prolonged nicotine administration was quite striking. The dose of nicotine given daily was approximately equivalent to the amount absorbed by a human subject who smokes 20 cigarettes daily, and the slow absorption vehicle permitted drug administration comparable to the effect of continuous smoking. Carefully controlled, long-term studies at the onset and cessation of smoking are necessary to determine whether serum cholesterol is similarly affected in human subjects. Disturbances of lipid metabolism are considered important factors in the pathogenesis of atherosclerosis. Since smoking changes the normal pattern of some aspects of fat metabolism, it may, on this basis, have etiological significance in atherogenesis.

SUMMARY

In dogs with coronary insufficiency, produced by coronary artery ligation or artificial gradual coronary artery narrowing, the nicotine-induced augmentation of the coronary flow was considerably less marked than in control animals, and it frequently dropped below normal values in the post-infusion period. The response of other parameters, such as cardiac output, oxygen consumption and coronary a-v difference was also altered.

The electrocardiogram showed transient elevations of the RT segment in dogs with artificial coronary insufficiency when nicotine was injected.

These findings would appear to have a bearing on the clinical problem relative to the effect of nicotine and of nicotine-liberated catecholamines in human subjects with established coronary artery disease.

Smoking in humans and nicotine in dogs caused a rapid and consistent rise in serum free-fatty acids. Patients with myocardial infarction developed an elevation more than twice that of normal subjects and noncoronary patients.

In dogs receiving nicotine daily for a six-week period, there was a gradual 50 per cent rise in the level of serum cholesterol. Since smoking and nicotine change the normal pattern of some aspects of lipid metabolism, they may have etiological significance in atherogenesis.

REFERENCES

1. BARGERSON, L. M., JR., EHMKE, D., GONLUBOL, F., CASTELLANAS, A., SIEGEL, A., and BING, R. J., Effect of cigarette smoking on coronary blood flow and myocardial metabolism. *Circulation, 15:* 251, 1957.
2. KIEN, G. A., LASKER, N., and SHERROD, T. R.: Action of cigarette smoke on cardiovascular hemodynamics and oxygen utilization in the dog. *J Pharmacol Exp Ther, 124:*35, 1958.
3. STEWART, G. N., and ROGOFF, J. M.: The action of drugs on the output of epinephrine from the adrenals: nicotine. *J Pharmacol Exp Ther, 13:* 193, 1919.
4. BELLET, S., WEST, J. W., MULLER, O. F., MANZOLI, U., TSITOURIS, G., and JUNG, M.: The effect of nicotine on the coronary blood flow and related circulatory parameters: A correlative study in the normal dog. *Circ Res, 10:*27, 1962.
5. BELLET, S., KERSHBAUM, A., MEADE, R. H., JR., and SCHWARTZ, L.: The effects of tobacco smoke and nicotine on the normal heart and in the presence of myocardial damage produced by coronary ligation. *Amer J Med Sci, 201:*40, 1941.
6. BELLET, S., *et al.*: Unpublished results.
7. KERSHBAUM, A., BELLET, S., DICKSTEIN, E. R., and FEINBERG, L. J.: Effect of cigarette smoking and nicotine on serum free-fatty acids: Based on a study in human subjects and experimental animals. *Circ Res, 9:*631, 1961.
8. KERSHBAUM, A., BELLET, S., CAPLAN, R. F., and FEINBERG, L. J.: Effect of cigarette smoking on free-fatty acids in patients with healed myocardial infarction. *Amer J Cardiol, 10:*204, 1962.
9. KERSHMAN, A., KHORSANDIAN, R., CAPLAN, R. F., BELLET, S., and FEINBERG, L. J.: Role of catecholamines in free-fatty acid response to cigarette smoking. *Circulation, 28:*52, 1963.
10. FOLTZ, E. L., SHELDON, W. F., PAGE, R. G., SAYEN, J. J., and FITTS, W. T.: Quantitative circulatory response to an acute anoxemia test in dogs with progressive experimental coronary narrowing. *Amer J Med Sci, 222:*115, 1951.
11. REGAN, T. J., FRANK, M. J., McGINTY, J. F., ZOBL, E., HELLEMS, H. K., and BING, R. J.: Myocardial response to cigarette smoking in normal subjects and patients with coronary disease. *Circulation, 23:*365, 1961.
12. HAVEL, R. J., and GOLDFEIN, A.: Role of sympathetic nervous system in metabolism of free-fatty acids. *J Lipid Res, 1:*102, 1959.
13. SHAFRIR, E., and STEINBERG, D.: Essential role of adrenal cortex in response of plasma free-fatty acids: cholesterol and phospholipids to epinephrine. *J Clin Invest, 39:*310, 1960.
14. RICHARDSON, J. A., WOODS, E. F., and BAGWELL, B. S.: Circulating epinephrine and norepinephrine in coronary occlusion. *Amer J Cardiol, 5:* 613, 1960.
15. FRIEDMAN, M., ST. GEORGE, S., BYERS, S. O., and ROSENMAN, R. H.: Excretion of catecholamines, 17-ketosteroids, 17-hydroxycorticoids and 5-hydroxyindole in men exhibiting a particular behavior pattern (A) associated with high incidence of clinical coronary artery disease. *J Clin Invest, 39:*758, 1960.

Chapter X

LIFE STRESS AND URINARY EXCRETION OF ADRENALINE AND NORADRENALINE

LENNART LEVI

(Stockholm, Sweden)

IT IS well established that conditions of stress are accompanied by reactions from the sympathoadrenomedullary system (1–4). If too often repeated or long lasting, stress has been claimed to result in permanent and structural changes of pathogenic significance (3, 5, 6, 31, 32). The sympathoadrenomedullary system can be activated by a wide variety of stimuli (7–12). Out of these, the emotional burdens of everyday living have been said to be specially pathogenic in predisposed individuals (13–15). Stress activity may be evaluated by measuring the output of catecholamines in urine (29, 30). We decided to investigate the question further as to whether and to what extent such stimuli affect sympathoadrenomedullary neurosecretory activity as reflected in the urinary excretion of adrenaline and noradrenaline.

Prior to the experiments reported here, other stimuli known or suspected to affect the catecholamines had been standardized (16, 17). They included diurnal variation, bodily posture, intake of food and fluid, smoking, alcoholic and caffeine-containing beverages, drugs, physical activity, night rest prior to the experiment, instructions, experimental stimuli and measurements.

The primary aim of the experiments to be reported here was to study the interrelationships between (a) type and intensity of stimuli as defined physically as well as psychologically; (b) reported subjective feelings; (c) observed behavior, and (d) a number of autonomic and endocrine responses in different types of personalities and patient groups.

The present paper centers exclusively on the catecholamine excretions of some 250 subjects of different categories, exposed to emotional stimuli judged to be of slight to moderate intensity. The stimuli were selected from among those we are most likely to encounter in our daily life. More than 1600 urine samples were obtained and analyzed fluorimetrically by the method of Euler and Lishajko (18).

INDUSTRIAL STRESS

The experiment "Industrial Stress I" involved a monotonous but attention-demanding task—the sorting of small, shiny steel balls of 4 very similar sizes in the presence of a realistic industrial noise (97-104 dB-C), variations in the intensity of illumination, a rush due to considerable lack of time, and critical observation. The experimental situation

85

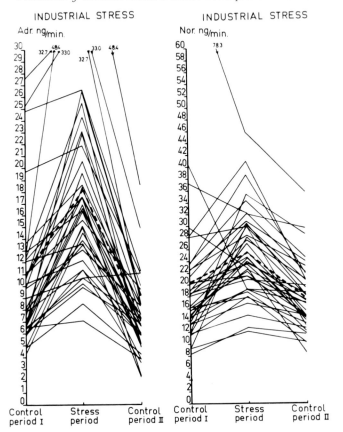

Figure 10–1. Urinary excretion of adrenaline (ADR) and noradrenaline (NOR) before, during, and after 2 hours of simulated industrial work in healthy soldiers. Short-dash line indicates mean values.

thus resembled conditions of work, to which millions of people in factories and workshops all over the world are being subjected every day during most of their lives (19).

One 2-hour control period preceded and one followed the 2-hour stress period. During the control periods of this experiment and all the experiments described in this paper, the subjects relaxed, reading a weekly magazine and listening to soft music. Urine samples were obtained and questionnaires and observation forms were completed from all periods.

An experimental group of 40 young healthy soldiers was divided into two

subgroups with clinically-rated high and low stress tolerance, respectively, within the range of normal psychological variation.

The two subgroups excreted very similar amounts of the catecholamines. When looking at the individual levels (Fig. 10–1) one may note the very high excretion of some of the subjects (20).

In the next experiment, "Industrial Stress II," the five most vulnerable subjects from the low-tolerance subgroup and the five least vulnerable ones from the high-tolerance subgroup were re-exposed to the experimental situation, which, however, was made somewhat

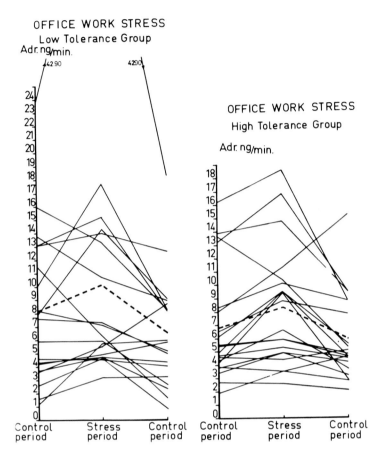

Figure 10–2. Urinary excretion of adrenaline (ADR) before, during, and after 2 hours of simulated office work in healthy office clerks. Short-dash line indicates mean values of low-tolerance group (*left*) and of high-tolerance group (*right*).

more severe. In spite of the objective increase in stressor intensity, the subjects this time appeared to be calmer, probably due to increased familiarity with the experimental setting, and the excretion levels were accordingly significantly lower than in the previous experiment, but again very similar in the two subgroups (20).

OFFICE WORK STRESS

In order to study the reactions of two groups with clinically different stress tolerance to what may be supposed to be a very weak stressor, the stress period of the next experiment, "Office work stress," was modified to include simple proof-reading with ordinary typewriter noise (79–83 dB-C). Thirty-nine healthy clerical and technical employees of both sexes were subdivided into a high tolerance group and a low tolerance group, as rated clinically. Again, both groups excreted very similar amount of the catecholamines. In spite of the weak stressors used, some of the subjects reacted with considerable increments in their adrenaline excretion (Fig. 10–2).

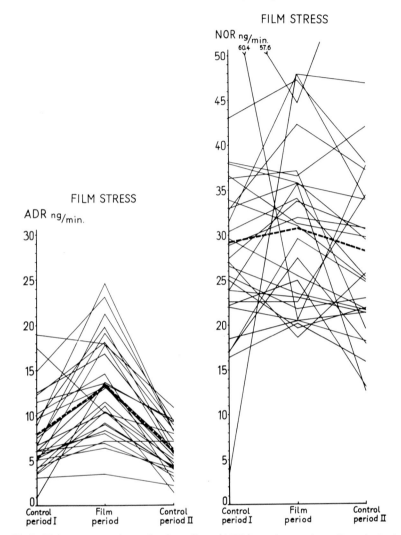

Figure 10–3. Urinary excretion of adrenaline (ADR) and noradrenaline (NOR) before, during, and after a two-hour film program depicting cruelty, violence and torture. Short-dash line indicates mean values of healthy soldiers.

PLEASANT AND UNPLEASANT EMOTIONAL STATES

In the following series of experiments different film programs were used in order to produce somewhat more specific emotional reactions, resembling those occurring in real life.

In "Film Stress I," 10 healthy male medical students were shown a program of 30 cuttings disapproved of by the Swedish Film Censor Board. The cuttings depicted murders, fights, torture, executions, and cruelty to animals. The primary aim was to study whether films as stimuli could activate the sympathoadrenomedullary system in subjects as relatively sophisticated as medical students. The stimulus proved potent enough, as the catecholamine output rose significantly, the mean rise being 70 per cent or adrenaline and 35 per cent for noradrenaline (21).

The reactions of subjects less sophisticated than medical students were studied in the similarly designed experiment "Film Stress II." The subjects were 30 young healthy soldiers, half of them with high clinically-rated stress tolerance, the others with low stress tolerance. As in the previous experiments, in which such subgroups were compared with each other, the levels and changes of both groups were very similar (20). The individual excretion levels are shown in Figure 10–3.

In the next experiment, "Film Stress II," 20 young healthy female office clerks, who served as their own controls, were shown 4 entirely different film programs of 90 minutes each on four consecutive evenings (17). The first program was composed of bland natural scenery films, produced by the Swedish National Railway Company. In spite of this experiment's character of "first experience" to the subjects, the group reacted (Figs. 10–4 and 5) with a significant lowering of the catecholamine excretion during the film period, apparently reflecting subjectively reported feelings of calmness and equanimity, induced by the films.

The next evening the subjects were shown Stanley Kubrick's tragic and agitating "Paths of Glory." During it, the subjects reported feelings of anger and excitement. Simultaneously, (Fig. 10–4) the adrenaline excretion rose significantly.

On the third evening, a charming and amusing comic film was shown, "Charley's Aunt," directed by Hans Quest. The subjects roared with laughter, and reported being very amused. In spite of the absence of any obvious anxiety or aggression-provoking elements in this film, and the pleasant feelings reported

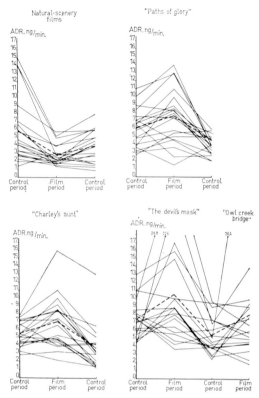

Figure 10–4. Urinary excretion of adrenaline (ADR) in healthy, female office clerks before, during, and after viewing bland natural scenery films, the agitating and aggression provoking "Paths of Glory," the comedy "Charley's Aunt" and the anxiety provoking "The Devil's Mask," and "An Occurrence at Owl Creek Bridge."

Short-dash line indicates mean values.

to be evoked by it, the catecholamine excretion (Figs. 10–4 and 5) rose significantly, possibly reflecting the intensity and not the quality of affective arousal.

The main film of the fourth evening was Mario Bava's gruesome ghost story "The Devil's Mask," during which the subjects screamed with fear and reported anxiety and dismalness. The concomitant catecholamine excretion (Figs. 10–4 and 5) rose markedly.

After the end of the second control period of this day, a short-length film

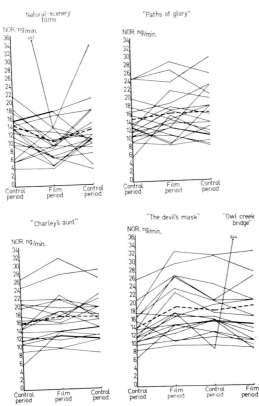

Figure 10–5. Urinary excretion of noradrenaline (NOR) in healthy, female office clerks before, during, and after viewing bland natural scenery films, the agitating and aggression provoking "Paths of Glory," the comedy "Charley's Aunt," and the anxiety provoking "The Devil's Mask," and "An Occurrence at Owl Creek Bridge." Short-dash line indicates mean values.

of 27 minutes was unexpectedly shown, Robert Enrico's highly dramatic and thrilling "An Occurrence at Owl Creek Bridge." Again, the subjects reported feelings of apprehensiveness. The mean catecholamine excretion rose, but not significantly so, possibly because of the short duration of the stimulus.

All but one of the subjects participated also in the next experiment, "Film Stress IV". The fim of this experiment was Lars Görling's and Vilgot Sjöman's "491," which was entirely forbidden by the Swedish Film Censor Board, among other things for mental hygienic reasons. This film was supposed by the film censors to cause strong emotional arousal. However, both the subjective reports and the catecholamine excretions point to emotional reactions less pronounced than during one of the preceding pictures, "The Devil's Mask" Fig. (10–6).

LOVE AND EROTICISM

Love and eroticism are essential elements in most people's emotional life. Their possible relation to the sympatho-adrenomedullary system (22, 23), however, has not been extensively studied (24, 25), probably because those feelings are not easily induced in controlled experiments. One way of dealing with this problem may be to make use of suitable parts of high quality love films, chosen to allow the subjects to identify themselves with the film characters. Thus, in the "Love Film Experiment", 15 of the female office clerks were shown a program composed of nine purely sensual love scenes. An attempt was made to isolate the love element, avoiding obvious elements of tragedy, comedy, aggressiveness, or anxiety. The emotional reactions reported were of a very moderate intensity and usually of a pleasant kind, and catecholamine reactions were small or absent.

Though being sensual, the films of the last mentioned experiment, of course, did not show openly and realistically the shape and function of the human sex organs. The films of the next experiment, however, did so, which made them unsuitable to show to the female office clerks. For this "Sex Film Experiment," therefore, a presumably less vulnerable sample of 103 healthy medical and phys-

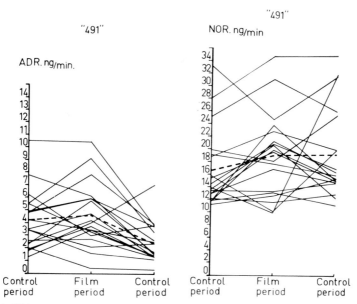

Figure 10–6. Urinary excretion of adrenaline (ADR) and noradrenaline (NOR) in healthy, female office clerks before, during, and after viewing the film "491." Short-dash line indicates mean values.

iotherapy students was chosen, 53 being females and 50 males. They were shown purely sexual films recently confiscated by the legal authorities and now put at the author's disposal by the public prosecutor. The subjects of this study, in contrast to the previously mentioned group, knew in advance what general type of program they were to be shown. In order to avoid the satiety likely to occur when viewing a substantial number of consecutive intercourses, each short-length sex film was preceded or followed by a bland natural scenery film of some 5 minutes duration. Sexual arousal was the main emotion reported by both sexes, the self-rating scores, however, being higher in the male group. This difference in reported subjective reactions was paralleled by a corresponding difference in noradrenaline excretion, the excretion levels as well as the increases over con-

trol levels being somewhat higher in the males (Fig. 10–7). Even more pronounced was the difference between sexes in adrenaline excretion, which increased by an average of 66 per cent in the males but remained largely unchanged in the females (Fig. 10–8). Some of the latter's individual excretion levels were quite high, however.

THE STRESS OF EVERYDAY WORK

In the last three experiments reported here, the stimuli used are no longer representations of real life situations, but the situations themselves.

In "Noise Stress," 22 young female IBM operators were studied in their usual work. In half of the group, the noise level produced by their own IBM machines was doubled from one day to the next during 4 consecutive days, the noise levels being 76, 82, 88 and 94 dB-C, respec-

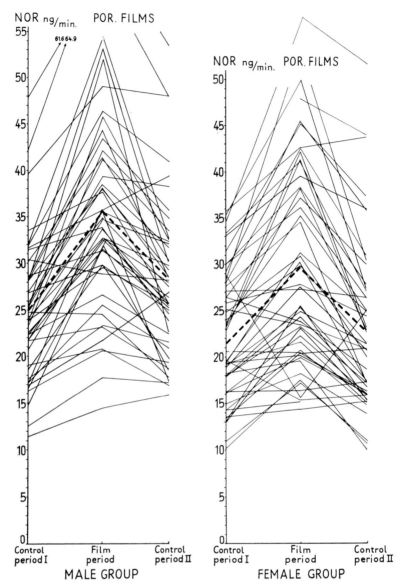

Figure 10–7. The urinary excretion of noradrenaline (NOR) in male and female students before, during, and after a 90-minute sex film program. Short-dash line indicates mean values.

tively. The other half were subjected to the same noise levels but in the opposite order (i.e., 94, 88, 82 and 76 dB-C, respectively). The noise level normally prevailing in this office was 76 dB-c.

Contrary to what might be expected, the subjects reported only minor emo-

tional reactions even during loudest noise levels. Accordingly, the changes in adrenaline and noradrenaline excretion occurring towards the end of the daily six-hour noise exposure were very small, and the absolute levels were relatively low. These inconsiderable emotional and

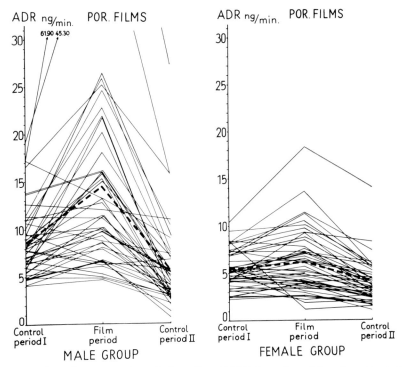

Figure 10–8. The urinary excretion of adrenaline (ADR) in male and female sutdents before, during, and after a 90-minute sex film program. Short-dash line indicates mean values.

sympathoadrenomedullary reactions to what is usually believed to be quite considerable noise levels might be explained as follows:

The subjects worked in their ordinary milieu, among their own fellow workers, performing their usual tasks. The noise was familiar to them as it emanated from their own machines. All the subjects had been properly informed about the purpose and the procedure of the investigation. In order to reduce apprehension and make sure that the experiment would run smoothly, the experiment was preceded by a "dress rehearsal" day. A good contact was established between the subjects and the experimenters. Both the managers and the employees' association encouraged the subjects to participate in the investigation. Those

who took part were liberally paid. This created a very favorable and positive attitude to the experiment and, hence, to the noise element in it. The results mentioned here illustrate objectively the everyday experience that the favorite program pouring from our own television set can be much less irritating than the soft, hardly audible music from the neighbor's piano. What really counts here—within certain limits—is the attitude, not the physical noise level.

During "Everyday Work Stress I," 9 female telephone operators were studied when performing their ordinary work on three Mondays during the same 8 hours of the day. The number of telephone calls to be connected varied considerably from hour to hour. In addition, several periods of rest, serving as control periods, were introduced. Urine was collected hourly. In general, the variations in the work load of these telephone operators clearly affected the noradrenaline and, though less markedly, the adrenaline output.

In the last experiment to be reported, "Everyday Work Stress II," 12 female invoicing clerks were studied during 4 consecutive days when performing their usual work. During the first and third of these days their usual mode of remuneration was changed from salary to extreme piece-wages. All other conditions were held constant. During piece-work days, their output of work rose significantly by 113 per cent. However, this very high output of work was accomplished at the expense of considerable feelings of mental and physical discomfort. Half of the group complained of feeling hurried, and all but two complained of fatigue, backache, and pain in their shoulders or arms during the piece-work days. During salaried days physical complaints were virtually absent.

This subjective state of stress during the piece-work days was paralleled by an objective one as reflected in the urinary catecholamines. During these days the noradrenaline excretion increased by 27 per cent, whereas adrenaline excretion increased by 40 per cent, as compared with the excretion levels of the two salaried days. The increases were statistically significant (26).

Further studies are in progress to examine the characteristics and the medical and psychological outcome of the catecholamine hyperexcretors, as well as the catecholamine output during the working hours in various professions. Statistical studies by other authors have demonstrated a high incidence of ischemic heart disease in high-strung, ambitious individuals with an elevated daytime urinary catecholamine excretion level (27), and in those exposed to intense professional occupational stressors (28).

SUMMARY

Emotional stimuli of a considerably smaller intensity than those occurring in everday life of most people are demonstrably potent in raising the catecholamine (adrenaline and noradrenaline) output of many subjects, whether emotionally vulnerable or not. There seems to exist a relationship between the individual's emotional arousal, whatever its quality, and his catecholamine output.

Experimental stimuli evoking responses of calmness and equanimity lower the catecholamine excretion significantly below control levels.

Pleasant stimuli, evoking amusement, are nearly as potent as unpleasant ones in provoking an increased catecholamine excretion.

Industrial and other occupational work performed under emotional tension, as well as experimentally-induced sexual arousal, are accompanied by a considerably increased excretion of urinary catecholamines.

The highest levels found in these experiments approach those usually considered to be diagnostic of pheochromocytoma. It appears reasonable to assume that they reflect a high activity level of the sympathoadrenomedullary system in the respective individuals.

REFERENCES

1. Cannon, W. B.: *Bodily Changes in Pain, Hunger, Fear and Rage.* 2nd Ed. Boston, C. T. Branford Co., 1929.
2. Selye, H.: *Stress.* Montreal, Acta Inc., 1950.
3. Raab, W., Stark, E., Macmillan, W. H., and

GIGEE, W. R.: Sympathogenic origin and anti-adrenergic prevention of stress-induced myocardial lesions. *Amer J Cardiol, 8:*203, 1961.

4. ALTSCHULE, M. D.: *Bodily Physiology in Mental and Emotional Disorders.* New York, Grune and Stratton, 1953.

5. ALEXANDER, F.: *Psychosomatic Medicine.* London, George Allen and Unmitt Ltd., 1952.

6. WOLFF, H. G.: *Stress and Disease.* Springfield, Thomas, 1953.

7. EULER, U. S. v.: *Noradrenaline.* Springfield, Thomas, 1956.

8. ELMADJIAN, F., HOPE, J. M., and LAMSON, E. T.: Excretion of epinephrine and norepinephrine in various emotional states. *J Clin Endocr, 17:*608,1957.

9. ELMADJIAN, F., HOPE, J. M., and LAMSON, E. T.: Excretion of epinephrine and norepinephrine under stress. *Recent Progr Hormone Res, 14:*513, 1958.

10. ROESSLER, R., and GREENFIELD, N. S.: *Physiological Correlates of Psychological Disorder.* Madison, University of Wisconsin Press, 1962.

11. SIMON, A., HERBERT, C., and STRAUSS, R.: *The Physiology of Emotions.* Springfield, Thomas, 1961.

12. SOURKES, T. L.: *Biochemistry of Mental Disease.* New York, Harper and Row, 1962.

13. WEISS, E., and ENGLISH, O. S.: *Psychosomatic Medicine.* Philadelphia and London, W. B. Saunders Co., 1950.

14. DUNBAR, F.: *Emotions and Bodily Changes.* New York, Columbia University Press, 1954.

15. TANNER, J. M.: *Stress and Psychiatric Disorder.* Oxford, Blackwell Scientific Publications, 1960.

16. LEVI, L.: The urinary output of adrenalin and noradrenalin during pleasant and unpleasant emotional states. *Psychosom Med, 27:*80, 1965.

17. LEVI, L.: Some principles and sources of error in psychophysiological research. Paper presented at Symposium on "Psychophysiological Reactions During Emotional Stress," Stockholm, 1965. (To be published as supplement to "Forsvarsmedicin.")

18. EULER, U. S. v., and LISHAJKO, F.: Improved technique for the fluorimetric estimation of catecholamines. *Acta Physiol Scand, 51:*348, 1961.

19. LEVI, L.: A new stress tolerance test with simultaneous study of physiological and psychological variables. *Acta Endocr, 37:*38, 1961.

20. LEVI, L.: The urinary output of adrenalin and noradrenalin during experimentally induced emotional stress in clinically different groups *Acta Psychother, 11:*218, 1963.

21. EULER, U. S. v., GEMZELL, C. A., LEVI, L., and STROM, G.: Cortical and medullary adrenal activity in emotional stress. *Acta Endocr, 30:*567, 1959.

22. KINSEY, A. C., et al.: *Sexual Behavior in the Human Male.* Philadelphia and London, W. B. Saunders. Co., 1948.

23. KINSEY, A. C., et al.: *Sexual Behavior in the Human Female.* Philadelphia and London, W. B. Saunders Co., 1953.

24. KLUMBIE, G., and KLEINSORGE, H.: Das Herz im Orgasmus. *Med Klin, 45:*952, 1950.

25. BARTLETT, R. G., JR.: Physiologic responses during coitus. *J Appl Physiol, 9:*469, 1956.

26. LEVI, L.: The stress of everyday work as reflected in productiveness, subjective feelings and urinary output of adrenaline and noradrenaline under salaried and piece-work conditions. *J Psychosom Res, 8:*199, 1964.

27. ROSENMAN, R. H., FRIEDMAN, M., STRAUS, R., WURM, M., KOSITCHEK, R., HAHN, W., and WERTHESSEN, N.: A predictive study of coronary heart disease: The Western Collaborative Group Study. *JAMA, 189:*15, 1964.

28. RUSSEK, H. I.: Emotional stress and coronary heart disease in American physicians, dentists and lawyers. *Amer J Med Sci, 243:*716, 1962.

29. EULER, U. S. v., and LUNDBERG, U.: Effect of flying on the epinephrine excretion in air force personnel. *J. Appl Physiol, 6:*551, 1954.

30. EULER, U. S. v.: Quantitation of stress by catecholamine analysis. *Clin Pharmacol Ther, 5:*398, 1964.

31. LEVI, L.: Sympathoadreno-medullary responses to emotional stimuli. Methodologic, physiologic, and pathologic considerations. Acta Endocr. Suppl. 100, 1965, p. 19. (Abstract.)

32. LEVI, L.: Stress: Sources, Management and Prevention. New York, Liveright Publ. Corp., 1966 (in press).

Chapter XI

PLASMA CATECHOLAMINES IN ANGINA PECTORIS AND MYOCARDIAL INFARCTION*

JAMES A. RICHARDSON

(Charleston, South Carolina, U.S.A.)

WITH the advent of accurate fluoro-metric methods for the assay of nor-epinephrine and epinephrine in body fluids and tissues (1, 2), general interest in the pathophysiological significance of these catecholamines has stepped into the foreground of clinical interest.

Their potentially pathogenic, hypoxi-ating and cardiotoxic properties had long been known (3). More recently it was found that even small doses of catechol-amines and electrical or reflectory stimu-lations of the cardiac sympathetic nerves are apt to elicit severe hypoxic and ne-crotizing manifestations in the heart mus-cle under certain accessory conditions such as artificial (4) or atherosclerotic (5) restrictions of the normal compensa-tory coronary dilatability, or the meta-bolically sensitizing influence of admin-istered adrenal mineralocorticoids (6).

In patients with coronary atherosclero-sis injections of epinephrine can elicit typ-ical attacks of angina pectoris (7), and the occurrence of such attacks under sym-pathetic stimulating circumstances (emo-tions, exercise) is well known. Antiadre-nergic measures and cardiac sympathec-tomy have been found therapeutically effective in the anginal syndrome (8).

In view of all these findings, and of earlier studies with a colorimetric assay method, which had indicated an abnor-mal elevation of total catecholamines in the blood of angina patients during exer-cise (9), it appeared of interest to in-vestigate the behavior of norepinephrine and of epinephrine in the blood plasma in ischemic heart disease (angina pectoris and myocardial infarction) with our own fluorimetric technique (2).

PATIENTS WITH ANGINA PECTORIS

Epinephrine and norepinephrine levels were determined in the plasma of 12 pa-tients with angina pectoris who were matched with 7 normal controls of similar age, diet habits, and body weight. Blood samples were taken before and after per-formance of a double 2-step Master test. When pain developed before completion of the test, a blood sample was taken at that point.

The results, shown in Tables 11–I and II, reveal an exercise-induced average increase of 119.3 per cent norepinephrine (p < .001) and 60.3 percent epinephrine

*This work was aided by research grants (HE-01846 and HTS-5200) from the U.S. Public Health Service, National Heart Institute, and from the American Heart Association.

TABLE 11–I

CATECHOLAMINES (µg/l plasma) IN NORMAL
SUBJECTS BEFORE AND AFTER EXERCISE

Subject No.	Before Exercise		After Exercise	
	Norepi-nephrine (µg/l)	Epineph-rine (µg/l)	Norepi-nephrine (µg/l)	Epineph-rine (µg/l)
1	3.09	.28	3.99	.21
2	2.86	.01	2.58	.15
3	2.43	.09	2.17	.01
4	2.55	.01	3.09	.00
5	3.35	.36	3.14	.15
6	1.35	.50	1.47	.68
7	1.40	.26	1.25	.45
Mean	2.43	.22	2.53	.24

TABLE 11–II

CATECHOLAMINES (µg/l plasma) IN CASES
OF ANGINA PECTORIS BEFORE AND
AFTER EXERCISE

Patient No.	Before Exercise		After Exercise	
	Norepi-nephrine (µg/l	Epineph-rine (µg/l)	Norepi-nephrine (µg/l)	Epineph-rine (µg/l)
1	2.46	.78	12.10	2.48
2	1.67	.29	1.27	.45
3	1.39	.51	1.43	.46
4	3.93	.11	8.33	.04
5	2.23	.80	5.17	.86
6	3.19	.44	7.43	1.28
7	3.55	.44	4.00	1.97
8	3.18	1.25	7.10	3.27
9	2.54	1.42	4.82	1.29
10	1.41	.74	1.49	.93
11	1.44	1.25	7.75	.02
12	3.40	.07	5.75	.10
Mean	2.53	.68	5.55	1.09

TABLE 11–III

CATECHOLAMINES (µg/l plasma) IN CASES
OF ACUTE MYOCARDIAL INFARCTION
DURING THE FIRST 36 HOURS AND
AFTER 72 HOURS

Patient No.	During First 36 Hours		After 72 Hours	
	Norepi-nephrine (µg/l)	Epineph-rine (µg/l)	Norepi-nephrine (µg/l)	Epineph-rine (µg/l)
1	9.10	1.00	2.26	1.07
2	6.34	.49	1.97	.19
3	3.48	.90	1.39	.51
4	7.50	.42	2.21	.81
5	4.32	.47	3.16	.63
6	4.90	2.84	3.60	.47
7	3.42	.45	1.12	.39
8	3.04	.59	1.04	.15
9	5.22	.11	1.73	.43
10	4.18	.78	2.19	.17
11	4.10	.05	1.39	.51
12	5.55	.70		
13	7.50	1.30		
Mean	5.28	.78	2.01	.48

myocardial infarction within the first 36 hour period, and in 11 cases 72 hours after the acute episode (Table 11–III). The average values for norepinephrine within the first 36 hours were considerably higher (61.9 per cent) than after 72 hours, and in all 13 cases the initial norepinephrine levels were significantly higher ($p < .001$) than in 7 normal subjects.

In 7 infarction cases the initial levels of epinephrine were higher than in the 7 normal controls ($p < .01$).

In order to evaluate the possible role of pain as a triggering stimulus for release of catecholamines into the blood stream, plasma catecholamines were determined in 6 instances of noncardiac painful conditions. All readings were within the normal range.

Determination of serum transaminase levels during the first 36 hours after infarction showed a significant linear relationship between the norepinephrine and transaminase values with a correlation

($p < .011$) in the angina pectoris patients, as compared with an increase of 4.1 per cent norepinephrine and 9.1 per cent epinephrine, in the normal controls.

In addition, 3 angina patients, tested before and during smoking, showed an average increase of 61.5 per cent norepinephrine and of 132.6 per cent epinephrine under the influence of nicotine.

PATIENTS WITH ACUTE MYOCARDIAL INFARCTION

Plasma catecholamine determinations were also carried out in 13 cases of acute

TABLE 11–IV

CATECHOLAMINE CONTENT OF TISSUE
FROM THE LEFT VENTRICLE OF NORMAL
AND OF EXPERIMENTALLY INFARCTED
HEARTS (in µg/g tissue)

Number of Hearts	Type of Material Studied	Norepi- nephrine (µg/l) (Average)	Epineph- rine (µg/l) (Average)
5	Normal hearts	1.18	0.06
3	Hearts after experi- mental coronary occlusion		
	Core of infarction	0.28	0.02
	Area adjacent to infarction	0.68	0.02
	Normal area	0.72	0.05

coefficient of 0.80 (p < .01). The cor- relation coefficient with epinephrine was not significant.

EXPERIMENTAL CORONARY OCCLUSION IN DOGS

In 33 dogs acute coronary occlusion was effectuated either by injection of glass microspheres into the coronary cir- culation or by ligation of the anterior descending coronary artery under pento- barbital anesthesia. Blood samples for the assay of catecholamines were withdrawn prior to occlusion and at daily intervals for several subsequent days. Electrocar- diograms and pulse pressure tracings were also taken, and the hearts were examined postmortem.

After coronary occlusion, the mean val- ues for plasma norepinephrine increased markedly with a maximum rise from 1.6 µg/1 to 10.5 µg/1 (p < .001), where- by the peak was usually reached during the first 24 to 36 hours following oc- clusion, with return toward normal in 48 to 72 hours.

Transaminase levels also reached their maximum within the first 24 to 36 hours, coinciding rather closely with the be-

havior of norepinephrine, whereas epi- nephrine remained nearly unchanged.

The electrocardiographic signs, pulse pressure curve tracings and autopsy find- ings were consistent with the appearance of large infarcts in each heart.

In 4 dogs which had been bilaterally adrenalectomized prior to coronary oc- clusion, the post-occlusion increments of plasma norepinephrine and of serum trans- aminase were in the same range as those ob- served in nonadrenalectomized dogs.

After administration of a sympatholytic drug (βTM 10) the initially elevated plas- ma norepinephrine level declined rapidly (within about 20 minutes) to its pre- occlusion level in 6 dogs.

Reserpine did not significantly reduce the postocclusion elevations of norepi- nephrine and transaminase in 11 dogs.

The average norepinephrine concen- trations in the tissue of the left ventricle of 3 infarcted dogs were somewhat lower than those in the hearts of 5 control animals. The lowest readings were ob- tained from the core of the infarct (Table 11–IV).

CLINICAL IMPLICATIONS

Our observations concerning exagger- ated discharges of both norepinephrine and epinephrine into the blood in pa- tients suffering from angina pectoris (10) are in agreement with earlier findings of Raab (9) (total catecholamines) and with those of Starcich and Ambanelli (11). The latter authors, and recently DiBiase and Labriola (12), recorded ab- normally high catecholamine levels in the plasma during deliberately provoked (ex- ercise, emotional disturbances), as well as spontaneous, attacks of anginal pain with considerable regularity, amounting to 100 per cent in individuals of age groups below 40 years (12).

The pain factor in itself does not seem to elicit any abnormally high elevations of the plasma catecholamines, as concluded from unchanged catecholamine levels in the plasma during episodes of noncardiac pain.

The fact that exogenous administration of catecholamines (8, 13) and the liberation of catecholamines from pheochromocytomas (14) can elicit anginal symptoms on the one hand, and that various forms of antiadrenergic therapy are effective in angina pectoris (13, 14) on the other, suggest that acute adrenosympathogenic neurohormone discharges play an important causal role in the origin of the anginal syndrome. This is further emphasized by the observation that even minute and otherwise innocuous doses of infused epinephrine can elicit marked electrocardiographic reactions of the hypoxic type in individuals with coronary sclerosis (15).

The basic background of the apparently characteristic overexciteability of the cardiac adrenosympathetic system in angina patients has not yet been clarified in detail. However, the generally augmented sympathetic tone, the increased urinary catecholamine excretion, and the accentuated adrenergic reactivity (8) of emotionally tense and irritable individuals, as well as the deficiency of antiadrenergic counterregulation, which has been found to result from habitual physical inactivity (8), may be considered as contributory elements.

The involvement of the adrenosympathetic neurosecretory system in the origin and sequelae of myocardial infarctions appears to be more complex. Our own findings concern exclusively animals with artificial coronary occlusions and patients in whom an infarction had already occurred. Thus, they cannot be applied to the now increasingly discussed problem of a causative participation of catecholamines in the origin of neurogenic myocardial necroses (3, 8, 16).

The regular occurrence of a marked hypercatecholemia during the first days following experimental as well as clinical myocardial infarctions, which was observed both by ourselves (10, 17) and by Starcich and co-workers (18), is reflected in an augmented urinary excretion of catecholamines (19, 20, 21). Vascular hypotension and shock, which frequently accompany myocardial infarction but were absent in our patients and experimental animals, cannot be made responsible for the postinfarction elevations of catecholamine liberation (19, 22).

Postganglionic sympathetic nerves may be regarded as a major source of the postinfarction hypercatecholemia since ganglionic blocking and sympatholytic drugs prevented or reduced it strikingly (17, 23). The adrenal medulla seems to be involved to a minor extent, concluding from the failure of bilateral adrenalectomy to modify the phenomenon (17) and from the less regular elevations, to plasma epinephrine (10, 17).

Reserpinization did not interfere with the post-occlusion hypercatecholemia in animals, probably because of inadequate depletion of the catecholamine stores. The mortality from coronary occlusion was actually higher in reserpine-pretreated dogs (39 per cent) than in the untreated group (15 per cent) (17).

A contribution of catecholamines deriving from the infarcted heart muscle to the high post-infarction catecholamine levels seems possible. The heart muscle is capable of releasing relatively large amounts of catecholamines under stimulation (24), and the catecholamine content of experimentally infarcted and necrotic hearts was found to be low (17, 25, 26), particularly in the damaged area, but also in the nonaffected portions of the myocardium (17, 25). The latter feature could be prevented by a monoamine oxidase inhibitor (25). In normal portions of human hearts with recent myocardial infarcts the norepinephrine content was likewise found reduced whereas epinephrine concentrations were relatively high (27). These findings, together with the observations of low norepinephrine concentrations in hearts with congestive failure (27, 28) and in other chronic cardiovascular ailments (27) suggest that metabolically and structurally deranged hearts lose their ability for normal production and/or accumulation of neurogenic and blood-borne norepinephrine. Similarly, low norepinephrine concentrations have been demonstrated recently in acute experimental conditions such as in hypovolemic shock (31).

Whether exogenously administered norepinephrine proves clinically either more useful (e.g., in post-infarction cardiogenic schock), or more detrimental by producing multiple myocardial necroses (29) depends presumably on the degree of its effectiveness or ineffectiveness, respectively, in augmenting vascular tone and myocardial contractile force (30), on the one hand, and in causing a pressoreceptor-mediated antiadrenergic limitation of myocardial oxygen-wastage (14) on the other.

CONCLUSIONS

⤳ A potential pathogenic significance of adrenosympathetic neurosecretory overactivity in the anginal syndrome is suggested by a growing number of observations, including our own. The international literature provides evidence of (a) a characteristic tendency of angina patients to discharge abnormally large quantities of catecholamines into the circulation during physical effort and under emotional stress; (b) an exaggerated sensitivity of individuals with coronary atherosclerosis to the myocardial hypoxiating and pain-producing effect of administered or reflex-discharged catecholamines, and (c) therapeutic benefits from a reduction of adrenosympathogenic neurosecretory activity and catecholamine action in angina pectoris.

A contributory role of adrenosympathetic overactivity in the origin also of myocardial necrotic lesions, especially in the presence of predisposing coronary atherosclerosis, is being postulated by some investigators. However, the elevated plasma catecholamine levels, observed by us after the establishment of myocardial infarctions, must be interpreted as a secondary post-infarction phenomenon with beneficial rather than detrimental implications in favoring the maintenance of vascular tone and myocardial contractile force.

Post-infarction catecholamine losses from the damaged heart muscle may contribute to the development of myocardial functional insufficiency and failure.

From the point of view of prevention of ischemic heart disease, it appears desirable to counteract all factors which are apt to aggravate the dangers inherent in coronary atherosclerosis. Such preventive measures should be directed toward a reduction in activity of the neurosecretory adrenosympathetic system.

SUMMARY

An abnormally high increase in the plasma catecholamine level during a standard exercise test was observed as a characteristic feature in patients suffering from the anginal syndrome.

Similar elevations, particularly of norepinephrine, and, less regularly, of epinephrine, occurred within the first 36 hours after acute myocardial infarction.

Experimental coronary occlusions in dogs were likewise followed by a marked increase of norepinephrine, but not of epinephrine in the blood plasma.

Adrenalectomy and reserpine exerted no definite influence. Sympatholytic and ganglionic blocking agents reduced the post-occlusion hypercatecholemia.

Circulatory shock and pain could be excluded as eliciting factors.

A positive correlation existed between the post-infarction rises of norepinephrine and transaminase levels.

Pathogenic and preventive aspects of adreno-sympathogenic neurosecretory overactivity are briefly discussed.

REFERENCES

1. WEIL-MALHERBE, H., and BONE, A. D.: The chemical estimation of adrenaline-like substances in blood. *Biochem J, 51:*311, 1952.
2. RICHARDSON, J. A., RICHARDSON, A. K., and BRODIE, O. J.: Fluorometric determination of epinephrine and norepinephrine in plasma. *J Lab Clin Med, 47:*832, 1956.
3. RAAB, W.: Neurogenic multifocal destruction of myocardial tissue. *Rev Canad Biol, 22:*217, 1963.
4. RAAB, W., VAN LITH, P., LEPESCHKIN, E., and HERRLICH, H. C.: Catecholamine-induced myocardial hypoxia in the presence of impaired coronary dilatability independent of external cardiac work. *Amer J Cardiol, 9:*455, 1962.
5. KIPSHIDZE, N. N.: Pathogenesis of myocardial infarction. *Ter Arkh, 29:*40, 1957. (See Chapter 8.)
6. SELYE, H.: *The Pluricausal Cardiopathies.* Springfield, Thomas, 1961.
7. LEVINE, S. A., ERNSTENE, A. C., and Jacobson, B. H.: The use of epinephrine as a diagnostic test for angina pectoris. *Arch Intern Med, 45:*191, 1930.
8. RAAB, W.: The nonvascular metabolic myocardial vulnerability factor in "coronary heart disease." *Amer Heart J, 66:*685, 1963.
9. RAAB, W.: The pathogenic significance of adrenalin and related substances in the heart muscle. *Exp Med Surg, 1:*188, 1943.
10. GAZES, P. C., RICHARDSON, J. A., and WOODS, E. F.: Plasma catecholamine concentrations in myocardial infarction and angina pectoris. *Circulation, 19:*657, 1959.
11. STARCICH, R., and AMBANELLI, U.: Importanza della determinazione delle catecolamine plasmatiche in patologia coronarica. *Giorn Clin Med, 40:*1, 1959.
12. DI BIASE, G., and LABRIOLA, E.: Contributo allo studio della catecolaminemia nell'insufficienza coronarica. *Cardiol Prat, 15:*511, 1964.
13. RAAB, W.: The sympathogenic biochemical trigger mechanism of angina pectoris. *Amer J Cardiol, 9:*576, 1962.
14. RAAB, W.: *Hormonal and Neurogenic Cardiovascular Disorders.* Baltimore, Williams and Wilkins, 1953.
15. AMBANELLI, U., and STARCICH, R.: Aspetti clinici ed elettrocardiografici da microdose di adrenalina in corso di insufficienza coronarica acuta. *Boll Soc Ital Cardiol, 8:*336, 1963.
16. MYASNIKOV, A. L.: Myocardial necroses of coronary and non-coronary genesis. *Amer J Cardiol, 13:*435, 1964.
17. RICHARDSON, J. A., WOODS, E. F., and BAGWELL, E. E.: Circulating epinephrine and norepinephrine in coronary occlusion. *Amer J Cardiol, 5:*613, 1960.
18. STARCICH, R.: Plasma catecholamines and urinary vanillyl mandelic acid in clinical ischemic heart disease. (See Chapter 12.)
19. KUSCHKE, H. J., and SCHNEIDER, K. W.: Die sympathiko-adrenale Reaktion beim Herzinfarkt. *Z Kreislaufforsch, 49:*261, 1960.
20. FORSSMAN, O., HANSSON, G., and JANSSEN, C. C.: The adrenal function in coronary thrombosis. *Acta Med Scand, 142:*441, 1952.
21. NUZUM, F. R., and BISCHOFF, F.: The urinary output of catechol derivatives including adrenaline in normal individuals, in essential hypertension and in myocardial infarction. *Circulation, 7:*96, 1953.
22. RICHARDSON, J. A.: Circulating levels of catecholamines in acute myocardial infarction and angina pectoris. *Prog Cardiov Dis, 6:*56, 1963.
23. RICHARDSON, J. A.: Plasma catecholamine concentrations in acute infarction. In: *Coronary Heart Disease.* Wm. Likoff and J. H. Moyer, Ed. Philadelphia, Hahnemann Medical College, 1962.
24. RICHARDSON, J. A., and WOODS, E. F.: Release

of norepinephrine from the isolated heart. *Proc Soc Exp Biol Med, 100*-149, 1959.

25. SERRANO, P. A., VILLANUEVA, S. A., LERDO DE TEJADA, L. A., CASTANEDA, Y., CHAVEZ, B., and BISTENI, A.: Catecolaminas cardiacas despues de la ligadura de la arteria coronaria. *Arch Inst Cardiol Mex, 31:*197, 1961.

26. RAAB, W., STARK, E., MACMILLAN, W. H., and GIGEE, W. R.: Sympathogenic origin and anti-adrenergic prevention of stress-induced myocardial lesions. *Amer J Cardiol, 8:*203, 1961.

27. RAAB, W., and GIGEE, W. R.: Norepinephrine and epinephrine content of normal and diseased human hearts. *Circulation, 11:*593, 1955.

28. CHIDSEY, C. A., HARRISON, C., and BRAUNWALD, E.: Augmentation of plasma norepinephrine response to exercise in patients with congestive heart failure. *New Eng J Med, 267:*650, 1962.

29. SZAKACS, J. E., and CANNON, A.: l-norepinephrine myocarditis. *Amer J Clin Path, 30:*425, 1958.

30. GAZES, P. C., GOLDBERG, L. I., and DARBY, T. D.: Heart force effects of sympathomimetic amines as a basis for their use in shock accompanying myocardial infarction. *Circulation, 8:*883, 1953.

31. RICHARDSON, J. A., and HIOTT, D. W.: Unpublished data.

Chapter XII

PLASMA CATECHOLAMINES AND URINARY VANILLYL MANDELIC ACID IN CLINICAL ISCHEMIC HEART DISEASE

RICCARDO STARCICH

(Parma, Italy)

THE following report concerns the involvement of neurohormonal activity in the pathogenesis of acute coronary insufficiency and resulting myocardial hypoxia.

Such an involvement is suggested by several elementary facts:

1. Sympathetic stimulation and the thereby liberated adrenosympathogenic catecholamines (sympathetic neurogenic norepinephrine, adreno-medullary epinephrine) cause a marked augmentation of myocardial oxygen consumption (1, 2).

2. Availability of adequate amounts of oxygen to the myocardial tissue depends simultaneously on the vascular oxygen supply (which is unevenly distributed in different areas of the heart muscle), and on the degree of myocardial oxygen consumption which varies with the degree of sympathetic tone and neurohormonal activity (2, 3).

3. The myocardial hypoxia-producing effects (ECG, necrotic lesions) of sympathetic stimulation and catecholamine action are greatly intensified when the compensatory coronary dilatation (which normally accompanies augmented cardiac oxygen consumption (4, 5, 6) is impaired by experimental coronary restriction (7, 8) or by atherosclerosis (9, 10).

4. Civilized, competitive living with its socioeconomic emotional tensions and stresses, sensory overstimulation, lack of physical activity, and abuse of nicotine, combines several factors which increase sympathetic neurohormonal activity and resulting interference in myocardial metabolism both in a sustained fashion and with acute exacerbations (2, 10-13).

5. No clear relation exists between the degree of existing atherosclerotic coronary vascular lesions on the one hand, and the occurrence of clinical manifestations of myocardial ischemia on the other (angina pectoris, ECG, multiple micro-infarctions) (10), except in cases of severe coronary stenosis or occlusion. It is no longer possible to ascribe myocardial ischemic structural changes to vascular factors alone without consideration of those contributory nonvascular mechanisms which interfere in myocardial oxygen metabolism (i.e., primarily the neuroendocrine system) (14–16).

Augmentations of the adrenergic catecholamines under emotional stress have been observed in the blood (12) and urine (11, 13, 17–19). Similar findings were obtained in the blood (20–23) and urine (24) during and after physical exertion.

Accumulations of catecholamines in the heart muscle occur under conditions of physical stress (25), and during central nervous (26), as well as peripheral cardiac, sympathetic nerve stimulation (27).

The development of focal necrotic lesions of the myocardium under the influence of injected catecholamines has been demonstrated since Josué (1907) (28) in numerous experimental series (10), and in clinical cases (29). Analogous changes were more recently found in animals as a result of stimulation of the midbrain (26, 30, 31) and of the cardiac sympathetic nerves (32). Multiple myocardial necroses were elicited in animals by intensive, sympathetic-stimulating emotional stresses (33–35).

A high incidence of ischemic heart disease has been reported in heavy smokers (36) and in population groups subjected to socioeconomic emotional stresses (11, 37–39). By contrast, carefree-living Italian immigrants in Roseto, Pennsylvania (40), and nomadic tribes of Somaliland (41) displayed a low incidence of ischemic heart disease, the latter also a low urinary catecholamine excretion (42).

In view of the thus apparent causal connections between myocardial oxygen-wasting adrenergic neurohormonal over-activity under various catecholamine-liberating and stressful situations, on the one hand, and the clinical syndromes of myocardial hypoxia on the other, the following study concerning blood catecholamines in clinical cases of ischemic heart disease, and in connection with emotional stresses was carried out.

MATERIAL AND METHODS

Thirty-eight "normal" subjects and a total of 133 cardiac patients were used in this study. The latter were subdivided in groups with (a) angina pectoris on effort and emotional excitement but without electrocardiographic abnormalities in the painless interval (26 cases); (b) angina pectoris with chronic coronary insufficiency identified by the electrocardiogram (36 cases); (c) myocardial infarction (51 cases), and (d) nonischemic cardiac conditions (20 cases).

Assay of catecholamines was carried out by means of the fluorometric method of Weil-Malherbe and Bone (43)*. The catecholamine metabolite vanillyl mandelic acid was determined in the urine with the method of Pisano et al. (44).

RESULTS

In patients with angina pectoris and with or without electrocardiographically manifest chronic coronary insufficiency, the plasma catecholamine levels (both epinephrine and norepinephrine) during pain-free intervals did not, in general, differ from the norm. However, during attacks of pain provoked either, by physical effort (Master test) or by emotional stimulation (disturbing interviews, financial worries, watching sports events in TV, sudden noises, dreams) the plasma catecholamines concentrations rose markedly (Table 12–I, Fig. 12–1). Epinephrine and norepinephrine were augmented in similar proportions both dur-

---

*More recently developed methodical modifications (H. WEIL-MALHERBE: The simultaneous estimation of catecholamines and their metabolites. *Klin Chem*, 2:21, 1964) yield lower readings for epinephrine and norepinephrine in plasma. Nevertheless, the values reported here appear sufficiently indicate of the deviations of plasma catecholamines for normal levels occurring under the conditions studied.

TABLE 12–I

PLASMA CATECHOLAMINES AND URINARY VANILLYL MANDELIC ACID IN
ISCHEMIC AND NONISCHEMIC HEART DISEASE

Patients Examined	Sex	Average Age	Diagnosis	Clinical Features	Adrenaline μg/l		Noradrenaline μg/l		Vanillyl Mandelic Acid	
					Min	Max	Min.	Max	μg/ml	μg/24 hrs
26	21 M. 5 F.	42 46	Angina pectoris on effort, emotion, etc.*	Painless	0,80	2,02	3,12	5,80	Normal range (see below)	
				Pain	2,10	6,73	4,95	21,03		
36	33 M. 3 F.	47 48	Angina pectoris in chronic coronary insuff.††	Painless	0,35	2,45	2,63	5,77	Normal range (see below)	
				Pain	2,05	11,71	7,40	20,60		
51	42 M. 9 F.	51 55	Myocardial infarction (without shock)	Acute stage	3,21	13,20	7,80	21,66	11,20 14,90 (in 30% of the cases)	
				Stationary stage	0,80	2,90	1,10	5,90		
20	12 M. 8 F.	50 45	Nonischemic heart disease (valvular, cardiac in-sufficiency without critical phenomena)		—	0,95	1,48	2,03	4,90	Normal range (see below)
38	34 M. 4 F.	40 45	Normal		—	1,28 ±0,88		4,75 ±1,39	3,10 ±1,90	2,80 ±1,22

†Without electrocardiographic abmornalities in the painless interval
*With electrocardiographic changes in the interval

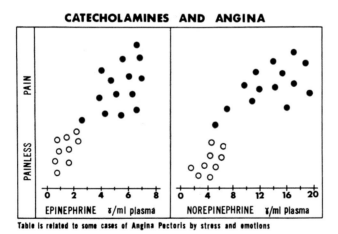

CATECHOLAMINES AND ANGINA

Table is related to some cases of Angina Pectoris by stress and emotions

Figure 12–1. Plasma catecholamines in patients with angina pectoris with pain (*black*) and without pain (*white*).

ing deliberately provoked, and during spontaneous attacks (Table 12–II). These elevations lasted for only limited periods of time. Some of the patients were highly emotional individuals between 35 and 45 years of age, with a labile blood pressure but without definite objective signs of coronary atherosclerosis, showing electrocardiographic changes only occa-sionally, and especially after exercise. In

TABLE 12–II

PLASMA CATECHOLAMINES IN 5 PATIENTS WITH ANGINA PECTORIS DURING
PAINFREE INTERVAL, AFTER EXERCISE, AND DURING PROVOKED AND
SPONTANEOUS ANGINAL ATTACKS

			Painless µg/l		Exercise (Master's Test) µg/l		Spontaneous Anginal Attack µg/l		Provoked Anginal Attack µg/l	
No.	Age	Sex	Adrenaline	Nor-adrenaline	Adrenaline	Nor-adrenaline	Adrenaline	Nor-adrenaline	Adrenaline	Nor-adrenaline
1	38	M.	1,10	3,85	1,47	8,38	2,80	9,30	4,80	15,38
2	40	M.	2,00	8,15	1,28	4,42	2,12	10,31	2,50	12,73
3	39	M.	1,15	7,69	1,56	5,60	1,60	12,21	7,18	12,31
4	45	M.	1,50	3,25	4,09	9,61	2,05	7,15	7,90	18,20
5	41	M.	0,35	0,80	1,04	3,61	1,49	3,45	2,66	13,76

TABLE 12–III

PLASMA CATECHOLAMINES AND URINARY VANILLYL MANDELIC ACID IN 5 PATIENTS
WITH MYOCARDIAL INFARCTION, FOLLOWED FOR 10 TO 12 DAYS AFTER ATTACK

Case No.	Age - Sex Diagnosis	Days Following Onset	Humoral Positivity	Blood Pressure	Plasmatic Catecholamines Adrenaline µg/l	Nor-adrenaline µg/l	Urinary Vanillyl Mandelic Acid µg/ml	mg/24h	mg/g Creatine
22	M. M.	3 hrs	–	100/60	3,21	9,65	4,01	–	3,43
	47 M.	2 hrs	++	80/60	–	–	4,06	–	2,98
	Posterior	24 hrs	++	90/60	3,10	8,51	4,15	–	3,20
	Myocardial	2 days	+++	90/60	2,50	7,90	2,96	2,57	2,41
	Infarction	3 days	+++	90/60	–	–	4,5	3,15	–
		4 days	+++	95/60	–	–	3,4	3,01	–
		10 days	++	100/60	1,80	5,12	2,96	2,98	–
23	B. E.	10 hrs	+	110/80	4,85	12,62	3,93	–	2,13
	52 M.	24 hrs	+++	145/80	–	–	9,93	–	5,30
	Anterior	2 days	+++	115/80	5,40	10,20	11,25	6,81	4,95
	Myocardial	3 days	+++	100/75	–	–	5,27	3,50	2,91
	Infarction	4 days	+++	160/80	4,80	8,91	11,85	12,90	16,53
		7 days	++	110/90	–	–	3,69	2,88	3,18
		10 days	++	105/80	–	–	3,54	2,47	2,24
24	M. V.	12 hrs	+	80/60	8,05	9,26	1,95	–	2,10
	38 M.	24 hrs	++	105/80	–	–	2,80	–	2,05
	Posterior	2 days	++	105/80	1,02	3,80	2,70	2,12	–
	Myocardial	10 days	++	100/60	–	–	2,36	2,15	–
25	S. S.	6 hrs	–	120/80	5,1	13,40	6,12	–	7,12
	38 M.	24 hrs	++	120/80	–	–	5,46	–	5,02
	Anteroseptal	2 days	+++	130/80	3,9	9,02	5,70	4,58	–
	Myocardial	5 days	+++	115/80	1,10	3,60	3,32	2,65	–
	Infarction	10 days	++	115/70	–	–	3,92	2,35	–
26	L. D.	1 day	–	155/100	4,06	12,20	11,3	6,84	-
	52 M.	2 days	++	160/90	1,8	13,10	27,3	14,96	–
	Anteroseptal	3 days	+++	150/80	1,25	4,60	8,16	4,89	–
	Myocardial Infarction	12 days	++	170/100	1,5	5,02	6,06	3,60	–

TABLE 12–IV

URINARY EXCRETION OF VANILLYL
MANDELIC ACID IN PATIENTS WITH
ANGINA PECTORIS

Cases No. 1–6: Without electrocardiographic abnormalities during painless intervals.
Cases No. 7–13: With electrocardiographic abnormalities during the painless intervals.

Case No. Age—Sex	Number of Crises During a Day	Vanillyl Mandelic Acid	
		μg/ml	mg/24 hrs
1 46 M	6	3,20	2,80
	1	2,95	2,85
2 58 M.	3	3,02	2,98
3 52 M.	3	2,03	2,40
	–	2,15	2,70
4 39 M.	2	1,98	2,28
5 53 M.	3	3,05	3,15
	–	3,10	3,08
6 45 M.	1	2,30	2,95
	–	1,98	2,45
7 49 M.	3	3,95	2,81
	–	3,28	3,01
8 42 M.	10	9,84	4,73
	2	4,89	3,66
9 48 M.	1	3,68	3,31
	1 with hyper- tension	4,88	4,48
10 40 M.	1	5,13	4,55
	–	3,80	2,95
11 49 F.	2	2,20	2,05
12 62 M.	1	2,74	1,89
13 46 M.	1	2,88	3,12

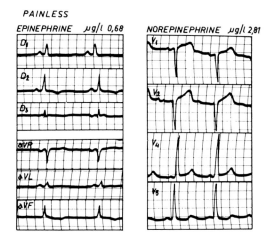

PAINLESS

EPINEPHRINE μg/l 0,68   NOREPINEPHRINE μg/l 2,81

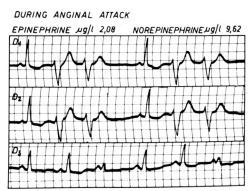

DURING ANGINAL ATTACK

EPINEPHRINE μg/l 2,08   NOREPINEPHRINE μg/l 9,62

Figure 12–2. Electrocardiogram and plasma catecholamine concentrations in a patient with angina
pectoris during painless interval (*top*) and during
an anginal attack (*bottom*).

a few instances, with attacks of angina
pectoris of long standing, significant increases, particularly of the epinephrine
level, were also observed during painfree
intervals.

In some of our patients in whom anginal symptoms were elicited by emotional interferences, the rise of the plasma
catecholamine level was accompanied by
electrocardiographic and electroenceph-
alographic responses and by cardiac arrhythmias (Fig. 12–2).

Marked increases of the plasma catecholamine level were also observed during the first hours and the first 2 days
following the occurrence of fresh myocardial infarctions without shock (Tables
12–I and III).

No comparably high catecholamine
concentrations appeared in the plasma
of patients with nonischemic cardiac pathology (valvular lesions) (Table 12–I).

The behavior of urinary vanillyl mandelic acid was far more irregular and
far less impressive than that of the plasma
catecholamines. The 24-hour excretion
values of this metabolite did not clearly
reflect the transient augmentations of the
plasma catecholamines, which accompany acute episodes of anginal pain.
Only in a few isolated instances of repeated anginal attacks during the day

did the values slightly exceed the normal range (Table 12–IV).

In cases of myocardial infarction, the discrepancy between the high plasma catecholamine levels of the first days and the usually near-normal excretion of vannilyl mandelic acid was also quite conspicuous with only a few exceptions, when unusually large amounts of the latter appeared in the urine.

Intravenous infusions of small doses of epinephrine (a total of 200 to 300 μg over 20 min which did not cause any increase of the 24-hour excretion of vanillyl mandelic acid, nor any electrocardiographic changes in normal individuals) were nevertheless sufficient to elicit, in patients with coronary atherosclerosis, severe anoxic alterations of the electrocardiogram.

Such microinfusions of epinephrine raised the level of the free-fatty acids in the blood in analogy to its elevations during anginal attacks which we observed in 8 cases.

DISCUSSION

Our observations (45, 46, 47) are in agreement with the early findings of Raab (20) and those of Gazes et al. (22), who reported abnormally high elevations of the blood catecholamines immediately after exercise in patients with angina pectoris. Gazes et al. (22) also observed unusually high blood catecholamine concentrations within 36 hours after myocardial infarction.

These and our own observations concerning rather regular and intense catecholamine discharges into the blood at the time of anginal attacks may be correlated with the well-known hypoxiating effect of the sympathogenic neurohormones on the myocardium, especially

when coronary compensatory dilatation is inadequate (7, 8).

The conclusion appears justified that adrenergic catecholamine discharges are causally involved in the pathogenic mechanism of the anginal attack, as repeatedly suggested by Raab (48) over the last 28 years. This hypothesis remained long disregarded despite the recognized therapeutic efficacy of cardiac sympathetic denervation (49) and various other antiadrenergic forms of treatment for angina pectoris (27), but is now gaining wide acceptance.

The objection that the rise of blood catecholamines in angina pectoris patients might be not a causal factor but merely a secondary phenomenon, evoked by the anginal pain, seems to be contradicted by our demonstration of a greatly augmented sensitivity of the human heart, afflicted with coronary sclerosis, to even minute does of epinephrine (50). This is in accord with similar observations of S. A. Levine (51), who used the provocation of anginal symptoms by injection of small doses of epinephrine as a diagnostic test for coronary atherosclerosis. Furthermore, Richardson et al. (52), found that painful sensations, other than those connected with angina pectoris, were not associated with significant augmentations of the blood catecholamines.

In the case of myocardial infarctions, it is more difficult to interpret the mechanism and meaning of the catecholamine augmentation in the plasma (22, 47). Even though the possibility of a causal participation of catecholamine discharges in the development of myocardial necroses is strongly suggested by numerous experimental observations (14, 15, 26, 28, 29, 30, 32–35), it is not possible a this time to assess the part played by the stress of an established infarction in the elevations of plasma catecholamines which continue for days after the acute event. Kuschke and Schneider (53) observed post-infarction augmentations of the catecholamine excretion in the urine which persisted for several days without a clear relation to clinical signs, such as high blood pressure or shock.

Increased plasma catecholamine levels have been recorded by Chidsey et al. (54) in patients with congestive heart failure in response to exercise. This too may be assumed to represent a secondary rather than a primary causative phenomenon.

The behavior of urinary vanillyl mandelic acid was too irregular and seemingly too unrelated to the fluctuations of the plasma catecholamines during attacks of angina pectoris and after infarctions to serve as an informative and clinically useful parameter. Apparently the transient and the more moderate rises of the plasma catecholamines are not sufficiently large for quantitative representation in the urinary levels of their metabolites. Analogous conclusions were recently reached by Raab and Gigee (55).

A profound and potentially toxic influence of circulating and intramyocardially liberated catecholamines upon the metabolism of the heart muscle is abundantly documented and, thus, can be regarded as a probably pathogenic factor in ischemic disease of the myocardium.

On the other hand, there is only little evidence so far in favor of a major participation of adrenosympathogenic catecholamine activity in the development of coronary vascular lesions.

Whether or not the influence of the sympathetic neurosecretory system upon blood lipid levels or blood coagulability contributes to coronary atherogenesis and, thus, to ischemic heart disease remains to be elucidated in the future.

In interpreting the origin of ischemic heart disease, it is important, in principle, to distinguish clearly between its two constituents, i.e., the vascular morphological element (coronary atherosclerosis,) on the one hand, and the complementary myocardial metabolic element (adrenergic catecholamine overactivity) on the other. Coronary atherosclerosis and ischemic heart disease overlap to a great extent but are not simply identical conditions, as the often indiscriminately misused term "coronary artery disease," instead of "ischemic heart disease," would imply.

SUMMARY

The plasma catecholamines (epinephrine and norepinephrine) usually rise to abnormally high levels in patients with coronary atherosclerosis and with angina pectoris during physical exertion or emotional excitement, and during anginal attacks.* They are also markedly elevated during the first hours and days after the occurrence of myocardial infarctions. By contrast, no increase of plasma catecholamine concentrations was found in patients with nonischemic heart disease.

Urinary excretion of the catecholamine metabolite vanillyl mandelic acid does not clearly reflect the fluctuations of the plasma catecholamines.

Patients with coronary atherosclerosis proved highly sensitive to the infusion even of small doses of epinephrine.

The presumable contributory patho-

---

*Analogous results were recently obtained by the author with the method of Crout, J. R., Creveling, C. R., and Udenfriend, S. J., *J. Pharmacol. and Exp. Therap.* 132:269, 1961.

genic role of the myocardial oxygen-wasting sympathoadrenal catecholamines in ischemic heart disease is discussed.

REFERENCES

1. Marchetti, G., Maccari, M., and Merlo, L.: Recherches expérimentales sur les effets de l'adrénaline et de la l-noradrénaline sur la circulation coronarienne. *Cardiologia, 42:*1, 1963.
2. Raab, W.: The neurogenic metabolic factor in ischemic heart disease. Pathogenesis and prevention. *Dis Chest, 46:*150, 1964.
3. Schimert, G., Schimmler, W., Schwalb, H., and Eberl, J.: Die Coronarerkrankungen (Coronarinsuffizienz, Angina pectoris und Herzinfarkt). In: Mohr, L., and Staehelin, R., Ed., *Handbuch d. Inn. Med.*, vol. IX, part 3, Ed. 4. Berlin-Göttingen, Heidelberg, Springer Verlag, 1960.
4. Alella, A., Williams, F. L., Bolene-Williams, C., and Katz, L. N.: Interrelation between cardiac oxygen consumption and coronary blood flow. *Amer J Physiol, 183:*570, 1955.
5. Gregg, D. E.: *Coronary Circulation in Health and Disease.* Philadelphia, Lea and Febiger, 1950.
6. Eckstein, R. W., Stroud, M., Dowling, C. V., Eckel, R., and Pritchard, W. H.: Response of coronary blood flow following sympathetic nerve stimulation. *Amer J Physiol, 162:*266, 1950.
7. Raab, W., Van Lith, P., Lepeschkin, E., and Herrlich, H. C.: Catecholamine-induced myocardial hypoxia in the presence of impaired coronary dilatability independent of external cardiac work. *Amer J Cardiol, 9:*455, 1962.
8. Bellet, S., West, J. W., Manzoli, U. C., Muller, O. F., and Rossi, P.: Effect of nicotine on the coronary blood flow in the presence of coronary insufficiency. An experimental study in dogs. *NY Acad Sci, 90:*317, 1960.
9. Kipshidze, N. N.: K voprosu o patogonese infarkta miokarda. *Ter Arkh, 29:*40, 1957.
10. Raab, W.: The nonvascular metabolic myocardial vulnerability factor in "coronary heart disease." *Amer Heart J, 66:*685, 1963.
11. Friedman, M., St. George, S., Byers, S. O., and Rosenman, R. H.: Excretion of catecholamines, 17-ketosteroids, 17-hydrocorticoids and 5-hydroxyindole in men exhibiting a particular behavior pattern (A) associated with high incidence of clinical coronary artery disease. *J Clin Invest, 39:*758, 1960.
12. Mason, J. W., Mangan, G., Brady, J. V., Conrad, D., and Rioch, D. McK.: Concurrent plasma epinephrine, norepinephrine and 17-hydroxycorticosteroid levels during conditioned emotional disturbances in monkeys. *Psychosom Med, 23:*344, 1961.
13. Levi, L.: The urinary output of adrenaline and noradrenaline during experimentally induced emotional stress in clinically different groups. *Acta Psychother, 11:*218, 1963.
14. Raab, W.: Neurogenic multifocal destruction of myocardial tissue. Pathogenesis mechanism and prevention. *Rev Canad Biol, 22:*217, 1963.
15. Selye, H.: *The Pluricausal Cardiopathies.* Springfield, Thomas, 1961.
16. Myasnikov, A. L.: Myocardial necroses of coronary and noncoronary genesis. *Amer J Cardiol, 13:*435, 1964.
17. Sulkovitch, H., Perrin, G. M., and Altschule, M. D.: Excretion of urinary epinephrines in psychiatric disorders. *Proc Soc Exp Biol Med, 95:*245, 1957.
18. Bergsman, A.: The urinary excretion of adrenaline and noradrenaline in some mental diseases. *Acta Psychiat Scand, 34:* Suppl. 133, 1959.
19. Ström-Olsen, R., and Weil-Malherbe, H.: Humoral changes in manic depressive psychosis with particular reference to the excretion of catecholamines in urine. *J Ment Sci, 105:*696, 1958.
20. Raab, W.: *Hormonal and Neurogenic Cardiovascular Disorders.* Baltimore, Williams and Wilkins, 1953.
21. Grey, J., and Beetham, W. P.: Changes in plasma concentration of epinephrine and norepinephrine with muscular work. *Proc. Soc Exp Biol Med, 96:*636, 1957.
22. Gazes, P. C., Richardson, J., and Woods, E. F.: Plasma catecholamine concentrations in myocardial infarction and angina pectoris. *Circulation, 19:*657, 1959.
23. Lovatt-Evans, C., Smith, D. F. G., and Weil-Malherbe, H.: The adrenaline and noradrenaline of venous blood of the horse before and after exercise. *J Physiol, 128:*58P, 1955.
24. Kärki, N. T.: The urinary excretion of noradrenaline and adrenaline in different age groups. Its diurnal variation and the effect of muscular work on it. *Acta Physiol Scand, 39:* Suppl. 132, 1956.
25. Raab, W.: The pathogenic significance of adrenaline and related substances in the heart muscle. *Exp Med Surg, 1:*188, 1943.
26. Shkhvatsabaya, I. K., and Menshikov, V. V.: K voprosu o znatchenii katekholaminov v patogeneze nevrogennykh izmenenii miokarda. *Kardiologiia, 2:*27, 1962.
27. Raab, W.: The sympathogenic biochemical trigger mechanism of angina pectoris. Its therapeutic suppression and long-range prevention. *Amer J Cardiol, 9:*576, 1962.
28. Josué, O.: Hypertrophie cardiaque cause pa

l'adrenaline et la toxine typhique. *Cpt Soc Biol,* (*Paris*), *63:*285, 1907.

29. SZAKACS, J. E., and CANNON, A.: l-Norepinephrine myocarditis. *Amer J Clin Path., 30:*425, 1958.

30. MELVILLE, K. I., BLUM, B., SHISTER, H. E., and SILVER, M. D.: Cardiac ischemia changes and arrhythmias induced by hypothalamic stimulation. *Amer J Cardiol, 12:*781, 1963.

31. NAKABAYASHI, Y.: The effect of the destruction of the brainstem on the function of the heart, with especial reference to change on electrocardiogram. *Iqaku Kenkyuu, 23:*14, 1953.

32. VEDENYEYEVA, Z. J.: Myocardial lesions due to sympathomimetic amines of endogenous and exogenous origin and their analysis. *Farmakol Toksik, 3:*286, 1962.

33. MIMINOSHVILI, D. J., MAGAKYAN, G. O., and KOKAYA, S. Ya: O korkovykh vliyaniyakh na vyenechnoye krovo-obrashcheniye. *Voprosy Fiziologii y Patologii Obyezyan,* Sukhumi, 1961.

34. CHERKOVICH, G. M.: Mikronekrozy v syerdtse obyezyany v resul'tate eksperimental'nogo nevroza. *Patologiicheskaya fiziologiya y eksperimental'naya terapiya.* Moscow, Medgiz, 1959.

35. RAAB, W., CHAPLIN, J. P., and BAJUSZ, E.: Myocardial necroses produced in domesticated rats and in wild rats by sensory and emotional stresses. *Proc. Soc Exp Biol Med, 116:*665, 1964.

36. DOYLE, J. T., DAWBER, T. P., KANNEL, W. B., HASLIN, A. S., and KAHN, H. A.: Cigarette smoking and coronary heart disease. *New Eng J Med, 266:*796, 1962.

37. RUSSEK, H. J.: Emotional stress and coronary heart disease in American physicians. *Amer J Med Sci, 240:*79–711, 1960.

38. PAUL, O., LEPPER, M. H., OSTFELD, A., MAC-MILLAN, A., and PHELAN, W. H.: Coronary heart disease in an industrial population; a prospective study. *Circulation, 26:*770, 1962.

39. ROSENMAN, R. H., FRIEDMAN, M., STRAUS, R., WURM, M., KOSITCHEK, R. J., HAHN, W., and WERTHESSEN, N. T.: A predictive study of coronary heart disease. The Western Collaborative Group Study. *JAMA, 189:*15, 1964.

40. BRANDT, E. N., JR., STOUT, S., HAMPTON, J. W., and WOLF, S.: Coronary heart disease in Roseto, Pennsylvania and among Italians and non-Italians in nearby communities. (See Chapter 27.)

41. LAPICCIRELLA, V., ABBONI, F., LAPICCIRELLA, R., and LIOTTA, S.: Una indagine epidemiologica sul pastore nomade della Somalia e un gruppo di pescatori delle isole Bagiuni, Ed. Mediche Italiane, 1962.

42. LAPICCIRELLA, R., MARRAMA, P., and Bonati, B.: Hormone excretion, diet and physique in Somalis. *Lancet,* p. 24, July 1, 1961.

43. WEIL-MALHERBE, H., and BONE, A. D.: The fluorimetric estimation of adrenaline and noradrenaline in plasma. *Biochem J, 67:*65, 1957.

44. PISANO, J. J., CROUT, J. R., and ABRAHAM, D.: Determination of 3-methoxy-4-hydroxymandelic acid in urine. *Clin Chim Acta, J:*285, 1962.

45. STARCICH, R., and AMBANELLI, U.: Importanza della determinazione delle catecolamine plasmatiche in patologia coronarica. *Giorn Clin Med, 40:*1, 1959.

46. STARCICH, R.: Fattori emozionali e variazioni p plasmatiche delle carecolamine nella insufficienza coronarica acuta critica, Acta III. *Europaei de Cordis Scientia Conventus.* Roma, Excerpta Medica, 1960, p. 155.

47. AMBANELLI, U., and STARCICH, R.: Comportamento delle catecolamine plasmatiche e urinarie nelle sindromi coronariche. Aspetti clinici e farmacodinamici dell' escrezione dell' acido vanilmandelico. *Giorn Clin Med, 46:*682, 1963.

48. RAAB, W.: Nebennieren und Angina pectoris: Pathogenese und Röntgentherapie. *Arch Kreislaufforsch, 1:*225, 1937.

49. WHITE, J. C., and BLAND, E. F.: The surgical relief of severe angina pectoris; methods employed and end results in 83 patients. *Medicine, 27:*1, 1948.

50. AMBANELLI, U., and STARCICH, R.: Aspetti clinici ed elettrocardiografici da microdosi di adrenalina in corso di insufficienza coronarica acuta. *Boll Soc Ital Cardiol, 8:*336, 1963.

51. LEVINE, S. A., ERNSTENE, A. C., and JACOBSON, B. H.: The use of epinephrine as a diagnostic test for angina pectoris. *Arch Intern Med, 45:*191, 1930.

52. RICHARDSON, J. A., WOODS, E. F., GAZES, P. C., and BAGWELL, E. E.: Plasma catecholamines in coronary occlusion and angina pectoris. *Fed Proc, I–18:*437, 1959.

53. KUSCHKE, H. J., and SCHNEIDER, K. W.: Die sympathiko-adrenale Reaktion beim Herzinfarkt. *Z Kreislaufforsch, 49:*261, 1960.

54. CHIDSEY, D., HARRISON, C., and BRAUNWALD, E.: Augmentation of plasma norepinephrine response to exercise in patients with congestive heart failure. *New Eng J Med, 267:*650, 1962.

55. RAAB, W., and GIGEE, W.: Urinary 3-methoxy-4-hydroxymandelic acid (VMA) in ischemic heart disease and in uremia. *Am J Med Sci, 250:* 99/547, 1965

Chapter XIII

EMOTIONAL STRAIN AFFECTING THE ELECTROCARDIOGRAM

LOUIS H. SIGLER

(Brooklyn, New York, U.S.A.)

ELECTROCARDIOGRAPHIC abnormalities may occur in some individuals with no demonstrable organic heart disease, but are more frequently encountered in the presence of coronary arteriosclerosis.

CLINICAL FEATURES

The patient is usually a neurotic, tense and worrisome individual with fear of impending danger to health and life. In some, there is underneath a surface appearance of calmness, a state of emotional upset at all times. Any trivial pain or ache may cause palpitation, dizziness, sweating, marked weakness and other disturbances. There is usually a history of severe psychic trauma at one time or another, with perpetual reminiscences of tragic experiences.

Some cases have demonstrable structural heart disease. In others, the heart is of normal size, configuration, rate and rhythm, and the sounds are of good quality. Most of these individuals are able to carry on normal activities if reassured that there is nothing wrong with the heart.

ELECTROCARDIOGRAPHIC MANIFESTATIONS *

The types and degrees of electrocardio-graphic changes appear to depend in part on the extent of psychic trauma in the given individual. Milder emotional disturbances may merely produce some changes in the terminal ventricular complex, ranging from diminished height to isoelectric or negative T waves in various leads where previously the T wave had been normal, or some changes in the appearance and direction of this wave when abnormal. There may also be depression or abnormal elevation of the ST segment in some leads. In more severe forms, there may be a greater or lesser degree of changes in the initial ventricular complex. These may consist of increase or decrease in its voltage, the appearance of a Q wave in some of the leads where it had previously been absent, or accentuation of that wave when present; changes in the direction of the components of the QRS complex in various leads from time to time; intermittent or more or less prolonged occurrence of bundle branch block; delayed intraventricular conduction time, and development of slurring or notching. The changes may occur in a transient form for very

---

*The illustrations used here are reproduced from a previous paper by the author (12). The case reports are brought up-to-date.

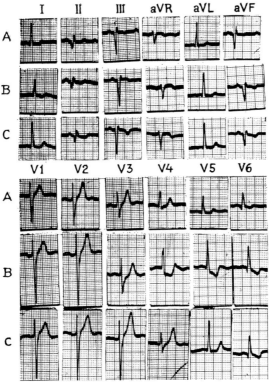

Figure 13–1. Case 1: *A.* Residual findings of posterior wall infarction. *B.* After emotional upset: marked depression of the ST segment in leads V3 to V6, diphasic T wave in V4, negative T wave in V5 and V6. *C.* After 15 minutes of relaxation: ST segment isoelectric in leads V3 to V6, tall positive T wave in V3, V4, and V5. Changes in voltage of the QRS complex in various leads.

short periods in one or more leads while the tracing is being taken, or they may persist a long time.

We must bear in mind that there are other conditions which may cause changes in the electrocardiogram resembling those caused by emotional stress. Thus, alterations in posture, acute tachycardia and arrhythmia, alkalosis, acidosis, electrolyte imbalance, hyperventilation, shock caused by embolization, trauma, vascular thrombosis, and hemorrhage may produce acute changes in the electrocardiogram. In such cases, the specific cause is readily recognizable and the changes in the electrocardiogram may have more or less specific appearances. The changes in the electrocardiogram under emotional strain, on the other hand, are erratic, unstable, unpredictable, and often transient in nature during the acute phase. Some features may change while the tracing is taken. Previous similar observations (1–11) and the possibly underlying neurogenic and neurohormonal mechanisms have been discussed elsewhere (12).

ILLUSTRATIVE CASES

Case 1. A male physician, 58-years-old, was highly irritable, emotional, and introspective since his escape from a Hitler concentration camp in 1944 where several members of his family were killed before his eyes. On arriving in this country, he obtained a position of resident physician in a home for the aged where he was required to interview and examine many senile, mentally defective individuals. During one prolonged interview of a demented individual he became highly emotional and excited because he could not obtain a coherent history, and he soon developed severe pain in the anterior chest, radiating to the left arm, and a fainting sensation. He was admitted to the hospital where he showed acute myocardial ischemia, followed a few days later by clinical and laboratory evidence of infarction of the posterior wall of the left ventricle.

Many electrocardiograms were taken during a period of 8 years following recovery from the myocardial infarction until his death at 66 years of age. The tracings were stable most of the time, but during episodes of emotional disturbance acute changes were frequently noted.

Figure 13–1A shows the residual findings of the posterior wall infarction as the usual pattern he presented.

Figure 13–1B shows that during an episode of extreme nervous excitement there is a greater negativity of the T wave in aVF, depression of the ST segment in leads V4 and V5, diphasic T wave in lead V4 and deeply negative T wave in V5 and in V6. The QRS complex in all leads, except in leads I and aVL, is of higher voltage.

Figure 13–1C, obtained 15 minutes later, after the subject had calmed down, shows a taller T wave in lead V3, an isoelectric ST segment and tall positive T wave in V4, and an isoelectric ST segment and positive T wave in V5, indicating a diminution in the acute ischemic pattern shown in Figure 13–1B. The QRS complex is of higher voltage in aVR and V3 and of lower voltage in V4 and V6.

Case 2. A woman, 53-years-old, complained of recurring attacks of black-outs, faintness, light-headedness, pinching in the left precordium, and a sensation as if the heart were "jumping." She was married 25 years and her husband died 5 years ago, compelling her to go to work. She constantly feared losing her job because of her age.

Although appearing cheerful, she often expressed fear of impending danger to her life. Following a radical mastectomy for carcinoma several years ago, there was an accentuation of the symptoms.

During a 2-weeks stay in the hospital, her heart was of normal size, the rate 96 beats per minute and regular, the sounds were somewhat accentuated, A2 being louder than P2. The blood pressure was 150/96 mm Hg. The transaminase was 18 units. The electrocardiogram on the day of admission (Figure 13–2A), showed an isoelectric T wave in lead I, depression of the ST segment and negative T wave in leads II, III, aVF, V4, V5 and V6, and tall R waves in leads V3, V5, and V6.

Four months later she felt better. The electrocardiogram (Figure 13–2B) showed a low, semi-inverted T wave in the conventional and unipolar extremity leads; the T wave was positive in V5 and in V6; a lower voltage QRS complex was seen in the con-

Figure 13–2. Case 2: *A.* During severe emotional disturbances: isoelectric T in lead I, positive T in aVR, depression of ST segment and negative T in leads II, III, aVF, V4, V5 and V6. *B.* During a more tranquil period: improvement of ST segment and T in leads II, III, aVR and V4; T in leads I and aVL is now slightly negative; directional changes of the QRS complex in V3 and V4; T is positive in V4 and V5 and slightly diphasic in V6. *C.* 3 months after *B:* marked abnormalities of the ST segment in V3, V4 and V5; QRS in V4 of lower voltage. *D.* 2 weeks after *C:* left bundle branch block. *E.* 2 months later: intraventricular conduction normal with marked directional and voltage changes of QRS. The T waves are normal.

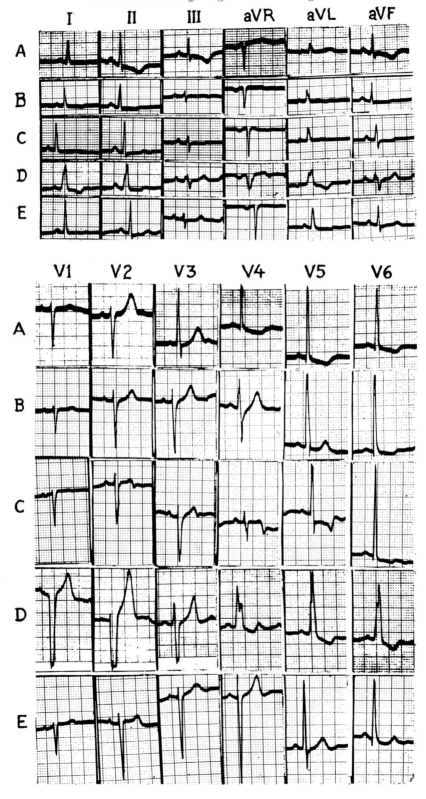

ventional and unipolar extremity leads, and a marked change in direction of the QRS complex in V3 and V4.

Three months later she complained of "pinching" pain in the left precordial region, not related to exertion, and "light-headedness." She experienced at that time a disturbing event, having been told by a physician that the remaining breast had a cyst. The electrocardiogram (Fig. 13–2C) showed little change in the conventional leads, but marked changes in the terminal ventricular complexes in V2 through V6, suggesting acute myocardial ischemia. She was readmitted to the hospital, and during a 3-weeks stay she had normal temperature, normal transaminase and normal blood count and sedimentation rate. She was symptom-free except for an occasional "groggy feeling" and slight palpitation. The physical findings were within normal limits. An electrocardiogram (Fig. 13–2D) now revealed left bundle branch block.

One month after discharge from the hospital, she was almost symptom-free. An electrocardiogram at that time (Fig. 13–2E) showed normal intraventricular conduction, with normal T waves in all precordial leads. At the present writing, at 58 years of age, her electrocardiogram still undergoes changes from time to time, with changes in moods.

Case 3. A woman, first seen in 1936 when she was 33-years-old, complained of recurring palpitation, dyspnea, headache, pressure in the precordial region, extreme weakness and at times a "fainting" sensation. The heart was of normal size, the rate was 90 beats per minute, with sinus arrhythmia; the heart sounds were accentuated. The blood pressure

was 150/100. Her reaction to exercise was greatly exaggerated. Thus, after a few knee bends she exhibited a frightful appearance of choking and complained of being "unable to catch her breath." The post-exercise electrocardiogram was normal.

She was not seen again until 11 years later, when she complained of spells of weakness and a tightening sensation in the left precordium on excitement or exertion. During the interval she had had her left breast removed for carcinoma in 1939, and the gall bladder was removed in 1946. The heart findings remained the same as in 1936, but the electrocardiogram (Fig. 13–3A) showed left bundle branch block. While the tracing was taken, there were periods when the intraventricular conduction was normal, as in lead aVR.

Since 1947 she was seen intermittently. The complaints were the same as when I first saw her 28 years ago. She considered herself an invalid and was afraid to venture out of the house because of a feeling that she was going to die if she carried on any exertion. She is an intelligent extrovert, desiring to make friends, and yet refusing to go out for fear of impending danger. During all these years the heart was persistently normal in size and shape, the rate varying between 75 and 85 beats per minute, and the blood pressure between 130/80 and 160/100. At no time was there any evidence of heart failure.

Many electrocardiograms were obtained during the last 17 years. Most of these showed left bundle branch block (Fig. 13–3B, C, D, F), but often normal intraventricular conduction was observed (Fig. 13–3E) for vari-

————————————>

Figure 13–3. Case 3: *A.* 1947: left bundle branch block except in aVR where conduction is normal. *B.* 1949: left bundle branch block with slight changes in appearance of QRS in some leads. *C.* left bundle branch block with marked changes in direction and amplitude of QRS complex and T wave in leads V2 through V5. *D.* 1954: left bundle branch block, deeper S wave in V2, and lower T in V1, V2 and V3 than in *A* and *B*. *E.* 1955: normal intraventricular conduction. *F.* 1959; left bundle branch block, changes in direction and amplitude of QRS in some precordial leads.

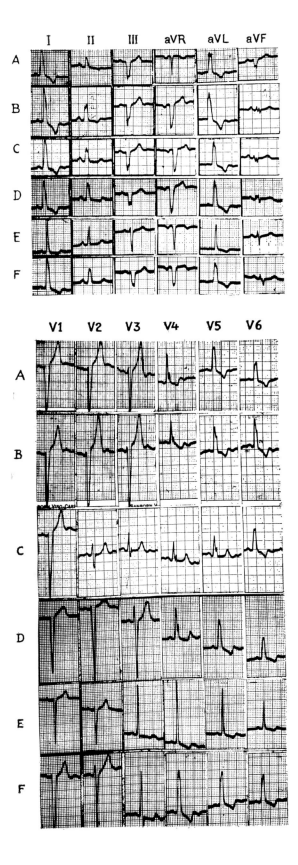

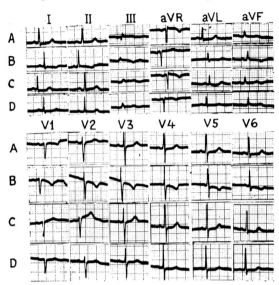

Figure 13–4. Case 4: *A.* normal tracing. *B.* after emotional upset: negative T in leads I, II, III and aVF; low T in aVL, positive T in aVR; depression of ST segment and negative T in all precordial leads. *C.* 5 months after *B*, normal tracing. *D.* 2 years later, after another emotional upset: lower T in all leads with slight depression of the ST segment in some.

able periods of hours or days. Even during the time when left bundle branch block was present, there were often marked variations in the appearance of the ventricular complexes and some variations in intraventricular conduction (Fig. 13–3C).

In 1951 she was hospitalized after an "acute heart attack," with complaints of severe, "agonizing" pain in the chest, and a "fainting" sensation. Repeated electrocardiograms showed left bundle branch block, with some variations in the appearance of the ventricular complexes from time to time.

Case 4. This was a woman, first seen on June 2, 1955, when she was 46-years-old. She complained of recurring pain in the anterior part of the chest of 3 years' duration, radiating to the left interscapular region and left arm, not related to physical exertion. She also complained of dizziness, numbness of hands and a "jittery" feeling. She was very apprehensive. The heart was normal in size and shape, the rate was 78 and regular. The blood pressure was 145/85. An electrocardiogram (Fig. 13–4A) showed complexes within normal limits in all leads.

In 1955, after an emotional upset due to a death in her family, she suddenly became dizzy and experienced cold sweat, a sensation of "needles in her toes and knees," and precordial pain, radiating to the left supraclavicular region. An electrocardiogram (Fig. 13–4B) showed negative T waves and slight depression of the ST segment in leads I, II, III, aVF and in all precordial leads. When the patient was admitted to the hospital, the pain in the anterior portion of the chest recurred intermittently. The temperature was persistently normal and the pulse rate varied between 75 and 90 beats per minute. The sedimentation rate and blood count were within normal limits. The blood pressure varied between 108/78 and 135/85. The heart and lungs were normal on physical and x-ray examinations. Cholecystography revealed a normally functioning gall bladder without stones. Gastrointestinal roentgenograms showed an esophageal hiatus hernia.

The electrocardiogram returned to normal after 2 weeks and has remained so since then (Fig. 13–4C). After reassurance she was practically symptom-free for 5 years, except

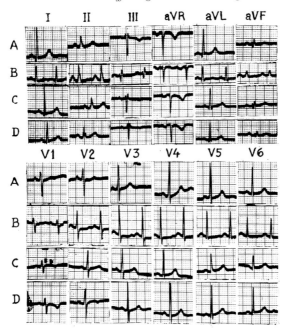

Figure 13–5. Case 5: *A.* normal tracing, horizontal electrical position. *B.* after a severe emotional upset: diminished voltage of QRS in leads I, III, aVL, V1, V5 and V6 with changes in direction; T almost isoelectric in all leads but less negative in aVR. *C.* 11 days after *B*, tracing normal. *D.* 2 months later, after another episode of milder emotional upset: T more negative in V1 and V2.

for occasional complaints of pain in the left scapular or precordial region on emotional upsets, at which time electrocardiographic abnormalities recurred. Thus, in 1957, when a friend had suddenly died, she reported numerous and unrelated symptoms. An electrocardiogram (Fig. 13–4D), obtained at that time, showed a decrease in voltage of the T wave in all leads with slight depression of the ST segment in leads V3 through V6.

Case 5. A woman, 58-years-old, a very emotional individual, complained of pain below the left breast, radiating to the left arm following emotional disturbances. One night she was awakened by a severe pain lasting about 2 hours. She was told by a physician that she had "a heart attack" and she rested in bed for a week, but the pain recurred intermittently. The heart was of normal size; rate 80 beats per minute, regular; sounds normal. The blood pressure was at first 170/110 but dropped to 136/90 after

relaxing. The retinal arteries showed slight sclerosis. An electrocardiogram (Fig. 13–5A) merely showed left axis deviation and a semihorizontal electrical position. She was reassured that there was nothing wrong with her heart and that the symptoms were due to emotional strain.

For 9 days she felt quite well, having only occasional slight pain in the anterior part of the chest, not aggravated by exertion. On the 10th day she had an argument with a neighbor who, she claimed, "spread malicious lies" about her. Soon she felt severe pain in the left scapular region, radiating to the shoulder and left arm, with pallor, sweating, vomiting, and a drop in blood pressure to 80/50. The heart rate was 110 beats per minute. She was admitted to the hospital. Oxygen therapy and meperidine gave relief. An electrocardiogram obtained that day (Fig. 13–5B) showed abnormal T waves in all leads. During a 3-weeks stay at the hospital the temperature was normal, the heart rate varied between 75 and 80 beats per minute, and the rhythm was regular. The blood pressure varied between 108/60 and 132/78. Transaminase on the second day was 24 units, on the third day 20 units, and on the fifth day 14 units. Reassurance and an occasional sedative progressively improved her condition and the electrocardiogram returned to normal (Fig. 13–5C).

After discharge from the hospital she continued to feel well, except for occasional mild pain in the chest on excitement. On one occasion she again had a nervous upset and the electrocardiogram (Fig. 13–5D) showed an inverted T wave in V1 and V2, and the T wave in the other precordial leads was of slightly lower voltage.

SUMMARY

Electrocardiographic changes have been observed under emotional strain and stress in neurotic, tense, and worrisome individuals who are fearful of impending danger to health and life. The changes may consist of alterations in the position of the ST segment in relation to the isoelectric line; changes of the T wave, ranging from diminished height to isoelectric or negative, where previously it had been normal, or changes in its appearance and direction when originally abnormal; increased or decreased voltage of the QRS complex; acute appearance of a Q wave; changes in direction of the components of the QRS complex; intermittent or prolonged bundle branch block; simple delay in intraventricular conduction time and appearance of slurring or notching.

Although acute changes in the electro-cardiogram may occur also in other abnormal constitutional states, the erratic, unstable, and usually transient nature of abnormalities appearing under emotional strain can be readily differentiated from those caused by other conditions.

REFERENCES

1. GRAYBIEL, A., and WHITE, P. D.: Inversion of the T wave in lead I or II of the electrocardiogram in young individuals with neurocirculatory asthenia, with thyrotoxicosis, in relation to certain infections and following paroxysmal ventricular tachycardia. *Amer Heart J, 10:*345, 1935.
2. LOGUE, R. B., HANSON, J. F., and KNIGHT, W. A.: Electrocardiographic studies in neurocirculatory asthenia. *Amer Heart J, 28:*574, 1944.
3. LOFTUS, T. A., GOLD, H., and DIETHELM, O.: Cardiac changes in the presence of intense emotion. *Amer J Psychiat, 101:*697, 1944–45.
4. HEYER, H. E., WINANS, H. M., and PLESSINGER, V. I.: Alterations in form of the electrocardiogram in patients with mental disease. *Amer J Med Sci, 214:*23, 1947.
5. MAGENDANTZ, H., and SHORTSLEEVE, J.: Electrocardiographic abnormalities in patients exhibiting anxiety. *Amer Heart J, 42:*849, 1951.
6. MAINZER, F., and KRAUSE, M.: The influence of fear on the electrocardiogram. *Brit. Heart J, 2:*221, 1940.
7. STEVENSON, I., DUNCAN, C. H., and RIPLEY, H. S.: Variations in the electrocardiographic changes in emotional state. *Geriatrics, 6:*164, 1951.
8. WINTON, S. S., and WALLACE, L.: An electrocardiographic study of psychoneurotic patients. *Psychosom Med, 8:*332, 1946.
9. GRAYBIEL, A., McFARLAND, R. A., GATES, D., and WEBSTER, F. A.: Analysis of the electrocardiogram obtained from 1000 young healthy aviators. *Amer Heart J, 5:*24, 1944.
10. GRAU, S.: The effect of the psyche upon the electrocardiogram. *Amer J Cardiol, 2:*184, 1958.
11. SIGLER, L. H.: Emotional disturbances as a cause of an acute cardiac insult. *Amer J Cardiol, 4:*557, 1959.
12. SIGLER, L. H.: Abnormalities in the electrocardiogram induced by emotional strain. *Amer J Cardiol, 8:*807, 1961.

Chapter XIV

CARDIAC SYMPATHETIC TONE AND STRESS RESPONSE RELATED TO PERSONALITY PATTERNS AND EXERCISE HABITS

(A Potential Cardiac Risk and Screening Test)*

WILHELM RAAB and HANS J. KRZYWANEK

(Burlington, Vermont, U.S.A.)

A SIGNIFICANT contributory role of socioeconomic emotional factors and of lack of physical exercise in the high morbidity and mortality rate from multicausal hypoxic † heart disease in industrialized prosperous nations has been made probable by numerous clinical statistical (1–13, 86, 87) and pathophysiological studies. Animal experiments suggest that intensive emotional stimuli per se are capable of eliciting myocardial necroses (14–17) (Fig. 14–1).

Both emotional tensions and habitual inactivity share as their common denominator a demonstrable augmentation of sympathetic adrenergic activity (18–26). In the case of emotional tensions, this is presumably due to exaggerated hypothalamic stimulation; in the case of physical inactivity, to a deterioration of sympathoinhibitory inotropic and vagal chronotropic antiadrenergic counterregulatory mechanisms at rest (23, 24, 27–29) (Fig. 14–2). (Another contributory

element in hypoxic heart disease, tobacco smoking, is likewise associated with adrenergic overactivity, in this case caused by nicotine-induced ganglionic stimulation.)

The long-known myocardial oxygen "wasting" and potentially anoxiating cardiotoxic properties of the adrenosympathogenic catecholamines (30–39), are being increasingly appreciated with respect to their clinical pathogenic significance (26, 33, 40–48).

Currently used objective criteria for the recognition of so-called "coronary-prone" individuals (high serum lipid level, obesity, hypertension, mesomorphy, low vital capacity) do not include any parameter which would reveal the subject's cardiac sympathetic nervous activity pattern.

To our knowledge, only 2 published statements mention a statistically faster heart rate in connection with "coronary-proneness" (49, 50). A high catecholamine and catecholamine metabolite excretion was observed in "coronary-prone" Americans (19, 20), and a low catecholamine excretion in Africans with a low incidence of hypoxic heart disease (51). Patients with angina pectoris react to

*This study was aided by Research Grant HE-02169 from the National Heart Institute.

†Preference of the term "hypoxic" over "coronary" or "ischemic" is explained in the Introduction of the book and is based on the present state of knowledge of myocardial pathophysiology.

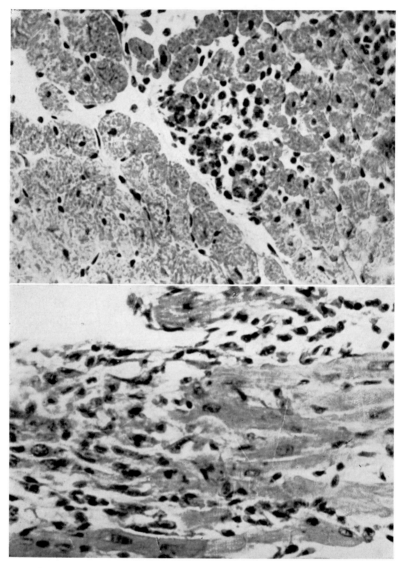

Figure 14–1. Degenerating and necrotic foci in the myocardium of rats which had been exposed to frustrating (obstacles in access to food) and frightening (tape recorded cat-rat fight) situations. (W. Raab *et al.: Proc Soc Exp Biol Med, 116:*665, 1964.)

exercise and to emotional stimuli with exaggerated rises of the blood catecholamines (22, 42, 52, 53, 84, 89-91).

In view of the fundamental role which an elevated sympathetic resting tone and stress response seems to play in the origin of hypoxic heart disease, particularly in the presence of impaired compensatory coronary dilatability (54, 55), the following study was carried out. It concerns the behavior of 2 cardiac functional parameters, directly representing autonomic nervous (neurohormonal) regulatory influences on the heart muscle (56, 57) and indirectly indicative of its oxygen economy (25, 58, 85), namely heart rate

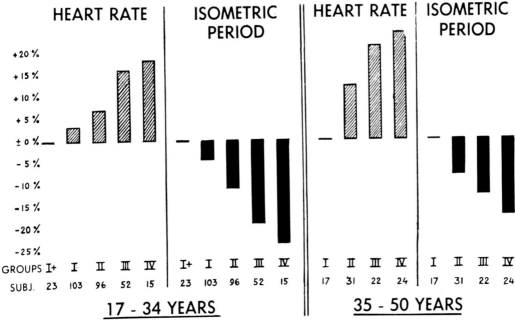

Figure 14–2. Increasing sympathetic-adrenergic preponderance in cardiac function (increasing resting heart rate and decreasing length of isometric period of left ventricle) occurs in proportion to decreasing exercise habits in 360 healthy men, ranging from competitive athletes (group I+) to completely sedentary individuals (group IV). The older age group does not include any competitive athletes. Group I are active but not competing sportsmen. (W. RAAB et al.: *Amer. J Cardiol*, 5:300, 1960.)

and length of the isometric tension period (TP) of the left ventricle at rest and under standardized sensory and mental stresses. (The heart rate is augmented, the tension period shortened by sympathetic adrenergic action [23, 57]). These parameters were measured jointly with blood pressure, serum cholesterol and free-fatty acids, and correlated with the emotional personality patterns and exercise habits of the test subjects.

PROCEDURE

Two hundred "normal" male subjects‡ (average age 44) were first instructed what to expect, and then exposed to the following procedure:

‡Including 12 with mild hypertension.

1. 30 minutes rest on a bed in semi-darkness;

2. 10 minutes noise of a rhythmically ringing telephone bell and a strong flickering light (thrown on a white screen at the foot of the bed by a projector with a fan rotating in front of the lens);

3. 10 minutes continued noise and flicker light plus mental arithmetic (2 successive problems were projected on the screen during two 5-minute periods each. Both periods were disturbed by the projected text "Are you sure of your result? Check it again!" Answers were asked for at the end of each calculating period and recorded without comment);

4. 10 minutes recovery period.

Electrocardiogram, phonocardiogram, and carotid pulse wave were registered simultaneously for measurement of the dynamic phases of the left ventricle (total systole, isometric tension period and ejection period, expressed in milliseconds) according to the method of Blumberger (59), as described elsewhere (57). The relative length of the ventricular systole in per cent of the total cardiac cycle was calculated by the formula " (Total Systole x Heart Rate per minute): 600." The heart rate was counted at the radial artery and the blood pressure measured by auscultation. Blood samples for cholesterol and free-fatty acids were taken from an indwelling cannula in a cubital vein.

Data on the degree of emotional irritability and tenseness were obtained from self-evaluation questionnaires, and scored by a cumulative point system ranging from +10 to −2.

Exercise habits were scored in a similar fashion with cumulated points ranging from +4 to ±0.

In view of the adrenergic implications of positive emotion scores and the anti-adrenergic implications of positive physical training scores, the mutual interference of both was integrated by subtracting the cumulated exercise habit scores from the cumulated emotion scores, and the result designated as adrenergic-anti-adrenergic "balance" score.

Examples: Em. (+8) minus Ex. (+2) = Bal. (+6); or Em. (−2) minus Ex. (+4) = Bal. (−6), etc.

All cardiovascular parameter readings and all questionnaire-derived scores were obtained and calculated independently of each other by the two authors.

Taking the inevitable inaccuracies of self-evaluation by questionnaire into account, conclusions regarding possible connections between emotional personality patterns and exercise habits on the one hand, and cardiovascular manifestations on the other, were based solely on data from subjects occupying the upper and lower sections of the various score spectra, respectively. Accordingly, subjects were grouped by (a) emotion scores from +5 up versus from −1 down; (b) exercise scores from +3 up versus ±0, and (c) balance scores from +3 up versus from −2 down.

Conversely, 2 groups, displaying maximal or minimal cardiac adrenergic and vasopressor activity, respectively, were correlated with their corresponding average emotion and exercise habit scores.

Further details concerning test subject material, measuring techniques, questionnaires, scoring points, and computing system can be found elsewhere (60).

RESULTS

The resting heart rate, isometric tension period (TP), and blood pressure, and their responses to sensory and mental stresses varied within wide ranges, whereby the average stress responses revealed a typical adrenergic reaction (cardiac acceleration, shortening of TP) which was more marked under combined sensory and mental stresses than under sensory stress alone (Table 14–I).

When the most and the least emotional subjects (average emotion scores +6.5 versus −1.6) were compared (Fig. 14–3), the former showed a higher heart rate and shorter TP at rest, as well as higher heart rates and shorter TPs in response to stress.

Comparison of the physically least active with the most active subjects (average exercise habit scores ±0 versus +3.3) showed an analogous relationship (Fig. 14–3).

TABLE 14–I

RANGES OF ABSOLUTE READINGS AND OF DEVIATIONS FROM RESTING VALUES IN RESPONSE TO SENSORY AND COMBINED SENSORY + PLUS MENTAL STRESS (200 SUBJECTS)

Phases of Test	Heart Rate Per Min.			Isometric Period (TP) of Left Ventr. (msec)			Systole in % of Cycle		Systolic Blood Pressure (mm Hg)			Diastolic Blood Pressure (mm Hg)			Serum Cholesterol (mg%)	
	Max.	Min.	Average	Max.	Min.	Average	Max.	Min.	Max.	Min.	Average	Max.	Min.	Average	Max.	Min.
Rest	100	46	66.3	135	61	93.9	58	32	170	90	114.9	110	50	73.9	350	131
Sensory stress	+18	−6	+4.6	−24	+16	−2.5			+25	−5	+5.7	+20	−5	+4.0		
Sensory plus mental stress	+52	−14	+15.3	−37	+10	−6.1			+45	−15	+15.3	+35	−5	+9.9		
Recovery	+10	−15	+0.1	−13	+16	+0.7			+30	−15	+2.2	+20	−10	+3.1		

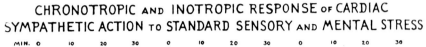

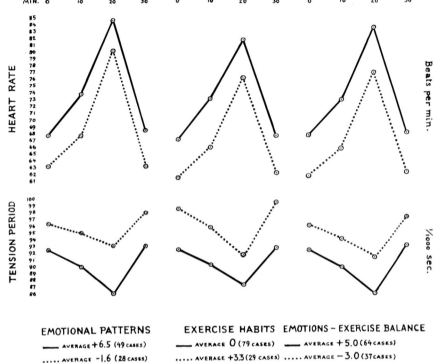

Figure 14–3. Drawn-out curves show a higher sympathetic cardiac resting tone and stress response level (higher heart rate and shorter isometric [tension] period) in emotionally excitable, sedentary, and "high balance" subjects, as compared with placid, physically active and "low balance" ones (*dotted curves*).

Comparison of the subjects with the highest and the lowest emotion minus exercise (= "balance") scores (averages +5.0 versus −3.0) again showed similar differences (Fig. 14–3).

The group differences of the resting values of heart rate and TP were statistically highly significant, except for TP in the emotion and "balance" groups. The group differences during stress exposure were also, for the most part, significant between "p" <005 and <.025.

The relative (percentile) length of the left ventricular systole was significantly greater in the highly emotional, physi-

cally inactive, and high "balance" groups than in their counterparts.

Thirty-two subjects displaying maximal adrenergic characteristics (highest heart rates and shortest TPs at rest and/ or under stress) had high average emotion and low exercise scores (Fig. 14–4). Thirty-two others with minimal adrenergic characteristics had lower average emotion and higher exercise scores (Fig. 14–4).

Differences of the systolic and diastolic blood pressure levels and stress responses in the various groups were not statistically significant (Fig. 14–5). The apparently

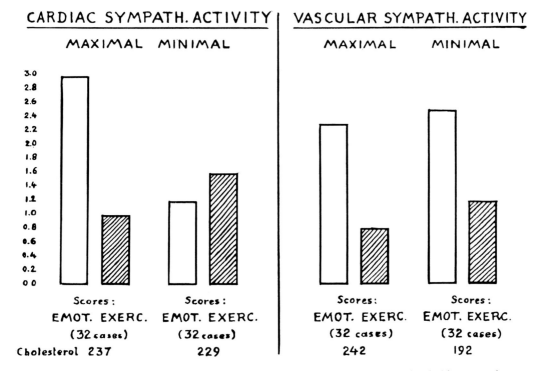

Figure 14–4. Relation between emotional excitability scores and exercise habit scores in subjects with maximal and minimal cardiac and vascular sympathetic tone and stress response, respectively.

higher resting and response level in the physically inactive group may have been influenced by inclusion of a few sedentary subjects with mild hypertension.

The two groups with maximal and minimal blood pressure resting and response levels respectively did not exhibit significant differences with regard to their corresponding emotion and exercise score proportions.

Serum cholesterol concentrations and the body height: weight ratios were practically identical in all groups (Table 14–II).

The mean serum free-fatty acid level was only little influenced by sensory stresses but rose markedly during combined sensory and mental stresses (88). Differences between the high and low emotion and exercise groups were statistically not significant.

Smoking habit scores were somewhat higher in the emotionally irritable, sedentary, and high "balance" groups (Table 14–II).

A hereditary predisposition (hypoxic heart disease and/or hypertension in one or both parents) seemed to be twice as common in the maximally cardiac adrenergic and maximally vasopressor groups as in their opposites.

DISCUSSION

In the great majority of our 200 subjects, mild sensory and mental stresses were accompanied by adrenergic chronotropic and inotropic responses of the heart, by a rise of the systolic and dia-

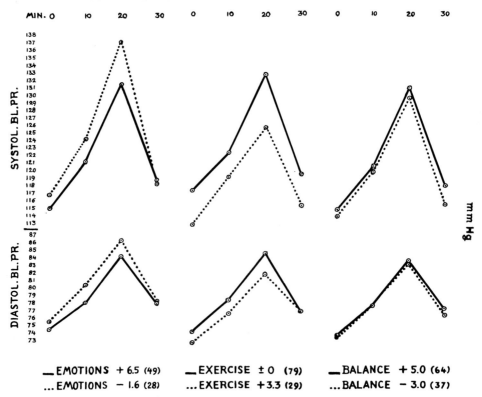

Figure 14–5. Reaction curves show no statistically significant difference of resting blood pressure and stress response levels between emotionally excitable and placid, sedentary and physically active, and high and low "balance" subjects, respectively.

stolic blood pressure, and by an elevation of the serum free-fatty acids, all of which reached their maximum during mental stress. These features reflect the augmented production of catecholamines during emotional arousal (18, 22, 61–66) and sensory annoyances (67).

Similar adrenergic cardiovascular reactions have been previously reported under the influence of noise and flicker light (68, 69) and during mental arithmetic (70, 71).

The cardiac adrenergic manifestations at rest, (including a relatively prolonged ventricular systole) and in response to

stress were more pronounced in emotionally irritable and in sedentary than in placid and in physically active individuals.

The occupations of the test subjects (intellectuals and professionals) varied in stressfulness but we grouped the subjects on the basis of their subjective stress awareness and resentment rather than by the magnitude of outward "stressor" circumstances. Accordingly, we ascribe the differences observed primarily to the respective personality patterns. No differences in heart rates were observed by Friedman et al. (72) between two rela-

TABLE 14–II

	(No. of Cases)		Serum Cholesterol (mg %)	Body Height-Weight Ratio	Smoking Habit Scores*	Heredity Scores†
Total	(200)	Ave.	228	2.3		
averages		S.D.	(42.2)			
Emotional	+6.5	Ave.	234	2.3	0.69	0.51
excitability	(49)	S.D.	(38.4)			
scores	−1.6	Ave.	238	2.2	0.61	0.64
	(28)	S.D.	(43.1)			
Exercise	±0	Ave.	232	2.3	0.86	0.52
habit	(79)	S.D.	(40.5)			
scores	+3.3	Ave.	229	2.2	0.76	0.48
	(29)	S.D.	(40.3)			
"Balance"	+5.0	Ave.	230	2.3	0.89	0.41
scores	(64)	S.D.	(38.7)			
	−3.0	Ave.	230	2.2	0.70	0.51
	(37)	S.D.	(46.8)			

*Smoking habits were scored with "1" for 9 cigarettes or less per day; with "2" for 10 to 20, and with "3" for more than 20 per day. Scores for pipe smoking were given one-half of the approximate equivalent in cigarette tobacco.
†Score "1" was given for each parent afflicted with hypertension or ischemic heart disease or both.

TABLE 14–III
ANTI-ADRENERGIC EFFECTS (SLOWER HEART RATE, PROLONGED ISOMETRIC PERIOD) INDUCED BY PHYSICAL ACTIVITY HABITS

Type of Subjects	No. of Subjects	Age Years (Average)	Heart Rate (Average)	Isometric Period (TP) (msec)(Ave.)	Authors
Average population	20	?	?	90	Emmrich et al. (80)
Highly trained sportsmen	10	?	?	106	" " "
Average population	?	?	72	80	Reindell et al (24)
Trained sportsmen	?	?	47	110	" " "
Highly trained sportsmen	107	44	50	115	Mellerowicz (25)
Average population	?	?	?	85	Blumberger (81)
Sedentary	39	36	75	88	Raab et al. (23)
Light, irregular activity	74	29	74	89	" " "
Regular sports; mountain troops	127	27	68	95	" " "
Strenuous sports and competition	120	25	65	102	" " "
Sedentary	79	44	67*	93†	Raab, Krzywanek (60)
Moderately trained	29	42	62	99	" " "
Average students	20	21	70	90	Raab et al. (23)
6–12 wks training	20	21	65	98	" " "
General fitness training	2	23	55	108	Raab, Krzywanek (60)
After 3400 miles cycling (across USA in 37 days)	2	23	46	129	" " "
"Physical culture" training	?	middle	low	prolonged	Letunov (82)
Before 4 weeks reconditioning	40	?	82	76	Nesswetha and
After 4 " " "	40	?	71	83	Nathusius (83)
After 23 days reconditioning	30	?	lower	longer	Marchet (27)
30 years voluntary uninterrupted bed rest	1	68	108	65	Raab et al. (23)

*Relative low heart rate, possibly because of 30 minutes complete rest in semi-darkness before test.
†Relative long isometric period for the same reason.

tively small groups exhibiting major and minor degrees of ambitious drive, but their exercise habits were not recorded.

The possibility to counterbalance an augmented cardiac sympathetic tone and emotionally exaggerated adrenergic response to sensory annoyances by the antiadrenergic effects of physical training is suggested by studies of Holmgren et al. (73), Heinecker (69), and Faulkner (74), and by the fact that among 29 of our own subjects with a high emotional irritability, 8 who exercised regularly displayed a lower average cardiac sympathetic resting tone and stress response than the sedentary ones.

Table 14–III shows earlier observations of ours, demonstrating the cardiac antiadrenergic effectiveness of intensive physical activity on the one hand, and an extraordinarily high cardiac sympathetic tone in a case of prolonged, voluntary, extreme immobility, on the other.

The lack of significant differences between the blood pressure resting levels and responses in the various groups may be due, in part, to the fact that the blood pressure is much less regularly influenced by physical training than the function of the heart muscle (12, 69). The same applies to serum cholesterol (12).

Tobacco smoking, although stimulating the sympathetic ganglia for a limited period, exerts no lasting influence on cardiac sympathetic tone. (75).

Elevated cardiac sympathetic adrenergic activity interferes in myocardial oxygen economy and contributes to potentially pathogenic myocardial hypoxia when coronary compensatory dilatability is impaired (26, 30, 54) (Fig. 14–6). Thus, the augmented cardiac sympathetic tone and stress response in emotionally irritable and tense, and in physically inactive in-

dividuals can be considered as an important contributory factor in the origin of hypoxic heart disease.

In conjunction with the conventional signs of "coronary-proneness" (76–78), none of which reveals myocardial functional and metabolic criteria, our test procedure (possibly limited to the initial and 20-minute readings) may provide an additional, epidemiologically useful criterion for risk factor screening, and for the evaluation of preventive cardiac reconditioning effects (79).

It should be specifically emphasized that this criterion concerns primarily the heart muscle and not the coronary arteries. Psychological factors and exercise habits have not yet been proven conclusively to influence arterial atherogenesis but they exert marked effects on myocardial metabolism and vulnerability via the autonomic nervous system.

SUMMARY

Cardiac sympathetic adrenergic manifestations (accelerated heart rate, shorter isometric period, relatively prolonged systole) at rest and during exposure to standard sensory and mental stresses (noise, flicker light, mental arithmetic) were more pronounced in emotionally irritable and in sedentary than in placid and in physically active individuals.

No definite differences between the respective groups were found concerning blood pressure, serum cholesterol, serum free-fatty acids, body height:weight ratio, and smoking habits. Parental cardiovascular morbidity was higher among subjects with exaggerated cardiac sympathetic activity.

In view of the potentially myocardial vulnerability-increasing implications of a higher sympathetic tone and stress re-

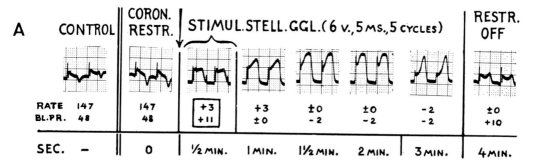

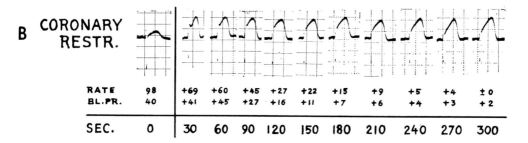

IN THE PRESENCE OF CORONARY NON-DILATABILITY (artificial restriction)

A: SYMPATHETIC stimulation (30 seconds)   B: EPINEPHRINE injection (2 seconds, i.v.)

CAUSES MYOCARDIAL ANOXIA (S-T elevation).

W. RAAB et al., Am.J.Cardiol. 9:455,1962

Figure 14–6. Otherwise innocuous, subthreshold catecholamine action (A: stimulation of cardiac sympathetic nerves; B: epinephrine injection) causes transient severe myocardial hypoxia (S-T elevation) when compensatory coronary dilatation is impaired by snugly fitting but not occluding pericoronary ligature. (W. RAAB *et al.: Amer. J Cardiol, 9:455,* 1962.)

sponsiveness, the above described test procedure (in a simplified form) may prove useful by providing additional early screening criteria of hypoxic heart disease-proneness, based on strictly myocardial functional parameters. It may also be suited for the immediate and long-range evaluation of preventive cardiac reconditioning effects.

REFERENCES

1. ROSENMAN, R. H., FRIEDMAN, M., STRAUS, R., WURM, M., KOSITCHEK, R. J., HAHN, W., and WERTHESSEN, N. T.: A predictive study of coronary heart disease. The Western Collaborative Group Study. *JAMA, 189:*15, 1964. (See also page 201 of this book.)

2. RUSSEK, H. I.: Emotional stress and coronary heart disease in American physicians, dentists and lawyers. *Amer J Med Sci, 243:*716, 1962. (See also page 190 of this book.)

3. WEISS, E., DLIN, B., ROLLIN, H. R., FISCHER, K., and BEPLER, C. R.: Emotional factors in coronary occlusion. *Arch Intern Med, 99:*628, 1957.

4. WARDWELL, W. I.: Stress and coronary heart disease in three field studies. *J Chronic Dis, 17:* 73, 1964.

5. LAPICCIRELLA, V., ABBONI, F., LAPICCIRELLA, R., and LIOTTA, S.: Una indagine epidemiologica sul pastore nomade della Somalia e un gruppo di pescatori delle isole Bagiuni. Ed. Mediche Italiane, 1962. (See also page 212 of this book.)

6. BRANDT, E. N., STOUT, C., HAMPTON, J. W., and WOLF, S.: Coronary heart disease in Roseto, Pennsylvania, and among Italians and non-Italians in nearby communities. (See Chapter 27.)

7. MORRIS, J. N., HEADY, J. A., RAFFLE, P. A. B.

ROBERTS, C. G., and PARK, J. W.: Coronary heart disease and physical activity of work. *Lancet*, 2:1053, 1111, 1953.

8. TAYLOR, H. L.: Coronary heart disease in physically active and sedentary populations. *J Sport Med*, 2:73, 1962.

9. BRUNNER, D., and MANELIS, G.: Myocardial infarction among members of communal settlements in Israel. *Lancet*, II:1049, No. 7159, 1960. (See also page 236 of this book.)

10. MYASNIKOV, A. L.: An epidemiology of atherosclerosis of heart coronary vessels in the Soviet Union. *Cardiol Prat*, 13:72, 1962.

11. McDONOUGH, J. R., HAMES, C., STULB, S., and GARRISON, G.: Coronary heart disease among Negroes and whites in Evans County, Georgia. *J Chronic Dis*, (in press).

12. KRAUS, H., and RAAB, W.: *Hypokinetic Disease.* Springfield, Thomas, 1961.

13. FOX, S. M., III, and SKINNER, J. S.: Physical activity and cardiovascular health. *Amer J Cardiol*, 14:731, 1964.

14. MIMINOSHVILI, D. J., MAGAKYAN, G. O., and KOKAYA, S. YA: O korkovykh vliyaniyakh na vyenechnoye krovoobrashcheniye. Voprosy Fiziologii y Patologii Obyezyan, Sukhumi, 1961.

15. CHERKOVICH, G. M.: Mikronekrozy v syerdtse obyezyany v resul'tate eksperimental'nogo nevroza. Patologeecheskaya fiziologiya y eksperimental'naya terapiya. Moscow, Medgiz, 1959.

16. GROOVER, M. E.: Myocardial infarction without atherosclerosis in the Kenya baboon. *Circulation*, 25:645, 1962.

17. RAAB, W., CHAPLIN, J. P., and BAJUSZ, E.: Myocardial necroses produced in domesticated rats and in wild rats by sensory and emotional stresses *Proc Soc Exp Biol Med*, 116:665, 1964.

18. LEVI, L.: The urinary output of adrenaline and noradrenaline during experimentally induced emotional stress in clinically different groups. *Acta Psychother*, 11:218, 1963.

19. FRIEDMAN, M., ST. GEORGE, S., BYERS, S. O., and ROSENMAN, R. H.: Excretion of catecholamines, 17-ketosteroids, 17-hydrocorticoids and 5-hydroxyindole in men exhibiting a particular behavior pattern (A) associated with high incidence of clinical coronary artery disease. *J Clin Invest*, 39:758, 1960.

20. BYERS, S. O., FRIEDMAN, M., ROSENMAN, R. H., and FREED, S. C.: Excretion of 3-methoxy-4-hydroxymandelic acid in man with behavior pattern associated with high incidence of coronary artery disease. *Fed. Proc*, 21:99, Suppl 11, 1962.

21. MASON, J. W., MANGAN, G., BRADY, J. V., CONRAD, D., and RIOCH, D. McK.: Concurrent plasma epinephrine, norepinephrine and 17-

hydroxycorticosteroid levels during conditioned emotional disturbances in monkeys.

22. STARCICH, R.: Fattori emozionali e variazioni plasmatiche delle catecolamine nella insufficienza coronarica acuta critica. Acta III., Europaei de Cordis Scientia Conventus, Excerpta Med., Roma, 1960, p. 155.

23. RAAB, W., DE PAULA E SILVA, P., MARCHET, H., KIMURA, E., and STARCHESKA, Y. K.: Cardiac adrenergic overactivity due to lack of physical exercise and its pathogenic implications. *Amer J Cardiol*, 5:300, 1960.

24. REINDELL, H., KÖNIG, K., ROSSKAMP, H., and KEUL, J.: Sport- und Schreibtischherz. *Die Aerztl Fortbildg*, 9:4, 1959.

25. MELLEROWICZ, H.: Oekonomieprinzip in Arbeit und Leistung des trainierten Kreislaufs. *Arch Kreislaufforsch*, 24:70, 1956.

26. SCHIMERT, G., SCHIMMLER, W., SCHWALB, H., and EBERL, J.: Die Coronarerkrankungen. *Handb. d. Inn. Med.*, Vol. IX, part 3. Mohr, L., and Staehlin, R., 4th Ed., Springer Verlag, Berlin-Göttingen-Heidelberg, 1960.

27. MARCHET, H.: Some early measurable circulatory parameters and their change during four weeks of reconditioning therapy in the Alps. Abstracts First International Conference on Preventive Cardiology, Queen City Printers, Burlington, Vermont, 1964, p. 34.

28. BROUHA, L. A.: *Science and Medicine of Exercise and Sports.* Johnson, W. R., (Ed.). New York, Harper and Bros., 1960.

29. KIRCHHOFF, H. W.: "Interne" Uebungsbehandlung bei Krankheiten des Herzens und der Gefässe. *München Med Wschr*, 105:1806, 1963.

30. RAAB, W.: Neurogenic multifocal destruction of myocardial tissue. *Rev Canad Biol*, 22:217, 1963.

31. ECKSTEIN, R. W., STROUD, M., ECKEL, R., DOWLING, C. V., and PRITCHARD, W. H.: Effects of control of cardiac work upon coronary flow and O₂ consumption after sympathetic nerve stimulation. *Amer J Physiol*, 163:539, 1950.

32. SELYE, H.: *The Pluricausal Cardiopathies.* Springfield, Thomas, 1961.

33. BÜCHNER, F.: Relative Durchblutungsnot des Herzmuskels. Akute Koronarinsuffizienz. *Deutsch Med Wschr*, 82:1037, 1957.

34. STARCICH, R., and AMBANELLI, U.: Importanza della determinazione delle catecolamine plasmatiche in patologia coronarica. *Giorn Clin Med.*, 40:1, 1959.

35. MELVILLE, K. I., BLUM, B., SHISTER, H. E., and SILVER, M. D.: Cardiac ischemic changes and arrhythmias induced by hypothalamic stimulation. *Amer J Cardiol.*, 12:781, 1963.

36. VEDENEYEVA, Z. J.: Myocardial lesions due to sympathomimetic amines of endogenous and

exogenous origin and their analysis. *Farmakol y Toksikol.*, 3:286, 1962.

37. SHKHVATSABAYA, I. K., and MENSHIKOV, V. V.: K voprosu o znachenii katekholaminov v patogeneze nevrogennykh izmenyenii miokarda. *Kardiologiya*, 2:27, 1962.

38. RAYSKINA, M. E.: *Biokhimiya Nyervnoy Regulyatsii Syerdtsa.* Moscow, Medgiz, 1962.

39. SZAKACS, J. E., and CANNON, A.: l-Norepinephrine myocarditis. *Amer J Clin Path*, 30:425, 1958.

40. ZBINDEN, G., and BAGDON, R. E.: Isoproterenol-induced heart necrosis, an experimental model for the study of angina pectoris and myocardial infarct. *Rev Canad Biol*, 22:257, 1963.

41. SOFIYEVA, J. E.: Znacheniye katekholaminov v patogeneze koronarnoy nyedostatochnosti. *Ter Arkh*, 43:3, 1962.

42. AMBANELLI, U., and STARCICH, R.: Comportamento delle catecolamine plasmatiche e urinarie nelle sindrome coronariche. Aspetti clinici e farmacodinamici dell'escrezione dell'acido vanilmandelico. *Giorn Clin Med*, 44:682, 1963.

43. RESNIK, W. H.: Pre-infarction angina. *Mod Conc Cardiov Dis*, 31:751, 757, 1962.

44. MYASNIKOV, A. L.: Myocardial necroses of coronary and noncoronary genesis. *Amer J Cardiol*, 13:435, 1964.

45. RUSSEK, H. I.: Emotional stress and the etiology of coronary artery disease. *Amer J Cardiol*, 2: 129, 1958.

46. BING, R. J., DANFORTH, W. H., and BALLARD, F. B.: Physiology of the myocardium. *JAMA*, 172:438, 1960.

47. GORLIN, R.: Physiologic studies in coronary atherosclerosis. *Fed Proc*, 21:93, 1962.

48. PAGE, I. H.: *The Heart and Circulation.* Second National Conference on Cardiovascular Diseases, Washington, D. C., 1964, p. 22.

49. LUONGO, E. P.: Health habits and heart disease—challenge in preventive medicine. *JAMA, 162:* 1021, 1956.

50. PAUL, O., LEPPER, M. H., OSTFELD, A., MAC-MILLAN, A., and PHELAN, W. H.: Coronary heart disease in an industrial population: a prospective study. *Circulation*, 26:770, 1962.

51. LAPICCIRELLA, R., MARRAMA, P., and BONATI, B.: Hormone excretion, diet and physique in Somalis. *Lancet*, p. 24, July 1, 1961.

52. RAAB, W.: The pathogenic significance of adrenalin and related substances in the heart muscle. *Exp Med Surg*, 1:188, 1943.

53. GAZES, P. C., RICHARDSON, J., and WOODS, E. F.: Plasma catecholamine concentrations in myocardial infarction and angina pectoris. *Circulation, 19:*657, 1959.

54. RAAB, W., VAN LITH, P., LEPESCHKIN, E., and HERRLICH, H. C.: Catecholamine-induced myocardial hypoxia in the presence of impaired coronary dilatability independent of external cardiac work. *Amer J Cardiol*, 9:455, 1962.

55. RAAB, W.: The nonvascular metabolic myocardial vulnerability factor in "coronary" heart disease. *Amer Heart J*, 66:685, 1963.

56. REEVES, T. J., and HEFNER, L. K.: Isometric contraction and contractility in the intact mammalian ventricle. *Amer Heart J*, 64:525, 1962.

57. RAAB, W., DE PAULA E SILVA, P., and STARCHESKA, Y. K.: Adrenergic and cholinergic influences on the dynamic cycle of the normal human heart. *Cardiologia*, 33:350, 1958.

58. KATZ, L. N.: Recent concepts of the performance of the heart. *Circulation*, 28:117, 1963.

59. BLUMBERGER, KJ.: Die Untersuchung der Dynamik des Herzens beim Menschen. Ihre Anwendung als Herzleistungsprüfung. *Ergebn Inn Med Kinderheilk*, 62:424, 1942.

60. RAAB, W., and KRZYWANEK, H. J.: Cardiovascular sympathetic tone and stress response related to personality patterns and exercise habits. A potential cardiac risk and screening test. *Amer J Cardiol*, 16:42, 1965.

61. EULER, U. S. VON, GEMZELL, C. A., LEVI, L., and STRÖM, G.: Cortical and medullary adrenal activity in emotional stress. *Acta Endocr*, 30:567, 1959.

62. BOGDONOFF, M. D., ESTES, E. H., HARLAN, W. R., TROUT, D. A., and KIRSHNER, N.: Metabolic and cardiovascular changes during a state of acute central nervous system arousal. *J Clin. Endocr*, 20:1333, 1960.

63. ELMADJIAN, F., HOPE, J. M., and LAMSON, E. T.: Excretion of epinephrine and norepinephrine in various emotional states. *J Clin Endocr*, 17:608, 1957.

64. SULKOVITCH, H., PERRIN, G. M., and ALTSCHULE, M. D.: Excretion of urinary "epinephrines" in psychiatric disorders. *Proc Soc Exp Biol Med*, 95: 245, 1957.

65. BERGSMAN, A.: The urinary excretion of adrenaline and noradrenaline in some mental diseases. *Acta Psychiat Scand*, 34:Suppl. 133, 1959.

66. STRÖM-OLSEN, R., and WEIL-MALHERBE, H.: Humoral changes in manic depressive psychosis with particular reference to the excretion of catecholamines in urine. *J Ment Sci.*, 104:696, 1958.

67. LEVI, L.: A new tolerance test with simultaneous study of physiological and psychological variables. *Acta Endocr*, 37:38, 1961.

68. JANSEN, J.: Wirkungen des Lärms auf das vegetative Nervensystem. *Acta Otorhinolaryng Belg*, 16:293, 1962.

69. HEINECKER, R., ZIPF, H. E., and LÖSCH, H. W.: Ueber den Einfluss körperlichen Trainings auf

Kreislauf und Atmung (parts I and II). *Z Kreislaufforsch, 49:*913, 924, 1960.

70. BROD, J., FENCL, V., HEJL, Z., and JIRKA, J.: Circulatory changes underlying blood pressure elevation during acute emotional stress (mental arithmetic) in normotensive and hypertensive subjects. *Clin. Sci, 18:*270, 1959.

71. ENGEL, B. J.: Stimulus response and individual response specificity. *Arch Gen Psychiat, 2:*305, 1960.

72. FRIEDMAN, M., ROSENMAN, R. H., and BROWN, A. E.: The continuous heart rate in men exhibiting an overt behavior pattern associated with increased incidence of clinical coronary artery disease. *Circulation, 28:*861, 1963.

73. HOLMGREN, A., JONSSON, B., LEVANDER, M., LINDHOLM, H., MOSSFELDT, F., SJÖSTRAND, T., and STRÖM, G.: Physical training of patients with vasoregulatory asthenia. *Acta Med Scand, 158:*437, 1957.

74. FAULKNER, J. A.: Effect of cardiac conditioning on the anticipatory, exercise and recovery heart rates of young men. *J Sport Med, 4:*79, 1964.

75. RAAB, W., MARCHET, H., and DEMING, H.: Tobacco smoking, smoking habits and the dynamic cycle of the left ventricle (chronodynogram). *Exp Med Surg, 18:*128, 1960.

76. DAWBER, T. R., and KANNEL, W. B.: Susceptibility to coronary heart disease. *Mod Conc Cardiov Dis, 30:*671, 1961.

77. STAMLER, J., BERKSON, D. M., YOUNG, O. D., HALL, Y., and MILLER, W.: Approaches to the primary prevention of clinical coronary heart disease in high-risk middle-aged men. *Ann N Y Acad Sci, 97:*932, 1963.

78. GERTLER, M. M., WHITE, P. D., CADY, L. D., and WHITER, H. H.: Coronary heart disease. A prospective study. *Amer J Med Sci, 248:*35/377, 1964.

79. RAAB, W.: *Organized Prevention of Degenerative Heart Disease.* Burlington, Vermont, Queen City Printers, 1962.

80. EMMRICH, J., KLEPZIG, H., and REINDELL, H.: Zur Frage der klinischen Bedeutung einer Unterteilung der Anspannungszeit des linken Ventrikels in Umformungszeit und Druckanstiegszeit, *Arch Kreislaufforsch, 24:*177, 1956.

81. BLUMBERGER, K. J.: Quoted by Emmrich *et al., Loc. cit.*

82. LETUNOV, S. P., and MOTYLYANSKAYA, R. E.: Profilakteecheskoye znatcheniye aktivnogo dvigatel'nogo rezhima v pozhilom vozraste. *Klin Med, 11:*115, 1964.

83. NESSWETHA, W., and NATHUSIUS, W. V.: Untersuchungen über die prophylaktische und therapeutische Bedeutung der Terrainkur bei Regulationsstörungen des Kreislaufes der Industriearbeiter. *Int J Prophyl Med, 4:*No. 6, 1960.

84. D'BIASE, G. and LABRIOLA, E.: Contributo allo studio della catecholaminemia nell' insufficienza coronarica. *Cardiol. pratica, 15:*511, 1964.

85. FRICK, M. H., KONTINEN, A., and SARAJAS, H. S. S.: Effects of physical training on circulation at rest and during exercise. *Amer J Cardiol, 12:*142, 1963.

86. RYBKIN, I. A.: Epidemiologeecheskye issledovaniya koronarnogo ateroskleroza v sovietskom soyuze. In: *Rasprostranyenye gipertoneecheskoy bol'yezni i koronarnogo ateroskleroza y usloviya zhizni.* Publ. "Meditsina," Leningrad issue, 1964, p. 9.

87. STEZHENSKAYA, E. I.: Vliyaniye kharaktera truda na porazhenost' syerdechno-sosudystoy sistemy lits 80 lyet y starshe. In: *Krovoobrashcheniye y starost'.* Institute of Gerontology of the Acad. of Med. Sci. of the USSR, Kieve, 1965 p. 166.

88. KRZYWANEK, H. J., RAAB, W., and BÖHLE, E.: Einfluss des sympathiko-adrenalen Systems auf Herz-Kreislauf—Regulation und unveresterte Fettsauren des Blutserums. *Deutsche med Wchnschr, 91:*193, 1966.

89. BOYCHEVA, M. S. and RATNER, N. A.: *Proc. Conf. Problems of Atheroscl. and Coron. Insuff.* Medgiz, Moscow, 1956, p. 58.

90. DUBINSKI, A. A. and PASHCHENKO, A. E.: *Vrachebnoye Dyelo,* no. 1, p. 43, 1958.

91. NESTEL, P. J., VERGHESE, A. and LOVELL, R. R. H.: Catecholamine secretion and sympathetic nervous responses to emotion in man with and without angina pectoris (in press).

Chapter XV

EXERCISE, TRAINING AND CARDIAC STROKE FORCE

ERNST JOKL and JOHN B. WELLS, JR.

(Lexington, Kentucky, U.S.A.)

Nervous Control of the Heart

THE part played by sympathetic and parasympathetic activity in cardiac control presented itself for consideration when it was discovered that the physiological adjustment of the heart to intensive physical training involves "inhibition" of its "rhythm" as well as "augmentation" of its "force" (Fig. 15–1). Bradycardia at rest, which is commonly found in outstanding athletes, is accompanied by an increased systolic stroke force.

Initial Ventricular Impulse

Ballistocardiography records "cardiac force" or "initial ventricular impulse." The latter is also a determinant of ventricular and aortic pressure, arterial pulse waves, the roentgen- and electro-kymogram, and of apical and precordial kinetograms (Fig. 15–2). According to Rushmer (2), during the early stages of ventricular systole, myocardial tension develops very quickly, ventricular pressure rises steeply to exceed arterial pressure, and momentum is rapidly imparted to the blood flowing out of the ventricles. The acceleration of blood out of the ventricles is an expression of the force being applied by the contracting myocardium, and the peak flow velocity can be regarded as the product of the net force applied over the time from the onset of ejection to the peak. The product of force and time, designated by the physical term impulse (I-Ft), is proportional to the tangent values computed from length of segments and height of amplitudes of the first systolic deflection of the ballistocardiogram. The ejection of blood from the ventricles (particularly the left) is more like striking a piston

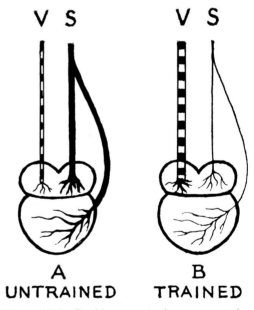

A **B**
UNTRAINED **TRAINED**

Figure 15–1. Raab's concept of neurovegetative regulatory patterns of the untrained and the trained heart, respectively. V = Vagus; S = Sympathetic. (A) Untrained heart: Adrenergic sympathetic preponderance; (B) Trained heart: Cholinergic vagal preponderance (1).

135

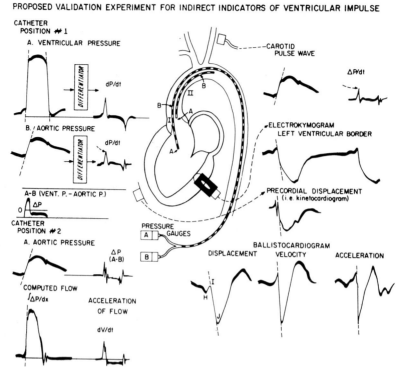

Figure 15–2. Rushmer's experimental design for the determination of the extent to which indirect clinical measures such as arterial sphygmography, electrokymography, precordial displacement records, and ballistocardiography might be employed to assess changes in initial ventricular impulse. (By means of a double-lumen catheter, positioned at 2 sites in the aorta, a number of derivatives of left ventricular ejection can be identified as indicated on left. Indirect methods allow evaluation in terms of changes in initial deflections on wave forms as indicated on right.) (R. F. Rushmer [2])

with a mallet than like squeezing blood out of a chamber.

It will be shown that modifications of the initial ventricular impulse occur as parts of parasympathetically, as well as of sympathetically, mediated adjustments of the autonomic system (e.g., during long-term adjustments of the heart to training, and during short-term adjustments of the heart to exercise).

Methodology

In our own studies, ballistocardiograms were taken singly as well as seriatim. Single tracings sufficed for the identification of the categorical differences of cardiac stroke force in champion athletes and sedentary subjects at rest while nature and magnitude of the modifications of cardiac stroke force under the influence of exercise were revealed in an experiment during which serial recordings were obtained from the same individual at rest and after exertion, with the first serving as norm for the evaluation of the second.

Correlations between cardiac stroke force and cardiac stroke volume are close enough to allow general conclusions to be drawn from the former as regards the latter. Though at the present stage of development of ballistocardiography, exact quantitative comparisons between *single* tracings taken from different subjects are

AV. BALLISTO AMPLITUDE

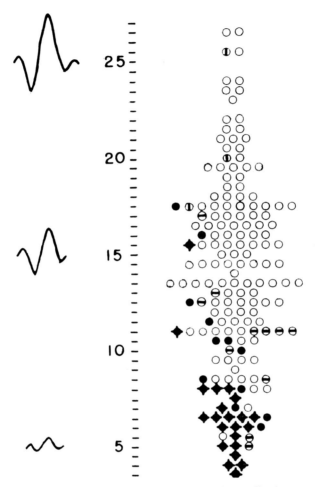

Figure 15–3. The prognostic relevance of ballistocardiographic amplitudes was demonstrated by I. Starr *et al.* (5), who found the incidence of heart disease 17 years after the recording of initial ballistocardiograms lowest in subjects whose tracings had shown the highest amplitudes at rest. *Circles*—no heart disease developed. *Dots*—those who developed undoubted heart disease. *Crosses*—superimposed indicate that they died from it. *Horizontal bars*—those who developed a doubtful cardiac status. *Vertical bars*—those who developed hypertension without evidence of heart disease.

not feasible, important insights have been obtained from statistical evaluations of measurements of ballistocardiograms collected in *group* studies (e.g., that resulting in the discovery of the enhancement of systolic stroke force in champion athletes, referred to presently, and Starr's analysis of the incidence of heart disease 17 years after the recording of first tracings) which revealed that subjects with the highest systolic deflections in their initial ballistocardiograms had been least afflicted (Fig. 15–3) (3).

We are aware that technical progress

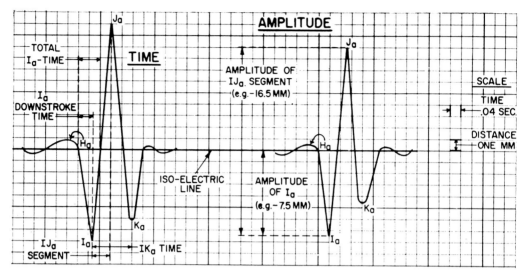

Figure 15–4. Identification of H, I, and J deflections of systolic complexes as well as of marks of reference for time and amplitude measurements of ballistocardiogram.

must and, we believe, will be made in respect to reliability and reproducibility of ballistocardiography as a means of providing data on cardiac output along the lines attempted in our study. Efforts are currently afoot to attain the same objective by recording ballistocardiograms through multiple strain gauge support or air jet suspension of platforms, in combination with computers to measure the shift of the center of gravity of the body during systole. Since the area under the I-wave of the ballistrocardiogram is proportionately correlated to the magnitude of initial ventricular stroke volume, the "code" which modifies the ballistocardiogram is likely to be deciphered in due course.

Time and amplitude analyses of the ballistocardiograms (the S. Arbeit direct-body-contact-acceleration-model (4) was used in our studies) were undertaken according to the scheme shown in Fig. 15–4 (5). The time analyses of the electrocardiograms followed the customary

procedure. Figure 15–5 indicates the values for the fastest and for the slowest performers in the 2.2 mile running test.

EFFECT OF TRAINING ON CARDIAC STROKE FORCE AND CARDIAC FREQUENCY

Cardiac Stroke Force

In 1958-59, attention was drawn to the fact that at rest the heart of highly trained athletes is characterized not only by bradycardia, but also by conspicuously forceful systolic contractions (6–8). I, J, and K deflections in ballistocardiograms from champion athletes are larger than in ballistocardiograms from sedentary subjects. Analyses of the tracings of the 2 groups yielded the following values: mean amplitudes for I waves: 7.1 versus 4.5 mm; for J waves: 11.5 versus 7.7 mm; and K waves: 12.3 versus 8.7 mm (Fig. 15–6).

The largest I, J, and K deflections at rest were seen in athletes who excelled in feats of endurance (9). Power training

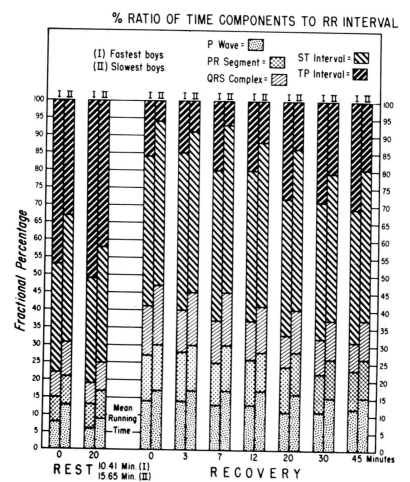

Figure 15–5. Time analysis of segments of electrocardiogram expressed as percentages of length of total cycle at rest and after 2.2 mile running test. Comparison of computations for "fastest" (mean running time 10 minutes 27 seconds) and "slowest" performers (mean running time 15 minutes 43 seconds). In the better runners, the "sledgehammer effect" of the systolic force impact is more marked, and the duration of diastole proportionately longer, at rest and after exercise.

also was found to cause an increase of cardiac force though of lesser magnitude (10). The I-J-K phase is shorter and the diastole, therefore, longer in ballisto-cardiograms from athletes than in trac-ings obtained from untrained subjects. The extent to which discontinuation of physical training causes a decline of car-diac force was shown by a comparison of ballistocardiograms taken at rest from

champion athletes at the height of their performance capacity, and from former athletes after prolonged periods of in-activity (Fig. 15–7).

In 1947, T. Cureton (11) reported that at rest brachial pulse waves of ath-letes are conspicuously high; that arterial sphygmograms of *trained* middle-aged and elderly subjects are similar to those obtained from *young* men and of *athletes*;

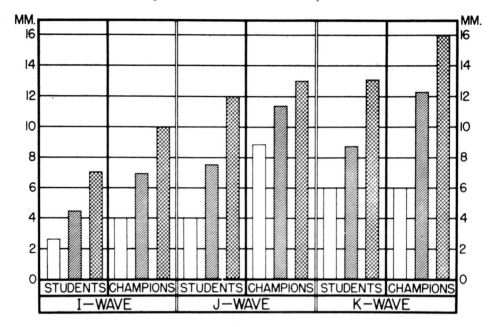

AMPLITUDE MEASUREMENTS OF I–J–K COMPLEXES OF
STANDARDIZED VELOCITY BALLISTOCARDIOGRAMS OF
YOUNG, HEALTHY STUDENTS COMPARED WITH RECORDS
OBTAINED FROM TRACK CHAMPIONS. (MINIMAL, MEAN
AND MAXIMAL VALUES COMPUTED FROM EACH TRACING)

☐ MINIMAL   ▨ MEAN   ▨ MAXIMAL

Figure 15–6. Amplitude measurements of I-J-K complexes of standardized velocity ballistocardiograms of young, healthy students taken at rest, compared with records obtained from
track champions. (Minimal, mean and maximal values were computed from each tracing.)

and that discontinuation of training causes
a diminution of pulse wave amplitudes,
irrespective of age.

In 1963, Frick et al. (12) conducted
an experiment with 14 young men with
sedentary habits who were studied before and after a 2 months course of intensive physical training. Their cardiac
stroke volumes at rest, determined with
Evans blue dye dilution technique, increased significantly with training.

In 1964, Skinner (13) presented ballistocardiographic evidence which confirmed the validity of the conclusion that
physical fitness enhances the power of
myocardial contraction at rest. Ampli-

tudes of I, J, and K deflections in tracings, obtained from sedentary middle-
aged subjects, increased significantly after 6 months of gymnasium training, consisting of interval running and calisthenic
exercises.

Cureton (14) obtained brachial spyhg-
mograms and ballistocardiograms from
the former champion runner Joie Ray,
who at age 70 adhered to a strict exercise
schedule: both tracings revealed typical
patterns of adaptation to training.

Evidently, each of the 3 manifestations
of cardiovascular adjustment which have
been observed in athletes at rest, viz.,
increased amplitude and steep ascent of

STUDENTS ATHLETES EX-ATHLETES

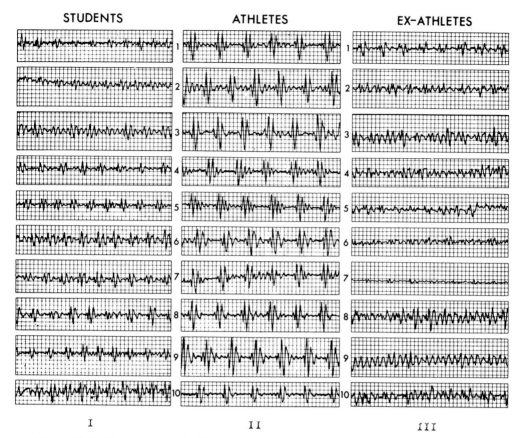

I II III

Figure 15–7. Three series of ballistocardiograms consecutively recorded: (I) from 10 untrained students, ages 18 to 21; (II) from 10 NCAA championship finalists in middle and long distance races in Austin, Texas, 1958; and (III) from 10 middle-aged ex-athletes who 8 and more years ago had performed on a level comparable to that of the men whose tracings are shown in (II).

I, J, and K waves in the ballistocardiogram, high brachial pulse waves, and large ventricular stroke volumes, reflects the enhancement of the initial ventricular impulse which sustained physical training engenders.

Cardiac Frequency

Mean resting pulse rates for the champion athletes studied in our investigation were 45, for the students 70. Fractional time analyses of electrocardiograms corroborated the validity of the conclusion drawn from the ballistocardiographic time-analyses that the diastole is significantly longer in the hearts of the athletes than in the hearts of the untrained subjects (Fig. 15–5). Correlations between cardiac rates, length of diastole, and amplitudes of I, J, and K deflections in ballistocardiograms recorded at rest, are statistically significant for highly trained athletes and for sedentary subjects* (Fig. 15–8).

*The results of the time analyses are related to the fact that the papillary muscles and the inner

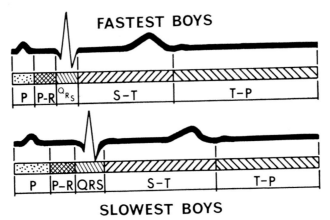

Figure 15–8. Effect of parasympathetic preponderance due to training upon proportionate representation of time components of electrocardiogram of athletes and nonathletes, obtained at rest.

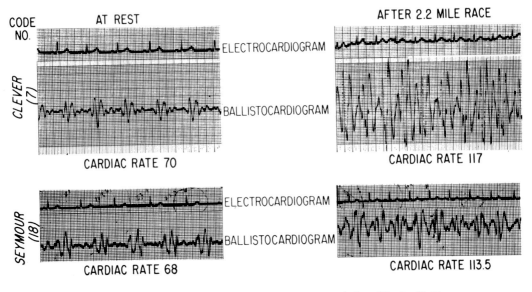

Effect of Exercise upon Ballistocardiographic Time and Amplitude Patterns.

Figure 15-9. Electrocardiograms and ballistocardiograms taken at rest and after 2.2 mile race from subjects Clever (running time: 10 minutes, 42 seconds) and Seymour (running time: 17 minutes, 52 seconds). Cardiac rates and stroke forces at rest as well as post-exercise stroke forces differed greatly: Clever's (*above right*) ballistocardiogram shows a much greater augmentation of amplitudes after the race than Seymour's (*below right*).

---

layers of the ventricular walls of the heart receive coronary artery blood only during diastole since intramyocardial pressure compresses the blood vessels of these regions during systole. The lengthening of the diastolic phase of the cardiac cycle brought about through training represents a facet of physiological adaptation whose significance relates immediately to the subject's physical performance capacity, as well as to the long-term problem of his resistance to certain degenerative influences upon the myocardium.

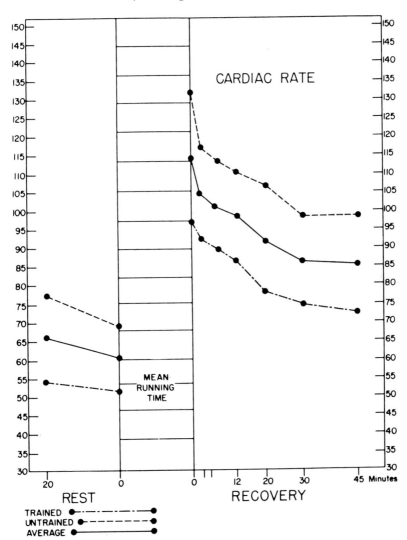

Figure 15–10. Cardiac frequency is distinctly slower at rest as well as after exercise in trained than in untrained subjects. The above diagram shows mean cardiac frequencies for the 10 fastest and the 10 slowest participants in the 2.2 mile running experiment (compare with legend to Fig. 15–5).

We took serial ballistocardiograms from 21 students at rest and after a run over a standardized distance of 2.2 miles. Running times reflected levels of physical performance capacity.

Significant increases of cardiac stroke force were found in the majority of subjects after the race though considerable varieties of responses were encountered.

No consistent relationship was found in respect to changes after exercise of cardiac stroke forces and of cardiac rates †;

—————

†Evidently, modifications of cardiac frequency and force during exercise are mediated, as well as integrated, as separate entities of the sympathetic system. In 1962, Fang *et al.* (15) showed that the principles of cardioacceleration" and of cardioaugmentation" are represented in the hypothalamus. Statistically different responses of cardiac frequency and force

an observation which reflects the extent to which the ergogenic augmentations of time and force parameters of the heart are independent of each other (Fig. 15–9). Cardiac frequencies after the 2.2 mile running tests were, however, significantly lower in the fastest performers (Fig. 15–10). Running times did not represent primary determinants of magnitudes of responses of cardiac stroke forces to the exercise.

HOMEOSTASIS AND HETEROSTASIS

We will now revert to consideration of the mechanisms by which the autonomic system mediates the adjustments of rhythm and force of cardiac action to exercise and to training. In discussing the functional adjustment to training, it was pointed out that a parasympathetic preponderance characterizes the homeostatic shift thus engendered; while a sympathetic preponderance signifies the heterostatic deployment of the ergogenic components of the autonomic system during exercise (16).

The sustained enhancement of cardiac stroke force which forms part of the working of the trained heart reflects a parasympathetic; the short-lasting increase of cardiac stroke force during exercise a sympathetic accentuation.

The autonomic changes which accompany the transformation from the resting state to activity have been described as "emergency function of the sympathico-

adrenal system" (Cannon), "alarm reaction" (Selye), "sympathicotonic as against vagotonic preponderance" (Eppinger and Hess), "ergotropy" (Atzler) (which W. R. Hess contrasted with "trophotropy") or "adrenergic liberation of catecholamines" (Raab) (16). Jokl has emphasized the bipolar nature of, and the integrative relationship between the deployment of autonomic levels during exercise and the homeostatic resting state and, therefore, called the former "heterostasis." Autonomic changes that occur during short lasting intensive physical exercise can be reproduced in human subjects by injection of epinephrine (17, 18).

Homeostasis and heterostasis are diametrically opposed states of the autonomic system. Both are activated and integrated on what the Pavlovian School calls the "higher functional level of the nervous system," as well as in the "vegetative centers" in midbrain and hypothalamus. During exercise, the nature of the motor act determines the heterostatic alignment of motor impulses as well as of their autonomic accompaniments. The former largely determine scope and duration of the latter.

The sustained enhancement of cardiac stroke force of the trained athlete at rest, and the sharp rise of cardiac power during exercise—notwithstanding the fact that both result in an augmentation of myocardial contraction—are corresponding opposites in that they involve, respectively, activation of the two different patterns of autonomic regulation which function in diametrical juxtaposition: the one forms part of a parasympathetically-directed homeostatic shift; the second is a facet of the sympathetically induced heterostatic deployment. The identifica-

---

can be elicited from separate points in the midbrain of vagotomized dogs (*Amer. J Physiol*, 203:147, 1962). The demonstration by Frick *et al.* (12) of an absence of correlation between percentile changes in stroke volume and heart volume during training suggests that correspondingly separate regulatory entities exist in respect to parasympathetic control (*Amer. J Cardiol*, 142, August 1962).

tion of these two modifications of cardiac force at rest and during exercise, respectively, as manifestations mediated by the counterregulatory divisions of the autonomic system, emphasizes the importance of analyzing the vegetative integration of complex functions in their entirety.

Since at rest the homeostatic alignment of the autonomic system of trained athletes is distinguished by a preponderance of the parasympathetic while the heterostatic alignment of the autonomic system during exercise is distinguished by a predonderance of the sympathetic system, it is reasonable to consider the increased initial ventricular impulse of the heart of the athlete at rest a component of the enhancement of vagal tone which characterizes "the trained state." In other words, strong systolic forces at rest reflect the same general trend which causes athletes' hearts to be larger, cardiac rates to be slower, myocardial capillarization to be greater, isometric (19, 20) and "isovolumetric" (21) contraction time to be longer, systolic blood pressure to be lower (19) pulse wave velocity to be less rapid, and arteriovenous oxygen utilization to be greater (22).

SUMMARY

Analyses of ballistocardiograms obtained at rest from trained and untrained subjects revealed enhanced systolic stroke forces and bradycardia as integrated components of the physiological syndrome of cardiac adaptation resulting from sustained physical activity. After a 2.2 mile run, the majority of contestants showed a significant augmentation of systolic stroke force together with a sharp acceleration of cardiac frequency, whereby the latter was less marked in trained than in untrained individuals.

Since the functional status of the autonomic system of trained athletes is distinguished by a generalized parasympathetic preponderance, the enhanced systolic stroke force at rest must be considered an integral component of the latter while the increase of systolic stroke force attending short-lasting strenuous exercise represents part of the "heterostatic deployment" mediated through the sympathetic division of the autonomic system.

REFERENCES

1. HERRLICH, H. C., RAAB, W., and GIGEE, W.: Influence of muscular training and of catecholamines on cardiac acetylcholine and cholinesterase. *Arch Int Pharmacodyn, 129*:201, 1960.
2. RUSHMER, R. F.: Initial ventricular impulse. *Circulation, 29*:268, 1964.
3. STARR, I., and WOOD, F. C.: Twenty year studies with the ballistocardiograph, the relationship between the amplitude of the first record of "healthy" adults and eventual mortality and morbidity from heart disease. *Circulation, 23*: 714, 1961.
4. ARBEIT, S. A.: A new full-frequency range calibrated ballistocardiograph. *Amer Heart J, 45*: 52, 1963.
5. ARBEIT, S., JOKL, E., KOSKELA, A., and McCUBBIN, W.: Ballistocardiographic changes during a thirty day physical training period. *Amer Heart J., 54*:556, 1957.
6. JOKL, E., KOSKELA, A., McCUBBIN, W., JOKL, P., and ARBEIT, S. R.: Proceedings of the ballistocardiography research society. *Amer J Cardiol, 1*:529, 1958.
7. JOKL, E., ARBEIT, S. R., McCUBBIN, W., GRENIER, G., KOSKELA, A., and JOKL, P.: Ballistocardiographic studies on Olympic athletes. *Amer J Cardiol, 1*:199, 1958.
8. JOKL, E.: Ballistocardiographic studies on athletes. *Amer J Cardiol., 4*:105, 1959.
9. Tracings obtained from outstanding middle- and long distance runners during the NCAA track championships held at Austin, Texas, in 1957.
10. Tracings obtained from members of the United States Weightlifting Team for the 1956 Olympic Games in Melbourne, Australia.
11. CURETON, T. K.: Physical Fitness, Appraisal and Guidance. London, Henry Kimpton, 1947.
12. FRICK, M., HEIKKI, A. K., and SAMULI SARAJAS, H. S.: Effects of physical training on circulation

at rest and during exercise. *Amer J Cardiol, 142:* 1963.

13. SKINNER, J. S.: The effects of a six-month program of endurance exercise on work tolerance, serum lipids and ULF ballistocardiograms of 15 middle-aged men. Proceedings Ninth Annual Meeting, Ballistocardiographic Research Society, Atlantic City, May 2, 1964.

14. CURETON, T. K.: A physical fitness case study of Joie Ray. *J Ass Phys Ment Rehab, 18:*64, 1965.

15. FANG, H. S., and WANG, S. C.: Cardioaccelerator and cardioaugmentor points in the hypothalamus of the dog. *Amer J Physiol, 203:*147, 1962.

16. JOKL, E.: *Heart and Sport.* Springfield, Thomas, 1964.

17. JOKL, E.: Vegetative Regulation des Blutes. *Z Neur, 142:*2, 1932.

18. JOKL, E.: Blutbild und Sauerstoffmangel. *Deutsch Med Wschr, 26:*1001, 1933.

19. MELLEROWICZ, H.: Vergleichende Untersuchungen über das Oekonomieprinzip in Arbeit und Leistung des trainierton Kreislaufs und seine Bedeutung für die rehabilitative Medizin. *Arch Kreislaufforsch, 24:*70, 1956.

20. RAAB, W., SILVA, P. DE, MARCHET, H., Kimura, E., and STARCHESKA, Y. K.: Cardiac adrenergic preponderance due to lack of exercise and its pathogenic implications. *Amer J Cardiol, 5:*300, 1960.

21. EMMERICH, J., KLEPZIG, H., and REINDELL, H.: Zur Frage der klinischen Bedeutung einer Unterteilung der Anspannungszeit des linken Ventrikels in Umformungzeit und Druckanstiegszeit. *Arch Kreislaufforsch, 24:*177, 1956.

22. REINDELL, H., KONIG, K., ROSSKAMP, H., and KEUL, J.: Sport- und Schreibtischherz. *Die arztl. Fortbildung, 9:*No. 4, 1959.

Chapter XVI

FUNCTIONAL AND METABOLIC FACTORS IN THE ORIGIN AND PREVENTION OF MYOCARDIAL ISCHEMIA*

GUSTAV C. SCHIMERT and HANS SCHWALB

(Munich, Germany)

AUTOPTIC findings reveal severe narrowing of the coronary arteries in uncomplicated angina pectoris in 92 to 100 per cent of the cases. The same is true in massive transmural myocardial infarctions.

These optically impressive morphological facts are the reason why most clinicians, in interpreting the origin of ischemic heart disease, overlook certain frequently participating functional pathogenic factors which, in our opinion, are of paramount importance. The customary one-sided over-estimation of merely anatomical findings which constitute, of course, the most common predisposition to ischemic heart disease, is based upon a conveniently over-simplifying, erroneous deduction. If we find an almost 100 per cent correlation between angina pectoris and myocardial infarction on the one hand, and coronary sclerosis on the other, it is only too tempting to overrate the importance of the vascular lesion as the one and only pathogenic factor.

In addition, it was generally believed in the past that functional factors consist solely in coronary spasms and a poor adaptability of the peripheral ramifica-

tions of the coronary system. It is practically impossible to prove the occurrence of these phenomena in man; neither are they clearly supported by animal experimentation.

The concept of those authors who stressed an unduly augmented oxygen demand in the myocardium as a possible accessory functional factor in ischemic heart disease, such as Raab (1) and ourselves (2, 3), had remained generally disregarded for decades but is now being increasingly appreciated. In the past, the adequacy of myocardial oxygenation used to be evaluated exclusively in terms of blood supply without any attention being paid to the elementary fact that, in considering the adequacy of the blood supply of any organ, it is mandatory also to take into account its fluctuating requirements. The oxygen requirements of the heart depend on the amount of external mechanical work performed by the heart muscle, on its mode, and on the specific neurohormonal metabolic influences under which this takes place.

THE "CORONARY RESERVE"

Years ago we introduced the term "coronary reserve" and we could demon-

---

*Translated by W. Raab.

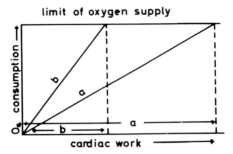

Relationship between myocardial oxygen consumption and coronary reserve

(Schimert G.)

Figure 16–1. If the rate of O_2 consumption by the heart muscle is high (*curve b*), the upper limit of the coronary reserve (= availability of adequate amounts of O_2 to myocardial tissue) is reached under a smaller workload than if the O_2 consumption rate is low (*curve a*).

strate its dependence on the heart's metabolism and mode of action. We interpreted the term "coronary reserve" as the range within which an adequate oxygen supply of myocardial tissue is guaranteed under circumstances of any given demands up to a maximum. The degree of availability of needed blood or oxygen to the myocardium is characterized by the formula:

$$\text{Oxygen economy} = \frac{\text{Blood (or Oxygen) supply}}{\text{Blood (or Oxygen) demand}}$$

If this ratio equals 1 or is greater than 1, the availability of oxygen to the myocardium is adequate. A diminution of the ratio below 1 is equivalent with myocardial ischemia.

The quotient becomes smaller as a result of a decrease in blood flow due to coronary stenosis, or due to a drop of blood pressure, or if the oxygen supply is reduced by anemia, or by a lowered arterial oxygen saturation. Physical stress, by way of neurohormonal influences which cause a potentially uneconomical mode of action of the heart, also reduces the quotient, unless coronary dilatation compensates for the increased oxygen demand of the myocardium. The

steepness with which the oxygen consumption of the heart muscle rises under an increasing work load exerts a significant influence upon the coronary reserve. Accordingly, the coronary reserve and, by the same token, the limit of work efficiency of the heart at which it reaches the state of myocardial ischemia, can be quite different in different subjects, having the same caliber of the coronary vessels (Fig. 16–1). Condition "b" shows a steep increase of oxygen consumption and a resulting earlier occurrence of coronary insufficiency than condition "a" where oxygen consumption rises in a flat curve.

FUNCTIONAL FACTORS WHICH DIMINISH THE CORONARY RESERVE

Heart Rate. As to the relation between heart rate and oxygen consumption, all investigations have uniformly shown that under a constant workload, oxygen consumption increases with an increase of the heart rate.

Experiments by Laurent et al. (4) (Fig. 16–2) demonstrate the gradual increase of oxygen consumption together

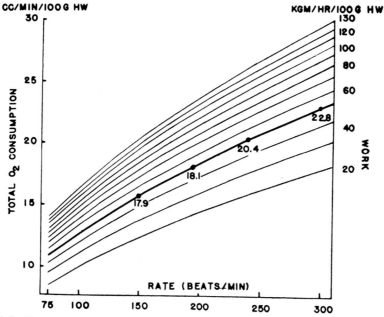

Figure 16–2. Nomogram of cardiac isowork lines relating total myocardial O_2 consumption to heart rate. The heavy line represents experimental points with work level of 50 kg m/hr/100 gm HW. The cardiac O_2 consumption values from one experiment at this work level are plotted on the nomogram and are found to lie close to (1_σ) what would be predicted. (Laurent *et al.* [4].)

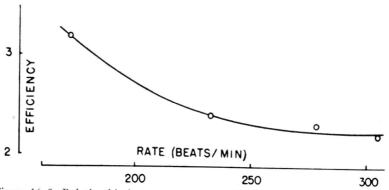

Figure 16–3. Relationship between per cent cardiac "efficiency" and heart rate.

with the acceleration of the heart rate when a constant workload is maintained. Tripling of cardiac work at a constant pulse rate is accompanied by a 33 per cent increase of the oxygen consumption. By contrast, tripling of the heart rate at a constant workload causes an increment of oxygen expenditure of more than 75 per cent. Thus, the heart works less economically and with lesser efficiency at a higher rate than at a lower rate and greater stroke volume. The decline of efficiency with increasing heart rate is also evidenced in Figure 16–3, which illustrates the experimental findings of Laurent, Bolene-Williams, Williams, and Katz (4).

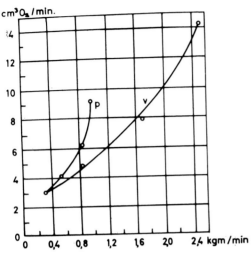

Figure 16–4.Increases of myocardial oxygen consumption by augmented work due to increasing aortic pressure (p) and to increasing cardiac output (v). (Kiese and Garan (16)).

The heart muscle is provided with arterial blood mainly during diastole and it is very likely that in a stenotic coronary system, tachycardia impairs the myocardial blood flow also by shortening the diastole. The blood flow through the subendocardial layers of the ventricles, the papillary muscles, and, probably, the septum is particularly endangered by tachycardia (5–8).

Mechanical Strain. The type of mechanical strain imposed on the heart also exerts a definite influence upon its oxygen consumption (9).

Figure 16–4 shows a steep increase of oxygen consumption connected with work against increasing pressure (curve p), whereas under conditions of augmented stroke volume (curve v) the increase is slow, indicating a significantly greater efficiency of the heart. Thus, economy of the cardiac work or, in other words, the coronary reserve, can be substantially improved by lowering the mean arterial pressure.

Adrenergic Activity. An augmentation of myocardial oxygen consumption is caused by adrenergic neurohormonal influences even without alteration of the workload and of the aortic pressure (1, 10–15). As long as the coronary arteries are intact and normally dilatable, this fact is not of any major pathogenic importance, since any increase in myocardial oxygen consumption is promptly followed by an adequate dilatation of the coronary arteries. Nevertheless, it has been shown by numerous investigators that repeated injections of epinephrine and stress-induced intensive stimulations of the sympathetic nervous system and the hypothalamus produce myocardial necroses even in healthy animals (1). If the coronary vessels are narrow, a rising sympathetic tone will endanger particularly the subendocardium by causing a lack of local oxygenation (1).

In contrast to the effect of the sympathogenic catecholamines, sympathetic inhibition and vagal stimulation exert an opposite, oxygen-preserving effect which enables the heart to work with a lesser oxygen consumption, as first shown by Gollwitzer-Meier (11), Bohnenkamp (17) and others.

Since heart rate and pressure work of the heart muscle are governed by the chronotropic and inotropic influences, respectively, of the autonomic nervous system, it follows that myocardial oxygen requirements are reduced by mechanisms inhibiting the sympathetic and augmenting the cardiac vagal tone.

A diminution of the oxygen demand of the myocardium, that is, a more economical performance of its work, enables the heart to do a greater amount of work at any given coronary caliber than a higher oxygen demand would permit without risk of oxygen deficit.

Conditions which impair the coronary reserve for reasons not primarily affecting the coronary flow prevail most commonly in those disorders which involve an acceleration of the heart beat and rise of the blood pressure, mostly as a result of an exaggerated cardiac sympathetic tone. Such conditions are characterized by a disproportionate increase of the cardiac output at rest as well as during stress and exercise, whereby the augmentation of the cardiac output is due chiefly to the inecrased heart rate. At the same time, the so-called oxygen pulse, that is, the uptake of oxygen per heart beat, which is the most important parameter for circulatory economy, is usually diminished.

Lack of Physical Activity. Another important factor in this respect is a disturbance of circulatory economy, resulting from lack of physical activity. Poor vascularization of the muscles, inadequate coordination of muscular action and of blood distribution during exercise, and a reduced effectiveness of muscular effort cause an augmented total oxygen requirement of the body as a whole, and thus impose an additional strain on the heart to which it responds primarily with acceleration of the rate.

In the presence of arterial hypertension, the heart performs pressure work of an exaggerated degree both at rest and during physical exercise. During the latter, the peripheral vascular resistance decreases less, as a rule, than cardiac output rises. Accordingly, the mean pressure during exercise is usually higher in hypertensive than in normotensive individuals.

A combination of arterial hypertension with other sympathogenic manifestations prevails especially in the early stages of essential hypertension and in angina pectoris, as we have shown in the past (18). In addition, the diffusion of oxygen into the enlarged cells of the hypertrophic heart of hypertensive individuals is partially impaired, and this aggravates the threat of myocardial ischemia.

Both therapy and prophylaxis of ischemic heart disease depend almost entirely on ameliorating modifications of myocardial functional and metabolic rather than of coronary vascular structural factors.

This is illustrated by the symptomatic effectiveness of drugs in angina pectoris. The nitrites do not produce their beneficial effects primarily by coronary dilatation (19), but rather by way of an improvement of the myocardial functional features of cardiac work, namely a reduction of the latter and of concomitant oxygen consumption. After administration of nitrities the cardiac work is reduced on an average by more than 63 per cent as shown by Schimmler (20).

AUGMENTATION OF THE CORONARY RESERVE BY PHYSICAL TRAINING

The most impressive and clinically most important augmentation of coronary reserve is achieved by physiological means, namely by physical training. It is known that systematic physical training or any form of persistent and vigorous muscular activity reduces the cardiac sympathetic tone and excitability, and raises the vagal tone (1, 21, 22). This is manifested by a slow heart rate, a decrease of cardiac output, and lowering of the systolic blood pressure at rest. Consequently, the oxygen consumption

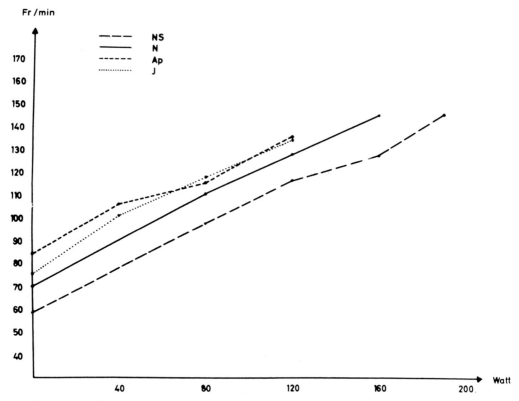

Figure 16–5. Heart rate at rest and during work on bicycle ergometer. Men between 50 and 59 years of age. NS: trained sportsmen; N: normal, nontrained; AP: patients with angina pectoris; I: post-infarction patients.

of the heart at rest can be assumed to be diminished. Under physical strain, the trained heart works with a lower frequency and ejects a larger stroke volume than the untrained heart. It requires, for a given workload, a lesser amount of oxygen than that of a sedentary individual.

Furthermore, experimental data by Eckstein (23) suggest that, in the presence of stenotic coronary arteries, the development and dilatation of preformed collaterals is being favored by physical exercise.

It may be assumed that regular physical training ameliorates the oxygen utilization in the body's muscle mass and

that, by improving the coordination of muscular activity during exercise, it increases muscular efficiency and with it facilitates an optimal distribution of blood in the body. All this should entail advantages also for the efficiency of the entire cardiovascular system.

PREVENTIVE AND THERAPEUTIC SIGNIFICANCE OF PHYSICAL TRAINING

The prophylactic value of physical training is already well established. If coronary stenosis develops, the coronary reserve remains, nevertheless, relatively large despite a reduction in coronary flow, and clinical symptoms are miti-

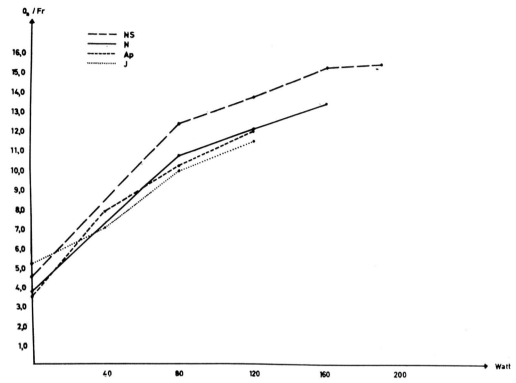

Figure 16–6. Oxygen pulse at rest and during work on bicycle erogmeter. Men between 50 and 59 years of age. NS: trained sportsmen; N: normal, nontrained; AP: patients with angina pectoris; I: post-infarction patients.

gated or remain altogether absent The improved development of preformed anastomoses, in turn, may contribute to an augmentation of the coronary reserve by increasing coronary blood supply.

We have measured cardiovascular parameters in healthy men of 50 to 59 years who were divided into two groups, one of which consisted of sedentary, and the other of physically-trained individuals. These parameters were compared with those of patients of comparable age level who either had angina pectoris or had suffered a myocardial infarction. Among other things, we determined the heart rate and the oxygen pulse. Figure 16–5 shows that both at rest and under

graded work loads on a bicycle ergometer, sportsmen have a lower heart rate than untrained subjects. The patients with angina pectoris, and those with old infarctions exhibit heart rates equivalent to those of untrained normal individuals. None of our patients were in a state of cardiac failure, and none were hypertensive.

Figure 16–6 demonstrates the oxygen pulse, that is, the amount of oxygen uptake per heart beat, in the same subjects as those just mentioned. The oxygen pulse increases in proportion with the stroke volume and the arteriovenous oxygen difference. Here again, a marked contrast distinguishes trained from physically inactive subjects. Our results show that regular systematic physical training is capable of improving circulatory economy even in the advanced years of life, as has also been pointed out by Jokl (24), Mellerowicz (21, 22), Hollmann (25), Cureton (25), and others.

An improvement of the coronary reserve can be achieved by regular physical exercise also in the presence of considerable vascular pathology. In our own patient material, the blood pressure, heart rate, oxygen uptake, oxygen pulse, and the respiratory equivalent were determined at rest and under different work loads.

In all cases, including those of older age groups, a reduction of the heart rate was achieved under identically repeated exercise conditions after training periods of several months. In a number of cases of hypertension, exercise treatment was followed by a lowering of the blood pressure at rest as well as under equal exercise loads. Nearly in all instances we observed a considerable increase of the oxygen pulse, suggestive of an improved coronary reserve. This was also true in several post-infarction patients without and with angina pectoris, who experienced a marked degree of subjective improvement and acquired the physical ability to take extended walks, to go hiking and even to climb mountains at altitude differences of 900 to 1,200 feet.

SUMMARY

The actual availability of oxygen to myocardial tissue is defined by the ratio:

$$\frac{\text{Vascular oxygen supply}}{\text{Myocardial oxygen consumption}}$$

Any fall of this quotient below 1.0 signifies myocardial ischemia. This oc-

curs (a) in case of a lowered oxygen supply, such as due to coronary stenosis, arterial hypotension, or low oxygen saturation of the blood; (b) in case of an augmented myocardial oxygen consumption under an exaggerated influence of sympathogenic catecholamines, and (c) in case of a combination of both factors.

The "coronary reserve" ranges between the coronary flow and oxygen consumption at rest, on the one hand, and their combined maximal augmentation to the point which still permits an adequate oxygen availability to myocardial tissue, on the other.

The trained, efficient heart with its lower sympathetic and higher vagal tone (augmented coronary reserve) requires less oxygen for a given amount of work than the inefficient faster beating heart of the sedentary individual. In addition, the trained body requires for a given physical performance a smaller myocardial energy expenditure.

These combined metabolic and dynamic effects of training, together with an improved development of collaterals, protect the heart against myocardial ischemia even in the presence of some degree of coronary atherosclerosis.

REFERENCES

1. RAAB, W.: (a) *Hormonal and Neurogenic Cardiovascular Disorders*. Baltimore, Williams and Wilkins, 1953. (b) The nonvascular metabolic myocardial vulnerability factor in "coronary heart disease." *Amer Heart J.*, 66:685, 1963.
2. SCHIMERT, G., SCHIMMLER, W., SCHWALB, H., and EBERL, J.: Die Coronarerkrankungen. *Handbuch der Inneren Medizin*. Berlin, Springer-Verlag, 1960.
3. SCHIMERT, G.: Körperbelastung und Coronarkrankheiten. *Munch Med Wschr*, 18:894, 1965.
4. LAURENT, D., BOLENE-WILLIAMS, C., WILLIAMS, F. L., and KATZ, L. N.: Effects of heart rate on coronary flow and cardiac oxygen consumption. *Amsr J Physiol*, 185:355, 1956.

5. JOHNSON, J. R., and DiPALMA, J. R.: Intramyocardial pressure and its relation to aortic blood pressure. *Amer J Physiol, 125:*234, 1939.

6. LASZT, L., and MULLER, A.: Der myocardiale Druck. *Helv Physiol Pharmacol Acta, 16:*88, 1958.

7. SCHÜTZ, E.: Ueber den Einfluss des intraventrikularen systolischen Druckes auf die Coronardurchblutung. *Z Kreislaufforsch, 45:*708, 1956.

8. SCHÜTZ, E.: *Physiologie des Herzens.* Berlin, Springer-Verlag, 1958.

9. EVANS, C. L., and MATSUOKA, Y.: The effect of various mechanical conditions on the gaseous metabolism and efficiency of the mammalian heart. *J Physiol, 49:*378, 1915.

10. GOLLWITZER-MEIER, K., KRAMER, K., and KRÜGER, E.: Der Gaswechsel des suffizienten und insuffizienten Warmblüterherzens. *Pflüger Arch Physiol, 237:*68, 1936.

11. GOLLWITZER-MEIER, K., KROETZ, CHR., and KRÜGER, E.: Sauerstoffverbrauch und Kranzgefässdurchblutung des innervierten Herzens in ihrer Beziehung zu Arbeit und Arbeitsform des Herzens. *Pflügers Arch Physiol, 240:*263, 1938.

12. GOLLWITZER-MEIER, K., and KRÜGER, E.: Zur verschiedenheit der Herzenergetik und Herzdynamik bei Druck- und Volumleistung. *Pflügers Arch Physiol, 238:*279, 1936.

13. ECKSTEIN, R. W., STROUD, M., DOWLING, C. V., ECKEL, R, and Pritchard, W. H.: Response of coronary blood flow following stimulation of cardiac accelerator nerves. *Fed Proc, 8:*38, 1949.

14. ECKSTEIN, R. W., STROUD, M., ECKEL, R., DOWLING, C. V., and PRITCHARD, W. H.: Effects of control of cardiac work upon coronary flow and O_2 consumption after sympathetic nerve stimulation. *Amer J Physiol, 163:*539, 1950.

15. GREMELS, H.: Ueber die Steuerung der energetischen Vorgänge am Säugetierherzen. *Arch Exp Path & Pharm, 182:*1, 1936.

16. KIESE, M., and Garan, R. S.: Mechanische Leistung, Grösse und Sauerstoffverbrauch des Warmblüterherzens. *Arch Exp Path Pharm, 188:* 226, 1938.

17. BOHNENKAMP, H.: *Lehrbuch der Speziellen Pathologischen Physiologie.* Jena, Gustav Fischer, 1944.

18. SCHIMERT, G.: Die Therapie der Coronarinsuffizienz im Lichte einer neuen Betrachtung der Pathogenese. *Schweiz Med Wschr, 81:*598, 1951.

19. GORLIN, R., BRACHFELD, N., McLEOD, C., and BOPP, P.: Effect of nitroglycerine on the coronary circulation in patients with coronary artery disease or increased left ventricular work. *Circulation, 19:*705, 1959.

20. SCHIMMLER, W.: Thesis, University of Munich, 1950.

21. MELLEROWICZ, H.: Vergleichende Untersuchungen über das Oekonomieprinzip in Arbeit und Leistung des trainierten Kreislaufs und seine Bedeutung für die präventive und rehabilitative Medizin. *Arch Kreislaufforsch, 24:*70, 1956.

22. MELLEROWICZ, H.: Ueber Trainingswirkungen auf Herz und Kreislauf und ihre Bedeutung für die präventive Cardiologie. *Preventive Cardiologie,* Berlin-Steglitz, Medicus Verlag, 1961.

23. ECKSTEIN, R. W.: Effect of exercise and coronary artery narrowing on coronary collateral circulation. *Cir Res, 5:*230, 1957.

24. JOKL, E.: Effect of sports and athletics on the cardiovascular system. *Cardiology,* Vol. 5, New York, McGraw-Hill, 1961.

25. HOLLMANN, W.: *Der Arbeits- und Trainingseinfluss auf Kreislauf und Atmung.* Darmstadt, Steinkopff, 1959.

26. CURETON, T. K.: *Physical Fitness Appraisal and Guidance.* St. Louis, 1947.

Chapter XVII

CIVILIZED PATTERN OF ACTIVITY, CARDIAC ADAPTATION AND ISCHEMIC HEART DISEASE

SALEK MINC

(Perth, West Australia)

PSYCHOLOGICAL studies conducted in the last few years demonstrated the prevalence of certain traits and behavior in subjects prone to ischemic heart disease. Osler (1) was the first to describe the type of person likely to suffer from "angiosclerosis," leading to ischemic heart disease, as a "man who has risen early and late taken rest, who has eaten the bread of carefulness, striving for success in commercial, professional or political life."

In more recent times Dunbar (2) states that "a coronary disease patient is a consistently striving person of great control and persistence, a long-term planner; he is self-disciplined and presents the "need to get to the top."

Miles et al. (3) suggested that features of "coronary personality" are personality characteristics due to cultural factors.

Forssman and Lindegard (4) found "high degree of occupational leadership" amongst a group of coronary patients. In their study they aimed at determination of fundamental personality traits, disregarding whenever possible the superimposition of a new pattern "suited to the subjects's age, social position and profession."

The tendency to disregard acquired characteristics (the ones due to social adaptation) may obscure the significance of psychological factors in coronary heart disease. The findings of Cady (5) illustrate such possibility; his coronary patients presented a constitutional cyclothymic temperament exuberant and driving; in the same time they presented inhibitory habits and showed acceptance of responsibilities induced by environmental influences.

The findings of Wardwell et al. (6) also indicate that the coronary patient exercises great control over his behavior, drives and impulses; while other patients depend on external control and authority, the coronaries carry their social monitoring system within themselves.

In a recent study of Cleveland and Johnson (7), a typical coronary patient is described as "a person who presents himself as success-driven and independent. The coronary group reveals in his responses great concern about behaving in a conventional manner, conforming to accepted ethical norms and presenting to the world a controlled, cautious front."

Cleveland and Johnson's "coronary profile" is nearly identical with the one outlined by Friedman and Rosenman (8) and also by Russek and Zohman (9).

156

The main traits are competitiveness, desire for recognition, multiple activities, and sustained drive. Upward mobility and striving towards high status was also noted by Hinkle (10).

Our own studies (11) brought further evidence showing that coronary disease patients possess a greater measure of rational control than the comparison group. In our study it appeared that at least some of the coronary patients were temperamentally unsuited to their inhibited behavior.

By putting together the major characteristics commonly encountered in "coronary candidates," we arrive at a definite image of a man who tends to become a "solid citizen" committed to high normative standards. The pillar of society, he means well and does well. Because of his concern with socially-accepted norms and eye to future achievements, the coronary patient exercises great control over his behavior, drives and impulses; his activities would be guided rationally rather than emotionally.

In a previous presentation (12) I tried to sum up "desirable" social qualities of the man of Western Society. Under the heading "The Typical Western Man," a tabulation was presented which apparently corresponds with most of the recent findings on coronary candidates.

The Typical Western Man

1. He has a broad time prospective and strong orientation to the future.

2. He seems to be self-directed and self-disciplined.

3. He is detached from strong desires for immediate gratification.

4. He selects activities for potential achievements, not for the pleasure of work itself.

5. Although in every choice there must be an emotional element, once this choice is made, further emotional influences are subordinated to rationally patterned behavior.

6. He is reliable. When necessary, he drives himself to work through rational self-imposition.

7. He has a conscious awareness of responsibility and is rarely motivated by actual enthusiasm.

The above characteristics based on rational control and related to social values are part of the precept and practice of civilized society. They are mostly self-imposed or socioeconomically imposed. I emphasize the fact that:

1. The "socially desirable" qualities of the typical Western man figure prominently in the psychological makeup of the coronary patient

2. The coronary personality is, at least in part, the product of "Western acculturation."

The immediate corollary of it is that the increase in coronary heart disease in the "Western culture" countries may be partly due to psychological factors inherent to this culture and reflected in patterns of behavior and activity. I defined this pattern as the "civilized pattern of human activity."

Great prominence has been given to "stress" as a causative or contributing factor in ischemic heart disease. Emotional stresses figure often in the history of coronary patients (9, 13, 14, 15). Chronic pyschic stress has been invoked by Wardwell (6); it is caused by rational control of the "drive discharge" which prevents the "acting out" of problems.

The suggested pathogenetic link occurs via neurohormonal pathways; sympathetic overactivity with increased production of catecholamines appears to be a major culprit, causing myocardial oxygen wastage (16). Selye (17) has shown that the cardiotoxicity of the adreno-sympathogenic catecholamines is greatly potentiated by adrenal corticoids. An increase in plasma cholesterol during stress was observed by Schneider (18), Wertlake (19), Rosenman and Friedman (20).

From the quoted studies one could conclude that the civilized pattern of human behavior leads to conflict and stress. Because of rational control, situation of "emotion without action" occurs frequently; its neurohormonal repercussions affect adversely the cardiovascular system, and eventually cause or contribute to ischemic heart disease.

These conclusions appear justifiable even if not definitely proven. But if instead of considering mainly the pattern of behavior we put the accent on civilized pattern of human activity, other aspects of neurohormonal functioning due to psychological influences may appear. The suggested new approach points out the following:

Although the major demands on cardiac performance (and on coronary blood supply) occur during neuromuscluar activity, the mechanism of cardiac adaptation to activity and its possible impairment has not received much consideration in the pathogenesis of ischemic heart disease.

Only the overactive neurohormonal influences have been considered and their noxious role emphasized. On the other hand, there is evidence of neurohormonal processes having a positive task in cardiac adaptation to activity. One has, therefore, to envisage the possibility that under civilized conditions the neurohormonal mechanism of cardiac adaptation to activity may lack the promoting boost of psychological (emotional) stimulus.

Psychological Links in Cardiovascular Adaptation to Activity

When in response to exercise the heart has to perform more work, it shows an increased mechanical efficiency (in other words, reduced oxygen consumption per unit of work) (21). Thus, a favorable balance can be maintained between the blood and oxygen supply. Cardiovascular adaptation manifests itself also with widespread vasomotor changes, including the coronary tree.

The regulating mechanism of this adaptation involves the autonomic nervous system and (known and possibly ununknown) hormonal factors.

If one considers that neuromuscular activity is psychologically determined, because it constitutes man's conscious response to environmental influences or inner stimuli, and that this activity calls for immediate cardiovascular adaptation, it will be obvious that psychological stimulus, activity, and adaptation to it are constantly linked. A definite relationship pattern must have been established for them through the phylogenetic history of the human race. One could expect, therefore, that psychological factors will influence cardiovascular adaptation to activity and this would occur via neurohormonal pathways.

The adjustment mechanisms were established at a primitive evolutionary stage of the history of the human species. At this stage, action or activity was either reflex or followed a stimulus capable of producing emotional charges, as for example, in case of hunger, of sexual desire, or in the necessity for fight or flight

The stimulus which leads to activity would provoke other physiological reactions, destined to bring the cardiovascular system into maximum efficiency during activity.

Many studies, in fact, demonstrate that emotional states affect cardiac and vasomotor centers (22). It is known that sympathetic tone affects cardiac contraction, and according to Wood (23), increased adrenergic activity is the first cardiac reserve. Matthes (24) observed that autonomic nervous system stimulation promotes cardiac adaptation prior to neuromuscular activity. Gregg (25) noted that during excitement, the same as during cardiac sympathetic nerve stimulation, the heart is able to augment its coronary circulation with an increased coronary flow per heart beat.

The recent work by Braunwald et al. (26), showed that "during the stress of muscular exercise the function of the adrenergic nervous system assumes greater importance." They found that "inhibition of the adrenergic system alone prevents the increase in stroke volume which normally occurs during exercise." They concluded that "the autonomic nervous system plays a significant role in stimulating the myocardium during exercise" to major efficiency.

Sarnoff and Mitchell (27) stress the important role of norepinephrine and sympathetic stimulation in cardiac performance. There is enhancement of myocardial contractility and the stroke work rises higher in relation to ventricular pressure. The increased myocardial contractility leads also to a shorter systole. Such shortening is of paramount importance in exertional or other tachycardias; it permits a relatively longer diastole with better muscular relaxation of myocardial fibers; there is a greater ventricular filling, and better coronary flow.

Recent studies have also demonstrated that even everyday emotional stimuli affect catecholamine excretion. Emotions provoked by fictitious phenomena (movie plays, etc.) could raise the amount of excreted catecholamines to the level observed in pheochromocytoma (28).

Studies of Rushmer (29) stress the importance of the central nervous system in the pattern of left ventricular response to exercise. Stimulation of certain areas of the hypothalamus would reproduce such response; similar response could also be induced by stimulation of sympathetic nerves to the heart.

Here again the governing power of the sympathetic nerves implies possible emotional influences; in the same hypothalamus which commands the sympathetic nerves and the cardiac response, the emotions are being translated into somatic repercussions. Manifold nervous influences not only of emotional but also of environmental or behavioral nature could alter cardiovascular response to exercise. It varies with individuals, and could also vary with the stimulus.

We learned then that the mode of cardiovascular adaptation to activity is governed by nervous processes and mediated by neurohormonal action. We realize also that these processes are subject to psychological influences. Such influences become more significant when the stimulus to activity is emotionally charged. Cannon's alarm reaction with readiness for fight or flight is an extreme example of it. This does not mean that every emotion favors cardiac adaptation; the autonomic nervous pattern varies with diverse emotional states. One could expect this pattern to become effective and to integrate with activity when the emotional stimulus for action is related to basic motivational drives. In these drives there is enhancement of activity with alertness of the organism; through the reticular facilitatory system a "high state of physiological efficiency is achieved." This activation controls cortical tone, muscular activity and sympathetic tone (30). The cardiovascular adjustment is part of this response.

While adaptation to activity is related to the motivation of drive, in diverse cultures different motivations will be selected as stimuli to action. We shall consider, therefore, the nature of the motivations which dictate the "civilized pattern of activity."

Human motivating forces have their hierarchy and range from the most primitive to the most refined. Engel (31) presents a summary of this hierarchy:

Hierarchy of motivating forces as related to the following:

a. drives rooted in the biology of the organism (based on fundamental biological needs);

b. the primitive systems to protect against bodily damage;

c. effects evolving in the course of development;

d. learned signals (symbolically or otherwise represented) which provide information about the environment (relevant to basic needs and to dangers);

e. highly derivative psychic processes related to all of the preceding but operating with less urgency in the service of self-realization, productivity, (creativity, play, work, etc.). The last operate with the greatest degree of autonomy and are the most accessible to control by will.

This hierarchy is one of biological development; it means that the primitive drives were established at the same early stage of human evolution when homeostatic mechanisms were being formed; the more recent has been the appearance of a drive or of a motivational force (as in (d) and in (e)), the less probable is the existence of an adaptive mechanism backing the execution of this drive.

In civilized society, the individual is taught not to select his stimulus to activity in the range of basic biological drives or in the immediate emotional impulses. By virtue of precept and practice of Western civilization, the "well-socialized" man" tends to act on cerebral orders only, well within the category (e); the one with the lowest motivational force.

I stress this "unemotional activity" as typical of the "Western Man." It still requires cardiovascular adaptation but has no boosting effect on it. "Action without emotion" may burden the heart more than "emotion without action" which has been often invoked as cause of disease.

Once we refer to the civilized man as acting on cerebral orders, guided by psychic processes and motivational forces partly controlled by will, we realize that we are well within the psychological traits of the "coronary personality"; the pillar of society is guided by rational judgement, by long-term program, and is self-disciplined. This does not mean that he has no emotions; his attitude and inner reactions to the outside world may be the same as of his primitive ancestor, but his active response to them has changed because he is "civilized."

The mechanism by which the presumably insufficient adaptation of cardiovascular system to activity leads to ischemic heart disease can be described so far only in general and oversimplified terms. Because the myocardium works uneconomically it becomes more vulnerable or ages quicker through wear and tear. The coronary system on the other hand is presented with the demand for extra supply. Minor coronary insufficiency leads to major myocardial damage or necrosis.

I would like also to emphasize that stresses or stressful situations requiring emergency action or bursts of activity vary vastly in their emotional implications. In some of them as in case of maternal duties with many children, or on the battlefield, or in case of outside aggression, there is a strong emotional stimulus arousing the autonomic nervous system and thus gearing the organism into activity. These situations are part of human history and are still with us. On the other hand, the business executive and the medical practitioner of today's society are pressed often into emergency action through a conventional signal and intellectual elaboration. Their motivation for action is only rationally and remotely related to basic drives; their cardiovascular adaptation will have no extra boost. The emergency activity will affect the maladapted heart of the doctor more than the "stirred" heart of the mother attending to her acutely ill child.

This to me appears the explanation of the controversy about stresses leading to ischemic heart disease; man has been biologically adapted to stresses of primitive society which carry with them the adequate stimuli for adustment. There is less adaptation when the environmental challenge is perceived and countered on the rational level, as it often happens in Western society.

In the exposition of my views, the main point has been that in the "Western Man" the emotional preamble to neuro-muscular activity is reduced to a minimum. It was stressed also that such "emotional preamble" has its biological purpose and is a prime mover of cardiovascular homeostasis in activity. I feel that the purposefulness of human emotions is worth emphasizing. For some reason (or is it also influence of civilization?) most medical thoughts concentrate usually on the negative value of emotions.

It may be that in our present society emotions have lost much of their purposefulness. We do not let them be of biological use in our everyday activities. We do not synchronize our actions with our emotions. But our constitution and physiological functioning are still as they were 25,000 years ago. We find that today, when the activity is rationally determined and not emotionally motivated, the heart "is not in it" and works less economically. It asks for more from its feeding channels. Ischemic heart disease comes as punishment for living in the age of reason, a "nemesis" for the man of today whose precept is to act as "homo sapiens" and not as "homo sentiens."

SUMMARY

The coronary patient tends to control intellectually his behavior and his activity. He is concerned with socially-accepted norms.

His cerebrally-planned activities mostly lack emotional backing. His "action without emotion" does not sufficiently favor the arousal of the autonomic nervous system.

Cardiac adaptation to exercise, which is governed by the autonomic nervous system, is less efficient in such "civilized pattern of activity."

This maladaptation, either by frequent recurrence or in combination with anatomical factors (coronary narrowing) may lead to myocardial degeneration or necrosis, classified today as ischemic phenomena.

REFERENCES

1. OSLER, W.: *Lectures on Angina Pectoris and Allied States.* New York, Appleton, 1897, p. 153.
2. DUNBAR, F.: *Psychosomatic Diagnosis.* New York, P. B. Hoeber, Inc., 1943.
3. MILES, N. N. W., WALDFOGEL, S., BARROBEE, E. L., and COBB, S.: Psychosomatic study of 46 young men with coronary artery disease. *Psychosom Med, 16:*455, 1954.
4. FORSSMAN, O., and LINDEGARD, B.: The post-coronary patient. *J Psychosom Res, 3:*89, 1958.
5. CADY, L. D., GERTLER, M. M., GOTTSCH, L. G., and WOODBURY, M. A.: The factor structure of variables concerned with coronary heart disease. *Behav Sci, 6:*37, 1961.
6. WARDWELL, W. I., BAHNSON, C. B., CARON, N. S., and EISENBERG, H.: Social and psychological factors in myocardial infarction. Submitted for publication, 1961.
7. CLEVELAND, S. E., and JOHNSON, D. L.: Personality patterns in young males with coronary disease. *Psychosom Med, 24:*600, 1962.
8. FRIEDMAN, R., and ROSENMAN, R. H.: Association of specific overt behavior pattern with blood and cardiovascular findings. *JAMA, 169:*1286, 1959.
9. RUSSEK, H. J., and ZOHMAN, B. C.: Relative significance of heredity, diet and occupational stress in coronary heart disease of young adults. *Amer J Med Sci, 235:*266, 1958.
10. HINKLE, L. E.: Social mobility, personality and coronary disease. Research plan submitted to the National Institute of Health, July 1, 1962.
11. MINC, S., SINCLAIR, G., and TAFT, R.: Some psychological factors in coronary heart disease. *Psychosom Med, 25:*133, 1963.
12. MINC, S.: The civilized pattern of human activity and coronary heart disease. *Med J Aust, 2:*87, 1960.
13. WEISS, E., DLIN, B., ROLLIN, H. R., FISHER, H. K., and DEPLER, C. R.: Emotional factors in coronary occlusion. *Arch Intern Med, 99:*628, 1957.
14. PEARSON, N. E. S., and JOSEPH, J.: Stress and occlusive coronary artery disease. *Lancet, 1:*415, 1963.
15. OLIVER, M. F., and BOYD, G. S.: Endocrine aspects of coronary sclerosis. *Lancet, 2:*1273, 1956.
16. RAAB, W.: Civilization-induced neurogenic degenerative heart disease. *Cardiologia, 41:*129, 1962.
17. SELYE, H.: *The Pluricausal Cardiopathies.* Springfield, Thomas, 1961.
18. SCHNEIDER, R. A.: *Res Publ Ass Nerv Ment Dis, 29:*818, 1950.
19. WERTLAKE, P. T., WILCOX, A. A., HALEY, M. I., and PETERSON, J. E.: Relationship of mental and emotional stress with serum cholesterol levels. *Proc Soc Exp Biol, 97:*163, 1958.
20. FRIEDMAN, N., ROSENMAN, R. H., and CARROLL, V.: Changes in the serum cholesterol and blood clotting time in men subjected to cyclic variations of occupational stress. *Circulation, 17:*852, 1958.
21. GORLIN, R.: Measurement of coronary flow in health and disease. In: *Modern Trends in Cardiology,* London, Butterworth, 1960.
22. WRIGHT, S.: *Applied Physiology.* Ninth Ed. London, Oxford Univ. Press, 1956, p. 663.
23. WOOD, P.: *Diseases of the Heart and Circulation.* London, Eyre and Spottiswoode, 1956, p. 266.
24. MATTHES, K.: Hemodynamics of the right and left ventricle in relation to circulatory needs. Circulation Proceedings of the Harvey Tercentennary Congress, Blackwell, Oxford, *92,* 1957.
25. GREGG, D. E.: Physiology of the coronary circulation. Abstracts 35th Scientific Session, Amer. Heart Assoc. *Circulation, 26:*679, 1962.
26. BRAUNWALD, E., CHIDSEY, C. A., HARRISON, C. D., GAFFNEY, T. E., and KAHLER, R. L.: Studies on the function of the adrenergic nerve endings in the heart. *Circulation, 28:*958, 1963.
27. SARNOFF, S. J., and MITCHELL, J. N.: The control of the function of the heart. In: *Handbook of Physiology,* Section 2, Circulation, *1:*489. Amer. Physiol. Soc., Washington, D. C., 1962.
28. LEVI, L.: A new stress tolerance test with simultaneous study of physiological and psychological variables. *Acta Endocr, 37:*38, 1961.
29. RUSHMER, R. F., SMITH, O., and FRANKLIN D.: Mechanisms of cardiac control in exercise. *Circ Res, 7:*602, 1959.
30. DELL, P.: Some basic mechanisms of the translation of bodily needs into behavior. CIBA Foundation Symposium on the Neurological Basis of Behavior. London, Churchill, 1958, p. 187.
31. ENGEL, G. L.: *Psychological Development in Health and Disease.* Philadelphia and London, Saunders Co., 1962, p. 27.

Chapter XVIII

THE ROLE OF STRESS IN THE PRODUCTION AND PREVENTION OF EXPERIMENTAL CARDIOPATHIES*

HANS SELYE

(Montreal, Canada)

THE principal object of this paper is to summarize the concept of pluricausal diseases and to report on some recent animal experiments which show that, depending upon circumstances, exposure to various stressors can either elicit cardiac necroses, when they would not otherwise occur, or prevent their development under circumstances normally conducive to fatal cardiac damage.

The belief is common, not only among physicians but also among laymen, that sudden exposure to a particularly stressful experience may elicit a cardiac infarct, at least in predisposed individuals. Almost every physician has seen patients in whom myocardial infarction followed soon after some unaccustomed, intense physical exertion or emotional shock. In such cases it is customary to assume that stress was the underlying cause of the cardiac lesion. Yet for various reasons many cardiologists seriously doubt that stress plays any role in the pathogenesis of cardiovascular disease in general and acute cardiac necrosis in particular because (a)

it is often impossible to identify any particularly stressful experience in the immediate past of a patient who died of cardiac infarction; (b) up to quite recently, it has not been possible to produce any parallel of a cardiac infarct in experimental animals by exposure to even lethal stress, and (c) there is considerable evidence in support of the view that certain stressful experiences (exercise, cold baths, etc.) can actually protect the heart against infarction.

By way of an introduction to our analysis of this problem, we must say a few words about the concept of "pluricausal diseases."

We have learned to distinguish between unconditionally and conditionally acting pathogens. The former type invariably produces disease under ordinary circumstances; their effect does not depend upon any special sensitization. Intense heat produces a burn, transection of motor nerves causes paralysis and complete occlusion of all renal vessels results in necrosis of the kidney. The body possesses no compensatory mechanisms able to abolish "susceptibility" to such agents nor can the physician hope to prevent their action by any prophylactic measures.

Conditionally-acting pathogens pro-

*This work was supported by the U.S. Army Medical Research and Development Command (Contract No. DA-49-193-MD-2039), the USPHS, National Heart Institute (Grant No. HE-06182-05) and the Canadian Heart Foundation.

duce disease only under special circumstances. Allergens, certain types of microorganisms and emotional stimuli cause lesions only in those who are susceptible to them. In other words, the former are obligatory, the latter potential, pathogens. The organism possesses natural defensive mechanisms with which to defend itself against the action of potential disease-producers and the physician can often give further assistance by stimulating or complementing these innate homeostatic mechanisms.

There are many gradations between the two extremes, the absolutely unconditional pathogen and the agent that never produces disease by itself. Yet we must distinguish between the two prototypes if we are to avoid one of the oldest and still most common errors of medical logic, namely that a given agent cannot be the cause of disease if it has been proved not to have produced lesions in many patients. The fallacy of this argument appears to be self-evident; yet our predecessors stubbornly rejected antiseptic measures because in many instances no infection occurred after operations performed with unwashed hands.

Let us remember also the frequently repeated contention that stress could not be responsible for the production of such diverse conditions as peptic ulcers, hypertension, cardiac infarcts, psoriasis or increased susceptibility to infection, for if it were, it would have to produce all of them in every patient exposed to any stressor. As we shall see, we have learned not only to direct the effect of stress upon the cardiovascular system selectively, but even to produce *or prevent* highly specific and qualitatively distinct cardiovascular lesions by exposure to the same stressor (e.g., forced muscular exercise).

EXPERIMENTAL CARDIO-VASCULAR LESIONS

Under normal conditions exposure to stress produces no serious cardiac damage in healthy young people. However, in animals conditioned by pretreatment with certain electrolytes (e.g., Na_2HPO_4, Na_2SO_4) and certain steroids (e.g., corticoids) in doses ineffective by themselves, subsequent exposure to stress invariably elicits massive infarct-like cardiac necroses.

This Electrolyte-Steroid-induced Cardiopathy characterized by Necrosis (ES CN) fails to occur if the animals are exposed to stress prior to the electrolyte-steroid conditioning (that is, at a time when the heart is not yet sensitized to this type of injury). This is so even if exposure to stress is repeated at the end of the conditioning period, that is, at a time when subjects not previously exposed to stress respond with an ESCN.

Rats pretreated with sodium acetate plus fluorocortisol for a few days, and then exposed to the stress of forced muscular exercise in a revolving drum, all died with massive infarctoid myocardial necroses within 24 hours after the exercise period. Another group of animals survived when similarly treated with sodium acetate and fluorocortisol but forced to run both before and after the conditioning treatment was given; indeed, in this case, even histologically no cardiac necrosis could be demonstrated (See Table 18–I.)

Here we have what in stress research we call a case of *simple resistance*, because the animals became insensitive to a certain stressor following pretreatment with the same agent.

This type of experimental arrangement may be schematically illustrated as:

TABLE 18–I

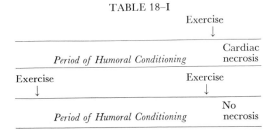

	Exercise ↓ Cardiac necrosis
Period of Humoral Conditioning	
Exercise ↓	Exercise ↓ No necrosis
Period of Humoral Conditioning	

Interestingly, cardiac necrosis can be prevented under such circumstances even by pretreatment with a stressor different from that used as an elicitor. For example, muscular exercise prior to the conditioning period can protect against the ESCN normally elicited by subsequent bone fractures in such electrolyte-steroid-conditioned animals. (See Table 18–II). This phenomenon of *cross resistance* may be illustrated as follows:

TABLE 18–II

	Bone fracture ↓ Cardiac necrosis
Period of Humoral Conditioning	
Exercise ↓	Bone fracture ↓ No necrosis
Period of Humoral Conditioning	

Conditioning with calcium salts and certain corticoids sensitizes for the production, by subsequent stress, of an entirely different lesion: the Electrolyte-Steroid Cardiopathy with Calcification (ESCC). This is characterized by the deposition of calcium salts in the coronary arteries and the myocardium itself. The development of this lesion—like that of the ESCN—is precipitated by exposure to stress following humoral conditioning, but prevented by pretreatment with a stressor.

It is particularly interesting that pretreatment with a stressor can protect the heart not only against diverse cardiopathies whose development is normally precipitated by stress, but also against myocardial and coronary lesions produced by purely humoral means. We have learned that, even without exposure to stress, treatment with certain vitamin D derivatives, such as dihydrotachysterol (DHT), produces calcification of the Mönckeberg-sclerosis type in the coronary arteries, while conjoint administration of Na_2HPO_4 and DHT results in a suppurating myocarditis in addition to the coronary calcification. Structurally quite different cardiac lesions can be produced—again without exposure to stress—by acute overdosage with plasmocid, an obsolete antimalarial, or papain, a proteolytic enzyme preparation. Yet pretreatment with a stressor (forced restraint, muscular exercise, ice-cold baths) can offer virtually complete protection against the induction of any of these experimental cardiopathies.

STRESS AND CARDIAC INFARCT IN MAN

Many observations have been cited in support of the view that stress can elicit cardiac infarcts in man (1–5). It has also been reported that stress significantly increases the blood level of lipids and lipoproteins, which are thought to participate in the pathogenesis of coronary disease (6–8).

From these and similar observations it was concluded that "the increasing occupational stresses unique to industrialized society play a dominant role in the high incidence of coronary heart disease" (9). It should be kept in mind, however, that the alleged contemporary increase in coronary heart disease, if real, may have other causes as well; for example, a "high living standard," that is, too much rich food and too little hard work.

The fact that high-fat, high-carbohydrate diets sensitize the myocardium for the production of acute necroses by stress has been experimentally demonstrated beyond question (10, 11). Furthermore, as we have just said, inurement to stress exerts an opposite, protective effect; hence, habitual inactivity could also be a potent predisposing agent for myocardial necrosis. In this respect, the current trend towards an increasingly softer, sheltered, sedentary life may be just as noxious as the "occupational stresses unique to industrialized society." The tendency to avoid even the shortest walk by using cars and elevators, our ever more perfect defenses against infection, malnutrition, exposure to extremes of temperature and other adversities may well have to be bought at the price of an increased susceptibility to sudden stresses to which our way of life cannot properly inure us (11). There is considerable evidence in support of the view that "men in physically active jobs have a lower incidence of coronary heart disease in middle age than have men in physically inactive jobs (12).

On the basis of these considerations, it is hardly necessary to point out that I am most enthusiastic about the possibilities of the reconditioning programs as organized in several countries abroad.

In addition, the experimental analysis of the role played by stress in the production and prevention of cardiovascular lesions suggests a number of new therapeutic and prophylactic possibilities that may have clinical applications. The most obvious among these is proper adjustment of the stress factor itself. The realization that stress can play a decisive role in both the prevention and the production of cardiovascular disease clearly shows that stressful activities should be neither peremptorily proscribed nor prescribed, but properly adjusted to the requirements of each patient. Much more clinical investigation will be necessary before we learn to do this well, but meantime other more immediately applicable therapeutic and prophylactic measures with drugs are suggested by the evidence just surveyed.

A great variety of the experimental pluricausal cardiopathies, and especially those enhanced by sudden exposure to unaccustomed stress, largely depend upon the simultaneous action of mineralocorticoids. In experimental animals, the induction of such lesions is greatly facilitated by dietary sodium supplements and inhibited by the oral administration of potassium salts and various chlorides.

It is highly probable that these electrolytes exert their respective pathogenic or beneficial actions by accentuating or antagonizing the effect of endogenous mineralocorticoids (10, 11). Clinical work along these lines has barely begun, but balanced therapeutic regimens based on the withdrawal of sodium (by low sodium diets, sodium diuretics, excess administration of water, etc.), preferably combined with an increased administration of KCl, $MgCl_2$ and other chlorides, have already given encouraging results (13–16) and deserve to be developed further.

Another interesting therapeutic possibility is suggested by the observation that some antimineralocorticoids are likewise extraordinarily effective in protecting the heart against the variety of experimental pluricausal cardiopathies just mentioned (11). Numerous clinical observations have shown that these substances are highly useful in combating excessive fluid retention in patients with cardiovascular decompensation and edema, even if these derangements are not due to a primary mineralocorticoid excess (17–29). Such observations strongly suggest not only that increased mineralocorticoid production can occur as an adaptive reaction to various pathologic or even physiologic stressors, but also that this hormonal response can be pathogenic in itself, since its blockade by an antimineralocorticoid improves the patient's condition. In such instances, the electrolyte and fluid derangements may well be considered to be "diseases of adaptation."

It is hoped that the experimental analysis of the pluricausal cardiopathies, and particularly the demonstration that stress can play a decisive part in both the production and the prevention of fatal cardiovascular lesions, will help the clinical investigator to develop new preventive and curative measures against cardiovascular disease.

SUMMARY

Experimental work on factors influencing the production of cardiac infarcts in animals is reviewed. Special attention is given to the role of hormones and electrolytes. However, perhaps the most important outcome of these investigations was the demonstration that certain types of acute experimental cardiac necroses can be prevented by pretreatment with such stressors as physical exercise and cold baths, etc. The possible implications of these findings in clinical medicine are discussed particularly in connection with the proposed establishment of physical reconditioning centers.

REFERENCES

1. ANDREEV, I., and DOSKOV, I.: Coronary disease with myocardial infarction following electrotrauma. *Savr Med*, 8:119, 1957. (*Abstract Bulgarian Scient Lit*, 1:50, 1958.)

2. ROBERTACCIO, A., and MARINO, A.: Fattore elettrico, traumatico ed emotivo nella patogenesi di un caso di infarto del miocardio. *Rass Int Clin Ter*, 38:913, 1958.

3. DAVIDSON, K., and SMITH, B. J.: Myocardial infarction after acute gastro-intestinal haemorrhage. Report of 3 cases. *Brit Med J*, p. 1400, May 7, 1960.

4. WEISS, E., DLIN, B., ROLLIN, H. R., FISCHER, H. K., and BEPLER, C. R.: Emotional factors in coronary occlusion. I. Introduction and general summary. *AMA Arch Intern Med*, 99:628, 1957.

5. RUSSEK, H. I.: Role of heredity, diet, and emotional stress in coronary heart disease. *JAMA*, 171:503, 1959.

6. GRUNDY, S. M., and GRIFFIN, A. C.: Relationship of periodic mental stress to serum lipoprotein and cholesterol levels. *JAMA*, 171:1794, 1959.

7. McCABE, W., HAMMARSTEN, J., SCHOTTSTAEDT, W., ADSETT, C. A., YAMAMOTO, J., and WOLF, S.: Elevations of serum cholesterol in man in association with life stress and independent of diet and exercise. *J Lab Clin Med*, 54:922, 1959.

8. ROSENMAN, R. H., and FRIEDMAN, M.: The effect of cyclic variation of occupational stress on the serum cholesterol and blood clotting time. *Clin Res*, 6:87, 1958.

9. ROSENMAN, R. H., and FRIEDMAN, M.: The possible relationship of occupational stress to clinical coronary heart disease. *Calif Med*, 89:169, 1958.

10. SELYE, H.: *The Chemical Prevention of Cardiac Necroses*. New York, Ronald Press, 1958.

11. SELYE, H.: *The Pluricausal Cardiopathies*. Springfield, Thomas, 1961.

12. MORRIS, J. N., HEADY, J. A., RAFFLE, P. A., ROBERTS, C. G., and PARKS, J. W.: Coronary heart-disease and physical activity of work. *Lancet*, p. 1111, Nov. 28, 1953.

13. DUSSERT, A.: Chlorure de potassium et coeur. *Sem Hop Paris*, 34:1390, 1958.

14. MICHON, P., LARCAN, A., and GAUCHER, P.: Potassium et energétique myocardique. *Sem Hop Paris*, 35:3289, 1959.

15. SODI-PALLARES, D., FISHLEDER, B. L., CISNEROS, F., VIZCAINO, M., BISTENI, A., MEDRANO, G. A., POLANSKY, B. J., and DE MICHELI, A.: A low sodium, high water, high potassium regimen in the successful management of some cardiovascular diseases. Preliminary clinical report. *Canad Med Ass J*, 83:243, 1960.

16. Bosse, J.: Vorsorgliche Behandlung infarkt-gefährdeter Patienten. *Landarzt, 36:*588, 1960.

17. Bolte, E., Verdy, M., Marc-Aurele, J., Brouillet, J., Beauregard, P., and Genest, J.: Studies on new diuretic compounds: spirolactone and chlorothiazide. *Canad Med Ass J, 79:*881, 1958.

18. Clowdus, B. F., Higgins, J. A., Rosevear, J. W., and Summerskill, W. H. J.: Diuretic effect of spirolactone SC-9420. *Lancet,* p. 598, March 12, 1960.

19. Gantt, C. L., and Dyniewicz, J. M.: Some effects of 17-spirolactosteroids on the edema of cirrhosis, with observations on a new spirolactone derivative. *Clin Res, 7:*298, 1959.

20. Kerr, D. N. S., Read, A. E., Haslam, R. M., and Sherlock, S.: The use of a steroidal spirolactone in the treatment of ascites in hepatic cirrhosis. *Lancet,* p. 1084, Nov. 22, 1958.

21. Kowlessar, O. D., Clarkson, B., and Sleisenger, M. B.: Use of an antialdosterone compound for fluid retention in hepatic disease. *Clin Res, 7:*37, 1959.

22. Liddle, G. W.: Sodium diuresis induced by steroidal antagonists of aldosterone. *Science, 126:*1016, 1957.

23. McCrory, W. W., and Eberlein, W. R.: The nature of the sodium diuresis produced by an "aldosterone antagonist," spirolactone. 50th Annual Meeting Amer. Society Clin. Invest., Atlantic City, p. 47, May 5, 1958.

24. Morrison, R. S., and Chalmers, T. C.: The effects of an aldosterone antagonist in decompensated liver disease. *Clin Res, 6:*300, 1958.

25. Morrison, R. S., and Chalmers, T. C.: Combined diuretic and steroid therapy in cirrhosis with ascites. *Clin Res, 7:*37, 1959.

26. Slater, J. D. H., Moxham, A., Hurter, R., and Nabarro, J. D. N.: Clinical and metabolic effects of aldosterone antagonism. *Lancet,* p. 931, Nov. 28, 1959.

27. Sleisenger, M. H., Richard, J., Kowlessar, O. D., Clarkson, B., Thompson, D., and Peterson, R. E.: Effects of spirolactones on excretion of water and electrolytes, and on aldosterone metabolism in cirrhosis. 51st Annual Meeting Amer. Society Clin. Invest., Atlantic City, p. 64, May 4, 1959.

28. Taylor, F. F., and Faloon, W. W.: The role of potassium in the natriuretic response to a steroidal lactone (SC-9420). *J Clin Endocr, 19:*1683, 1959.

29. Vesin, P.: Diuretic effect of spirolactone SC-9420. *Lancet,* p. 774, April 2, 1960.

Chapter XIX

EFFECT OF PHYSICAL EXERCISE ON ADRENAL 17-HYDROXYCORTICOSTEROID SECRETION RATE IN THE DOG

TATUZI SUZUKI

(*Nagasaki, Japan*)

IT HAS been demonstrated that sensory and emotional stresses which are accompanied by an increase in adrenal cortical and sympathoadrenal activity can produce myocardial necrosis (1). On the other hand, regular physical exercise within reasonable limits is believed to be of great value in preventing ischemic, degenerative heart disease and is now widely advocated for practical prevention. In view of these observations, it appeared worthwhile to investigate as to how physical exercise affects the adrenal cortical secretion.

More than 10 years ago, when we started studies of the physiology of the adrenal cortical secretion, little information was available on the resting secretion rate of the corticosteroids. It was suggested by a number of investigations using indirect indices, such as the depletion of the adrenal ascorbic acid, that the adrenal cortical activity was increased by various stressful stimuli. However, direct evidence on these points was lacking. The pioneer work of Vogt (2), reported as early as 1943, showed that a considerable amount of corticosteroids was continuously secreted from the adrenal gland, but, as was suggested by herself, this high level of basal secretion rate may have been due chiefly to the special conditions, such as anesthesia and severe abdominal operation, under which her experiments were performed. The history of the physiological studies of the adrenal medullary secretion suggested to us that there was a need to carry out experiments under more physiological conditions.

In our experiments, adrenal venous blood was collected by a modification of the method of Satake, Sugawara, and Watanabe (3). In order to obtain the adrenal venous blood from unanesthetized dogs without provoking any pain, the dorsal spinal roots through which the sensory nerve fibers from the lumbar region run (i.e., Th_{11}-L_3 dorsal spinal roots), were cut under anesthesia with sodium pentobarbital (Nembutal, 25 mg/kg body weight, i.v.). Three or more weeks later, the lumboadrenal vein was exposed by the lumbar approach and a small glass cannula, connected with a short rubber tube, was inserted into the vein at the site just distal to the adrenal gland. The cannula and the rubber tube were filled with heparin-saline solution and the end of the tube was clamped. A loop of silk thread was loosely placed around the adrenal vein between the inferior vena cava and the adrenal gland.

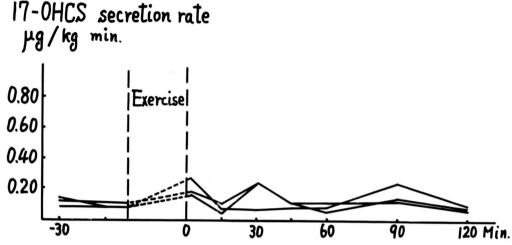

Figure 19–1. Effect of nonexhausting exercise on the adrenal 17-hydroxycorticosteroid secretion rate in 3 dogs.

The silk thread was pulled gently at the time of blood collection so as to direct adrenal blood flow to the exterior through the cannula and the rubber tube. As a rule, observations were started about 18 hours after cannulation of the adrenal vein. Adrenal venous blood was collected without anesthetizing the animals. After collection, it was analyzed for 17-hydroxycorticosteroids (17-OHCS) by the method of Nelson and Samuels (4).

The resting secretion rate of 17-OHCS of one gland in conscious dogs, obtained in 133 assays, ranged from 0.01 to 0.30 μg/kg body wt/min and the mean value was 0.10 ± 0.0053 μg/kg/min (Mean ± s.e.).

Effect of exercise on the adrenal cortical activity was estimated by some investigators by using indirect indices (5, 6, 7). They found in the rat a definite adrenal ascorbic acid depletion or adrenal cholesterol depletion. A direct evaluation was made in our previous study (8). Five dogs, paced by an attendant on a bicycle, were run 5.1 to 14.7 km at speeds of 109-276 m/min. At the end of the running all dogs except one were completely exchausted. After running, a marked increase in 17-OHCS secretion rate was observed in those dogs. Thus exhausting exercise was found to accelerate the adrenal cortical secretion. More recently, we have attempted to compare the adrenal cortical secretion in response to nonexhausting and exhausting exercise. This study is still in progress. A preliminary report will be given here.

Three dogs were run 1.2 to 1.4 km at speeds of 106 to 138 m/min. During and after running no signs of exhaustion were observed. Timed collections of adrenal venous blood samples were made before and after running. The results of nonexhausting exercise are shown in Figure 19–1. The secretion rates of 17-OHCS after running were 0.03 to 0.25 μg/kg/min (i.e., values within the range of variations of resting 17-OHCS secretion). Four dogs were run at speeds of 121 to 175 m/min until they fell down 2 or 3 times and refused to run further. After such exhausting exercise the adrenal 17-OHCS secretion rate increased markedly and reached 1.11 to 2.14 μg/kg/min. Experimental results in one rep-

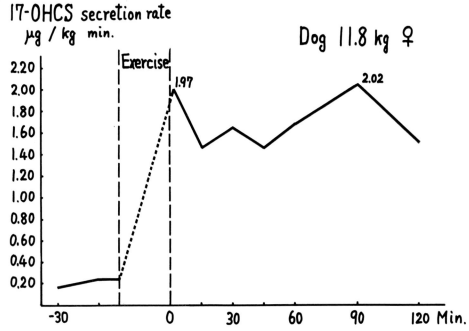

Figure 19–2. Effect of exhausting exercise on the adrenal 17-hydroxycorticosteroid secretion rate in the dog.

resentative case are shown in Figure 19–2. In this case the dog was run 3.5 km at an average speed of 158 m/min.

After completion of this study the details will be reported elsewhere.

SUMMARY

In unanesthetized dogs, whose dorsal spinal roots (Th_{11}-L_3) had been sectioned previously, adrenal venous blood was collected and analyzed for 17-hydroxycorticosteroids (17-OHCS). The animals, paced by an attendant on a bicycle, were run at speeds of 106 to 175 m/min. After nonexhausting exercise no definite changes in 17-OHCS secretion rate were observed. On the other hand, a definite increase in 17-OHCS secretion rate was always observed after exhausting exercise.

REFERENCES

1. Raab, W., Bajusz, E., and Chaplin, J. P.: Myocardial necroses produced in domesticated rats and in wild rats by sensory and emotional stresses. *Proc Soc Exp Biol Med, 116:*665, 1964.
2. Vogt, M.: The output of cortical hormone by the mammalian suprarenal. *J Physiol, 102:*341, 1943-44.
3. Satake, Y., Sugawara, T., and Watanabe, M.: A method for collecting the blood from the suprarenal gland in the dog, without fastening, narcotizing, laparotomy or provoking any pain. *Tohoku J Exp Med, 8:*501, 1927.
4. Nelson, D. H., and Samuels, L. T.: A method for the determination of 17-hydroxycorticosteroids in blood: 17-hydroxycorticosterone in the peripheral circulation. *J Clin Endocr, 12:*519, 1952.
5. Ratsimamanga, R.: Variations de la teneur en acide ascorbique dans la surrénale au cours du travail. *C R Soc Biol., 131:*863, 1939.
6. Knouff, R. A., Brown, J. B., and Schneider, B. M.: Correlated chemical and histological studies of the adrenal lipids. 1. The effect of extreme muscular activity on the adrenal lipids of the guinea pig. *Anat Rec, 79:*17, 1941.
7. Božović, Lj., and Kostial-Živanović, K.: Muscular work and adrenocortical activity. *Arch Int Physiol, 60:*459, 1952.
8. Suzuki, T., Yamashita, K., and Mitamura, T.: Muscular exercise and adrenal 17-hydroxycorticosteroid secretion in dogs. *Nature, 181:*715, 1958.

Chapter XX

THE DETERIORATIVE TRENDS IN THE CARDIOVASCULAR SYSTEM

GEORGE C. GRIFFITH

(Los Angeles, California, U.S.A.)

THE art of detecting deteriorative trends in the cardiovascular system was a cherished dream 40 or more years ago. Medical science was concerned with anatomy, histology, physiology, biochemistry and pathology. Accordingly, it gave very little thought to the recognition of disease at its basic inception. In recent years numerous new facts have been learned, but these have served only to open the door to more unsolved problems. Today, many fundamental questions regarding the cardiovascular system remain unanswered. For example, what initiates the heart beat? What determines the rhythm? What are the intricacies of smooth muscle metabolism? When does deterioration begin? At conception? In utero? In the neonatal period, or in early adolescent life? How shall we define deterioration? Is it a decrease in the ability of the organism to deal effectively with environmental stress? Is it a loss of functional cellular units in key organ systems associated with the reduction in the functional capacities of the remaining cells, thus causing a slow deterioration of the integrative functions? Does the cardiovascular system die a bit every day? Deterioration must include involutional as well as abiotrophic changes.

The roles of heredity, environment, nutrition, disease, trauma, abuse and disuse all need to be clarified.

Tissue culture studies of the heart cells have raised many questions. The heart and the major blood vessels develop almost entirely between the third and eighth weeks of life, the pacemaker being the last area to appear. However, these structures begin to function before innervation takes place. Isolated myocardial cells in a culture medium demonstrate rhythmic beating at a rate varying from 10 to 150 times per minute. These isolated heart cells assume various shapes and emit long finger-like filaments. Eventually the cells make contact, form a network of cells, and multiply. Then an amazing event takes place: the cells no longer maintain an individual rate of beating, but they begin to beat in rhythmic unison with the pace apparently being set by the most rapidly beating cell or group of cells in the network. What constitutes the autorhythmicity of the isolated cell? What is the source of energy for the activity of these cells? May any cell act as a pacemaker? Why does a cell die if it does not unite with its neighbor? Why do certain of these cells form a rosette and act as a pacemaker? These tissue culture cells are extremely sensitive to changes in temperature and alteration in nutrients. Would the smooth muscle cell live indefinitely if bathed in the proper milieu of nutrients? What is it that causes maldevelopment of these cells in the first 90 days after fertilization of the ova? Is there a viral etiology as many believe? Is the deformity a basically faulty cytoplasm, or is it the result of some autoimmune reaction which interferes with the normal development of the heart and its great vessels at this very early period? Is a heart or great vessel which is deformed at birth not only a deformed heart, but are the heart cells already old? Is it a heart with altered cytoplasm? Today there is neither an answer to the problem of the etiology of congenital heart deformities, nor an accepted answer to the state of the myocardial cell cytoplasm.

The Lysosome Granule

A smooth muscle cell is characterized by automaticity, rhythmicity, irritability, and contractility. Such substances as ribonucleic acid, mucin, and actin are within the cell. The nucleus contains desoxyribonucleic acid. The cell carries an electrical charge. Before we can determine when deterioration begins, we need to know the biochemistry of the normal functioning cell in detail. Is the life span of a normal cell three score and ten, or may it be six score years? The study of the ultrastructure of cells with the electron microscope, coupled with enzyme study, has yielded valuable information. Mitochondria conduct the primary energy transformation of the cell, and the smaller organelles, called ribosomes, are the centers of enzyme production. The lysosomes, which are as yet undefined

are the latest addition to the list of organelles. Many believe that they are the first evidences of deterioration. Does their appearance indicate diminished function, or the very beginning of myocardial cell death? The lysosomes have been separated from other subcellular particles by fractional centrifugation. Electron microscopic studies show that they may assume a variety of shapes and sizes. The particular contours are apparently a function of the concentration in the stage of the disintegration of the variety of substances and objects that are being digested within the lysosome. The lysosome granules are believed to contain powerful hydrolytic enzymes such as ribonuclease, desoxyribonuclease, phosphatase, cathepsin, glycosidase and sulfatase. How do these substances function? It is believed that three different modes of activity are apparent. First, in the white cells and other scavenger cells that aggregate in areas of cellular destruction, the lysosomes are engaged in normal digestive functions inside the cell. Second, a process termed "autophagy" appears to occur, during which particular portions of a cell somehow gain entrance into the lysosomes and are broken down— the lysosomes functioning as intracellular disposal units. A third mode of action involves the rupture of the lysosomal membrane inside the cell, and the autodigestion of the entire smooth muscle cell. This raises the challenging question of the nature of the lysosome membrane which enables the organelle to contain enzymes which, upon liberation, are capable of digesting the entire smooth muscle cell.

Some recent studies indicate that cortisone and hydrocortisone have a stabilizing influence on the lysosome membrane. It is known that the endocrine glands regulate a large number of biological processes from cellular metabolism to the regulation of the diameter of small blood vessels. Measurements suggest a decrease in the functional capacity of the adrenal cortex, advancing with age, and there is a reduction in the level of adrenal steroids in the plasma and urine with increasing age. What effect, if any, does the decrease of adrenal hormones have upon the function of the smooth muscle cell? May a decrease in circulating steroids promote myocardial cell death through altered action of the lysosomes? These are problems concerning the early detection of degeneration.

The Age Pigment

How is aging related to the accumulation within the cell of age pigment? Is this pigment derived from the lysosome? Myocardial pilofuchsin (that is, age pigment) is absent in the very young, and universally present in the myocardial cells of older subjects. One study of hearts in individuals under the age of 10 years reported no age pigment in the myocardial cell, and an increase in age pigment concentration linearly with age. Age pigment may represent as much as 30 per cent of the total solid of a muscle fiber as late maturity is reached. Thus, age pigment appears to be associated with the basic biologic process of smooth muscle cell deterioration.

Myocardial Biopsies

When individuals aged 100 to 120 die from injury, infection, or carcinoma, do their hearts appear old biochemically and structurally? It has been noted that there was a progressive grey-white thickening which develops within the first decade, primarily in the right atrium and then in the ventricle. With advancing age these lesions become more and more prominent. In the elderly, endocardial thickening appears to be a relatively constant finding. Is this thickening of the endocardium due to direct mechanical stress of a hydrostatic nature, or may it be due to nonsuppurative inflammatory disease, caused by hypersensitivity or autoimmunity?

In the hypersensitivity state which, for example, is rheumatic fever, there appears to be a faulty antigen antibody reaction which first results in a cloudy swelling of the myocardial cell, a breakdown of the collagen and the adhesive substances affecting the nutrient arteries of the heart.

Autoimmunity suggests the development in the smooth muscle cell of a pathological reaction to its own tissue. Autoimmunity implies that, for some unknown reason, a response resulting in a change in tissue structures, which is perhaps pathological, occurs. Autoimmunity is an ill-defined reaction which may in itself lead to deterioration, or, on the other hand, it may be a protective mechanism. There are scientists who adhere to the hypothesis that, as a consequence of spontaneous somatic mutations or other genetic alterations, the cells of the individual gradually undergo increasing immunogenic diversification during his lifetime. This diversification in turn leads to prolonged minor degrees of cellular incompatability or immune reaction in the tissue, and such reactions may be pathogenetically related to the aging process. As of this moment, autoimmunity, like hypersensitivity, presents basic unsolved problems as far as the heart and blood vessels are concerned.

Objective Evidence of Age-Induced Deterioration

There is a reduction in the reserve capacity of the body which appears with age. A general pattern emerges, consisting of a constant decrease in organ function, clinically recognizable at about 30 years of age. For example, in comparing the vital functions of the average 30-year-old man with a man 75 years of age, the blood flow to the brain of the 75-year-old man is 80 per cent of the 30-year-old control. The resting cardiac output is 70 per cent. The kidney plasma flow is 42 per cent. For a given exercise the blood pressure will increase more in the older person when compared with a 30-year-old counterpart; but, with maximal exertion the overall heart rate of the older person is less than that of the younger person and the cardiac output of the older subject is progressively less. The basal metabolic rate of the 75-year-old man is 84 per cent of the 30-year-old control. The maximal work capacity is 70 per cent. The vital capacity of the lungs is 56 per cent. Body water content falls to 82 per cent and the glomerular filtration rate is 69 per cent of the control. What effect does the reduction in vital function have upon the work of the cardiovascular structures? Will such changes accelerate the degenerating process? Such factors as blood glucose, protein-bound iodine, plasma and blood volume, and hemoglobin concentration all remain fairly constant throughout life. However, striated muscle mass decreases by 50 per cent due to a replacement of the cells by fat and fibrous connective tissue. From these facts we can conclude that a key characteristic of deterioration is a reduction in the reserve capacities of the body, and that there is a loss of functional

tissue resulting from the complex interplay of different organ systems.

Electrocardiogram

Does the electrocardiogram yield any information regarding degeneration? The coexistence of diseases in elderly patients creates difficulty in attempting to pinpoint electrocardiographic changes which are completely and solely due to the primary process of degeneration. In one study of 347 patients over the age of 70, who had no clinical evidence of organic disease, 34 per cent of the electrocardiograms were abnormal. In another study among Japanese over the age of 80, who had no other demonstrable evidence of cardiovascular disease, 84 per cent had abnormal electrocardiograms. The most common abnormalities were those of left ventricular hypertrophy, low voltage, prolonged Q-T interval and myocardial ischemia.

Hypertension

There is some evidence which suggests that essential hypertension may be a disease of single or multiple enzymatic defects. What role these enzymes play in hypertension, and what influence their derangements and the resulting hypertension have in early deterioration of myocardial tissue is not specifically known. We do know, however, that hypertension accelerates the atherosclerotic process.

Baroceptors

What is the role of the baroceptor mechanism in preventing or accelerating early degenerative changes in the cardiovascular system? We do know that the baroceptor system may divert adequate blood supply to vital organs where such a supply is needed; but, what are the degenerative results in those organs which are deprived of an adequate blood supply at the times of such diversion?

Atherosclerosis

Atherosclerosis is the challenge of this era. It is to be found in all decades of life even though much more prominent in the aged. As a disease which interferes with the blood and oxygen supply of tissues, particularly in the heart muscle, it must be considered as a potent factor in the development of degenerative changes in the myocardial cells.

The consequences of total vascular occlusion are obvious but, apart from this extreme situation, the common coincidence of atherosclerotic vascular rigidity or narrowing with an overactivity of the oxygen-utilization-augmenting sympathoadrenal system (induced by all kinds of stresses, nicotine action, and lack of exercise) entails detrimental and often fatal discrepancies between oxygen supply and demand. Hypoxic degeneration of the heart muscle is thus promoted in a large number of instances by combined vascular hemodynamic and neurogenic metabolic factors. In addition, it has been shown many times that, even in the absence of vascular abnormalities, an excess of sympathoadrenal neurohormones is apt to produce multiple degenerative and necrotic lesions in the myocardium.

Sex and Genetic Factors

Cardiovascular defects and disease claim 35 per cent more male than female infants in the first year of life. This difference remains true throughout a lifetime, and today we believe that the female hormone provides a protective mechanism against the degenerative process. However, we cannot say, conversely, that the male hormone accelerates degenerative processes.

Metalloenzymes

Alterations occurring in the metalloenzyme complexes apparently influence degenerative processes and accelerate atherosclerosis. At present, the relationship between enzymes and substrate in the genesis of degeneration is a matter of conjecture. The role which metalloenzyme complexes play in preventing or accelerating the degenerative process is unknown.

SUMMARY

In conclusion, it may be stated that a human being who has a favorable family background, remains normal in weight, has a normal fat metabolism, is free from hypertension, and avoids the excesses of life while possessing the habits of adequate exercise and rest, is in a favorable position to prevent the early development of cardiovascular degeneration.

The era of molecular medicine is upon us. Future biophysicochemical investigations will possibly unlock some of the cell's secrets, and provide us with a fuller understanding of the basic factors which control the degenerative processes in cardiovascular structure, and which must be counteracted for effective prevention.

But can we afford to wait for decades, until all theoretical problems are solved, and ignore already available, though fragmentary, knowledge, before taking positive preventive action without paralyzing timidity?

SECTION II
EPIDEMIOLOGIC DATA

Chapter XXI

EARLY RECOGNITION OF COVERT ISCHEMIC HEART DISEASE*

MENARD M. GERTLER and HARVEY H. WHITER

(New York, New York, U.S.A.)

THE Coronary Research Project, organized in 1946 at the Massachusetts General Hospital, set out to study and classify the clinical clues associated with ischemic heart disease. As early as 1949, a presentation based upon preliminary findings was given to the New York Heart Association which outlined the so-called "coronary profile" (1). This coronary profile demonstrated that patients with ischemic heart disease have several features which could distinguish them from the putative normal population. This was the first attempt to delineate individual differences in the "coronary-prone" individual in an effort to differentiate him from other members of his society before the overt symptoms of the disease occurred. It was followed by several further publications (2–8), and as a result of these studies it is generally accepted today that there exists in the putatively normal male populations a group of men who are singularly candidates for ischemic heart disease.

Some variables, associated with proneness to ischemic heart disease, are the following:

Cholesterol. There is abundant evidence which indicates that the level of serum cholesterol is intimately associated with the presence of ischemic heart disease, but although it is one of the best single predictors of the disease, it is far from perfect (2).

Phospholipids. In many biological systems where cholesterol and phospholipids are present, there is a biologic antagonism between them (9). In ischemic heart disease and in normal adults, there is almost a fixed relationship between total cholesterol and lipid phosphorus (3). The linear regression formula was able to recognize the protective action of the phospholipids against coronary heart disease and placed a negative value on the phospholipids in the formula.

Uric Acid. Previous studies have shown that uric acid is correlated with weight $+0.23 \pm .10$ and $+0.26 \pm .10$ in both a coronary group and a control group, respectively. There is also a negative correlation with ponderal index in both groups $-0.22 \pm .10$ and $-0.25 \pm .10$ (6). It becomes apparent, therefore, since uric acid tends to increase positively with weight and negatively with the ponderal index, that the more compact the individual (that is, endomorphic or mesomorphic), the higher will be the uric

*Supported by a grant from the John A. Hartford Foundation, Inc., New York City, and the Vocational Rehabilitation Administration, Grant RD 1715-M-65.

acid, statistically speaking. Hence, uric acid determinations may, on theoretical grounds, prove useful in the detection and classification of ischemic heart disease.

Body Weight and Body Build. The author and his colleagues suggested in 1951 that "overweight" had little or no bearing on the presence or absence of ischemic heart disease (10). The publication at that time revealed that in comparing a control group and a coronary group to the army height-age-weight standards, the control group deviated +19.13 pounds while the coronary group deviated +18.49 pounds. In a recent series, the actual mean weight of a noncoronary group was 171 pounds while the mean weight of the coronary group was 173 pounds.

Body build was of prime interest to our research project and it demonstrated beyond any doubt that the young "pure" coronary individual was predominantly mesomorphic and showed a paucity of ectomorphy. This observation has been confirmed by several groups (11). Recent data have shown that in the coronary patient of average 53 years, mesomorphy was again dominant, and, in comparison with a noncoronary group, the values were $4.6 \pm .16$ and $4.2 \pm .05$. The coronary patient and the noncoronary control weighed almost the same but the coronary patient is shorter and hence a more compact individual of different body build.

Height. A negative correlation between height and ischemic heart disease exists in the U.S.A. It is more inexplicable than any other of the factors involved in ischemic heart disease.

†x: 46.56 years; Range: 23.00 to 79.00; St. Dev.: 10.91; St. Error: .49.

of the coronary-prone individual was documented in a prospective study of 490 men †, 32 of whom were coronary-prone. It was found that the incidence

Family History. The importance of positive family histories in the selection of ischemic heart disease was significantly greater (p < .001) in the parents and siblings of the men in the coronary-prone group than in the parents and siblings of the men in the noncoronary-prone group. Fathers with a positive history of coronary heart disease were noted in 12 (38 per cent and 58 (13 per cent) of the individuals from the prone and nonprone groups, respectively; mothers with a positive history of coronary heart disease were noted in 12 (38 per cent) and 27 (6 per cent) of the individuals from the prone and nonprone groups, respectively; siblings with a positive history of coronary heart disease were noted in 11 (34 per cent) and 14 (3 per cent) of the individuals from the prone and nonprone groups, respectively (8).

Data in support of the familial nature of coronary heart disease were also obtained from a study on young adults (6).

Smoking. Cigarette smoking has been considered by some groups to be an important etiologic factor in the genesis of ischemic heart disease.

In reporting the results of the Coronary Research Project in 1951, it was noted that, on the average, the ischemic heart disease group smoked more cigarettes daily than did the control group (19.4 ± 1.6 and 13.8 ± 1.1 cigarettes daily, respectively). There were, also, proportionately more people in the ischemic heart disease group who smoked (90 per cent versus 77 per cent for the coronary and noncoronary groups, respectively) (5). There is no doubt that this and other

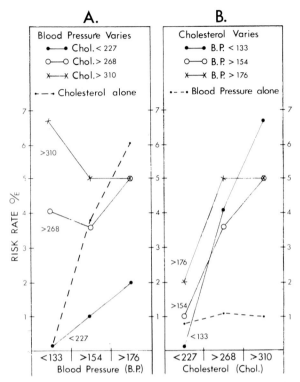

Figure 21–1. This figure shows the interrelationships of changing blood pressure values and changing serum cholesterol levels on the risk rate of coronary artery disease in healthy men. Note the effects of serum cholesterol levels alone (1A) and the effects of blood pressure values alone (1B).

published data indicate an association between cigarette smoking and coronary heart disease, but this does not prove a causal relationship. It is, therefore, not surprising that the inclusion of cigarette smoking as an additional variable in the linear discrimination analysis increased precision only by a negligible 0.05 per cent.

Blood Pressure. No significant differences between coronary-prone and non-prone men were found with respect to either systolic or diastolic blood pressure in a prospective study of 490 men (8), whereby 18.8 per cent and 15.1 per cent of the prone and non-prone groups, respectively, had systolic blood pressures above x + σ (154 mm of Hg) and 15.6

per cent and 13.5 per cent of the prone and non-prone groups, respectively, had diastolic pressures above x + σ (94 mm of Hg), the differences being nonsignificant.

It has been claimed that hypertension and hypercholesterolemia act synergistically to increase the risk rate of coronary artery disease. This hypothesis was tested by determining the risk rates (number observed/number expected x 100) of elevated cholesterol alone, and the combination of elevated blood pressure and cholesterol. Of 79 individuals with cholesterol values above x + σ (268 mg%), 19 were coronary-prone, where 5.15 were expected, giving a risk rate of 369. Of the 79, 17 also had systolic pressures above x+σ (154 mm of Hg), and 4 individuals in this group were coronary-prone, where 1.11 were expected, giving a risk rate of 360. Performing the same analysis with diastolic pressures, a risk rate of 385 was found for the group with both elevated cholesterol (above 268 mg%), and elevated diastolic pressures above x+σ (94 mm of Hg). The addition of elevated pressures, then, resulted in no change in risk rate (Fig. 21–1) (8, 12).

Electrocardiographic Information.

The electrocardiogram is valuable as an indicator of apparent ischemic heart disease but its usefulness is confined to this area, for electrocardiographic abnormalities indicate pathology already directly apparent in the heart. Thus, for predictive purposes, the resting electrocardiogram has no value, while the exercise electrocardiogram may be helpful in classifying covert ischemic heart disease (13).

THE MULTIPLE VARIABLE APPROACH

The published data from the Coronary Research Project showed that the coronary and noncoronary populations studied possessed distinguishing characteristics along biochemical, anthropometrical, and inheritance dimensions, among others, with respect to mean values. However, in reporting the results of the study, attention was called to the considerable area of overlap exhibited by the distribution of the variables in the coronary and noncoronary groups (2, 4). In such a situation, reliance on a single variable for classificatory purposes is not indicated, but it is possible to find a linear combination of measures on the various dimensions whose distributions for the

coronary and noncoronary populations possess very little overlap. This linear discrimination function takes the many relevant variables and yields one index number, or profile score, which summarizes the information contained in all the variables with respect to proneness to ischemic heart disease.

The profile score gives mathematical expression to individual differences, for it is the result of a linear combination of all the relevant factors, with each factor weighted according to the importance of its contribution to the picture of coronary-proneness. This profile score, as developed by this group, is calculated from the equation published previously in detail (7).

THE INDIVIDUAL VARIABLE VERSUS THE MULTIPLE VARIABLE IN THE EARLY RECOGNITION OF COVERT CORONARY HEART DISEASE

In the Prospective Study of Coronary Heart Disease (8), it was found that 78 per cent of individuals may be identified as coronary-prone if their stature is below the mean value of the group (69.17 inches). Cholesterol values above x+σ (268 mg%) identified 59 per cent of individuals as coronary-prone. Lipid phosphorus values above x+σ (12.03 mg%), uric acid values above x+σ (6.80 mg%), and a mesomorphic rating above x+σ (5.24) identified 44 per cent, 28 per cent and 16 per cent of the individuals, respectively, as coronary-prone. The comparable identification value of the various variables is summarized in Figure 21–2.

An examination of the risk rates of the various variables is helpful in assessing their identification value for detecting

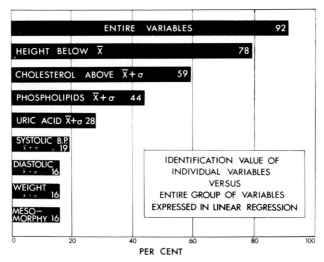

Figure 21–2. This figure summarizes the identification value of each variable independently in comparison with all variables together, expressed as a linear regression value.

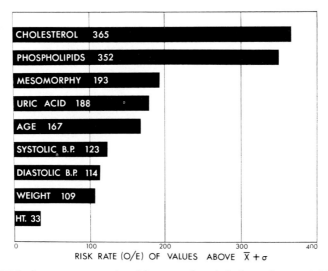

Figure 21–3. This figure expresses the risk rates of each independent variable when their values are above the mean plus one standard deviation (i.e., $\bar{X} + \sigma$).

the coronary-prone individual. In Figure 21–3, most of the variables which enter the linear discrimination formula are listed with their specific risk rates. Cholesterol serum values above $x + \sigma$ (268 mg%), have a risk rate of 365, whereas height values above $x + \sigma$ (71 inches) have a risk rate of 33. Weight values over $x + \sigma$ (195 pounds) have a risk rate of 109. Systolic blood pressures over $x + \sigma$ (154 mm mercury) have a risk rate of 114 and 123, respectively.

Proof of the superior accuracy of the multiple-variable technic is found in the data of the prospective study. Using the entire combination of relevant variables:

height, cholesterol, lipid phosphorus, uric acid, body build, and family history, each with the proper weighting as expressed in the linear discrimination function, maximal identification value is achieved. Of the 490 men in the sample population at the beginning of the study, 32 were designated coronary-prone on the basis of their profile score. Of these 32 originally symptom-free men, 22 have experienced myocardial infarction (2 recently), 5 of whom have expired, 8 have angina pectoris proven by clinical symptomatology or electrocardiogram, or both, and 2 are now free from any disease. This gives a prospective prediction of 94 per cent.

It should be noted that only one individual from the 458 designated as noncoronary-prone has experienced a myocardial infarction.

SUMMARY

Evidence has been presented to demonstrate that individual variables such as height, cholesterol, uric acid, phospholipids, heredity, body build, weight, blood pressure and tobacco have a certain value with regard to the prediction of ischemic heart disease.

However, the combination of relevant variables, each with the proper weighting as expressed in the linear discrimination function, was shown to have maximal identification value for selecting, prospectively, the coronary-prone individual. Furthermore, this multiple-variable approach gives mathematical expression to individual differences along biochemical, anthropometrical and inheritance dimensions.

Weight has been shown to be useful only as it reflects mesomorphy; otherwise it has no real meaning. Blood pressure

has been shown to make no significant contribution towards detecting the coronary-prone individual. Furthermore, hypertension and hypercholesterolemia do not act synergistically to increase the risk rate of ischemic heart disease.

Evidence has been presented which lends support to previous findings that individuals classified as coronary-prone are older, shorter, have higher values for serum cholesterol, uric acid, and phospholipids, are more mesomorphic, and show more positive family histories.

REFERENCES

1. GERTLER, M. M.: Some morphological, hormonal and biochemical aspects of the young coronary patient. New York Heart Assn., Science Session, New York, Feb., 1949.
2. GERTLER, M. M., GARN, S. M., and LERMAN, J.: The interrelationships of serum cholesterol, cholesterol esters and phospholipids in health and in coronary artery disease. *Circulation*, 2:205, 1950.
3. GERTLER, M. M., and GARN, S. M.: Lipid interrelationship in health and in coronary artery disease. *Science*, *112*:14, 1950.
4. GERTLER, M. M., DRISKELL, E. F., BLAND, E. F., GARN, S. M., LERMAN, J., SPRAGUE, H. B., LEVINE, S. A., and WHITE, P. D.: Clinical aspects of coronary heart disease. *JAMA*, *146*:1291, 1951.
5. GERTLER, M. M., GARN, S. M., and WHITE, P. D.: Young candidates for coronary heart disease. *JAMA*, *147*:621, 1951.
6. GERTLER, M. M., and WHITE, P. D.: Coronary heart disease in young adults. A multidisciplinary study. Harvard University Press and Commonwealth Fund, Massachusetts, 1954.
7. GERTLER, M. M., WOODBURY, M. A., GOTTSCH, L. G., WHITE, P. D., and RUSK, H. A.: The candidate for coronary heart disease. *JAMA*, *170*:149, 1959.
8. GERTLER, M. M., WHITE, P. D., CADY, L. D., and WHITER, H. H.: Coronary heart disease. A prospective study. *Amer J Med Sci*, *248*:377, 1964.
9. BROWDER, A.: The effect of lecithin and cholesterol upon the division rate of paramecium. Univ. of California Publishers, *Physiol*, *5*(1): 1, 1915.
10. GARN, S. M., GERTLER, M. M., LEVINE, S. A.,

and WHITE, P. D.: Body weight versus weight standards in coronary artery disease and a healthy group. *Ann Intern Med, 34:*1416, 1951.

11. SPAIN, D. M., NATHAN, D. J., and GELLIS, M.: Weight, body type and the prevalence of coronary atherosclerotic heart disease in males. *Amer J Med Sci, 245:*63, 1963.

12. GERTLER, M. M., and WHITER, H. H.: Individ-

ual differences relating to coronary artery disease. *Ann N Y Acad Sci.,* in press.

13. ROBB, G. P., MARKS, H. H., and MATTINGLY, T. W.: The value of the double standard 2-step exercise test in the detection of coronary heart disease. A clinical and statistical follow-up of military personnel and insurance applicants *Trans Ass Life Ins Med Dir Amer, 40:*52, 1957.

Chapter XXII

TOBACCO AND CARDIOVASCULAR DISEASE

JOSEPH T. DOYLE

(Albany, New York, U.S.A.)

ALTHOUGH tobacco was first introduced into Europe nearly 400 years ago under ecclesiastical and medical auspices, opposition to its use as a hazard to health promptly arose. Objections were based primarily on moralistic and anecdotal evidence, although in the nineteenth century a relationship between pipe smoking and oropharyngeal carcinoma was convincingly shown (1). In the early twentieth century European clinicians were much concerned with tobacco angina, an entity no longer considered to exist (2). In 1908 Bürger described thromboangiitis obliterans, a syndrome ascribed to unusual sensitivity to tobacco. Recently, however, the specificity of this disorder has been questioned by Wessler (3, 4). Save for Bürger's disease, no histologic lesions attributable to tobacco have ever been found in human subjects or experimentally induced in animals.

The combustion products of tobacco are irritant to the oral and bronchial mucosa and some are carcinogenic. The circulatory responses to tobacco smoking or chewing, however, are entirely due to the speed and quantity with which nicotine is absorbed. The pharmacologic effect of nicotine is to stimulate the secretion of epinephrine and norepinephrine from the walls of blood vessels, from myocardial ganglia and from the adrenal medulla. No convincing effects of tobacco or of nicotine on the coagulation mechanism have yet been demonstrated (5).

The first strong evidence that the use of tobacco, specifically in the form of cigarettes, has an adverse effect on cardiovascular mortality, was incidental to the large retrospective studies of bronchiogenic carcinoma. (6, 7, 8, 9). These data showed a more than twofold higher death rate from cardiovascular disease in heavy cigarette smokers compared with nonsmokers and pipe and cigar smokers. The majority of these deaths were, of course, due to coronary heart disease. It is of interest that at about the same time the initial experience of two large prospective studies of coronary heart disease, in Framingham, Massachusetts, and in Albany, New York, showed little apparent association between smoking habit and the various manifestations of coronary heart disease (10, 11). The strength of this association in the retrospective cancer studies, however, was so great as to compel further scrutiny of the question. It was therefore decided in 1961 to pool the information on male participants in these two studies in the expecta-

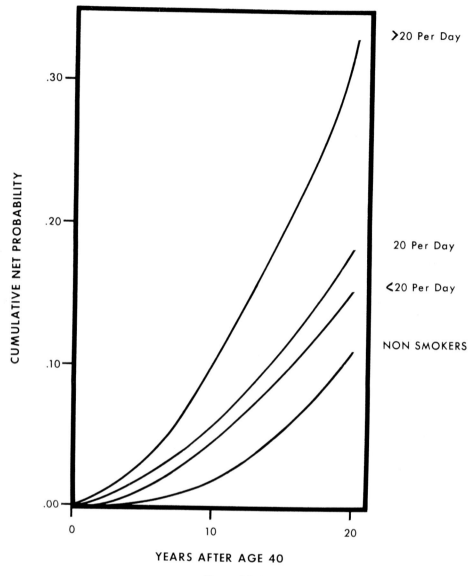

Figure 22–1.

tion that the numbers would be large enough to permit statistically significant inferences as to the association between smoking habit and cardiovascular morbidity and mortality (12).

Figure 22–1 shows the probability of developing coronary heart disease after age 40 related to smoking habit.

In brief, the pooled data showed that in 4,120 men ranging from 30 to 62 years of age, those who smoked 20 or more cigarettes daily experienced myocardial infarction two to three times more frequently than nonsmokers, ex-smokers, or pipe and cigar smokers. The adverse effect of cigarette smoking is independent of obesity and of arterial blood pressure, and apparently of serum total cholesterol concentration except perhaps at levels above 275 mg/100ml. There is some suggestion that the smoking effect is related to the length and intensity of exposure, while cessation of cigarette smoking is followed rather promptly by a reduction in risk. On the other hand, no association appears to exist between smoking habit and angina pectoris, an observation also made 3 decades earlier by White and Sharber. The findings of these two studies after 8 and 10 years, respectively, show the same trends (13).

The manner in which smoking cigarettes adversely influences morbidity and mortality from cardiovascular diseases is unclear (14). Heavy smokers die sooner of all causes, so the effect in cardiovascular diseases may be nonspecific. On the other hand, the powerful lipid-mobilizing effects of the catecholamines mobilized by nicotine suggest that atherogenesis, and particularly its occlusive features, might be favored by this mechanism. Moreover, an already ischemic myocardium is especially vulnerable to catecholamines. The negative association between smoking habit and angina is puzzling. It may well be that the pathogenesis of this syndrome is different and perhaps unrelated to the thrombotic-occlusive aspects of atheroslcerosis.

While no causal relationship between cigarette smoking and acute myocardial infarction is claimed, the therapeutic inference is clear *viz* cigarette smoking is a major risk factor in coronary heart disease and should be vigorously discouraged. The psychosocial and economic factors which reinforce the cigarette habit, however, are so powerful as to discourage and frustrate efforts to abolish even this blatant threat to good health and longevity.

SUMMARY

The cardiovascular effects of tobacco smoke are due to the amount and rate of nicotine absorption. All acute circulatory responses are accounted for by the powerful mobilization of catecholamines effected by nicotine. No tissue changes are caused by nicotine. Death from all causes occurs at an increased rate in heavy cigarette smokers. Most of these excess deaths are due to sudden cardiac death and to acute myocardial infarction.

Cessation of cigarette smoking is followed by a reduction in risk.

REFERENCES

1. HAMMOND, E. C.: The effects of smoking. *Sci Amer*, 207:39, 1962.
2. VON AHN, B.: Tobacco smoking, the electrocardiogram, and angina pectoris. *Ann N Y Acad. Sci.*, 90:190, 1960.
3. BÜRGER, L.: Thrombo-angiitis obliterans: study of vascular lesions leading to presenile spontaneous gangrene. *Amer J Med Sci*, 136:567, 1908.
4. WESSLER, S., MING, S., GUREWICH, V., and FREIMAN, D. G.: A critical evaluation of thrombo-angiitis obliterans. The case against Bürger's disease. *New Eng J Med*, 262:1149, 1960.
5. Cardiovascular effects of nicotine and smoking. *Ann N Y Acad Sci*, 90:1–344, 1960.
6. DOLL, R., and HILL, A. B.: Lung cancer and other causes of death in relation to smoking: second report on mortality of British doctors. *Brit Med J*, 2:1071, 1956.
7. DORN, H. F.: Tobacco consumption and mortality from cancer and other diseases. *Public Health Rep*, 74:581, 1959.
8. HAMMOND, E. C., and HORN, D.: Smoking and death rates—report on forty-four months of followup of 187,783 men. I. Total mortality. *JAMA*, 166:1159, 1958; II. Death rates by cause. *Ibid.*, p. 1294.
9. *Smoking and Health.* Report of the Advisory Committee to the Surgeon General of the Public Health Service. Washington, Public Health Service, Publication No. 1103 (1964).
10. DAWBER, T. R., MOORE, F. E., and MANN, G. V.: II. Coronary heart disease in the Framingham study. *Amer J Public Health*, 47:No. 4, April, 1957.
11. DOYLE, J. T., HESLIN, A. S., HILLEBOE, H. E., FORMEL, P. F., and KORNS, R. F.: III. A pros-

pective study of degenerative cardiovascular disease in Albany: report of three years' experience. I. Ischemic heart disease. *Amer J Public Health*, 47:No. 4, April, 1957.

12. DOYLE, J. T., DAWBER, T. R., KANNEL, W. B., HESLIN, A. S., and KAHN, H. A.: Cigarette smoking and coronary heart disease. Combined experience of the Albany and Framingham studies. *New Eng J Med*, 266:796, 1962.

13. DOYLE, J. T., DAWBER, T. R., KANNEL, W. B., KINCH, S. H., and KAHN, H. A.: The relationship of cigarette smoking to coronary heart disease. The second report of the combined experience of the Albany and Framingham studies. *JAMA*, 190:886, 1964.

14. WILENS, S. L., and PLAIR, C. M.: Cigarette smoking and arteriosclerosis. *Science*, 138:975, 1962.

Chapter XXIII

EMOTIONAL STRESS, TOBACCO SMOKING AND ISCHEMIC HEART DISEASE

HENRY I. RUSSEK

(Staten Island, New York, U.S.A.

THE finding that occupation-related emotional stress may play an even more significant role in the causation of ischemic heart attacks in young persons than heredity, dietary fat, tobacco consumption, or obesity, or lack of vigorous physical activity (Table 23–1), had led to the expectation of an unequal distribution of the disease among various occupational categories in the United States. To determine whether or not such a gradient in ischemic heart disease prevalence does indeed exist, it was decided to conduct a survey in selected types of employment which differ significantly with respect to "tensions" created by routine demands of the job. Although the claim is undoubtedly valid that "stress" cannot be measured by the "dimensions of the load" in the individual case, experience does permit us to identify certain occupational classes that are subject to strain more than others. By such vocational comparisons, we have sought to test the hypothesis that stress is an important trigger variable in the etiology of ischemic heart disease in populations subsisting on a "high fat" diet.

In this approach, we have also attempted to elicit possible interrelationships among job stress, tobacco consumption, and ischemic heart disease preval-ence. Current acceptance of a causal relationship between smoking and ischemic heart disease rests primarily on statistical correlation and on the fact that nicotine causes transient discharges of potentially cardiotoxic catecholamines via ganglionic stimulation. Besides, excessive smoking, like overeating and failure to obtain adequate exercise, is widely recognized as a common manifestation of emotional stress.

METHOD OF STUDY

After careful consideration, it was decided to seek data on various categorie-of practice within the professions of medicine, dentistry and law. In each professional class, general practice was assigned to the highest level of occupational stress while selected specialties were ranked in order of stressfulness according to our own personal appraisals. In addition to these groups, comparison was to be made between stock exchange security analysts and security traders. In order to determine whether or not our judgement of occupational demands is in agreement with the findings of others, qualified judges were requested to submit their independent evaluations. By this means we sought to provide assurance that our judgment was in no way influenced by

TABLE 23–I

INCIDENCE OF VARIOUS FACTORS IN YOUNG SUBJECTS WITH ISCHEMIC HEART
DISEASE AND IN CONTROL GROUPS

	No.	*Heredity (Positive)*	*High-Fat Diet*	*Stress and Strain (Occupational)*	*Obesity*	*Tobacco (30 cigs.)*	*Exercise*
Ischemic Heart Disease Group	100	67%	53%	91%	26%	70%	58%
Control Group	100	40%	20%	20%	20%	35%	60%
Ratio		1.7:1	2.7:1	4.6:1	1.3:1	2:1	1:1

TABLE 23–II

RESULTS OF RANKINGS OF SELECTED OCCUPATIONAL FIELDS
BY DEGREES OF STRESSFULNESS

	Occupational Field			
Composite Stress Rank	Medicine	Dentistry	Law	Securities
Least	Derm.	Perio.	Patent law	
Next Least	Path.	Ortho.	Various sp.	Analysts
Next Most	Anesth.	Or. surg.	Trial Law	
Most	G P	G P	G P	Traders
Judges	8 Physicians	7 Dentists	11 Attorneys	6 Experts
Coefficient of Concordance	.850	.951	.907	1.00
Statistical Significance	P<1%	P<1%	P<1%	P<1%

anything we had already known of ischemic heart disease and hypertension
among professional persons in the categories under consideration. The dimensions of stress which the judges employed
in formulating their rankings were regularity of working hours, variety of activities, frequency and importance of
"deadlines" and decisions, amount of
"hard work," opportunities for rest, and
others. Their judgements are summarized
in Table 23–II. It was found that there
was very high agreement with regard to
the "ranking by stressfulness" of the selected categories within each professional
group. The sums of ranks indicated that
the consensus rated the classes of work
within each profession in the following
order of increasing stressfulness:

Medicine: dermatology, pathology, an-
esthesiology, and general practice.

Dentistry: periodontia, orthodontia,
oral surgery, and general practice.

Law: patent law (nontrial), other specialties, trial law, general practice.

Securities: security analysis and security trading.

Questionnaires were sent out to 12,000
persons in the 14 professional categories
under consideration. Names of physicians
were selected at random from alternate
pages of the Directory of Medical Specialists of the American Medical Association and from the Membership Directory
of the American Academy of General
Practitioners. Names of attorneys were
obtained by random selection from the
Martindale-Hubbell Law Directory and
the Roster of the American Academy of
Trial Lawyers. Security analysts and
traders were also selected from national
association directories. The questionnaire
was primarily designed to determine the
hereditary background and prevalence
of ischemic or hypertensive heart disease,
or both, in the persons of the respective

TABLE 23–III
HEALTH SURVEY

1. Present Age_____   Height (in shoes)_____   Weight _____

2. Did a doctor ever tell you that you had any of the following?

Type of Ailment	Yes	No	Year of Onset
a) High Blood Pressure			
b) Angina Pectoris			
c) Heart Attack (coronary)			
d) Other Heart Condition (specify)			
e) Ulcer of Stomach			
f) Other Conditions (specify)			

3. Did illness (es) develop before or after entry into your present occupation?

Before _____   After _____   How Long Before or After _____

Remarks: _____

4. Smoking Data: Do You Smoke Now?   Yes_____   No_____

If 'Yes," how many . . .   Per Day   Age when smoking began:

Cigarettes _____
Cigars _____
Pipefuls _____   _____
    Age

If No," did you ever smoke?   Yes_____   No_____

If Yes," how many . . .   Per Day   Age when smoking began

Cigarettes _____   _____
Cigars _____   Age when smoking
Pipefuls _____   stopped: _____

5. Do you consider your work unusually stressful?   Yes_____   No_____

6. Signature: _____   Date: _____
    (not essential)

Code: CPA

groups, and the time of onset of these disorders in relation to commencement within the selected class of work (Table 23–III). In more than one-half of the total series, information was requested concerning smoking habits. Replies were received from 7,655 of the 11,881 surveyed (64.5 per cent), of which 4,981 were found usable (65.0 per cent) (Table 23–IV). The reasons for eliminating 35.0 per cent of the returns were as follows:

1. Owing to a negligible prevalence of ischemic heart disease in persons under the age of 40 and the relatively small number of returns in the age group 70 years and over, only persons from 40 through 69 years of age were included in the study.

2. Women were eliminated from the analysis because of the paucity of their numbers.

3. Failure to specify age or other perti-

TABLE 23–IV
QUESTIONNAIRE REPLIES

Occupational Field	Sent Out	Answered	No.	Used in Study % of Answered
Medicine:				
Anesthesiology	1,000	650	303	46.6
Dermatology	1,000	622	409	65.8
General practice	1,000	647	544	84.1
Pathology	1,000	668	581	87.0
Subtotal	4,000	2,587	1,837	71.0
Rate of response: 64.7%				
Dentistry				
General practice	1,000	657	418	63.6
Oral surgery	350	252	192	76.2
Orthodontia	650	412	304	73.8
Periodontia	251	198	186	93.9
Subtotal	2,251	1,519	1,100	72.4
Rate of response: 67.5%				
Law:				
General practice	1,000	634	337	53.2
Patent law	1,000	621	356	57.3
Trial law	1,000	658	354	53.8
Other specialties	750	468	245	52.4
Subtotal	3,750	2,381	1,292	54.3
Rate of response: 63.5%				
Securities:				
Traders	1,000	639	374	58.6
Analysts	880	529	378	71.5
Subtotal	1,880	1,168	752	64.4
Rate of response: 62.0%				
Total	11,881	7,655	4,981	65.0
Overall rate of response: 64.5%				

nent data was responsible for the elimination of a small number of questionnaires.

4. In a relatively small group, letters were returned because of death or the absence of forwarding addresses.

It is recognized that certain weaknesses are inherent in the questionnaire method of survey; most important is the unknown prevalence of disease among nonrespondents. The existence of unsuspected disease detectable only by careful medical examination is also not revealed by this technique of study. It seems probable, however, that the generally high educational level of persons in the study groups would appreciably lessen the likelihood that such disease would long remain unrecognized. The main advantage of the questionnaire method is that it affords an opportunity to obtain data on a large number of persons at low cost of time, effort, and expense.

RESULTS

Table 23–V shows the prevalence of ischemic heart disease and hypertension reported in respondent subjects by age decade and stress group. The most striking finding in the study was the tendency of ischemic heart disease prevalence rates to increase with advance in stress rank (Fig. 23–1). The observed gradient was

TABLE 23–V

ISCHEMIC HEART DISEASE AND HYPERTENSION
PREVALENCE BY AGE AND STRESS GROUP

Age	Stress Group*	HD	%HD	Hyp.	%Hyp.	Total
40–49	Low	4	0.70	18	3.17	568
	Medium	14	2.09	34	5.07	670
	High	33	4.20	39	4.96	786
	Total (40–49)	51	2.52	91	4.50	2,024
50–59	Low	24	5.42	26	5.87	443
	Medium	45	6.42	64	9.12	701
	High	84	11.40	62	8.41	737
	Total (50–59)	153	8.13	152	8.08	1,881
60–69	Low	18	7.38	23	9.43	244
	Medium	51	13.46	43	11.35	379
	High	88	19.43	48	10.60	453
	Total (60–69)	157	14.59	114	10.59	1,076
All Ages	Low	46	3.68	67	5.34	1,255
	(Age-Adjusted)		(3.91)		(5.59)	
	Medium	110	6.29	141	8.06	1,750
			(6.30)		(7.96)	
	High	205	10.37	149	6.98	1,976
			(10.31)		(7.49)	
	Total (40–69)	361	7.25	357	7.17	4,981
			(7.33)		(7.18)	

*Low: Dermatologists, orthodontists, patent lawyers and periodontists.
Medium: Oral surgeons, other lawyers, pathologists, security analysts and trial lawyers.
High: Anesthesiologists, GP dentistry, GP law, GP medicine and security traders.

found to be remarkably consistent within the age groups; statistical tests between high and low stress groups within decades were consistently significant beyond the .001 level. Whether the professional groups were classified collectively into low, medium, and high stress categories or considered separately, the same basic trend emerged. Thus, general practitioners in each of the fields of medicine, dentistry, and law showed prevalence rates for ischemic heart disease 2 to 3 times those of the specialists selected for the survey. These findings have been reported in detail previously (1, 2). Without exception, the prejudged ranking by stressfulness correlated remarkably with the relative prevalence of ischemic heart disease in the respective categories. As anticipated, the highly stressed security

trader was found to have a significantly higher prevalence of ischemic heart disease than his less stressed colleague, the security analyst, but this finding only emerges statistically within the 40 to 50 age span (P < .05).

The prevalence rates for hypertension were found to increase uniformly with advance in age (Table 23–V). In contrast with the pattern observed for ischemic heart disease, the trend of the prevalence rates for hypertension was significantly nonlinear (P < .05).

Usable data on smoking and ischemic heart disease history were received from 2,787 respondents, Table 23-VI shows coronary prevalence in relation to smoking incidence, stress group and age level. It is clearly apparent that the proportion of cases reported either to have been

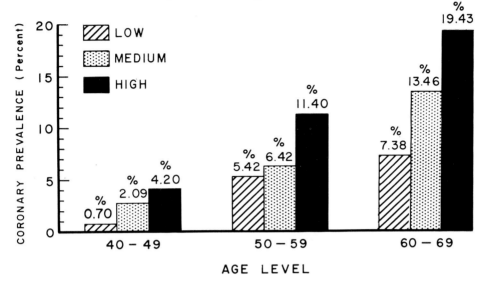

Figure 23–1. Incidence of ischemic heart disease by age and stress group.

TABLE 23–VI

ISCHEMIC HEART DISEASE PREVALENCE BY SMOKING INCIDENCE,
STRESS GROUP† AND AGE LEVEL

Age	Stress Group†	Never Smoked			Smoking Preference Stopped Smoking			Total Nonsmokers		
		HD	Total	%HD	HD	Total	%HD	HD	Total	%HD
40–49	Low	1	113	0.88	–	69	–	1	182	0.55
	Medium	1	57	1.75	–	45	–	1	102	0.98
	High	3	82	3.66	1	67	1.49	4	149	2.68
	Total 40–49	5	252	1.98	1	181	0.55	6	433	1.39
50–59	Low	6	78	7.69	1	80	1.25	7	158	4.43
	Medium	8	79	10.13	1	111	0.90	9	190	4.74
	High	6	80	7.50	2	107	1.87	8	187	4.28
	Total 50–59	20	237	8.44	4	298	1.34	24	535	4.49
60–69	Low	3	28	10.71	1	51	1.96	4	79	5.06
	Medium	4	46	8.70	6	72	8.33	10	118	8.47
	High	8	49	16.33	4	81	4.94	12	130	9.23
	Total 60–69	15	123	12.20	11	204	5.39	26	327	7.95
All	Low	10	219	4.57	2	200	1.00	12	419	2.86
Ages	Medium	13	182	7.14	7	228	3.07	20	410	4.88
	High	17	211	8.06	7	255	2.75	24	466	5.15
	Total 40–69	40	612	6.54	16	683	2.34	56	1,295	4.32

†Low Stress—Orthodontists, patent attorneys.
Medium Stress—Oral surgeons, security analysts, trial lawyers.
High Stress—GP dentists, general lawyers, security traders.

smoking during the years preceding a heart attack, if any, or else to be smoking at the time of the questionnaire survey, tends to rise with advance in occupation-related emotional stress (Figure 23–2). Even within the individual professions the trends in the data are consistent with the expectation of increase in smoking with advance in occupational stress. From Figure 23–3 and Table 23–VII, it

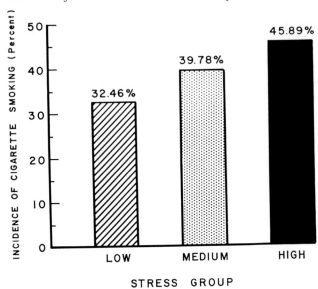

Figure 23–2. Smoking incidence by stress group.

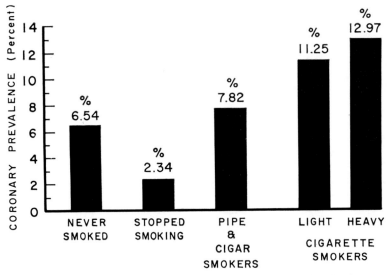

Figure 23–3. Incidence of ischemic heart disease by smoking habits.

is evident that prevalence of ischemic heart disease tends to increase with tobacco consumption. However, since comparisons among the 3 smoker classes (pipe and cigar, light cigarette, heavy cigarette) do not show that they are statistically distinct (Table 23–VII), it cannot be said that there is sufficient evidence in these data for the view that differential smoking habits are associated with "real" differences in prevalence of ischemic heart disease. Nevertheless, the dimension of smoking appears to contain 3 groups which exhibit parametrically distinct prevalences. The statistical probability is thus better than 99 per cent that a real difference in cardiac ischemic prevalence distinguishes the "Total Smoker" (10.86

TABLE 23–VII

ISCHEMIC HEART DISEASE PREVALENCE BY TYPE AND DEGREE OF SMOKING

Age	Stress Group*	Pipe and Cigar			Cigarettes						Total Cigarettes			Total Smokers and Nonsmokers		
					Light Smokers			Heavy Smokers								
		HD	Total	%HD	HD	Total	%HD	HD	Total	%HD	HD	Total	%HD	HD	Total	%HD
40–49	Low	1	37	2.70	2	76	2.63	–	24	–	2	100	2.00	4	319	1.25
	Medium	3	39	7.69	1	67	1.49	1	46	2.17	2	113	1.77	6	254	2.36
	High	3	41	7.32	5	109	4.59	3	63	4.76	8	172	4.65	15	362	4.14
	Total 40–49	7	117	5.98	8	252	3.17	4	133	3.01	12	385	3.12	25	935	2.67
	Low	2	40	5.00	10	73	13.70	3	27	11.11	13	100	13.00	22	298	7.38
	Medium	2	64	3.13	12	116	10.34	7	66	10.61	19	182	10.44	30	436	6.88
	High	5	49	10.20	18	136	13.24	18	99	18.18	36	235	15.32	49	471	10.40
	Total 50–59	9	153	5.88	40	325	12.31	28	192	14.58	68	517	13.15	101	1,205	8.38
60–69	Low	2	20	10.00	9	34	26.47	2	14	14.29	11	48	22.92	17	147	11.56
	Medium	4	32	12.50	9	41	21.95	7	24	29.17	16	65	24.62	30	215	13.95
	High	7	49	14.29	15	68	22.06	11	38	28.95	26	106	24.53	45	285	15.79
	Total 60–69	13	101	12.87	33	143	23.08	20	76	26.32	53	219	24.20	92	647	14.22
All Ages	Low	5	97	5.15	21	183	11.48	5	65	7.69	26	248	10.48	43	764	5.63
	Medium	9	135	6.67	22	224	9.82	15	136	11.03	37	390	10.28	66	905	7.29
	High	15	139	10.79	38	313	12.14	32	200	16.00	70	513	13.65	109	1,118	9.75
	Total 40–69	29	371	7.82	81	720	11.25	52	401	12.97	133	1,121	11.86	218	2,787	7.82

*See Table 23–VI.

TABLE 23–VIII

PREVALENCE OF ISCHEMIC HEART DISEASE BY SMOKING INCIDENCE

	Never Smoked	Stopped Smoking	Pipe and Cigar	Cigarette Smokers			Total Smokers
				Light*	Heavy	Total	
HD	40	16	29	81	52	133	162
Total	612	683	371	720	401	1,121	1,492
%HD	6.54	2.34	7.82	11.25	12.97	11.86	10.86

*Light—less than 30 cigarettes per day.
Heavy—more than 30 cigarettes per day.

per cent), "Never Smoked" (6.54 per cent), and "Stopped Smoking" (2.34 per cent) groups from each other (Table 23–VIII). The difference between smokers and those who never smoked is in accord with expectation. The paradox in the observed difference between "Never Smoked" and "Stopped Smoking," however, is entirely unexpected and, in view of the consistency and magnitude of the differences, warrants further study and explanation.

DISCUSSION

It is widely recognized that there is an interplay of many factors in the causation and progression of ischemic heart disease. Among those currently receiving special emphasis are heredity, diet, tobacco, other diseases, electrolyte derangements, hormonal patterns, anatomical configurations, factors influencing the autonomic nervous regulation of myocardial dynamics and metabolism, such as personality traits, social practices, and adaptations to life situations. Although the proportional contribution of each cause varies from case to case, there is mounting evidence that in the American male emotional stress of occupational origin is a major influence in the etiologic spectrum of ischemic heart disease. Certainly, the findings in the present studies appear to indicate that a marked gradient in the prevalence of this malady

exists among professional groups in the United States. This unequal distribution of the disease among various categories of professional practice in the fields of medicine, dentistry, law, and securities, respectively, does not appear to be related to heredity or diet but shows a striking association with the relative stressfulness of occupational activity. Thus, a highly statistically-significant finding throughout the present study, and one which was shown to be remarkably consistent by age, was the increase in prevalence rate with advance in stress. These observations lend support to clinical and experimental studies which suggest that emotional stress is (a) an accelerating factor in atherogenesis when the diet is relatively high in animal fat, and (b) that it also increases myocardial vulnerability by inducing a hypothalamosympathogenic (catecholamine-mediated) augmentation of myocardial oxygen consumption (3, 4). The elevation of catecholamine toxicity-increasing (5) adrenal hydroxycorticosteroid production under emotional stress (6) may possibly provide an additional pathogenic element.

There is not much reason to believe that occupational emotional stresses and their autonomic nervous plus hormonal corollaries possess any major significance in cardiac pathogenesis as long as coronary vascular compensatory dilatability remains intact. However, experiments by

Gunn (7) in cholesterol-fed rabbits, and other studies (8) strongly suggest the existence of a hypothalamic and adrenergic involvement also in the process of atherogenesis, so that both coronary atherosclerosis and myocardial vulnerability to it may be considered as being enhanced by emotional stress mechanisms.

When dietary factors essential to atherosclerotic impairment of coronary dilatability prevail, emotional stress can be assumed not only to accelerate the organic vascular lesions, but also to contribute to myocardial hypoxia through neurogenic catecholamine action. It appears clear, therefore, that in Western society where prodigious amounts of fat are ingested and coronary atherosclerosis is virtually omnipresent, greater attention must be focused on the role of stress in the clinical development of ischemic heart disease.

It is well-known that smokers increase their consumption of tobacco when exposed to increasing degrees of psychological stress. The present study appears to show that the prevalence of the tobacco habit itself varies in different vocational categories with the degree of occupation-related stress. Smoking patterns in the individual or in the group, therefore, appear to provide a barometer by which inner tensions may be estimated in a relative manner. Inasmuch as smoking varies with stress while both factors show a similar correlation with the clinical manifestations of ischemic heart disease, either or both of these elements could be causally related to its development.

One finding of the present study, however, casts doubt upon the alleged specific role of smoking in the genesis of ischemic heart disease. If a noxious agent exists in tobacco which is responsible in large measure for coronary attacks, the prevalence of the disease should bear a clear relationship to exposure to this harmful element. On the contrary, however, we have found a higher prevalence of ischemic heart disease among the professional persons in our series who had never smoked than those who had once smoked but subsequently discontinued the practice. The Albany and Framingham studies similarly have shown that persons who have stopped smoking do not show higher coronary heart disease prevalence than persons who have never smoked (9). From these considerations, it would appear possible that tobacco by itself may be without major etiologic significance in predisposing to ischemic heart attacks. To test this notion, further analysis of the data was undertaken.

Table 23–VI shows the relationship between smoking and prevalence of ischemic heart disease within each occupational category. Obviously, if smoking is symptomatic of emotional stress and not of itself a prevalent etiologic factor, we would expect smokers and nonsmokers within each "homogeneous" occupational stress category to have similar ischemic heart disease prevalence rates. Instead, we find that ischemic heart disease prevalence is higher for the smokers in each occupational subgroup than for the nonsmokers. Thus, it appears from the data that each of the pair-wise relationships among these 3 variables may be statistically real. On the other hand, the existence of a significant stress gradient among members of the same occupational category could account for the higher prevalence of ischemic heart disease among smokers even in the absence of an etiologic relationship. Further studies are needed to clarify this point.

For the present, the anomaly remains of a lower cardiac ischemia prevalence observed for former smokers than for nonsmokers. Recognition of the importance of emotional factors in the initiation and progression of clinical ischemic heart disease may permit a logical explanation for the unexpectedly low prevalence of this disorder in former smokers. The ability of such individuals to terminate the smoking habit may reflect an unusual capacity for adaptation to stress and thereby offer an explanation for their diminished susceptibility to heart attacks. Alternative hypotheses must assume that the noxious effects of years of smoking can be reversed, and protection conferred simply by the cessation of smoking.

SUMMARY

1. Emotional stress may be an important accelerating factor in ischemic heart disease when the diet is high in atherogenic animal fat.

2. Smoking patterns in the individual or group may provide an index by which emotional tensions may be relatively assessed.

3. While the smoking of tobacco may be implicated in the pathogenesis of ischemic heart disease, the relationship is not a simple one. No clear explanation is at hand to account for the low prevalence of the disease among persons who formerly smoked.

4. Discontinuance of the smoking habit may cause not only complete reversal of deleterious effects, but also a relative "immunity" to heart attacks. Alterna-

tively, the ability to stop smoking may imply a resilient personality response to stress, and thereby a diminished vulnerability to environmental influences. Further studies are in progress in an effort to interpret these findings.

5. It is of interest that no correlation was observed between lack of exercise and prevalence of ischemic heart disease in young subjects whose primary susceptibility (due to hereditary and/or vascular factors) may have been relatively greater than that of large, older age groups where a protecive influence of physical activity seems to have been well established.

REFERENCES

1. RUSSEK, H. I.: Emotional stress and coronary heart disease in American physicians. *Amer J Med Sci*, 240:711, 1960.
2. RUSSEK, H. I.: Emotional stress and coronary heart disease in American physicians, dentists and lawyers. *Amer J Med Sci*, 243:716, 1962.
3. RAAB, W.: The nonvascular metabolic myocardial vulnerability factor in "coronary heart disease." *Amer Heart J*, 66:685, 1963.
4. RAAB, W.: Myocardial necroses produced in domesticated rats and in wild rats by sensory and emotional stresses. *Proc Exp Biol Med*, 116:665, 1964.
5. SELYE, H.: *The Pluricausal Cardiopathies*. Springfield, Thomas, 1961.
6. MASON, J. W., MANGAN, G., BRADY, J. V., CONRAD, D., and RIOCH, D. McK.: Concurrent plasma epinephrine, norepinephrine and 17-hydroxycorticosteroid levels during conditioned emotinal disturbances in monkeys. *Psychosom Med*, 23:344, 1961.
7. GUNN, C. G., FRIEDMAN, M., and BYERS, S. O.: Effect of chronic hypothalamic stimulation upon cholesterol-induced atheroclerosis in the rabbit. *J Clin Invest*, 39:1963, 1960.
8. RAAB, W.: Neurohormonal atherogenesis. *Amer J Cardiol*, 1:113, 1958.
9. DOYLE, J. T., DAWBER, T. R., KANNEL, W. B., HASLIN, A. S., and KAHN, H. A.: Cigarette smoking and coronary heart disease. *New Eng J Med*, 266:796, 1962.

Chapter XXIV

THE ROLE OF A SPECIFIC OVERT BEHAVIOR PATTERN IN THE GENESIS OF CORONARY HEART DISEASE

RAY H. ROSENMAN

(San Francisco, California, U.S.A.)

SOME years ago Dr. Friedman and I (1) had occasion to review various data relating the increased incidence of clinical coronary heart disease observed in American males to their relatively high intake of dietary fats, with the conclusion that such a relationship was unproved. In surveying (1, 2) experimental and epidemiological data bearing upon this possible relationship, it became apparent to us that such data all too frequently were collected with little or no consideration of differences among the populations under study of such possibly important variables as the prevalence of diastolic hypertension, the incidence of myocardial infarction as opposed to coronary atherosclerosis per se, the qualitative nature of the dietary fats, the methods used to estimate the actual ingested diet, blood coagulability and changes in the incidence of thrombotic complications, and differences in smoking and exercise habits. Thus, for example, primitive natives were compared to American executives, with only their difference of ingested fat being accorded any serious relevance to the observed differences of coronary morbidity and mortality. In the intervening years since these earlier surveys, considerably more evidence has

accumulated to strengthen our belief that none of the classic culprits such as diet, exercise, smoking, or serum lipids or lipoproteins is the sine qua non of the increasing coronary morbidity of the middle-aged American male. Indeed, the very nature of the present conference emphasizes our own conviction (3, 4) that clinical coronary heart disease (CHD) results from the interaction of multiple causal factors operating within the framework of time.

In these earlier surveys (1–4) it was particularly striking to us that available epidemiological studies of CHD almost entirely had failed to assess the possible influence of differences of socioeconomic stresses among the groups under investigation, the more surprising in view of the evidence that a better correlation could be obtained between the presence of certain socioeconomic stresses and the incidence of CHD than between the latter and a high fat intake (1, 2). It was thus about a decade ago that our group began to wonder if the rising incidence of CHD among middle-aged American males might stem from some emotional interplay induced by the stresses imposed by our industrialized civilization, acting in conjunction with high fat diet, diminished physical activity, relatively high serum lipids, and so forth. Stress has always been an integral part of life, but as our most noted historians have pointed out, Western societies are fraught with stresses which not only are restricted to the industrialized groups but are uniquely new, having never previously been witnessed in any age of history.

This suspicion was strengthened by two observations. First, it could be noted in epidemiological surveys that CHD was scarce in groups and civilizations free of such socioeconomic stresses, no matter what their dietary, smoking or exercise habits were. Second, we found in a reexamination of our own patients that the younger and middle-aged victims of CHD very frequently exhibited a personality structure which we have since termed Behavior Pattern Type A (5). Pattern A primarily is characterized by certain personality traits, including aggressiveness, ambition, drive, competitiveness, and a profound sense of time urgency. The man with Pattern A thus exhibits traits which are variously present in most normal men, but he possesses them to an excessive, and often inordinate, degree. In association with these emotional facets he also frequently exhibits certain typical muscular or motor phenomena; these include forceful, rather rapid, and often explosively uneven speech, sudden gestures such as fist-clenching, desk-pounding, taut facial grimaces, and rapid movements and locomotion, reflecting his chronic sense of restlessness and impatience. In particular the man with Pattern A appears often to be excessively driven to achieve and to get things done, while being unable to overcome the inflexible factor of time itself, and frequently struggling against

the competing and obstructing influences of other persons and things. He thus appears habitually to be living under time pressure. Pattern A then is an interplay of certain personality or endogenous and certain environmental or exogenous factors. It exists in the milieu which characterizes our modern, urban civilization and, being so much an accompaniment of the socioeconomic stresses which are both unique and new to our industrialized and mechanized society, is increasingly prevalent in our American population. The man with Pattern A appears to be immersed habitually in these new stresses, often content with his commitments, whether demanded by his environment or self-imposed.

We have designated the relative absence of Pattern A as Behavior Pattern Type B, but it would be erroneous to think of this as being a sharply demarcated cleavage. As already pointed out, the man possessing Pattern A simply exhibits to an excessive degree certain specific emotional traits which may be absent or are present to a much lesser degree in the man with Pattern B. My associate (6) has likened the facets of Behavior Pattern A to an elevated body temperature or blood pressure, both of which are present in lesser degree in all men, or to metabolic disorders characterized only by an excess of some physiological substance which is normally present. Socioeconomic stresses and the interplay of such behavioral traits cannot be quantitated by some electronic device, but we have found that the presence of Pattern A usually can be identified by means of a suitable psychological interview (5, 7, 8), as well as by a provocative, psychophysiological test (9).

Thus, in comprehensively surveying

our own younger coronary patients, we were impressed that they could very frequently be distinguished by exhibition of a specific overt behavior pattern, but could not be differentiated by heredity, blood pressure, serum lipids, or habits of diet, exercise or smoking. We therefore considered it important to ascertain what might happen when a group of 42 tax accountants were faced with a situational challenge, such as the April 15 tax deadline, that clearly imposed an acute sense of time urgency upon most of the subjects. The men were bled bi-weekly for over five months for serum cholesterol and blood clotting determinations and were closely questioned at such times concerning their sense of time urgency. We were surprised in those early days of study to find that fluctuations of considerable and occasional marked degree occurred in their serial cholesterol levels. However, when the stimulus of work deadlines occurred and imparted a sense of acute time pressure, a significant rise of serum cholesterol and acceleration of blood clotting almost invariably was observed (10). Moreover, these changes could not be ascribed to alterations of diet, weight, or exercise patterns since these were closely controlled. The cholesterol results of this study have now been widely confirmed (11-13). This study also taught us that whatever emotional facets comprised Behavior Pattern Type A, it did not consist of fear, anxiety, or other simple neurosis, and it is unfortunate that this often has been confused by others, as has the seemingly obvious difference between the uniquely new socioeconomic stresses of the industrialized world and such age-old stresses of other civilizations as pestilence or famine.

In view of these observed responses to an environmental stimulus associated with an acute sense of time urgency, we considered it important to study a group of men who habitually exhibited Behavior Pattern A and who were immersed in vocational situations imparting a chronic sense of time urgency. Two additional groups of men also were studied, one group being free of significant competitive or time pressures and failing to exhibit the facets of Pattern A (i.e., they exhibited Behavior Pattern B), while the third group consisted of men blind from early age and exhibiting an attendant chronic anxiety state. The men with Pattern A were found (5) to exhibit significantly higher serum cholesterols and more rapid blood clotting, a threefold greater prevalence of arcus senilis, and most significant, a sevenfold higher prevalence of already present CHD. Yet on careful investigation these striking differences could not be attributed to any differences of stature, diet, smoking or exercise habits.

Our curiosity extended to the female who had entered the business world or a profession, thereby variously assuming the facets of Behavior Pattern A. As in the former study among men, female lay selectors chose two groups of women for us, solely on the basis of whether they exhibited Behavior Pattern A or B, respectively. Again, the women exhibiting Pattern A also exhibited strikingly higher serum cholesterols and markedly higher prevalence of diastolic hypertension, arcus senilis and clinical CHD (7), which could not be ascribed to any differences of stature, diet, smoking or exercise habits, or "femininity."

The above results appeared clearly to indicate that the possession of Behavior

Pattern A accelerated the advent of clinical CHD. We were well aware, however, that an epidemiological correlation does not fulfill Koch's postulates with regard to cause and effect relationships, and we therefore embarked on a series of experimental and clinical investigations aimed at determining the biophysicochemical pathways by which Pattern A might accelerate coronary atherogenesis and the advent of clinical disease, thereby engendering the observed higher prevalence of CHD in middle-aged subjects with Behavior Pattern A.

The earlier studies (5,710) had indicated that Pattern A is associated with an acceleration of blood clotting and with relatively elevated serum cholesterol levels that cannot be ascribed to dietary differences, and possibly with higher blood pressure levels (7). The emotional traits of subjects with Pattern A also suggested to us that neurohumoral pathways might be involved. Urine samples were collected repetitively from groups of men with well-defined Behavior Pattern A and B, respectively. Separate aliquots were purposefully collected during the working milieu and at other times. Although the two groups failed to exhibit any differences in excretion of ketosteroids, hydroxycorticoids, or serotonin metabolites, the men with Pattern A excreted, hence secreted, during their working day far more norepinephrine than did the subjects with Pattern B (14). The nocturnal urinary excretion of these hormones, on the other hand, was the same in the two groups.

In view of this, a study was initiated in collaboration with Dr. C.G. Gunn of the University of Oklahoma in which rabbits fed a fat-enriched diet were concurrently subjected to repetitive electrical stimulation of the hypothalamus by means of implanted electrodes (15). The stimulated animals exhibited considerably enhanced hypercholesteremia and intensified aortic and coronary atherosclerosis compared to control animals given a similar diet. The results of this study appeared clearly to indicate that central nervous system mechanisms exist which under certain conditions are capable of markedly influencing the hypercholesteremic response to a lipid-enriched diet and its atherogenic consequents.

Our next study was prompted by the finding of various investigators that men with clinical CHD exhibit elevated serum levels of triglycerides and beta-lipoproteins and by the belief that this is of causal importance in the genesis of coronary atherosclerosis. Thus, if Behavior Pattern A is "coronary-prone," then it might be expected that well men with this behavioral complex also would exhibit such elevated serum lipid levels, similar to the man with already existing clinical CHD. Therefore, we undertook an investigation of this in collaboration with Drs. R. Furman and R. P. Howard of the University of Oklahoma. Fasting blood samples were obtained from groups of men with well-defined Behavior Patterns A and B, respectively, and sent "blind" to Drs. Furman and Howard, who found that the men with Pattern A indeed did exhibit significantly higher serum content of triglycerides and of beta-lipoproteins than did the men with Pattern B (16).

We then became concerned with determining whether the heart of the man with Behavior Pattern A was being subjected to greater physical stress than was that of the man with Pattern B. Two rather crude indices were utilized in our first study of this phenomenon. Continuous heart rates were recorded over 4 separate 24 hour periods by means of a specially devised watch, and ballistocardiograms were obtained from the above same two groups of subjects, but the results failed to show any differences (17). These rather crude indices of hemodynamic stress thus failed to show that the heart of the subject with Pattern A was being subjected to any greater physical strain than was that of the men with Pattern B.

The finding of elevated serum triglycerides in men with Pattern A (16) and the rather uniform finding of other investigators that men with clinical CHD exhibit a delay in the removal of postprandial triglycerides from their blood prompted our next investigation. Thus we would again expect that if Pattern A indeed is "coronary-prone", then men exhibiting this behavioral complex also should exhibit the same delayed fat-tolerance curve of men with already existing clinical CHD. Accordingly, groups of men with Patterns A and B, respectively, were bled before, and serially after, feeding of a single fat-rich meal. At the same time that blood samples were collected, their conjunctival capillary circulation was examined and photographed through a microscope viewing barrel attached to a slit-lamp apparatus. The results of this study clearly indicated (18) that most of the subjects with Pattern A did exhibit a striking delay in the clearance of the fed triglyceride from their serum, compared to the men with Pattern B.

It was even more dramatic to observe that most of the men with Pattern A, but only a few of those with Pattern B, also exhibited marked postprandial sludging of red blood cells with considerable slowing of forward blood flow, and partial obliteration of the bulbar conjunctival capillary vasculature, and that these changes persisted often for more than nine hours after ingestion of a single, fat-enriched meal (18). The significance of this finding remains to be evaluated, but suggests among other things a mechanism by which prolonged ischemia might be induced in the subject whose myocardial blood flow already was significantly compromised as a result of narrowing of the larger coronary arterial vasculature. It was of interest that this postprandial sludging readily could be abolished by injection of heparin.

We have attempted thus to ascertain the possible biochemical pathways by which Behavior Pattern A might lead to the higher prevalence of clinical CHD which we observed in our earlier investigations. At the same time that we began this systematic series of studies, we were concerned with determining whether this observed higher prevalence of CHD was merely an associative relationship or whether Pattern A might also bear predictive, hence causal, relationship to the incidence of new clinical disease among initially well men. Accordingly, we began in 1960 an epidemiological investigation of 3,500 well men, aged 39 to 59 years, employed in 11 participating organizations (8). This study was initiated in collaboration with two other groups of investigators whose views differed from ours about the relative importance of various factors in coronary atherogenesis; Drs. Reuben Straus, M. Wurm, and R. Kositchek of St. Joseph Hospital, Burbank, being concerned with the serum lipid-lipoprotein spectrum, and Drs. N. Werthessen and W. Hahn, then of the

Southwest Foundation for Research and Education, San Antonio, being concerned with the blood clotting mechanism. At the outset each group independently "predictively" classified each of the 3,500 well men with regard to future proneness to clinical CHD, and submitted these classifications to a distinguished Data Repository Committee. Detailed studies of their socioeconomic status, smoking, dietary and exercise habits, family history, anthropometric factors, and many other parameters bearing possible relevance to the occurrence of CHD also were accomplished, with a view to determining a comprehensive profile of the man prone to coronary heart disease.

Extensive follow-up studies also have been obtained at annual intervals, revealing among other things that new clinical CHD had occurred in 69 men during the first two years since the initial investigation had been accomplished (19). Seventy three per cent of these 69 men had been classified initially as coronary-prone on the basis of their Type A Behavior Pattern, compared to 42 per cent on the basis of their serum beta/alpha lipoprotein ratio. The incidence of new CHD in all men originally classified as exhibiting Behavior Pattern A was 143 percent greater than in the men adjudged to exhibit Pattern B. Among the men aged 39 to 49 years, the incidence of new clinical CHD was over 4 time greater in the subjects initially "predictively" classified as coronary-prone on the basis of their exhibition of Pattern A than among the men classified as non-coronary-prone based on their adjudged exhibition of Pattern B.

The above studies appear to us to have shown 4 groups of findings: first, that younger and middle-aged men with clinical CHD very frequently possess a particular overt behavioral complex that we have designated as Behavior Pattern Type A; second, that a population of male and female subjects exhibiting Behavior Pattern A also exhibit a considerably higher prevalence of clinical CHD than does an otherwise comparable population without these behavioral characteristics; third, that new clinical CHD occurs strikingly more frequently in middle-aged men exhibiting Behavior Pattern A than it does in otherwise similar men largely free of such characteristics and fourth, that various physiological and biochemical mechanisms probably concerned with coronary atherogenesis are significantly altered by Behavior Pattern A in such fashion that permanent alterations of the coronary vasculature can ensue. Much more remains to be elucidated in this field and it is admittedly far more difficult to assess and to quantitate such factors than it is to determine the serum cholesterol. Nevertheless, the results of the above studies have led us to believe that a certain emotional interplay, probably increasingly associated with the socioeconomic stresses uniquely new to our industrialized society, may bear a dominant pathogenetic relevance to the increasing coronary morbidity in the middle-aged American male. These observations also have constrained us to believe that any future epidemiological study may not reach relevant conclusions concerning the genesis of CHD unless it includes a thorough investigation of these factors.

SUMMARY

An emotional interplay, designated as Behavior Pattern Type A, was found to be exhibited frequently by younger subjects with clinical coronary heart disease. New clinical coronary heart disease has been found to occur significantly more frequently in middle-aged men exhibiting Pattern A than among otherwise comparable men free of such behavioral characteristics. Various biochemical pathways are altered by Pattern A in such fashion as probably to enhance and accelerate atherogenesis and the advent of clinical disease.

REFERENCES

1. FRIEDMAN, M., and ROSENMAN, R. H.: Comparison of fat intake of American men and women. *Circulation, 16:*339, 1957.
2. FRIEDMAN, M., ROSENMAN, R. M., and BYERS, S. O.: Deranged cholesterol metabolism and its possible relationship to atherosclerosis: a review. *J Geront, 10:*60, 1955.
3. ROSENMAN, R. H., and FRIEDMAN, M.: *The Possible Relationship of the Emotions to Clinical Coronary Heart Disease in Hormones and Atherosclerosis.* New York, Academic Press, Inc., 1959.
4. ROSENMAN, R. H., and FRIEDMAN, M.: The role of a specific overt behavior pattern in the occurrence of ischemic heart disease. *Cardiol Prat, 13:* 42, 1962.
5. FRIEDMAN, M., and ROSENMAN, R. H.: Association of specific overt behavior pattern with blood and cardiovascular findings. *JAMA, 169:* 1286, 1959.
6. FRIEDMAN, M.: Behavior pattern and its pathogenetic role in clinical coronary artery disease. *Geriatrics, 19:*562, 1964.
7. ROSENMAN, R. H., and FRIEDMAN, M.: Association of specific behavior pattern in women with blood and cardiovascular findings. *Circulation, 24:*1173, 1961.
8. ROSENMAN, R. H., FRIEDMAN, M., STRAUS, R., WURM, M., KOSITCHEK, R., HAHN, W., and WERTHESSEN, N.: A predictive study of coronary heart disease: The Western Collaborative Group Study. *JAMA, 189:*15, 1964.
9. FRIEDMAN, M., and ROSENMAN, R. H.: Overt behavior pattern in coronary disease: detection of overt behavior pattern A in patients with coronary disease by a new psychophysiological procedure. *JAMA, 173:*1320, 1960.
10. FRIEDMAN, M., ROSENMAN, R. H., and CARROLL, V.: Changes in serum cholesterol and blood clotting time in men subjected to cyclic variations of occupational stress. *Circulation, 17:*852, 1958.
11. WERTLAKE, P. T., WILCOX, A. A., HALEY, M. J., and PETERSON, J. E.: Relationship of mental and emotional stress to serum cholesterol levels. *Proc Soc Exp Biol Med, 97:*163, 1958.
12. THOMAS, C. G., and MURPHY, E. A.: Further studies on cholesterol levels in Johns Hopkins medical students: Effects of stress at examinations. *J Chronic Dis, 8:*661, 1958.
13. DREYFUSS, F., and DZACZKES, J. W.: Blood cholesterol and uric acid of healthy medical students under stress of examination. *Arch Intern Med, 103:* 708, 1959.
14. FRIEDMAN, M., ST. GEORGE, S., BYERS, S. O., and ROSENMAN, R. H.: Excretion of catecholamine, 17-ketosteroids, 17-hydroxycorticoids and 5-hydroxyindole in men exhibiting a particular behavior pattern (A) associated with high incidence of clinical coronary artery disease. *J Clin Invest, 39:*758, 1960.
15. GUNN, C. G., FRIEDMAN, M., and BYERS, S. O.: Effect of chronic hypothalamic stimulation upon cholesterol induced atherosclerosis in the rabbit *J Clin Invest, 39:*1963, 1960.
16. ROSENMAN, R. H., and FRIEDMAN, M.: Behavior patterns, blood lipids and coronary heart disease. *JAMA, 184:*934, 1963.
17. FRIEDMAN, M., ROSENMAN, R. H., and BROWN, A. E.: The continuous heart rate in men exhibiting an overt behavior pattern associated with increased incidence of clinical coronary artery disease. *Circulation, 28:*861, 1963.
18. FRIEDMAN, M., ROSENMAN, R. H., and BYERS, S. O.: Changes in serum lipids and conjunctival circulation after fat ingestion in men exhibiting a behavior pattern (Type A) associated with a high incidence of clinical coronary artery disease. *Circulation, 29:*874, 1964.
19. ROSENMAN, R. H., FRIEDMAN, M., STRAUS, R., WURM, M., KOSITCHEK, R., HAHN, W., and WEETHESSEN, N.: Western Collaborative Group Study: A study of predictive factors in the occurrence of coronary heart disease (interim report). *Circulation, 28:*792, 1963.

Chapter XXV

SITUATIONAL STRESSES AS CAUSE OF CARDIOVASCULAR DISEASE

("The Nutcracker Syndrome")

JOSEPH B. WOLFFE

(*Norristown, Pennsylvania, U.S.A.*)

SITUATIONAL stresses which the individual is unable to cope with are common environmental causes of various functional and organic forms of cardiovascular disease. It was our impression that they constituted the predominating factor in many patients of the younger age group suffering from ischemic heart disease.

From this point of view we surveyed the medical records of 102 patients, 36 to 46 years of age, whose histories and electrocardiographic findings revealed evidence of myocardial and/or coronary disease.

The personal histories of 24 were clinically inadequate. However, the effect of situational stresses on the individual patient could be evaluated from the records of the remaining 78 (76 males and 2 females). Judging from roentgenographic studies of the large arteries and particularly of the abdominal aorta of this group, 42 showed the presence of atherosclerosis (1, 2, 3).

The 78 patients whose records comprise the basis of this presentation, were carefully interrogated for no less than 6 daily periods (approximately 1 hour each) during their hospital stay. Members of their immediate family were also interviewed. An evaluation was made of their social, economic, and particularly interpersonal relationships with those whom their lives were closely interwoven. Fifty-two of this group, approximately 60 per cent, revealed life dramas and situations in which they were irretrievably caught in a "nutcracker" squeeze between opposing forces, entrapped without respite—at home and/ or at work. Most of them had a high sense of responsibility and considered their status in the community of great importance. The type of situational impacts varied from one individual to another.

In the following, a few examples of such situations which apparently contributed to the manifestations of ischemic heart disease will be cited without entering into a discussion of clinical details.

A man of 40, who thought himself aging, was acting as vice-president—in name only—in a large firm owned by his successful father-in-law, who constantly countermanded his orders and blocked the young man's undertakings. The father-in-law did not limit his sphere of influence to the factories, but extended it to his daughter's home and children. The patient was trapped between the need of economic security on the one hand and, on the other, his inability to assert his rightful position in his home. After a number of exhaustive interviews, the patient finally concluded "I am a target for ridicule and criticism in my office, and a stranger in my own home."

A man, 45 years of age, well established in his community and church, escaped from "marital incompatability" by becoming deeply involved in an extramarital relationship. He discovered that his teenage daughter was promiscuous, and she, in response to his angry censure, pointed out the example he set. Unwilling to give up what he considered "his only haven," and grieved by his ineffectual father-daughter relationship, a sense of guilt, and his estrangement at home, he was caught in a "nutcracker" situation.

An underpaid accountant in a busy office was expected to flout the law to save taxes for the office clients. He had pangs of conscience because of this, but in addition was tormented by lack of appreciation from both client and employer. "This is bad enough," he stated, "but I am also very unhappy at home. My wife, by actions and words, belittles me, rubs it in, and tells me I have no guts."

(The patient's cardiac symptoms were most severe during and immediately following the filing of income tax returns.)

A 53-year-old man who sells seeds, fertilizer, and other farm needs is another "nutcracker" victim. He acts as the local representative for the State Cooperative Agency. Due to many financial reverses as the result of crop failures, his business, which had taken a lifetime to build, is now heavily mortgaged by this cooperative agency. Although the farmer cannot always pay, he must sell on credit. Between the cooperative agency and the farmer, this man is in a constant squeeze.

(This patient's first attack of myocardial infarction occurred during a severe emotional upheaval when the creditors insisted on payment and the farmers, as he stated, "were taking my life's blood on credit.")

(The patient showed no clinical or roentgenological evidence of atherosclerosis. However, the electrocardiographic pattern was typical of myocardial ischemia.)

A 43-year-old man, a draftsman in a large steel company, was given a job as a janitor, though maintained on the same salary, when the company curtailed the work in the drafting department. He was not laid off but was assigned to sweep floors in the department where he formerly worked. For economic reasons he could not leave—the security and the benefits to which he was entitled in case of sickness or death were too important to give up. Yet, he could not accept the degradation of his status.

(Severe attacks of angina pectoris occurred mainly at work. Within a few weeks, electrocardiographic evidence of coronary insufficiency developed. He was taught to accept the situation; his condition improved but he still had to resort frequently to nitroglycerin for relief of anginal pain. Later, as a result of policy changes, he was reassigned to his former duties. Since then he was relieved of pain, and within several weeks his pre- and post-effort ECGs were normal.)

It is rare that patients will readily disclose intimate personal experiences during their first interview with the physician. The failure to relate such environmental stresses was most often due to a lack of appreciation of their relevance or a reluctance to reveal what patients considered too personal.

Without exception, all of the 52 patients in whom noxious, situational impacts played an important role in their illness had symptoms referable to other body systems as well as the heart.

General extracardiac manifestations of an autonomic nervous upheaval in the sense of the concept of vagotonia and sympathicotonia, according to Eppinger and Hess (4), consisted of nervous agitation, insomnia, dizziness, headaches, vasomotor rhinitis, various allergies, occasional paresthesias, symptoms of peptic ulcer (8 of the patients had either active or healed ulcers shown roentgenologically), hyperirritability of the colon, mild diarrhea, and in some instances attacks due to hypoglycemia.

As far as the cardiovascular system was concerned, nearly all patients experienced heart consciousness or some ill-defined pain over the precordium, except in cases of acute myocardial infarction, when the pain distribution became more or less typical. Many were conscious of ectopic beats, and some felt a pounding in the chest and/or throbbing in the neck. Paroxysmal tachycardia, auricular fibrillation, and elevations of the blood pressure were not infrequently observed.

Weiss and English in a study of 43 patients suffering from myocardial infarction found that 21 (49 per cent) showed gradually mounting tension of emotional origin for months and years prior to the onset of myocardial infarction. Analyzing the incidence of mounting tension in different age groups in men, they found that it occurred in 2 out of 8 (25 per cent) over the age of 60, but in 18 out of 27 (67 per cent) under the age of 60.5.

The relationship of tension to myocardial and coronary disease in our group was very similar to theirs.

The term "nutcracker syndrome" is introduced to denote a chain of events resulting from suppressed, crushing environmental circumstances from which the patient cannot extricate himself. He is caught in a dilemma between what he ought to do and what circumstances compel him to do—the tyranny of the "should" over the "would."

Recent investigations indicate that the cerebral cortex plays an important role in evaluating stressful experiences. It is capable of recording, analyzing and sifting such experiences through thus far unknown pathways to affect favorably and unfavorably what MacLean refers to as the "visceral brain" (6). This in turn gains expression through the hypothalamus and affects the entire vegetative system, producing focal or systemic diseases in the vulnerable individual when the stresses are overwhelming.

The effect of stress on the sympathetic component of the autonomic nervous system has been widely studied. Emotional stress is frequently associated with an adrenergic response especially in the cardiovascular sphere (accelerated heart rate, shortened isometric period, elevation of the diastolic blood pressure). The majority of our patients showed, in addition, extracardiac parasympathetic responses as a result of continuous, overtaxing, stressful situations.

We are in agreement with those clinicians who take exception to the term "psychosomatic disturbance." Shanon aptly expressed it as follows:

". . . 'psychosomatic' embodies the concept of the immaterial 'psyche' instead of material 'brain.' The mind (psyche) cannot directly send impulses to body tissues (soma). . . . The sequence (of the two portions of the word) psychosomatic is often taken to imply that a disturbance of the psyche is the initial or even the only determining factor and that the somatic disturbance is the consequence" (7).

Strecker states: "The accomplishments of psychosomatic medicine are note-worthy. Its objective magnificent, but the name unfortunate. Its comparative recent usage makes it sound like the announcement of a marriage between the body and the mind with sub-divisions of medicine and psychiatry in the bridal party" (8).

Cooperation of the patient in a mutual search for the possible cause of the stress-ful situations and for ways and means to ameliorate them is often improved if the nature of the "nutcracker syndrome" is explained to him in simple terms. Members of the family can aid at least in relieving the squeeze of the emotional dilemma. This, however, proved in our experience to be only temporary unless major adjustments were effected. It was surprising, nevertheless, that after a few interviews numerous patients were re-lieved of many of their symptoms. Today, modern psychiatrists call for greater em-phasis on short-term, intensive interviews. While one cannot hurry the management of the mentally ill, this does not hold true with most of the victims of situational disturbances which cause the somatic manifestations seen by internists and car-diologists. Only in rare instances was it necessary to refer the patient to a psy-chiatrist for further evaluation and ther-apy.

Definite evidence of arteriosclerosis, atherosclerosis, or other etiologic factors does not absolve the physician from look-ing for situational stresses which may be closely interwoven in the causation and aggravation of existing pathology.

Dr. Norman A. Welsh, the late Presi-dent of the AMA, in his inaugural ad-dress wisely pointed out that "this out-standing progress in medicine as evi-denced by increased specialization con-stitutes one of the crucial problems of our times" (9). He also quoted from Dr. Ignacio Chávez's address at the World Congress of Cardiology when he warned ". . . that specialization can mean frag-mentation, partial vision and limitation

of our horizon. What is gained in depth is lost in breadth," and he concluded ". . . that preeminence of specialization is fertile in valuable achievement, but also pregnant with risks" (10).

SUMMARY

The "nutcracker syndrome" is caused by the crossfire of environmental stresses.

Persons with a vulnerable cardiovas-cular system may develop ischemic myo-cardial disease if the situational stresses are not relieved.

Manifold symptoms involving effects of the autonomic nervous system on vari-ous body functions are characteristic of this syndrome.

Functional disturbances precede the development of organic disease.

The holistic approach to the patient's problem should prove an important step in the prevention of irreversible cardio-vascular disease.

REFERENCES

1. WOLFFE, J. B., and SIEGAL, E. I.: X-ray of the abdominal aorta in the detection of athero-sclerosis. *Clin Med, 69:*401, 1962.
2. WOLFFE, J. B.: Roentgenologic test for the ante-mortem diagnosis of atherosclerosis. *Angiology, 16:*99, 1965.
3. WOLFFE, J. B.: Arteriosclerosis at present—a melting pot of arteropathies. *Geriatrics, 2:*296, 1947.
4. EPPINGER, H., and HESS, L.: *Vagotonia Nervous and Mental Disease*. New York, Pub. Co., 1915, p. 4.
5. WEISS, E., and ENGLISH, O.: *Psychosomatic Medi-cine*. Philadelphia-Boston, W. B. Saunders Com-pany, 1957, p. 213.
6. MACLEAN, P. D.: Psychosomatic disease in the "visceral brain." *Psychosom Med, 11:*338, 1949.
7. SHANON, J.: Considerations regarding the term psychosomatic disease. *Psychosomatics, 4:*302, 1963.
8. STRECKER, E. A.: *Fundamentals of Psychiatry*. Philadelphia, J. B. Lippincott Co., 1944.
9. WELSH, N. A.: Inaugural Address. *JAMA, 189:*224, 1964.
10. CHÁVEZ, I.: Grandeur and poverty of medical specialization; aspiration toward a new human-ism. *Circulation, 20:*481, 1959.

Chapter XXVI

EMOTION-INDUCED CARDIAC DISTURBANCES AND POSSIBLE BENEFITS FROM TRANQUIL LIVING

VINCENZO LAPICCIRELLA*

(Florence, Italy)

IT IS being increasingly recognized that views on a supposedly purely atherosclerotic origin of ischemic degenerative heart disease are no longer tenable.

Myocardial necrotic foci and infarctions occur frequently in the complete absence of vascular occlusions (1, 2, 3), and coronary atherosclerosis is not infrequently found at autopsy in clinically and structurally normal hearts.

Thus it has become obvious that some accessory nonvascular factors must be involved, the superimposition of which over widely varying degrees of coronary atherosclerosis would create the ultimately decisive pathogenic background for actual myocardial injury. Common experience had for a long time suggested a causal role of emotional tensions, anxieties and excitements in the origin of anginal pain as well as of death from a "broken heart."

Selye's (4) demonstration of stress-induced myocardial necroses (without coronary arterial lesions) provided a powerful impetus for the study of nonvascular hormonal and neurohormonal metabolic elements in myocardial pathology. The well-known participation of liberated adrenomedullary and sympathagenic cate-

cholamines in the immediate autonomic nervous reaction to all stresses, and their potentially cardiotoxic properties (5) make the appearance of severe cardiac disturbances under emotional and other stresses intelligible. This applies particularly to the frequently occurring coincidence of stress-induced hypothalamic and sympathetic stimulations with pre-existing atherosclerotic limitations of the "coronary reserve" (6).

Necroses of the heart muscle have been produced by electrical and mechanical stimulation of the central nervous system (7, 8), as well as of the peripheral cardiac sympathetic nerves (9), and by the experimental induction of intensive emotional and sensory stresses in animals (10, 11). The first observations of electrocardiographic changes in man in states of anxiety were made by Mainzer (12).

In the following a brief resumé will be given of our own investigations concerning the contribution of emotional factors to cardiac disturbances.

ELECTROCARDIOGRAM UNDER ACUTE AND SUBACUTE EMOTIONAL STRESSES

1. *Emotional Stress of Imprisonment.*

In generally healthy young men, electrocradiograms were taken during the first

---

*With the collaboration of Drs. F. Abboni, R. Lapiccirella, S. Liotta, and M. Fanfani.

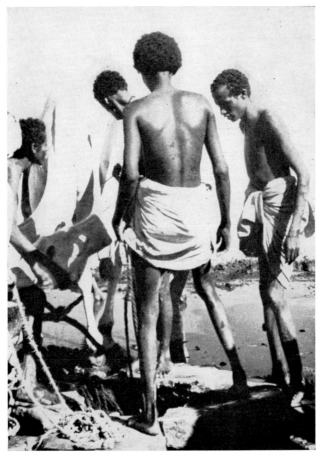

Figure 26–1. Somali herdsmen whose nutrition consists of at least 350 g of fat daily from camel's milk.

24 hours of detainment in prison, then subsequently (13, 28). Transient, upward concave elevations of the ST interval were an almost constant finding on the first day but disappeared during the following days. Unfortunately, Italian prison regulations do not permit the reproduction and publication of these tracings.

2.*Emotional Stress of Impending Surgery, Sports Competition and Critical Professional Situations.* Three groups of persons with quite different occupations and personality types showed essentially analogous temporary changes of the electrocardiogram when exposed to situations associated with anxiety and tension (14).

In 50 per cent of the persons expecting surgery, alterations of the electrocardiogram (mostly depression of the ST interval) were observed, but disappeared promptly under preanesthetic tranquilizing medication. In bank employees, the electrocardiogram showed similar abnormalities during the days preceding periodic inspection of their accounts. In about 40 per cent of competing sportsmen, immediately before athletic contests, the voltage of the T wave was augmented.

TABLE 26–I

DATA FROM SOMALI HERDSMEN (16)

Age	Weight	Blood Pressure	Serum Proteins Total %	Protein A.G. Ratio	Total Urinary 17-ketosteroids (mg per 24 hrs)	Total Urinary Catecholamines (μg per 24 hrs)
45	57	110/80	5.8	1.08	3.85	190
23	55	120/80	6.0	0.85	6.71	175
25	56	140/100	5.7	0.88	4.21	140
40	60	125/96	5.5	0.61	8.92	180
25	54	120/80	5.5	0.96	5.73	215
30	47	130/100	6.1	1.04	4.18	120
52	47	120/70	5.3	0.69	5.98	156
23	50	135/90	5.3	0.66	4.80	85
22	56	120/100	5.4	0.68	9.70	135
50	55	105/70	6.1	0.49	5.15	225
34	50	115/80	5.5	0.69	6.00	174
40	48	115/75	6.2	0.69	3.95	110
50	47	100/65	6.3	0.81	4.65	98

The above mentioned observations agree with those made by other investigators under comparable conditions, such as students facing examinations and patients before annual checkups.

Experiences of this kind caution against an unwarranted overrating of the diagnostic clinical significance of only temporarily abnormal electrocardiograms recorded under emotionally disturbing circumstances.

POSSIBLE CARDIAC BENEFITS FROM TRANQUIL LIVING CONDITIONS

A group of 203 Somali herdsmen were examined (15), originally in anticipation of a high incidence of atherosclerotic heart disease because of the fact that their nutrition consists almost entirely of camel's milk (5 or more liters per day). The fat content of camels milk is greater than that of cow's milk and the daily fat intake amounts to at least 350 g.

Against expectation, we found no clinical evidence of atherosclerotic heart disease. Only in two individuals did the electrocardiogram reveal signs of myo-cardial hypoxia. A few showed conduction disturbances and extrasystoles.

These nomadic people lead very active physical lives and have a lean body build (Fig. 26–1). Their primitive, patriarchal, pastoral living habits have remained practically unchanged for many centuries, and they are almost free of any serious psychological tensions and stresses.

Urinary catecholamines were determined in 13 individuals (16) and the 24-hour excretion was found uniformly low (average 154 μg), compared with the range of 200 to 500 μg reported as being normal for Caucasians (Table 26–I). The serum cholesterol level never exceeded 153 mg%; the beta/alpha lipoprotein ratio was high. Hypoproteinemia was marked with a low albumin:globulin ratio and low hemoglobin values.

DISCUSSION

Extensive statistical studies (17, 18) strongly suggest an important contributory role of emotional tensions and anxieties in the pathogenesis of ischemic heart disease. Animal experimentation has provided indirect evidence that the endocrine (4) and autonomic nervous neurosecretory systems (7, 8), especially through exaggerated liberation of cardiotoxic adrenomedullary and sympathogenic catecholamines (5, 8, 11), are fundamentally involved in the development of emotion-induced lesions of the heart muscle.

Our own observations and those of others in persons under emotional stress (19) revealed electrocardiographic patterns analogous to those provoked by catecholamine action (20). They correspond to the increased catecholamine liberation under emotional stimulations which are reflected in an augmented urinary catecholamine output (21, 22).

By contrast, the fact that, despite an enormously high intake of animal fat, the incidence of ischemic heart disease was found to be low among emotionally well equilibrated, carefree living, primitive people with a low catecholamine production, may be tentatively ascribed, at least in part, to these latter psychosomatic peculiarities.

Apart of a possible specific racial factor, the high degree of physical activity of the Somali nomads must be taken into consideration as an additional cardioprotective element (23).

At this point, it may be mentioned that studies of our own have long suggested a connection between *inadequate diaphragrmatic respiration of civilized man*, prematue atherosclerosis of the mesenteric vessels, and a predisposition to ischemic heart disease (24). A statistically demonstrated diminution of the vital breathing capacity in so-called "coronary-prone," physically inactive individuals (25) and its improvement after reconditioning periods with physical training (26, 27), seem to support this concept.

SUMMARY

Modern concepts of the pathogenesis of pluricausal degenerative heart disease ascribe an important contributory role to emotional tensions and anxieties which cause autonomic nervous interferences in myocardial metabolism.

This view seems to be supported by our observations of transient electrocardiographic changes under emotional stress (imprisonment, presurgery, etc.) on the one hand, and by the apparently low incidence of ischemic heart disease among carefree living, primitive Somali nomads, on the other, despite their extraordinarily high consumption of animal fats.

Catecholamine production was found uniformly low in the Somali herdsmen.

Avoidance of emotional stresses appears to be an important cardioprotective element in the prevention of ischemic disease of the heart muscle.

REFERENCES

1. MASTER, A. M., JAFFE, H. L., FIELD, L. E., and DONOSO, E.: Acute coronary insufficiency; its differential diagnosis and treatment. *Ann Intern Med*, *45:*561, 1956.
2. BLUMGART, H. L., SCHLESINGER, M. J., and ZOLL, P. M.: Angina pectoris, coronary failure and acute myocardial infarction; the role of coronary occlusion and collateral circulation. *JAMA*, *116:*91, 1941.
3. EHRLICH, J. C., and SHINOHARA, Y.: Low incidence of recent thrombotic coronary occlusion in hearts with acute myocardial infarction studied by serial block technique. *Circulation*, *26:*710, 1962.
4. SELYE, H.: *The Pluricausal Cardiopathies*. Springfield, Thomas, 1961.
5. RAAB, W.: Neurogenic multifocal destruction of myocardial tissue. *Rev Canad Biol*, *22:*217, 1963.
6. SCHIMERT, G., SCHIMMLER, W., SCHWALB, H., and EBERL, J.: Die Coronarerkrankungen. In: Mohr, L., and Staehelin, R., Ed.: *Handbuch der Inn Med.*, 9/III, Berlin-Göttingen-Heidelberg, Springer Verlag, 1960.
7. MELVILLE, K. I.: Cardiac ischemic changes induced by central nervous system stimulation.

First International Conference on Preventive Cardiology, Burlington, Vermont, Queen City Printers, 1964.

8. SHKHVATSABAYA, I. K., and MENSHIKOV, V. V.: Significance of catecholamines for the pathogenesis of neurogenic lesions of the myocardium. *Kardiologiia*, 2:27, 1962.

9. VEDENYEYEVA, Z. I.: Myocardial injury produced by sympathomimetic amines of endogenous and exogenous origin and its analysis. *Farmakol Toksik*, 3:286, 1962.

10. MIMINOSHVILI, D. J., MAGAKYAN, G. D., and KOKAYA, G. YA.: Cerebral cortical influences on coronary circulation. *Voprosy Fiziologii y Patologii Obyezyan.* Sukhumi, USSR, 1961.

11. RAAB, W., BAJUSZ, E., and GIGEE, W. R.: Myocardial necroses produced in domesticated rats and in wild rats by emotional stresses. *Proc Soc Exp Biol Med*, 116:665, 1964.

12. MAINZER, F., and KRAUSE, M.: The influence of fear on the electrocardiogram. *Brit Heart J*, 2:221, 1940.

13. LAPICCIRELLA, V., and ABBONI, F.: Prison stress; clinical and electrocardiographic observations on men during the first 24 hours of imprisonment. Third World Congress of Cardiology, Brussels, Sept., 1958.

14. LAPICCIRELLA, V., ABBONI, F., and FANFANI, M.: Studio elettrocardiografico del cuore atletico (calciatori e canottieri) e del cuore da emozione (emozione preoperatoria). Proc. XV Congresso della Soc. Ital. di Cardiol., Viareggio, June, 1953.

15. LAPICCIRELLA, V., LAPICCIRELLA, R., ABBONI, F., and LIOTTA, S.: Enquête clinique, biologique et cardiographique parmi les tribus nomades de la Somalie qui se nourissent seulement de lait. *Bull Org Mond de Santé (Bull. WHO)*, 27:681, 1962.

16. LAPICCIRELLA, R., MARRAMA, P., and BONATI, B.: Hormone excretion, diet and physique in Somalis. *Lancet*, July 1, 1961, p. 24.

17. RUSSEK, H. I.: Emotional stress and coronary heart disease in American physicians. *Amer J Med Sci*, 240:79/711, 1960.

18. ROSENMAN, R. H., FRIEDMAN, M., STRAUS, R., WURM, M., KOSITCHEK, R. J., HAHN, W., and WERTHESSEN, N. T.: Western collaborative group study: a study of predictive factors in the occurrence of coronary heart disease. *Circulation*, 28: 792, Part II, 1963 (abstract).

19. SIGLER, L. H.: Emotional strain affecting the electrocardiogram. See Chapter 13.

20. LEPESCHKIN, E.: *Modern Electrocardiography.* Baltimore, Williams and Wilkins, 1951.

21. LEVI, L.: The urinary output of adrenaline and noradrenaline during pleasant and unpleasant emotional states. *Psychosom Med*, 27:80, 1965.

22. FRIEDMAN, M., ST. GEORGE, S., BYERS, S. O., and ROSENMAN, R. H.: Excretion of catecholamines, 17-ketosteroids, 17-hydroxycorticoids and 5-hydroxyindole in men exhibiting a particular behavior pattern (A) associated with high incidence of clinical coronary artery disease. *J Clin Invest*, 39:758, 1960.

23. FOX, S. M., III, and SKINNER, J. S.: Physical activity and cardiovascular health. *Amer J Cardiol*, 14:731, 1964.

24. LAPICCIRELLA, V., and WEBER, G.: La claudicazione mesenterica, sindrome di allarme della malattia coronarica. *Arch De Vecchi Anat Pat*, 19: 1123, 1953.

25. DAWBER, T. R., KANNEL, W. B., and FRIEDMAN, G. D.: Vital capacity, physical activity and coronary heart disease. (See Chapter 31.)

26. NESSWETHA, W., and NATHUSIUS, W. V.: Untersuchungen über die prophylaktische und therapeutische Bedeutung der Terrainkur bei Regulationsstörungen des Kreislaufes der Industriearbeiter. *Int J Prophyl Med*, 4:No. 6, 1960.

27. SCHMIDT-KESSEN, W., GROH, W., and GROSS, W.: Ergebnisse eines Vergleiches von gymnastischen und Kneipp-Kuren bei vegetativer Dystonie. *Aerztl Forsch*, 18:347, 1964.

28. LAPICCIRELLA, V.: Stati ansiosi, aritmia respiratoria, malattia coronarica. *Med Psicosom*, 2:102, 1958.

Chapter XXVII

CORONARY HEART DISEASE AMONG ITALIANS AND NON-ITALIANS IN ROSETO, PENNSYLVANIA, AND IN NEARBY COMMUNITIES*

EDWARD N. BRANDT, JR., CLARKE STOUT, JAMES W. HAMPTON, THOMAS N. LYNN, and STEWART WOLF

(Oklahoma City, Oklahoma, U.S.A.)

EPIDEMIOLOGICAL studies of coronary disease in various ethnic groups have yielded a variety of interpretations. Keys, in several studies, has presented data suggesting that diet is important in the pathogenesis of myocardial infarction. He has inferred, for example, that there is more atherosclerosis among Japanese living in California or Hawaii than Japanese living in Japan because the former habitually eat more saturated fat than the latter (1). Similar studies of Italians have also led to the implication that a high fat diet is important in the genesis of atherosclerosis (2). Ethnic factors, on the other hand, were found by Dawber et al. not to be associated with differences in coronary heart disease in Framingham where there are substantial numbers of British, Irish and Italians (3). Danaraj reports a much higher mortality from coronary disease in Indian males than in Chinese males living in Singapore under superficially similar socioeconomic conditions (4). Whatever the relevant factors, it is evident that differences in the incidence of coronary heart disease do exist among different ethnic groups as well as among ethnically similar groups in different localities. The present study was undertaken in a nearly pure Italian community in the United States, hoping to minimize some of the variables inherent in a study involving widely differing geographical areas. The town of Roseto, Pennsylvania, was selected because it contains almost exclusively first, second and third generation Italian-Americans. The first objective of the study was to ascertain the death rate from myocardial infarction in this community as compared with other communities in the vicinity.

MORTALITY STATISTICS

The survey covered the 7-year period from 1955-1961. The communities included were, first, Nazareth, with a population of 6,209, predominantly German, descendants of Moravians who settled there before the American Revolution. The people continue to speak German in the home and eat a fairly typical German diet. They work mainly in steel and cement factories and on farms, but also make musical instruments and other

*This study was supported in part by a research grant, No. HE-06286-04, from the National Heart Institute and PHS grant FR 00005.

TABLE 27–I

POPULATION DISTRIBUTION BY AGE AND SEX OF THE FIVE COMMUNITIES STUDIED

Town	Sex	<5	5–14	15–24	25–34	35–44	45–54	55–64	<65	Total
Roseto	M	83	151	74	109	121	102	69	71	780
	F	70	153	83	118	143	145	63	75	850
Bangor	M	243	494	296	293	380	430	307	305	2748
	F	226	414	367	323	477	458	348	405	3018
Nazareth	M	289	536	321	400	406	410	307	314	2983
	F	276	512	388	405	454	440	365	386	3226
Stroudsburg	M	243	488	261	305	370	374	309	395	2745
	F	279	479	422	328	378	443	415	581	3325
East Stroudsburg	M	351	653	748	403	439	399	347	347	3687
	F	366	632	774	423	495	428	408	461	3987

items requiring specialized craftsmanship.

The second community was Roseto, population 1,630, which was settled in 1882 by immigrants from Roseto, Valfortore, in the province of Foggia, Italy. More than 95 per cent of the people of Roseto, Pennsylvania, are Italian and many of the original Italian customs are maintained. Vigorous and fun loving, the people eat a great deal, including much animal fat, and drink much wine. They are relatively prosperous financially due to hard work and ingenuity. Originally, most of the Rosetan men worked in the neighboring slate quarries. Today, most of the women and some of the men either own or work in small factories that manufacture shirts and blouses. Other men work in nearby steel mills and electrical industries, while only a few remain in the quarries.

Bangor, which is immediately adjacent to Roseto, was the third community studied. Its population is 5,766. Bangor was originally settled by Welsh quarriers who worked the nearby slate deposits. The town now contains a mixture of several ethnic types, including many of German and Italian origin. The inhabitants serve the surrounding farmers as merchants and tradesmen and work in nearby construction and steel industries. The fourth community was Stroudsburg, with a population of 6,070, and the fifth, East Stroudsburg, with a population of 7,674. Both of them are composed of mixed ethnic groups. Their work is mainly to supply the nearby mountain resorts with goods and services, although many men work in nearby cement, steel and state-operated industries.

Table 27–I shows the population distribution by age and sex in the 5 communities according to the 1960 census.

Death certificates of all people dying in the 5 towns between 1955 and 1961 were reviewed and verified whenever possible from physicians' and hospital records. The resulting values indicated a much lower death rate from myocardial infarction in Roseto than in the other 4 towns. This low death rate was particularly striking among Rosetan males (Table 27–II). Preliminary observations on the living indicated that Rosetans were obese and consumed approximately 40 per cent of their calories in the form of fat (5). The death rates from arteriosclerotic heart disease (without evidence of myocardial infarction), hypertensive heart disease, and other cardiovascular

TABLE 27–II

AVERAGE ANNUAL DEATH RATES PER 100,000 FROM MYOCARDIAL INFARCTION
BY AGE AND SEX FROM 1955 THROUGH 1961
(Proven Anatomically, Established Clinically and Presumed)

Town	Sex	Under 35	35–44	45–54	55–64	65–Up	Age Adjusted*
Roseto	M	—	—	144	—	813	109
	F	—	—	—	—	801	89
Nazareth	M	—	—	253	1049	2545	423
	F	—	—	134	234	1309	186
Bangor	M	—	35	305	1082	1866	363
	F	—	58	64	368	1431	212
Stroudsburg	M	42 (25–34)	74	373	910	1980	378
	F	—	—	—	140	695	92
East Stroudsburg	M	—	32	284	705	2344	374
	F	—	—	33	144	689	96

*Age-adjustment performed by the direct method (7) using the combined 1960 census male populations for the 5 communities as the standard population.

TABLE 27–III

AVERAGE ANNUAL AGE-ADJUSTED DEATH RATES PER 100,000 FROM
ARTERIOSCLEROTIC HEART DISEASE (EXCLUSIVE OF MYOCARDIAL INFARCTION),
HYPERTENSIVE HEART DISEASE AND OTHER CARDIOVASCULAR DISEASES
BY SEX FROM 1955 THROUGH 1961

Town	Sex	ASHD	HCVD	Other
Roseto	M	158	0	112
	F	89	22	44
Nazareth	M	161	31	97
	F	170	25	59
Bangor	M	137	5	114
	F	142	16	127
Stroudsburg	M	121	21	80
	F	66	29	37
East Stroudsburg	M	128	24	79
	F	98	25	56

causes were essentially similar for the 5 towns (Table 27–III) (5). The death rate from all causes (1955-63), however, was considerably lower in Roseto than in the other 4 towns, especially among males between the ages of 35 and 64, and males and females under age 55 (Table 27–IV).

STUDIES ON SURVIVORS

The second objective of the study was to determine the prevalence of myocardial infarction and related factors in Roseto and Bangor since they are immediately adjacent geographically, yet ethnically and culturally different (Table 27–V). Subjects over age 21 were examined, weighed, tested for serum cholesterol concentration, and questioned concerning dietary and social patterns. Also obtained on each person was a 12-lead ECG, a blood sugar, an assay for blood fibrinolytic activity, hematocrit, serum lipoprotein electrophoresis, clotting time, prothrombin time and fibrinogen concentration. In addition, with the collab-

TABLE 27–IV

AVERAGE ANNUAL DEATH RATES PER 1,000 FROM ALL CAUSES BY AGE AND SEX FOR
ROSETO, BANGOR, NAZARETH, STROUDSBURG AND EAST STROUDSBURG
1955 THROUGH 1963

Age Group	Roseto Pop.*	Roseto Ave. Rate	Bangor Pop.*	Bangor Ave. Rate	Nazareth Pop.*	Nazareth Ave. Rate	Stroudsburg Pop.*	Stroudsburg Ave. Rate	East Stroudsburg Pop.*	East Stroudsburg Ave. Rate
Males										
<5	83	1.34	243	6.86	289	7.69	243	9.60	351	6.96
5–14	151	.74	494	.67	536	.41	488	.23	653	.68
15–24	74	1.50	296	1.88	321	1.38	261	2.13	748	.59
25–34	109	–	293	2.66	400	.56	305	2.19	403	1.93
35–44	121	1.83	380	3.51	406	3.01	370	5.10	439	2.53
45–54	102	3.26	430	6.46	410	7.32	374	11.29	399	10.30
55–64	69	14.49	307	24.61	307	21.36	309	26.97	347	25.62
>65	71	64.17	305	70.68	314	95.89	395	75.95	347	79.73
Age-Adjusted Rates		9.72		13.00		15.22		14.83		14.24
Females										
<5	70	1.58	226	4.92	276	3.22	279	7.17	366	6.98
5–14	153	–	414	.54	512	.43	479	.23	632	.88
15–24	83	1.34	367	.60	388	.57	422	.53	774	.57
25–34	118	–	323	.34	405	1.10	328	1.35	423	2.36
35–44	143	.78	477	2.33	454	2.94	378	3.23	495	2.69
45–54	145	3.83	458	3.88	440	6.82	443	5.27	428	3.89
55–64	63	10.58	348	11.81	365	12.18	415	12.32	408	12.25
>65	75	47.41	405	59.53	386	68.22	581	53.74	461	56.88
Age-adjusted Rates		7.27		9.22		10.68		9.28		9.59

*Population: U.S. Census—1960.

TABLE 27–V

DISTRIBUTION OF SAMPLE BY TOWN, AGE, SEX AND RACE

Age Group	Roseto Italians	Bangor Italians	Bangor Non-Italians	Other Italians
0–34	52	37	54	46
35–44	51	40	60	47
45–54	54	44	98	43
55–65	33	26	58	20
65 & over	37	17	59	16
Total	227	164	329	172
Females				
0–34	54	27	61	43
35–44	66	44	102	48
45–54	80	57	111	30
55–64	47	19	98	25
65 & over	23	26	97	11
Total	270	173	469	157

oration of a sociologist, the communities were visited and families and individuals were interviewed at length. These data have been reported separately (8), but it may be said here that Roseto was found to be a closely-knit and mutually supporting community, where the family relationships are relatively stable, the man being the dominant figure. Close and supporting relationships exist also among collateral relatives.

Prevalence figures were then worked out for the Italian population of Roseto, their relatives and some other Italians scattered in various communities classified under "Other," and Italians in Bangor, and non-Italians in Bangor. Age-adjusted prevalences were obtained by the direct method of adjustment (7), using the combined sample figures for the five communities as the standard population.

Diabetes Mellitus. The diagnosis of diabetes was made according to the following criteria:

1. History of diabetes treated with insulin, oral hypoglycemics or diet.

2. Fasting blood sugar of 130 mg% or greater, 1 hour postprandial blood sugar of 180 mg% or greater, 2 hour postprandial blood sugar of 150 mg% or greater, 3 hour postprandial blood sugar of 130 mg% or greater, or any blood sugar of 200 mg% or greater.

Obesity. The diagnosis of obesity was made if the weight exceeded 120 per cent of the ideal weight for the given age, height, and sex (6).

Hypertension. Since the diagnosis of hypertensive cardiovascular disease could not be established on a single examination, a classification of hypertension was based on the following criteria:

a) Diastolic blood pressure 95 > mmHg.,
b) History of hypertension.

1) Definite hypertension: Both of the criteria present.

2) Probable hypertension: Criterion (a) only present.

3) Questionable hypertension: Criterion (b) only.

Myocardial Infarction. The diagnosis of myocardial infarction was divided into the following categories:

a) Definite myocardial infarction: This electrocardiographic diagnosis was based on the following criteria:

I. Q/R ratio of 1/5 to 1/3 in any of the leads I, II, V_2 through V_6, or in V_1 in the absense of right ventricular hypertrophy and right bundle branch block;

II. Q wave (1 mm. or more) lasting at least 0.04 sec. in any leads I, II, V_1 through V_6 or in aVL if an R of 3 mm. or more is present.

III. Q wave duration of 0.04 to 0.05 sec. in lead aVF (some Q must be present in II);

IV. Q amplitude of 5 mm. or greater in lead aVF when an R wave is present (some Q must be present in II);

V. QS pattern in V_1 - V_3 in the absence of left bundle branch block and left ventricular hypertrophy;

VI. Posterior infarction was read on the basis of a slurred R in lead V_1 with a duration greater than 0.04 sec. in the absence of right ventricular hypertrophy.

b) Probable myocardial infarction: An electrocardiogram was read as probable if it failed to meet the criteria for definite by 0.01 seconds or less or by 1 mm. or less.

TABLE 27–VI

PREVALENCE PER 1000 OF DIABETES MELLITUS BY TOWN, RACE, AGE AND SEX

Age Group	Roseto Italians Sample	Prev.	Bangor Italians Sample	Prev.	Non-Italians Sample	Prev.	Other Italians Sample	Prev.
Males								
0–34	52	19.2	37	–	54	–	46	21.7
35–44	51	–	40	–	60	33.3	47	21.3
45–54	54	18.5	44	22.7	98	91.8	43	–
55–64	33	30.3	26	192.3	58	120.7	20	100.0
65 & over	37	54.1	17	–	59	288.1	16	187.5
Age Adjusted	227	21.9	164	39.5	329	93.3	172	49.6
Females								
0–34	54	–	27	–	61	32.8	43	–
35–44	66	–	44	–	102	39.2	48	–
45–54	80	37.5	57	35.1	111	99.1	30	–
55–64	47	85.1	19	157.9	98	153.1	25	–
65 & over	23	87.0	26	115.4	97	216.5	11	90.9
Age Adjusted	270	33.3	173	52.9	469	98.5	157	128.9

TABLE 27–VII

PREVALENCE PER 1000 OF OBESITY BY TOWN, RACE, AGE AND SEX

Age Group	Roseto Italians Sample	Prev.	Bangor Italians Sample	Prev.	Non-Italians Sample	Prev.	Other Italians Sample	Prev.
Males								
0–34	52	365.4	37	378.4	54	277.8	46	391.3
35–44	51	411.8	40	350.0	60	233.3	47	255.3
45–54	54	296.3	44	227.3	98	173.5	43	139.5
55–64	33	151.5	26	38.5	58	172.4	20	100.0
65 & over	37	270.3	17	235.3	59	101.7	16	437.5
Age Adjusted	227	308.0	164	253.5	329	197.3	172	250.5
Females								
0–34	54	92.6	27	74.1	61	82.0	43	69.8
35–44	66	212.1	44	227.3	102	137.3	48	187.5
45–54	80	200.0	57	193.0	111	108.1	30	333.3
55–64	47	340.4	19	210.5	98	234.7	25	240.0
65 & over	23	391.3	26	538.5	97	185.6	11	272.7
Age Adjusted	270	234.1	173	230.5	469	143.2	157	223.4

RESULTS

Tables 27–VI, VII, VIII and IX summarize the findings with respect to the prevalence of diabetes, obesity, hypertension, and myocardial infarction. The sample sizes in each table indicate the number of subjects on which the information necessary to establish the diag-

TABLE 27–VIII

PREVALENCE PER 1000 OF HYPERTENSION (DEFINITE AND PROBABLE)
BY TOWN, RACE, AGE AND SEX

Age Group	Roseto Italians Sample	Prev.	Bangor Italians Sample	Prev.	Non-Italians Sample	Prev.	Other Italians Sample	Prev.
Males								
0–34	52	153.8	37	108.1	54	111.1	46	43.5
35–44	51	196.1	40	200.0	60	166.7	47	106.4
45–54	54	351.9	44	159.1	98	204.1	43	186.0
55–64	33	333.3	26	307.7	58	224.1	20	150.0
65 & over	37	489.2	17	–	59	186.4	16	250.0
Age Adjusted	227	293.2	164	162.5	329	178.4	172	142.6
Females								
0–34	54	–	27	–	61	32.8	43	23.3
35–44	66	106.1	44	45.5	102	98.0	48	41.7
45–54	80	162.5	57	228.1	111	99.1	30	233.3
55–64	47	340.4	19	157.9	98	214.3	25	240.0
65 & over	23	217.4	26	192.3	97	226.8	11	272.7
Age Adjusted	270	156.9	173	123.7	469	124.4	157	154.4

TABLE 27–IX

PREVALENCE PER 1000 OF MYOCARDIAL INFARCTION (DEFINITE AND PROBABLE)
BY TOWN, RACE, AGE AND SEX

Age Group	Roseto Italians Sample	Prev.	Bangor Italians Sample	Prev.	Non-Italians Sample	Prev.	Other Italians Sample	Prev.
Males								
0–34	52	–	37	–	54	–	46	–
35–44	51	–	40	25.0	60	16.7	47	–
45–54	54	–	44	45.5	98	51.0	43	46.5
55–64	33	151.5	26	38.5	58	34.5	20	100.0
65 & over	37	81.1	17	176.5	59	135.6	16	125.0
Age Adjusted	227	38.0	164	49.3	329	42.2	172	47.0
Females								
0–34	54	–	27	–	61	–	43	–
35–44	66	–	44	–	102	–	48	–
45–54	80	12.5	57	17.5	111	9.0	30	66.7
55–64	47	63.8	19	–	98	20.4	25	–
65 & over	23	43.5	26	–	97	113.4	11	90.9
Age Adjusted	270	20.5	173	4.5	469	21.9	157	29.9

N.B. The above figures differ from those published earlier by Bruhn (*J Chronic Dis*, *18:*353, 1965) in which electrocardiographic abnormalities not meeting the criteria stated here were included. In addition, the numbers of subjects differ slightly because some subjects initially gave addresses of family members rather than their own.

nosis was available. The prevalence of diabetes among Italian men in Roseto is substantially less than that of the non-Italian inhabitants of Bangor, and even less than the Bangor Italians. Among females, the Roseto inhabitants also had a relatively low prevalence, although their relatives living elsewhere gave no evidence of diabetes at all. More of the Italians in Roseto and Bangor were obese than were Bangor non-Italians. This difference held for both men and women. The differences in the prevalence of hypertension among the groups were not striking except that Roseto Italian men showed the highest prevalence. Electrocardiographic evidence of myocardial infarction was absent among Roseto men below the age of 55, although the prevalence among Italian men below age 55, living outside Roseto, was not strikingly different from that among non-Italians. The age-adjusted prevalences for men were all very similar except for the "other" Italians, the very small sample which included mainly relatives of Rosetans living elsewhere in Pennsylvania, New Jersey and New York.

DISCUSSION

The low incidence of death from myocardial infarction in Roseto is matched by a low incidence of ECG evidence of the disease in men below the age of 55. The fact that prevalence figures for those older than 55 do not strikingly differ from the groups outside Roseto may be a reflection of the relatively low mortality from myocardial infarction among Roseto men. The relatively high prevalence of ECG evidence of myocardial infarction among male relatives of Rosetans who live elsewhere suggest that the low death

rate and low prevalence of myocardial infarction among men under 55 in Roseto is not explained by genetic factors, or indeed by ethnic factors. Simply being an Italian does not appear to confer significant protection against myocardial infarction. Sociologic factors offer more promise. The investigators were impressed by the way of life of the people of Roseto, particularly by their adaptability, their energy for work and fun, their hospitality, the stability of their families, and the cohesive quality of their community.

SUMMARY

An unusually low death rate from myocardial infarction, less than half that of the surrounding communities, was observed in the Italian-American community of Roseto, Pennsylvania, during the 7-year period from 1955 to 1961. The low death rate, observed in both sexes, was particularly striking among the males. Preliminary studies of the living in Roseto and in one of the nearby communities indicate that the prevalence of coronary heart disease, as reflected in the ECG, is lower among Roseto Italian men under age 55 than among Italians from other communities, including the relatives of Roseto families. Over age 55 the prevalence of ECG changes indicative of coronary artery disease was not significantly different among the various groups. These data suggest not only a low incidence of myocardial infarction in Roseto in men under age 55, but a low death rate from myocardial infarction in the older age group. Whether the relative freedom of Rosetans from death from myocardial infarction is related to their way of life remains to be determined. At present, however, correlations with social patterns are more impressive than those with genetic or ethnic factors.

ACKNOWLEDGMENT

We wish to acknowledge the continued assistance of the Commonwealth of Pennsylvania, Department of Health, Division of Statistics and Records in our studies.

REFERENCES

1. KEYS, A., KIMURA, N., KUSUKAWA, A., BRONTE-STEWART, B., LARSEN, N., and KEYS, M. H.: Lessons from serum cholesterol studies in Japan, Hawaii, and Los Angeles. *Ann Intern Med, 48:* 83, 1958.
2. KEYS, A., FIDANZA, F., SCARDI, V., BERGAMI, G., KEYS, M. H., and DI LORENZO, F.: Studies on serum cholesterol and other characteristics of clinically healthy men in Naples. *Arch Intern Med, 93:*328, 1954.
3. DAWBER, T. R., KANNEL, W. B., REVOTSKIE, N., STOKES, J., KAGAN, A., and GORDON, T.: Some factors associated with development of coronary heart disease. *Amer J Public Health, 49:*1349, 1959.
4. DANARAJ, T. J., ACKER, M. S., DANARAJ, W., ONG, W. H., and YAM, T. B.: Ethnic group differences in coronary heart disease in Singapore. *Amer Heart J, 58:*516, 1959.
5. STOUT, C., MORROW, J., BRANDT, E. N., and WOLF, S.: Unusually low incidence of death from myocardial infarction. *JAMA, 188:*845, 1964.
6. SUNDERMAN, F. W., and BOERNER, F.: *Normal Values in Clinical Medicine.* Philadelphia, W. B. Saunders Co., 1950, p. 633.
7. HILL, A. BRADFORD: *Principles of Medical Statistics.* New York, Oxford University Press, 1961.
8. BRUHN, J. G.: An epidemiological study of myocardial infarction in an Italian-American Community—a preliminary sociological study. *J Chron Dis, 18:*353, 1965.

Chapter XXVIII

SUBMAXIMAL WORK CAPACITY OF A FRENCH CANADIAN MALE POPULATION*

CLAUDE ALLARD, CLAUDE GOULET, GASTON CHOQUETTE, and PAUL DAVID

(Montreal, Canada)

THE French Canadian population can probably be considered the most homogeneous among the white races in North America (1). To the student of human biology this "homogeneity" is a great advantage. Though much is known about the history and sociology of the French Canadians, the biological characteristics of this population are less known.

Our group is now pursuing at the Institut de Cardiologie de Montreal an extensive study of this ethnic group. The physical work capacity appears of importance in a research program on reconditioning as being set up in this Institute for coronary and coronary-prone subjects. Norms or base-line values for work capacity are not available in our population.

POPULATION

The population under study consists of 1000 French Canadian males, aged 20 to 70 years, and working for the City of Montreal. They were selected at random among the entire male population of

10,612 employees of French Canadian origin as shown in Figure 28–1. Our test population is composed of 450 policemen and firemen and 550 white collar and other workers. A total of 236 different occupations is represented among the white collar and other workers. With respect to age, the civic employees were a representative sample of the total French Canadian male population of the City of Montreal. Results on the first 399 subjects investigated are discussed in the present paper.

METHODS

The subjects were seen once, in groups of 3, at 8:30am, following an overnight fast. Fasting was controlled by a routine determination of the triglyceride concentration in the chylomicron portion and supernatant fraction of the fresh sera, isolated by differential centrifugation. After blood collection (60 ml) and an ECG at rest, breakfast was served, which consisted of 1 or 2 buns with coffee (sugar and cream to taste). Then smoking was permitted, but the subjects did not smoke during the rest of the evaluation period (3 to 4 hours). One subject was seen by the cardiologist, the other

*Supported by a grant (No. 604-7-397) from the Department of National Health and Welfare (Canada), according to a Provincial-Federal arrangement.

SAMPLING

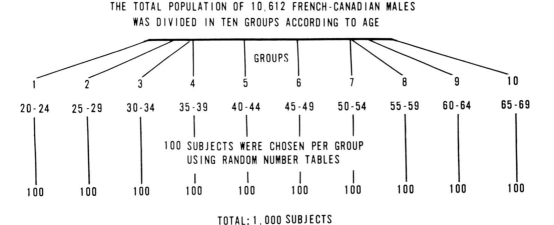

Figure 28–1. Description of the method employed for sampling the subjects under investigation.

TABLE 28–I

APPLICABILITY OF THE PHYSICAL WORK CAPACITY TEST

| | | *Number of Subjects* | | |
| | | | *Test Incomplete But Valid Capable of Two Loads (12 Min Work)* | *Test Completed Capable of Three Loads (18 Min Work)* |
Age	*Total*	*No. Refused for Medical Reasons*		
20–24	37	0	6	31
25–29	41	1	10	30
30–34	40	3	8	29
35–39	43	4	7	32
40–44	47	2	14	31
45–49	38	5	7	18
50–54	29	10	8	11
55–59	30	15	9	6
60–64	31	19	8	4
65–69	26	22	2	2
All ages	354	81	79	194
Percentage	100	23	22	55

by the anthropologist, and the third by the dietitian. At about 10:15 to 10:30 am, the first subject was ready for the work test on a bicycle ergometer (a model AM-368, manufactured in Stockholm by Elema-Schonander). This model maintains a preset load within the limits of 45 to 75 rev/min, regardless as to whether the subject is able to keep up a constant pedalling rate. The room temperature varied from 21 to 26 °C.

The work test was performed following a 30-minute rest on a comfortable lounge chair. The subject was taught how to

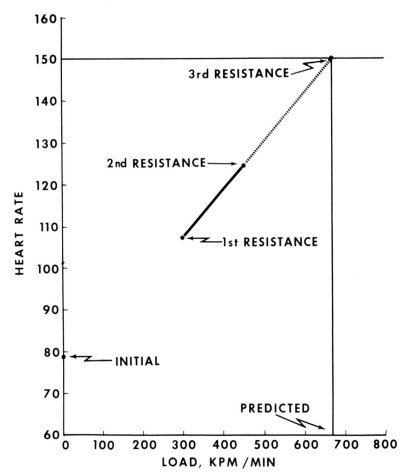

Figure 28–2. Prediction of the third ergometer resistance to be applied as calculated from the heart rates observed at the first two previous loads of 300 and 450 kpm/min, respectively.

perform on the ergometer and was then idle for 5 minutes. The heart rate (determined by measuring on the ECG the time for 30 beats) was determined during that time. The heart rate during the last minute of this period was considered as the initial or the anticipatory rate. Three consecutive loads were then imposed for 6 minutes each. The heart rate as well as the ECG and blood pressure were taken at each minute. The mean heart rate of the fifth and the sixth minutes of each load was regarded as that corresponding to this particular load. It was

considered in a steady state when the variation was less than 10 beats per minute between the fourth and the sixth minute.

The first load was 300 kg/meter/minute (kpm/min). The second load was 450 kpm/min. Following this second work load, the subject remained idle for 4 minutes and the heart rate was recorded at every minute. During this intermittent stop, the performance of the subject was quickly evaluated in such a manner as to decide which load to apply to obtain, in a steady state, a heart rate

TABLE 28–II

MEAN HEART RATE ±1 S.D.
DURING WORK TEST
(ALL AGES)

	RATE*		
	Loads, kpm/min for 6 Min.		
0	300	450	>450
79 ±10	107 ±16	119 ±17	141 ±11
(299) †	(299)	(264)	(191) ‡

*Measured at one minute before test, at minute 6 (300 kpm); at minute 12 (450 kpm); at minute 18 (>450 kpm).
†Number of subjects.
‡63 per cent of the population.

TABLE 28–III

MEAN PHYSICAL WORK CAPACITY 150

Age	No. of Subjects (All Ages)	kpm/150	kpm/150/M²†
Group A. White Collar and other workers:			
20–69	113	642 ±181	351 ±95
Group B. Policemen and firemen:			
20–69	143	719 ±167‡	365 ±87

*The mean kpm/170 extrapolated from the kpm/150 would be 891 ±203 for group A and 962 ±170 for group B.
†kpm/150 beats/min/meter² of body surface.
‡The difference between group A and B for the kpm/150 was significant (P<0.001) but the difference for the kmp/150/M² was not.

of 140 to 150 beats/min. This was done instantly by plotting on a peg board, instead of graph paper (having as coordinates heart frequency versus load in kpm/min), the two heart rates observed in a steady state. These rates corresponded to the two consecutive loads of 300 and 450 kpm/min. Extrapolation on a straight line to about 140 to 150/min was done to obtain the predicted kpm/min, as illustrated in Figure 28–2. This predicted load was then applied for 6 minutes. In 22 per cent of the subjects it was not necessary to apply the third load since they had reached a heart rate of about 150 during the second load. (See Table 28–I.)

To calculate the exact work capacity or performance at 150 beats per minute, the 3 experimental values were plotted on graph paper and a straight line was extra- or intrapolated to a heart rate of exactly 150. This result was expressed as the kpm/150. To compare with some data in the literature, extrapolation to 170 beats/minute was made. The physical work capacity being known for a submaximal work, the maximal oxygen consumption (Max VO²) or aerobic capacity was calculated according to a procedure prosposed by Åstrand and Ryh-

ming, using their correction factor for age (2). The Max VO² could then be expressed in liters of oxygen per minute or in milliliter of oxygen per kilogram of body weight per minute.

RESULTS

Table 28–II shows that the mean heart rate at minute 17 to 18 (last minute of the test) was 141 ±11. The number of subjects for each load was not the same because some had reached either during the first, second or third load a heart rate of 140 to 150.

The work capacity test described above was found to be appropriate for evaluating large groups of subjects since 77 per cent of 354 subjects could perform this test (Table 28–I). Most of the subjects not accepted for the test because of medical reasons were 50 years and older.

In the population sample under investigation, two groups of subjects (policemen and firemen) might bias the results of the general group because minimum height and weight are prerequisites for hiring policemen and firemen at the City of Montreal. Consequently, the results obtained with these subjects are presented separately (Table 28–III).

TABLE 28–IV
MEAN AEROBIC WORK CAPACITY 150

Age	No. of Subjects	Max. VO2, l/min.	Max. VO2, ml/kg/min.
Group A. White collar and other workers:			
20–24	12	2.54 ±0.63	35.4 ±8.7
25–29	13	2.24 ±0.43	33.9 ±6.6
30–34	11	2.67 ±0.49	34.5 ±8.9
35–39	15	2.25 ±0.51	30.5 ±8.4
40–44	22	2.02 ±0.48	27.8 ±4.9
45–49	12	1.72 ±0.29	27.3 ±7.3
50–54	10	2.02 ±0.44	28.8 ±4.9
55–59	10	1.57 ±0.41	25.6 ±5.7
60–64	6	1.60 ±0.11	21.8 ±2.9
65–69	2	1.95 ±0.07	27.5 ±7.8
All ages	113	2.10 ±0.56	29.8 ±7.6
Group B. Policemen and firemen:			
All ages	143	2.41 ±0.52	30.6 ±7.5

In confirmation of the results of Åstrand (3), the physical working capacity did not vary with age. This is the reason why only the mean values for all ages appear in Table 28–III. They were greater for policemen and firemen than for white collar and other workers (p < 0.001). Extrapolation of the physical work capacity at 150 to the work capacity at 170 beats per minute yielded an average value of 891 kpm for the white collar and other workers and a value of 962 kpm for the policemen and firemen.

A comparison with similar studies by Frisk et al (4) suggests that the physical working capacity of our population in Montreal was about the same as that in Stockholm. On the other hand, Cumming and Cumming in Winnipeg observed in young Canadian adults a value of 964 kpm/170/min (5). When the physical working capacity was expressed per unit body weight, a mean value of 351 ±95 kpm/min/M² was observed for the white collar and other workers, and 365 ±87

for the policemen and firemen; the difference between both groups was not significant.

Table 28–IV shows the mean predicted aerobic work capacity by age.

An attempt at classifying subjects according to their aerobic work capacity was made, using the classification table suggested by Åstrand (3).

Table 28–V shows that about 69 per cent of all subjects would fall into the low aerobic capacity class, whereas 17.7 per cent would fall into the fair, 12.8 per cent into the average and 0.8 per cent into the good aerobic capacity class. Not one subject was observed to have a high aerobic capacity according to the criteria used in that classification (3). The proportion of subjects in each category was about the same for the group aged 20 to 49 years. In older age groups the proportion of subjects classified as fair and average was greater; probably because only clinically healthy subjects were tested on the ergometer, which meant an increasing selection of healthy subjects with age (See Table 28–I.)

After using the work capacity test, described in this paper, to screen a large group of subjects, one is inclined to think that the anticipatory heart rate of the subject is somewhat related to his performance. Figure 28–3 shows the relationship between these two variables. The correlation coefficient was −0.45 with a p value of < 0.01. These results suggest that the anticipatory heart rate was related to performance but not in a consistent manner.

In the present project an attempt was made to relate the physical performance to anxiety. The suggestion was made by Cattell (6) that "correlation should be worked out between personality and

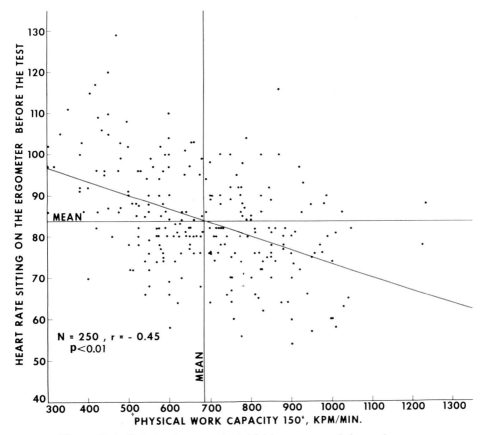

Figure 28–3. Relation between the initial heart rate and the performance.

TABLE 28–V

DISTRIBUTION OF SUBJECTS ACCORDING TO THE
AEROBIC WORK CAPACITY (VO₂, ML/KG)

Age	Low		Fair		Classification* Average		Good		High	
	VO_2	$N\dagger$ (%)	VO_2	N (%)	VO_2	N (%)	VO_2	N (%)	VO_2	N (%)
20–29	≤ 38	51 (73.9)	39–43	12 (17.4)	44–51	6 (8.7)	52–56	0	≥ 57	0
30–39	≤ 34	51 (76.1)	35–39	5 (7.5)	40–47	9 (13.4)	48–51	2 (3.0)	≥ 52	0
40–49	≤ 30	51 (72.9)	31–35	10 (14.3)	36–43	9 (12.9)	44–57	0	≥ 58	0
50–59	≤ 25	12 (44.4)	26–31	10 (37.0)	32–39	5 (18.5)	40–43	0	≥ 44	0
60–69	≤ 21	2 (20.0)	22–26	6 (60.0)	27–35	2 (20.0)	36–39	0	≥ 40	0
All ages 243 subjects (100%)		167 (68.7)		43 (17.7)		31 (12.8)		2 (0.8)		0 (0.0)

*Based on the evaluation of the aerobic work capacity made by Åstrand (3).
†Number of subjects. Percentage distribution by age groups in parentheses.

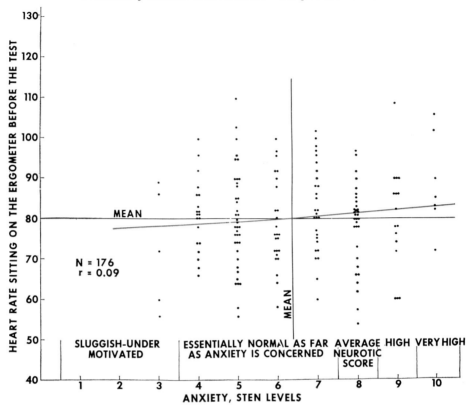

Figure 28–4. Relation between the initial heart rate and the level of anxiety.

physical fitness in the normal range and without the competitive situation."

The psychological test employed here was devised by Scheir and Cattell (7) and adapted to our population by Dr. D. Cormier (8) from the University of Montreal.

The results indicate that no correlation existed between the anticipatory heart rate and the anxiety level (Fig. 28–4). Nevertheless, when the mean initial heart rates at a sten level of 3 were compared with the other extreme, that is, at a level of 10, the difference was found to be significant with a p value of .06.

With respect to the performance on the ergometer, the relationship between anxiety and physical work capacity was more apparent. Table 28–VI shows that at a sten level higher than 7 the percentage of subjects who could not complete the test was higher than at a sten level corresponding to normalcy.

Surprisingly, the physical work capacity of those men who could complete the test was independent of their anxiety level. These results suggest that the physical work capacity among anxious individuals is a question of all or nothing (i.e., they either perform like normals or they fail the performance test). It would seem necessary to qualify anxiety better and to correlate personality factors with performance to see whether those whose performance was nil have characteristic personality traits with respect to the other anxious group whose physical perfor-

TABLE 28–VI

ANXIETY AND PERFORMANCE

Anxiety, Sten Levels	Anxiety, Description	No. of Subjects	Percentage of Subjects Who Failed the Test*	Mean KPM/150 Values for Those Whose Test Was Valid
1	Sluggish	0	0	–
2	Undermotivated	0	0	–
3		4	0	769
4		20	0	735
5	Essentially	29	0	733
6	Normal	26	8	715
7		25	4	713
8	Average neurotic score	30	16	760
9	High	14	28	700
10	Very high	8	75	690

*Because a heart rate of 150 or higher was reached during the first, or before the second load period was terminated.

mance was normal. This is being investigated.

DISCUSSION

In this preliminary epidemiological study of physical work capacity, it has been observed that about 75 per cent of the subjects could perform the multilevel work test on the bicycle ergometer and reach a heart rate of 140 to 150 beats/min. The refusals were mostly among people above 50 years of age. The number of subjects which were not accepted for the test might appear high, but since the object of this work is to establish base-line values, it seemed essential to exclude subjects carrying pathologies theoretically apt to alter their performance. In future studies, subjects presenting abnormalities will be examined and compared to the norms established in the present study. A significant difference was noted between the mean physical work capacity of the policemen and firemen group and that of the white collar and other workers' group. When expressing the physical work capacity per body surface or when the aerobic capacity was calculated per kilogram body weight or in ml/min, the results were similar for the policemen, firemen, and the white collar and other workers. These results suggested that, in general, policemen and firemen could work harder than the rest of the population (greater kpm/150), but that their physical fitness might not be superior. Even though the physical work capacity (kpm/150 or kpm/170) should be recognized as an important parameter, either for job classification or other purposes (sports), it would seem of limited value in epidemiological studies of physical working capacity or in comparing populations or groups of normals or pathological subjects (9, 10) because differences in work capacity between such groups might reflect, among other factors, a difference in weight and/or height as well as in training. The physical work capacity divided by the surface area permits a more valid comparison (5).

In our epidemiological project the

direct determination of the O^2 consumption and of the maximal aerobic capacity is not feasible. On the other hand, the prediction of the maximal oxygen consumption with the use of the nomogram of Åstrand and Ryhming (2) would appear applicable for screening large groups of subjects. It is of interest to note that Luft et al. (11), who compared the direct method of measuring the O^2 consumption with that of using the nomogram of Åstrand and Ryhming (2), found the nomogram valid.

The present investigation showed that the predicted maximal oxygen consumption was low in our population. These results are in accord with those in other populations (10) and also with the fact that at 25 years or older, only 2 per cent of our population was engaged in intense physical activity off the job. This information was obtained by questioning each subject on its past and present history of physical activity. The attempt to classify subjects according to their predicted aerobic work capacity showed moreover that only 0.8 per cent of our population could be considered as having a good aerobic capacity, whereas about 69 per cent had a low aerobic capacity. It is remarkable that the proportion of subjects in each category (low, fair, average, good) was about the same from 20 to 49 years. These results support the hypothesis that young males in our population are not more "fit" than healthy older ones.

The association of performance with anxiety revealed that the proportion of individuals who failed the work test was much higher in the anxious group than in the others.

Results given here on 399 subjects or less are considered preliminary and should be re-evaluated at the end of this study when nearly 1000 subjects will have been investigated.

SUMMARY

As a first phase in a "reconditioning" research program for coronary-prone-men, base-line values for various biological parameters are being sought in a randomly chosen population consisting of 1000 males working for the City of Montreal.

Among the parameters studied, the ability to perform a multilevel exercise tolerance test was assessed, using a bicycle ergometer. Essentially, this test consisted in applying 3 consecutive loads, each of 6 minutes duration, in order to obtain at the end of the third load a heart rate of about 150 beats/min in a steady state. Out of the nearly 400 subjects, aged 20 to 70, 78 per cent could perform the test. The refusals were mostly among subjects over 50 years.

The mean "physical work capacity 150" was 685 ± 177 kpm/min. The mean oxygen consumption calculated from a nomogram constructed by Åstrand and Ryhming was 2.27 ± 0.56 liters/min. The mean aerobic capacity was 30.3 ± 7.4 ml kg/min.

According to the evaluation of the aerobic capacity made by Åstrand, about 69 per cent of the population would have a low aerobic working capacity. The proportion of subjects who failed to complete the exercise test was greater among anxious subjects than among normal or undermotivated subjects.

REFERENCES

1. Langlois, G.: *Histoire de la Population Canadienne Française.* Ed. A. Lévesque, Montreal, 1934.
2. Åstrand, P. O., and Ryhming, I.: A nomogram for calculation of aerobic capacity (physical fit-

ness) from pulse rate during submaximal work. *J Appl Physiol*, 7:218, 1954.

3. ÅSTRAND, I.: Aerobic work capacity in men and women with special reference to age. *Phys Scand*, *49:*48, Suppl. 119, 1960.

4. FRISK, A. R., WERKÖ, L., HOLMGREN, A., and STRÖM, G.: Stockholm's city health survey 1954. *Acta Med Scand*, *163:*1, 1959.

5. CUMMING, C. R., and CUMMING, P. M.: Working capacity of normal children tested on a bicycle ergometer. *Canad Med Ass J*, *88:*351, 1963.

6. CATTEL, R. B.: Some psychological correlates of physical fitness and physique. In: *Exercise and Fitness*. The Univ. of Illinois College of Physical Education and the Athletic Institute, 1959, pp. 138–151.

7. SCHEIER, I. A., and CATTELL, R. B.: The IPAT anxiety scale, Champaign, Illinois: Institute of Personality and Ability Testing, 1959.

8. Echelle d'anxiété IPAT. Institut de Recherches Psychologiques, Montreal, 1962.

9. HIRSCH, E. Z., HELLERSTEIN, H. K., and HORNSTEN, T. R.: Study of an unfit coronary prone population. *Circulation, 26:*730, 1962.

10. BERNSTEIN, J. I., HIRSCH, E. Z., and HELLERSTEIN, H. K.: True test of exercise tolerance and physical work capacity in myocardial infarction patients. *Circulation, 28:*690, 1963.

11. LUFT, V. C., CARDUS, D., LIM, T. P. K., ANDERSON, E. C., and HOWARTH J. L.: Physical performance in relation to body size and composition. *Ann. N. Y. Acad. Sci.: 110:*795, 1963.

Chapter XXIX

THE INFLUENCE OF PHYSICAL ACTIVITY ON INCIDENCE AND PROGNOSIS OF ISCHEMIC HEART DISEASE*

DANIEL BRUNNER

(Tel Aviv-Jaffa, Israel)

THE relationship between occupation and the frequency and course of ischemic heart disease has received increasing attention during the last decade. Epidemiological studies in England, Sweden, USA, and Isreal have provided suggestive but still ambiguous and sometimes contradictory results (1–9).

This paper comprises the results of two studies:

Our observations regarding the frequency of clinical ischemic heart disease as related to physical activity at work in people living in Israeli Kibbutzim and the influence of type of work in the predisease period on the prognosis in patients after initial myocardial infarction.

The members of the Israeli collective settlements (kibbutz; plural, kibbutzim) are engaged in different types of work (e.g., agriculture, fishing, building, light industry, teaching, accounting, clerking, managerial work), but neither their success in, nor the importance of their particular job have any bearing on their income or standard of living. Food is prepared in a single kitchen and served in a communal dining room. Members of the old, established kibbutzim have shared the same environmental conditions for at least the last 20 years. Therefore, more than in any other society, it is possible to single out the factor of physical activity at work and to estimate its influence on the development of the clinical manifestation of ischemic heart disease. We surveyed the incidence rates of anginal syndrome, acute myocardial infarction, and fatalities due to ischemic heart disease in middle-aged males and females in the collective settlements during a 15-year period.

PLAN OF STUDY

Table 29–I shows the composition of the population at risk at the end of the surveyed 15-year period. There were 5,279 men and 5,229 women, 40 to 64 years old. The people included in this survey are Jews of European origin. The population statistics were obtained from the "Official Voter's Role," which was used as the basis for the 1961 general elections (10).

Three clinical forms of ischemic heart disease were distinguished: myocardial infarction, angina pectoris, and fatal cases

*This study was supported by grant OVR-ISR-21-62 from the Vocational Rehabilitation Administration, and grant HE-04520 (RI) from the National Heart Institute, U.S. Public Health Service.

TABLE 29–I

COMPOSITION OF THE POPULATION
AT THE END OF THE SURVEY

Age Range	Men	Women
40–44	878	891
45–49	1375	1601
50–54	1550	1485
55–59	883	725
60–64	420	350
65–69	173	177
Total	5279	5229

due to ischemic heart disease. The diagnosis of myocardial infarction was based on a clearly documented history, convincing laboratory data and confirmatory serial ECG findings, demonstrating the development of pathological Q-waves and/or deep "coronary" T-waves.

As regards angina pectoris, only cases of "definite anginal syndrome" as defined by the Princeton Conference were included in this study (11).

Patients who died within two months after initial myocardial infarction were included in the group of fatal cases. Likewise, patients whose angina pectoris appeared only as a prodromal syndrome, not more than two months before acute

myocardial infarction, were included in the group of myocardial infarctions. The exact type of work performed by every patient was established. In order to obtain unambiguous definitions, we differentiated only between sedentary and nonsedentary workers, and did not try to distinguish between heavy and light physical work. A sedentary worker was defined as one who is seated for at least 80 per cent of his/her time at work. This includes teachers, managers, clerks, treasurers, bus drivers, cobblers, and people engaged in light industry. On the other hand, all those engaged in light physical labor (gardeners, workers in the kitchen and kindergarten) are included in the group of nonsedentary workers.

It was established that approximately 70 per cent of the male workers of the kibbutzim over 40-years-old are nonsedentary workers, the remaining 30 per cent being sedentary. Corresponding figures for the female workers are 60 per cent and 40 per cent, respectively (12).

The incidence rates were related to

TABLE 29–II

ANGINAL SYNDROME AND SURVIVING CASES OF MYOCARDIAL INFARCTION
IN MALE KIBBUTZ MEMBERS (15-YEAR PERIOD)

Age Range	Total No.			Anginal Syndrome No. of Cases	Anginal Syndrome Per 1000/Year	Myocardial Infarct. No. of Cases	Myocardial Infarct. Per 1000/Year
			Sedent. w.	6,006	7	1.2	10	1.7
40–44	20,022	Nonsed. w.	14,016	15	1.1	7	0.5
		Sedent. w.	6,228	28	4.5	22	3.5
45–49	20,660	Nonsed. w.	14,432	24	1.7	25	1.8
		Sedent. w.	4,860	20	4.2	30	6.3
50–54	16,202	Nonsed. w.	11,342	12	1.1	20	1.8
		Sedent. w.	2,544	8	3.2	8	3.2
55–59	8,481	Nonsed. w.	5,937	6	1.0	10	1.7
		Sedent. w.	1,047	4	4.0	7	7.0
60–64	3,490	Nonsed. w.	2,443	4	1.6	7	2.9
		Sedent. w.	20,685	67	3.2	77	3.7
Total	68,855	Nonsed. w.	48,170	61	1.2	69	1.4

Sedentary versus Nonsedentary Workers—Incidence Rate per 1000/year

TABLE 29–III

ANGINAL SYNDROME AND SURVIVING CASES OF MYOCARDIAL INFARCTION
IN MALE KIBBUTZ MEMBERS (15-YEAR PERIOD)

				Anginal Syndrome		Myocardial Infarct.	
Age Range	Total No.			No. of Cases	Per 1000/Years	No. of Cases	Per 1000/Years
40–54	56,729	Sedent. w.	22,684	29	1.3	8	0.35
		Nonsed. w.	34,045	14	0.41	4	0.12
55–64	10,238	Sedent. w.	4,092	12	3.0	2	0.50
		Nonsed. w.	6,146	4	0.65	1	0.16
Total	66,967	Sedent. w.	26,776	41	1.5	10	0.37
		Nonsed. w.	40,191	18	0.45	5	0.12

Sedentary versus Nonsedentary Workers—Incidence Rate per 1000/year

the total number of man-years (woman-years) observed for each age group, which is obtained by adding the number of years spent by the total number of people passing through that particular age group during the course of the surveyed 15-year period.

RESULTS

Table 29–II presents the incidence rate of new cases of both anginal syndrome and myocardial infarction in the male patients.

ANGINAL SYNDROME

Males. In the youngest age group (40 to 44 years) during the 15-year period, the annual incidence rate of new cases per 1,000 men was about identical in the sedentary and the nonsedentary group. In the age group 45 to 49 years, the incidence rate for sedentary workers was 2.6 times higher than the respective figure for the nonsedentary workers. This difference is even more striking in the age range 50 to 54 years (4.2 versus 1.1). In the two oldest age groups, the incidence rate was about 3 times greater in the sedentary than in the nonsedentary group.

Females. Since, as is also the general experience, there were fewer women than

men suffering from IHD, we found it convenient to subdivide women into only two brackets, viz. 40 to 54 years and 55 to 64 years (Table 29–III). In these two groups, the annual incidence rates of new cases of angina pectoris per 1,000 women were 3.1 and 4.6 times higher, respectively, in the sedentary than in the nonsedentary women.

For the males in all age groups the annual incidence rates of the anginal syndrome per 1,000 in sedentary workers was 3.2 and in nonsedentary workers 1.2. For women of all age groups the corresponding figures were 1.5 and 0.45, respectively.

Myocardial Infarction (Surviving Cases)

Males. In males the incidence rate of new cases of myocardial infarction in each one of the 5-year age groups was 2 to 3.5 times greater in sedentary than in nonsedentary workers (Table 29–II) (3.4, 2.0, 3.5, 1.9 and 2.4 times for the individual groups). For the entire group of males the incidence rate of new cases of myocardial infarction was 3.7 per annum per 1,000 males for the sedentary group, whereas for the nonsedentary group the corresponding figure was 1.4.

Females. Females showed a very low

TABLE 29–IV

FATAL CASES IN KIBBUTZ MEMBERS (MEN AND WOMEN)

	Sedentary versus Nonsedentary Workers—Incidence Rate per 1000/year									
		Men—Years					*Women—Years*			
Age Range	*Total No.*			*No. of Cases*	*Per 1000/ Year*	*Total No.*			*No. of Cases*	*Per 1000/ Year*
40–54	56,884	Sedent. w.	17,094	11	0.64		Sed. w.	22,684	–	–
		Nonsed. w.	39,790	16	0.4	56,729	Nonsed. w.	34,045	–	–
55–64	11,971	Sedent. w.	3,591	14	4.0		Sed. w.	4,092	2	0.5
		Nonsed. w.	8,380	11	1.3	10,238	Nonsed. w.	6,146	1	0.16

TABLE 29–V

ISCHEMIC HEART DISEASE

		Incidence Rate per 1000/year—Male/Female Ratio					
		Anginal Syndrome			*Myocardial Infarction**		
Age Range		*Incidence per 1000/year Male*	*Female*	*Male/Female Ratio*	*Incidence per 1000/year Male*	*Female*	*Male/Female Ratio*
40–54	Sedentary workers	3.2	1.3	2.4	4.9	0.3	16.0
	Nonsed. workers	1.3	0.41	3.1	1.7	0.1	17.0
55–64	Sedentary workers	3.0	3.0	1.1	8.3	0.5	16.0
	Nonsed. workers	1.2	1.8	1.8	3.3	0.16	20.0

*Surviving and fatal cases.

incidence rate (Table 29–III). In both age groups, the incidence in the sedentary women was about 3 times higher than in the nonsedentary.

Fatal Cases

Table 29–IV presents the incidence rates of fatal cases due to coronary artery disease in both sexes. Because of the relatively small number of fatal cases, men also were subdivided into only two groups. In these two groups, the incidence in sedentary men was 1.6 and 3.1 times higher, respectively, in sedentary than in nonsedentary men.

In females the mortality rate was low; no fatalities were reported among the females under 54 years of age. In the age group 55 to 64 years, there were only 2 fatalities among the sedentary females; and among the nonsedentary group of this age range there was only 1 fatality. For the females as a group, the annual incidence rate per 1,000 was 0.07 in the sedentary group, and 0.02 in the nonsedentary group.

Sex Differences in the Clinical Expression of Ischemic Heart Disease

The incidence of ischemic heart disease in men is many times higher than in women of the same age range but there are considerable differences with regard to the anginal syndrome and myocardial infarction (Table 29–V). In the age group 40 to 54 years, angina pectoris is 2.4 times more common in sedentary men than in females with similar occupations, and 3.1 times more common in the nonsedentary group. In the age group 55 to 64 years this difference between males and females is even smaller. On the other hand, the incidence of myocardial infarction (surviving and fatal

TABLE 29–VI
CLINICAL MANIFESTATION OF IHD
DURING 15 YEAR PERIOD

	Male		Female	
	No. of Cases	%	*No. of Cases*	%
All cases of IHD	281	100%	75	100%
Anginal syndrome	83	30%	57	76%
Myocardial infarction	146	52%	15	20%
Myocardial infarction with precedent angina pectoris	19		3	
Myocardial infarction with precedent angina pectoris	127		12	
Fatal cases	52	18%	3	4%
Fatal cases with precedent angina pectoris	12		2	
Fatal cases without precedent myocardial infarction	22		1	
Sudden death without previous clinical IHD	18			

cases) is 16 to 20 times more common in males than in females, in both the sedentary and nonsedentary groups.

Thus, there is a sex-linked difference as regards the clinical expression of ischemic heart disease. Table 29–VI presents only "unduplicated cases" (i.e., patients who had suffered from angina pectoris and who later developed an infarct are included only in the infarction group). Similarly, all fatalities resulting from proven myocardial infarction, or sudden deaths in patients not known to have been suffering previously from ischemic heart disease (included in the survey only if an autopsy was performed), were included only in the subgroups of fatal cases.

Of the male patients, 30 per cent of all cases of ischemic heart disease were suffering from angina pectoris. Fifty-two per cent had had a myocardial infarction, and fatalities accounted for 18 per cent, of which less than one-half (i.e., 8 per cent of the total) had previously suffered from myocardial infarction (Table 29–VI).

Amongst the female patients, angina pectoris accounted for 76 per cent of the cases of ischemic heart disease, and myocardial infarction for 20 per cent. The remaining 4 per cent were accounted for by fatal cases.

In women there were no sudden deaths without previous clinical ischemic heart disease. Similar figures were reported in the Framingham study, where 69 per cent of all the women afflicted with coronary artery disease, but only 30 per cent of all the males similarly afflicted, developed angina pectoris as the predominant clinical manifestation (13).

Comments

In Western society, the differences in socioeconomic status are mainly determined by different occupations and salary levels. This socioeconomic differentiation does not exist in the kibbutz society where the population includes many people of superior intelligence and high educational levels who, because of idealistic motivation, have continued to be manual laborers. In addition, this unique form of life has eliminated many of those emotional and mental factors which are

TABLE 29–VII
MORTALITY RATES IN PATIENTS AFTER INITIAL MYOCARDIAL INFARCTION

Professions	No. of Persons	Hospital Mortality %	6 Years Follow-up Mortality of Patients After Discharge from Hospital	Total Mortality After 6 Years
Workers	48	4.2%	18.9%	23.1%
Skilled workers	41	12.2%	33.4%	45.6%
Clerks and office Workers	58	22.6%	36.4%	59.0%
Free professions and Merchants	79	17.7%	36.7%	54.4%
Women	49	24.5%	29.5%	54.0%
Not working	7	1 patient	3 patients	4 patients

often invoked as causative factors in the increasing incidence of ischemic heart disease. On the one hand, such personal problems as stagnation in the salary scale because of inherent inability, or as a result of inequality of previous educational opportunities, have been largely eliminated in the kibbutz society, whereas, on the other hand, many more people than in an industrialized private economy have to accept direct responsibility for work and production. Thus the only major differentiating environmental factor in the kibbutz society is the nature of one's work, and it appears justifiable to consider this factor as being responsible for the difference in incidence rates of IHD in every one of the investigated groups.

The results of this study suggest a favorable influence of physical activity at work on the incidence of ischemic heart disease in middle-aged men and women, living under otherwise equal social and environmental conditions.

The Influence of Type of Work in the Pre-disease Period on the Prognosis in Patients After Initial Myocardial Infarctions

This study comprises 233 male and 49 female patients less than 65 years old, who had been admitted consecutively to our department for initial myocardial infarction at least 6 years before the recent follow-up examinations. The further fate of only 27 patients (9.9 per cent) could not be traced. The diagnosis of initial myocardial infarction was based on the lack of a preceding clinical history, absence of electrocardiographic signs of previous infarctions, and the appearance of signs typical for recent infarction as defined above.

The male patients were subdivided according to professions. There were 48 laborers, 41 skilled workers, 58 clerks and office workers and 79 professionals and merchants. Seven men were not working. This study includes also 49 women. The hospital mortality (e.g., the mortality in the first 4 weeks after the acute event) was 4.2 per cent in workers, 12.2 per cent in skilled workers, 22.6 per cent in clerks and office workers and 17.7 per cent in members of free professions and merchants. It seems remarkable that women had the highest mortality rate, 24.5 per cent (Table 29–VII).

There exists also a distinct difference in the mortality rate of patients after their discharge from the hospital. Thirty-six per cent of professionals, merchants and office workers died within 6 years after leaving the hospital. The respective figure for workers is only one-half (i.e., 18.9 per cent). The corresponding figure for women is rather high: 29.5 per cent.

Thus, the cumulative figures obtained in the hospital and during the 6-year follow-up period show a striking difference in total mortality rates. Of the workers, 23.1 per cent were dead at the end of the 6-year period. The respective total mortality rate of clerks and office workers is 2.6 times higher (59 per cent), and that of professionals and merchants is 2.3 times higher (54.4 per cent). The mortality rate of skilled workers is in between with 45.6 per cent. Women had a high total mortality rate of 54 per cent.

Comment

These findings indicate a beneficial effect of physical activity at work in the premorbid period with regard to the later course and prognosis of initial myocardial infarction. Five times more office workers and clerks, and 4 times more professionals than laborers succumbed in the first 4 weeks after initial myocardial infarction. After 6 years the survival rate of laborers is about 2.5 times higher than of people who had been engaged in sedentary work in the premorbid period.

CONCLUSIONS

Ischemic heart disease is clearly a multietiological disease. Our data indicate that the incidence, as well as the course and prognosis of the established disease, is affected by such environmental factors as occupational physical activity in the premorbid period. The mechanism of its apparent favorable influence is not yet fully elucidated.

Raab et al. (14) have provided evi-

dence for a reduction by habitual physical exercise of the exaggerated cardiac sympathetic tone and reactivity which results from sedentary living and which endangers myocardial oxygen economy, especially in the presence of coronary atherosclerosis. Eckstein (15) found that in dogs exercised after they had survived partial surgical ligation of one of their coronary arteries, the coronary collateral circulation was greater than in dogs restricted to their kennels following the same operation.

Whatever the final explanation may be, it appears advisable to utilize the empirical results emerging from our and other similar studies as valuable guide posts for the development of active prevention programs to forestall ischemic heart disease in middle-aged people, and for the rehabilitation of patients suffering from the established disease.

SUMMARY

The frequency of IHD in a 15-year period was retrospectively surveyed in 5,279 men and 5,229 women, aged 40 to 64, living in Israeli collective settlements (kibbutzim) under uniform environmental conditions.

The incidence of the anginal syndrome, myocardial infarction and fatalities due to IHD was 2.5 to 4 times higher in sedentary workers than in nonsedentary workers. Women who in the kibbutz society do a full day's work, show a very low incidence rate of fatal IHD.

The male/female ratio for angina pectoris for sedentary as well as physically active workers was between 1.1 to 3.1, but myocardial infarction occurred 16 to 20 times more frequently in men than in women.

In a 6-year follow-up study of 233 men

and 49 women, 40 to 64 years old, after initial myocardial infarction, we found that the mortality in the first 4 weeks was 4.2 per cent in nonsedentary workers, and 22.6 per cent in clerks and office workers. The total mortality 6 years after the acute event was 23.1 per cent in nonsedentary workers and 54 to 59 per cent in clerks, merchants and professionals.

It is concluded that habitual physical activity should be considered a valuable principle in the primary and secondary prevention of ischemic heart disease.

REFERENCES

1. MORRIS, J. N., RAFFLE, P. A. B., ROBERTS, C. G., and Parks, J. W.: Coronary heart disease and physical activity of work. *Lancet*, 2:1053, 1953.
2. MORRIS, J. N., and CRAWFORD, M. C.: Coronary heart disease and physical activity of work. *Brit Med J*, 2:1482, 1958.
3. BIÖRCK, G., BLOMQUIST, G., and SIEVERS, J.: Studies on myocardial infarction in Malmö 1935–1954. II. Infarction rate by occupational group. *Acta Med Scand*, 21:159, 1958.
4. BERKSON, D. M., STAMLER, J., LINDBERG, H. A., MILLER, W., MATHIES, H., LASKY, M., and HALL, Y.: Socio-economic correlates of atherosclerotic and hypertensive heart diseases. *Ann N Y Acad Sci*, 84:835, 1960.
5. PAUL, OGLESBY, LEPPER, M. H., PHELAN, W. H., DUPERTUIS, G. W., MACMILLAN, A., McKEAN, H., and PARK ,H.: A longitudinal study of coronary heart disease. *Circulation*, 28:20, 1963.
6. TAYLOR, H. L.: The mortality and morbidity of coronary heart disease of men in sedentary and physically active occupations. Colloquim on the Scientific Aspects of Exercise and Fitness. University of Illinois, 1959.
7. ZUKEL, W., LEWIS, R., ENTERLINE, P., PAINTER, R., RALSTON, L., FAWCETT, R., MEREDITH, A., and PETERSON, B.: A short-term community study of the epidemiology of coronary heart disease. *Amer J Public Health*, 49:1630, 1959.
8. BRESLOW, L., and BUELL, P.: Mortality from coronary heart disease and physical activity of work in California. *J Chronic Dis*, 11:421, 1960.
9. BRUNNER, D., and MANELIS, G.: Myocardial infarction among members of communal settlements in Israel. *Lancet*, 2:1049, 1960.
10. sraeli Government, Ministry of Internal Affairs: General Election Register, 1962/63.
11. American Heart Association, National Heart Institute, *Amer J Public Health*, Vol. 50, No. 10, Supplement, 1960.
12. Statistical Reports, Cooperative Agricultural Supervision Inc., Ltd., Tel-Aviv, Vol. 38, April 1959.
13. KANNEL, W. B., DAWBER, TH. R., KAGAN, A., REVOTSKIE, N., and STOKES, J.: Factors of risk in the development of coronary heart disease. Six-year follow-up experience. *Ann Intern Med*, 55:33, 1961.
14. RAAB, W., SILVA, P. DE P., MARCHET, H., KIMURA, E., and STARCHESKA, Y. K.: Cardiac adrenergic preponderance due to lack of physical exercise and its pathogenic implications. *Amer J Cardiol*, 5:300, 1960.
15. ECKSTEIN, R. W.: Effect of exercise and coronary arterial narrowing on growth of interarterial coronary anastomoses. *Fed Proc*, 15:54, 1956.

Chapter XXX

PHYSICAL ACTIVITY AND ISCHEMIC HEART DISEASE AMONG NEGROES AND WHITES IN EVANS COUNTY, GEORGIA*

CURTIS G. HAMES, JOHN R. McDONOUGH, SARAH C. STULB
and GLEN E. GARRISON

(Claxton, Georgia, U.S.A.)

TEN years of clinical observation in Evans County, Georgia (C. G. Hames) suggested that ischemic heart disease was much less prevalent among Negroes than whites.

METHODS

The complete findings of an epidemiologic study for the prevalence of ischemic heart disease (IHD) in this area, including census, sampling techniques, examination response rate and other pertinent findings, have been published (1–7) and will only briefly be reviewed here. The study population was identified by census which included all persons of age 40 to 74, and a 50 per cent random sample of those aged 15 to 39. There were 3,377 persons eligible, 3,102 or 92 per cent were examined. The examination consisted of a history, physical examination, urinalysis, serum cholesterol determination, 12-lead ECG, and 14 in x 17 in,

7-foot posterior-anterior chest x ray. Two physicians, J. R. McDonough and G. E. Garrison, performed the examination. Alternate subjects were examined by each examiner as they came into the examination center. A diagnosis of IHD was made when angina pectoris, and/or a history of myocardial infarction or ECG evidence of myocardial infarction was present. World Health Organization criteria were used for defining angina pectoris and a history of myocardial infarction (8). Criteria used for evaluation of the ECG were essentially the class IQ and QS patterns of Blackburn and Keys (9). ST and T patterns were not used. IHD was classified as "definite" when both physicians agreed that the criteria for angina and history or ECG evidence of myocardial infarction were present; as "probable" when there was some disagreement between physicians, but the evidence was clearly in favor of IHD; as "possible" when the evidence was suggestive but not adequate to be placed in the "probable" category. Serum cholesterol was determined by the Abell et al. method (10).

*Supported by U.S. Public Health Service grant H-3341, a contract from the Georgia State Health Department Cardiovascular Disease Control Service, and the Heart Disease Control Program of the Public Health Service.

TABLE 30–I
PREVALENCE OF IHD BY AGE GROUP, SEX AND RACE

		Definite	Probable	Possible	Negative	Total	Ratio*
White Males	40–49	6	—	6	242	254	24
	50–59	10	3	6	200	219	59
	60–69	14	5	10	110	139	137
	70–74	3	3	5	41	52	115
	Total	33	11	27	593	664	68
Negro Males	40–49	1	—	1	148	150	7
	50–59	—	2	3	128	133	15
	60–69	2	2	3	78	85	47
	70–74	—	1	4	22	27	37
	Total	3	5	11	376	395	21
White Females	40–49	—	—	3	236	239	—
	50–59	1	1	7	198	207	10
	60–69	2	3	5	169	179	28
	70–74	—	2	1	57	60	33
	Total	3	6	16	660	685	12
Negro Females	40–49	—	1	2	178	181	6
	50–59	2	1	3	139	145	21
	60–69	—	—	5	96	101	—
	70–74	1	—	—	44	45	22
	Total	3	2	10	457	472	11
Total	40–49	7	1	12	804	824	10
	50–59	13	7	19	665	704	28
	60–69	18	10	23	453	504	56
	70–74	4	6	10	164	184	54
	Total	42	24	64	2086	2216	30

*Definite plus probable cases per 1000 examined. Ratios for the age group 40 to 74 are age-adjusted (indirect method).

The laboratory team was one of several which participated in a national cholesterol standardization program conducted by the Heart Disease Control Laboratory, Communicable Disease Center, Public Health Service, Atlanta, Georgia. The standard deviation of laboratory error was shown to be 2.8 mg/100 ml for within-day variation, and 3.0 mg/100 ml for between-day (including within-day) variations. Interlaboratory differences were within acceptable range when compared with 6 other participating laboratories.

Diet. A nutrition history was obtained by the nutritionist, S. C. Stulb. Each subject was asked to recall the 24-hour food intake for the previous day. He was then asked to estimate the frequency and amount of food eaten during the previous 2 weeks. Foods were recorded in household measures, converted to gram weight per week, and transposed to dietary constituents, using standard food conversion tables (11–14). The dietary survey was conducted on a 10 per cent random sample of the Evans County study population. Social status was evaluated by using a modification of the Warner scale which consisted of occupation, source of income and educational attainment of the head of the household (4).

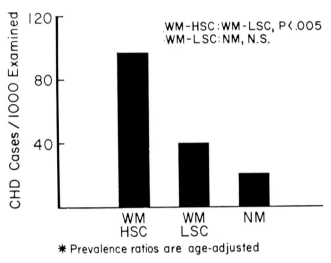

Figure 30–1.

RESULTS

Distribution of IHD by Age-Group, Sex and Race

IHD ratios were age-adjusted by the indirect method, using the total Evans County population (15). Distribution by age group, sex and race are shown in Table 30–I. A highly significant difference in IHD prevalence was found when comparing white males with Negro males, with white males having the higher rates. The differences between white and Negro females and Negro males were not significant.

Distribution of IHD by Social Class

Differences in social class between Negroes and whites have been measured and were found to be large (4). To further examine the relationship of social class and IHD, the two racial groups were classified by their social class scores. White males were dichotomized at the median of white social class scores into high and low social class groups. Negroes as a group were found to be most comparable to low social class whites, since 95 per cent of the group were below the white social class median. Again, the difference in IHD between high social white males and Negro males was highly significant. Low social white and Negro males, when compared for IHD, showed no significant difference (Fig. 30–1).

Distribution of IHD by Occupation

The distribution of IHD was next examined by occupation. The rarity of IHD among the Negroes excluded a biracial comparison. Therefore, only whites were included in this analysis. Among nonfarm occupations, IHD was highest among professionals, proprietors and managers, and lowest among laborers. Among farmers, IHD was highest for farm owners and lowest for sharecroppers

TABLE 30–II

IHD PREVALENCE AMONG WHITE MALES FARM OWNERS AGED 40–74 YEARS
BY TYPE OF OCCUPATION

	Farm Size	Examined	Cases/1000 Cases	Examined*
	Professionals, proprietors, managers	113	10	96
	Clerks, office workers	41	3	77
Nonfarm	Trades, service workers	121	5	48
	Manual laborers	89	3	41
	Unemployed	26	2	55
	Owners	181	17	87
Farm	Sharecroppers, laborers	76	2	31
	Unemployed	17	2	74
	Nonfarm	390	23	64
Total	Farm	274	21	73
	Both	664	44	68

*Prevalence ratios are age-adjusted (indirect method).

TABLE 30–III

IHD PREVALENCE AMONG WHITE MALE FARM OWNERS AGED 40–74 YEARS
BY FARM SIZE (DIVIDED AT THE MEDIAN)

Farm Size	Examined	Cases	Cases/1000 Examined*
20–188 acres	82	4	47
189–10,750 acres	83	11	127
Total	165	15	87
Small:Large farm, P< .05 (one-tailed test).			

*Age-adjusted (indirect method). Farm size was unknown for
16 examined, including 2 IHD cases.

and laborers (Table 30–II). This fact suggested that the association between IHD and occupation occurs among both farm and nonfarm workers. Further, a major difference between those occupations associated with high IHD prevalence and those with low IHD prevalence appeared to be *physical activity*.

In general, small farm owners are more physically active than large farm owners because of less mechanization and less hired help. Therefore, to investigate physical activity further, farm size by acres was evaluated and it was found that owners of small farms had significantly lower IHD prevalence than owners of large farms (Table 30–III). Even

more striking differences were found when farm owners were classified according to the kinds of activity they habitually performed (i.e., those doing fulltime physical work had considerably lower ratios than those doing no physical work, while the group engaged in physical work parttime had a ratio that was intermediate [Table 30–IV]).

When IHD prevalence among all white males was compared by exercise levels (job classification), the lowest exercise group had the highest prevalence rates and the highest exercise group had the lowest prevalence rate. The intermediate exercise group had an intermediate prevalence rate (Fig. 30–2).

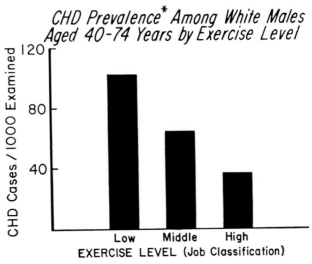

CHD Prevalence* Among White Males Aged 40-74 Years by Exercise Level

EXERCISE LEVEL (Job Classification)

* Prevalence ratios are age-adjusted

Figure 30–2.

TABLE 30–IV

IHD PREVALENCE AMONG WHITE MALE FARM OWNERS AGED 40–74 YEARS
BY CHARACTERISTICS OF WORK

	Examined	Cases	Cases/1000 Examined*
No supervision			
No physical work	49	9	132
(Rent farm land to others)	(10)	(2)	
All supervision			
No physical work	40	5	116
(All farm work done by others)	(1)		
Part supervision			
Part physical work	34	2	61
(Some farm work done by others)			
No supervision			
All physical work	56	1	20
(No farm work done by others)	(3)		
Total	179	17	87

*Age adjusted (indirect method). Characteristics of work were unknown for
2 examined. Numbers in parenthesis represent 14 examined, and 2 cases for
whom there is doubt concerning the accuracy of the census classification of
farm ower.

Distribution of Serum Cholesterol Values by Age-Group, Sex, Race and Social Class

Variations in cholesterol values for various groups can best be seen from examining mean values in Figure 30–3. Both Negro and white females had higher values than males of both races beyond the age group 35 to 44. When cholesterol was examined by social class, the high social class white male had significantly higher values than low social class white or Negro. No significant difference was found between low social class whites and Negroes (Fig. 30–4). Significant differences in serum cholesterol also occurred

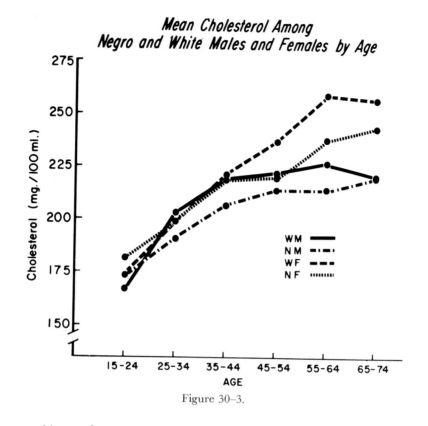

Figure 30–3.

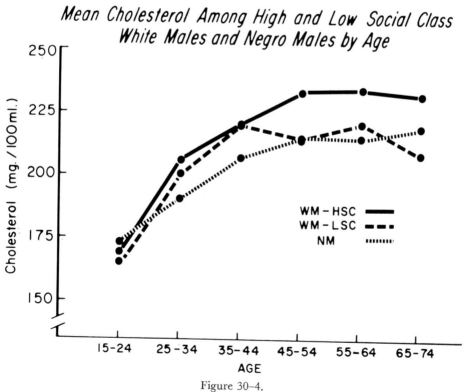

Figure 30–4.

TABLE 30–V

SERUM CHOLESTEROL OF WHITE AND NEGRO MALES
AGED 40–74 YEARS BY OCCUPATION
(Mean and Standard Deviation)

			White Males				*Negro Males*			*Significance of the Difference (P)*
		N	*Mean Age*	*Cholesterol Mean*	*S.D.*	*N*	*Mean Age*	*Cholesterol Mean*	*S.D.*	
	Professional	112	54.2	237.7	40.9	4	50.8	185.8	37.7	–
Non-	Clerks	39	56.5	228.4	41.3	5	68.2	202.4	23.9	–
farm	Trades	120	52.8	225.7	39.2	24	51.3	230.9	32.5	>.40
	Laborers	89	52.0	218.7	39.7	116	54.2	214.3	42.1	>.40
	Unemployed	26	61.7	219.7	45.0	10	56.1	209.7	46.7	–
	Owners	178	56.8	223.5	39.4	53	60.3	206.5	36.6	<.01
Farm	Sharecroppers	75	53.5	205.2	31.0	167	53.3	214.2	36.5	>.05
	Unemployed	16	69.3	199.3	34.9	9	73.1	226.7	30.1	–
	Nonfarm	386	54.0	227.4	41.4	159	54.2	215.4	41.6	<.01
Total	Farm	269	56.6	217.0	38.6	229	55.7	212.9	36.8	>.20
	Total	655*	55.1	223.1	40.6	388*	55.1	213.9	38.3	<.001

Significance of the differences between occupations:
Whites—Professional: clerks P>.20, Professional: trades P<.05, Professional: laborers P<.001,
farm-owners: sharecroppers P<.001.
Negroes—Trades: laborers P<.05, farm-owners: sharecroppers P>.10.
*Cholesterol was not determined on 9 white and 7 negro males.

among whites when professionals, proprietors, managers and clerks were compared with laborers and when farm owners were compared with sharecroppers and laborers. In both comparisons, occupations associated with higher levels of physical activity had the lower cholesterol levels (Table 30–V).

Among Negroes, the pattern is difficult to interpret because of inadequate numbers in the more sedentary occupations; however, tradesmen and service workers had significantly higher mean cholesterol levels than laborers. The Negro farm owners, as a group, engage in physically more demanding work. This might account for the absence of a significant difference when this group was compared to sharecroppers and laborers. Levels were similar for tradesmen, nonfarm laborers and sharecroppers, while for farm owners, cholesterol was significantly higher among whites. This might be accounted for by the greater amount of physical work demanded of Negro farm owners since Negro farms are, for the most part, small and not mechanized as fully as the whites. The data suggested that the association of IHD and serum cholesterol was not as prominent for Negro males and low social class whites as for high social class whites.

Dietary Patterns among Those with High and Low IHD Prevalence

Dietary patterns were compared between the various groups with high and low IHD prevalence. Heights, weight, body surface area †, daily caloric intake, and caloric intake related to body surface were studied (Table 30–VI). None of the differences between high and low social class white males was significant. However, Negroes differed significantly from whites in weight and body surface. The high social class "coronary-prone" white

---

†Calculated from height and weight, using a nomogram based upon the DuBoise-Meech formula (16).

TABLE 30–VI

BODY SIZE AND DAILY CALORIC INTAKE AMONG A RANDOM SAMPLE
HIGH AND LOW SOCIAL CLASS WHITE MALES AND NEGRO MALES AGED 40–74 YEARS
(Mean and Standard Deviation)

	WM-HSC $N \leq 33$	WM-LSC $N \leq 34$	NM $N \leq 23$	Significance (P)		
				HSC:LSC	HSC:NM	LSC:NM
Height (inches)	67.0	66.5	66.3	NS	NS	NS
	(2.67)	(2.67)	(2.97)			
Weight (pounds)	163	161	144	NS	.02	.05
	(32.4)	(35.3)	(26.6)			
Body surface area	1.85	1.83	1.73	NS	.02	.05
(sq. meters)	(0.18)	(0.21)	(0.16)			
Calories	3032	3118	3535	NS	.02	.05
	(630)	(644)	(803)			
Cal/M² body surface area	1639	1714	2046	NS	.001	.01
	(300)	(359)	(464)			

TABLE 30–VII

DAILY DIETARY INTAKE OF SELECTED NUTRIENTS AMONG RANDOM SAMPLE
HIGH AND LOW SOCIAL CLASS WHITE MALES AND NEGRO MALES AGED 40–74 YEARS
(Mean and Standard Deviation)

		WM-HSC $N \leq 33$	WM:LSC $N \leq 34$	NM $N \leq 23$	Significance (P)		
					HSC:LSC	HSC:NM	LSC:NM
	carbohydrate	44.8	42.6	47.0	NS	NS	.001
		(5.38)	(4.70)	(4.73)			
Calories	protein	12.9	12.4	11.3	NS	.01	.05
As		(1.77)	(2.15)	(1.85)			
Per cent	total fat	42.4	45.0	41.5	NS	NS	.01
		(6.8)	(4.9)	(4.1)			
	animal fat	25.8	30.6	30.1	.02	.05	NS
		(7.7)	(7.4)	(6.1)			
Saturated fatty acids (grams)		49.1	51.9	50.1	NS	NS	NS
		(17.7)	(13.4)	(10.6)			
Linoleic acid (grams)		17.2	15.5	13.8	NS	.05	NS
		(7.0)	(5.8)	(5.2)			
Saturated FA/Linoleic acid		3.37	3.75	3.96	NS	NS	NS
		(1.83)	(1.40)	(1.13)			
Cholesterol (milligrams)		608	650	527	NS	NS	.05
		(220)	(214)	(190)			

male weight approximates 19 pounds more than the low social class, less "coronary-prone" Negro male who consumed approximately 500 calories a day more. Dietary constituents were examined next. They included carbodydrate, protein, total fat, animal fat, saturated fatty acids, linoleic and saturated/linoleic fatty acid ratio and cholesterol. None of the differences comparing high with low social class white males were significant except that animal fat in the low social class had higher values. Negroes ate more carbohydrate, less protein, less total fat, but more animal fat, less linoleic acid and less cholesterol than either high or low social class white males, or both (Table 30--VII).

DISCUSSION

Factors which might influence the findings in the study are as follows: (a) misclassification of IHD cases; (b) less IHD cases because of nonresponse; (c) the use of cross-sectional rather than prospective data, and (d) selectivily; these have been analyzed in detail and were found not to affect the end results (1).

The difference in IHD prevalence between Negro and white males was found to be large and highly significant. Social class was shown to be an adequate explanation for the Negro-whites difference since low social class white males had an IHD prevalence ratio which was similar to the ratio for Negro males, while being significantly lower than the ratio for high social class white males. The pattern for serum cholesterol was also exactly the same. In turn, the social class difference for both IHD and serum cholesterol was found to be related to occupation.

Physical activity seemed to be the feature most likely to be associated with occupation and social class. Therefore, physical activity was looked at in several different ways and the pattern was invariably the same: the highly significant difference in IHD prevalence was found with the more active groups having the lower prevalence. Significant differences in prevalence were found among farming as well as nonfarming occupations.

Within-occupation differences were also found. Small farm owners had a significantly lower prevalence than large farm owners. This could possibly be attributed to less mechanization and hired help on the smaller farms. When data were gathered on work habits of individual farm owners, the pattern was even more striking. IHD prevalence ratios of those doing none of their own physical work were 6 to 7 times higher than of the group doing all of its own work (132 and 110 compared to 20; see Table 30–IV). Thus, it is reasonable to suppose that differences in physical activity could account for the differences in IHD and serum cholesterol which were observed between the various occupations, social classes and racial groups.

SUMMARY

An epidemiologic study has been carried out on various segments of the population of Evans County, Georgia.

The incidence of ischemic heart disease (IHD) and serum cholesterol levels were found to be significantly higher in white than in Negro males. A significantly higher incidence of IHD and higher cholesterol levels were also found in high, as compared with low, social class white males.

The differences between Negro and white males were attributed to social class because low social class white males and Negro males did not differ significantly in either IHD prevalence or cholesterol level. The social class difference could be explained by differences in occupation.

An important aspect of occupation appeared to be physical activity, as suggested by data on activity obtained for at least one occupation group.

Dietary fat intake could not explain the differences in IHD prevalence between Negroes and whites or high and low social class.

It is concluded that differences in IHD and serum cholesterol, observed between various racial, social class, and occupational groups of males, appear explainable by differences in physical activity.

Thus, a low level of physical activity appeared to be a possible major determinant of IHD prevalence in this study population.

REFERENCES

1. McDONOUGH, J. R., HAMES, C. G., STULB, S. C., and GARRISON, G. E.: Coronary heart disease among negroes and whites in Evans County, Georgia. *J Chronic Dis, 18:*443, 1965.
2. HAMES, C. G., and GREENBERG, B. G.: A comparative study of serum cholesterol levels in school children and their possible relation to atherogenesis. *Amer J Public Health, 51:*374, 1961.
3. McDONOUGH, J. R., HAMES, C. G., GREENBERG, B. G., GRIFFIN, L. H., JR., and EDWARDS, A. J., JR.: Observations on serum cholesterol levels in the twin population of Evans County, Georgia. *Circulation, 25:*962, 1962.
4. McDONOUGH, J. R., HAMES, C. G., STULB, S. C., and GARRISON, G. E.: Cardiovascular disease field study in Evans County, Georgia. Characteristics of the study population. *Public Health Rep, 78:*1051, 1963.
5. McDONOUGH, J. R., GARRISON, G. E., and HAMES, C. G.: Blood pressure and hypertensive disease among negroes and whites. *Ann Intern Med, 61:*208, 1964.
6. STULB, S. C., McDONOUGH, J. R., GREENBERG, B. G., and HAMES, C. G.: The relationship of nutrient intake and exercise to serum cholesterol levels in white males in Evans County, Georgia. *Amer J Clin Nutr, 16:*238, 1965.
7. LICHTMAN, M. A., HAMES, C. G., and McDONOUGH, J. R.: Serum protein electrophoretic fractions among negro and white subjects in Evans County, Georgia. *Amer J Clin Nutr, 16:* 492, 1965.
8. Hypertension and coronary heart disease: Classification and criteria for epidemiological studies. World Health Organization Technical Report, Serial No. 168, 1959.
9. BLACKBURN, H., KEYS, A., SIMONSON, E., RAUTAHARJU, P., and PUNSAR, S.: The electrocardiogram in population studies. *Circulation, 21:*1160, 1960.
10. ABELL, L. L., LEVY, B. B., BRODIE, B. B., and KENDALL, F. E.: A simplified method for the estimation of total cholesterol in serum. *J Biol Chem, 1:*357, 1952.
11. Composition of Foods, U.S. Dept. of Agriculture Handbook No. 8, Washington, D. C., 1950.
12. Nutritive Value of Foods, U.S. Dept. of Agriculture, *Home and Garden Bull,* No. 72, 1960.
13. HAYES, O. B., and ROSE, G.: Supplementary food composition tables. *J Amer Diet Assoc, 33:* 26, 1957.
14. Food Tables, Harvard University, School of Public Health, Dept. of Nutrition (unpublished).
15. LINDER, F. E., and GROVE, R. D.: Vital Statistics in the United States, 1900–1940. U.S. Government Printing Office, Washington, D. C., 1947.
16. CONSOLAZIO, C. F., JOHNSON, R. E., and PECORA, L. J.: *Physiological Measurements of Metabolic Functions in Man.* New York, McGraw-Hill, 1963.

Chapter XXXI

VITAL CAPACITY, PHYSICAL ACTIVITY AND CORONARY HEART DISEASE

THOMAS R. DAWBER, WILLIAM B. KANNEL and GARY D. FRIEDMAN

(Framingham, Massachusetts, U.S.A.)

THE benefits of physical activity in preventing heart disease and in improving cardiac function in patients with heart disease have been accepted for many years, although proof of such benefits is hard to find. In relation to coronary (ischemic) heart disease (CHD), the value of increased physical activity might result from possible prevention of, or delay in, the development of atherosclerosis or from changes in clotting tendency, with possible prevention of thrombotic complications of coronary atherosclerosis. Increased physical activity might also delay some of the adverse effects of coronary thromboatherosclerosis by improving cardiac function and/or collateral coronary circulation so that impaired coronary flow can be better tolerated. That any of the above mechanisms actually occur in human subjects has not been clearly established.

Physical activity was one of the factors which it was planned to study in the long-range epidemiologic investigation of CHD originally undertaken in 1949 by the National Heart Institute in Framingham, Massachusetts. Methodology developed to quantitate relative degrees of physical activity was not applied until several years had elapsed. Meanwhile, in the followup of 5,127 men and women, age 30 to 59, initially free of CHD, several personal characteristics were observed to be associated with an increased risk of subsequent CHD development. The most important of these were age, male sex, serum levels of cholesterol and other lipids, blood pressure, cigarette smoking, obesity, certain electrocardiographic abnormalities and the vital capacity.

The methods and findings of the Framingham Study have been described in previous publications (1–5). In brief, the diagnosis of CHD was based on the development of at least one of the following manifestations: (a) myocardial infarction was diagnosed only in the presence of unequivocal QRS changes in the electrocardiogram or elevation of the serum glutamic oxaloacetic transaminase (SGOT) above sixty units in the absence of another explanation for this phenomenon; (b) the diagnosis of angina pectoris required the finding by two physicians of repeated episodes of substernal discomfort brought on by exertion or excitement and relieved by rest; (c) coronary insufficiency was diagnosed if there were a clinical episode with prolonged chest pain accompanied by transient ST-T,

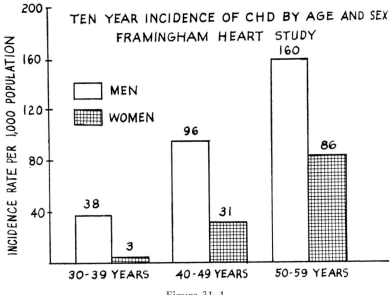

Figure 31–1.

but not QRS changes in the electrocardiogram, and (d) sudden death was also attributed to CHD, if documented to have occured within minutes and no other cause was suggested by prior medical history. The vital capacity was measured on all subjects in the seated position using a Collins Vitalometer. The Physical Activity Index, determined by interview at the fourth biennial examination, was a weighted sum of the number of hours per day ordinarily spent in various types of activity. The weights, reflecting relative energy expenditure, were assigned as follows: rest, 1.0; sedentary, 1.1; slight, 1.5; moderate, 2.4; heavy, 5.0.

The longitudinal data of the Framingham Study indicated that the incidence of CHD increased with age in both men and women. The incidence in women was similar to that noted in men who were ten years younger (Fig. 31–1). The serum concentrations of cholesterol, phospholipid and various lipoprotein fractions were found to be related to CHD inci-

dence. Persons with higher levels of these substances, measured at entry to the Study, showed a greater risk of subsequent CHD development (Fig. 31–2). A clear-cut relationship between the height of the blood pressure, both systolic and diastolic, and CHD incidence was noted (Fig. 31–3). Persons with certain electrocardiographic abnormalities (intraventricular block, left ventricular hypertrophy and nonspecific ST-T changes) when the study began were more prone to develop clinical manifestations of CHD.

Cigarette (but not cigar or pipe) smoking was also found to be a CHD risk factor related to some, but not all manifestations of CHD (Fig. 31–4). Cigarette smokers were about twice as prone as other persons to develop myocardial infarction and sudden death while their risk of angina pectoris was not significantly different from that of others. In addition, ex-smokers had about the same low risk as nonsmokers suggesting that the deleterious effect of smoking is not

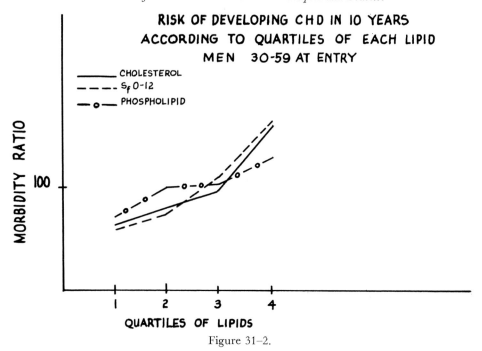

Figure 31–2.

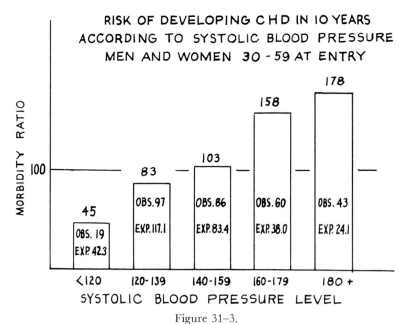

Figure 31–3.

the acceleration of atheroma formation but rather alteration of cardiac function or increase of the tendency to form thrombi. Obesity also appeared to act more by affecting cardiac function or

the work of the heart in that it was related to angina pectoris and sudden death, but not to myocardial infarction.

Persons with more than one "abnormality" in these characteristics were noted

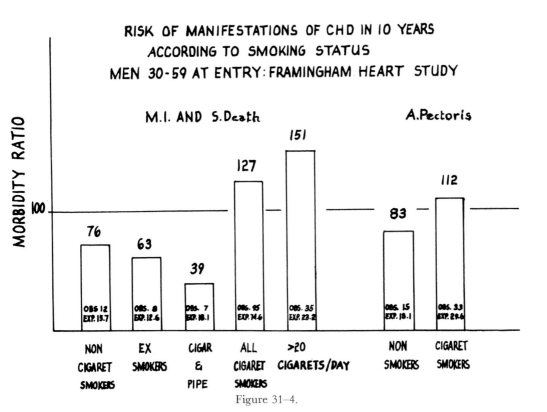

Figure 31–4.

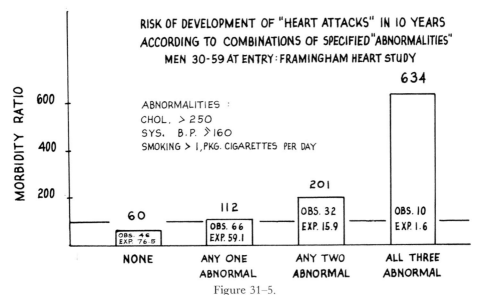

Figure 31–5.

to be a highly susceptible group to which, it would seem, the greatest preventive efforts should be directed (Fig. 31–5).

The relationship of the foregoing factors to CHD development by and large substantiated rational hypotheses. One factor investigated proved to relate to CHD development in the absence of any such hypothesis. This particular personal characteristic, the vital capacity, was

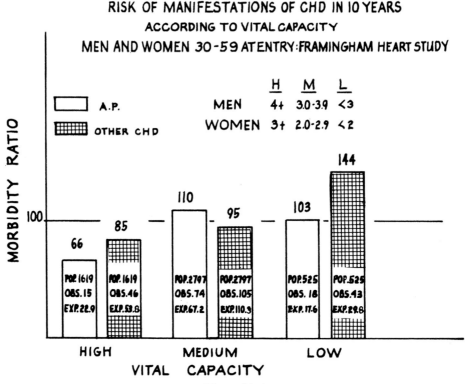

Figure 31–6.

measured because of its possible value as an indicator of impending congestive heart failure and not because of any belief that it might predict development of CHD. Examination of the study population classified according to initial vital capacity level revealed that the lower the vital capacity, the greater was the risk of subsequent CHD (Fig. 31–6). "Low" vital capacity made a contribution to risk regardless of the levels of blood pressure and cholesterol.

In contrast to the other risk factors for which possible pathogenetic mechanisms could be readily postulated, the mechanism relating level of vital capacity to subsequent CHD has remained obscure. Search for an explanation of this relationship was the original focal point of this

investigation. It did not seem reasonable that vital capacity could be directly related to pathogenesis, but rather that the vital capacity reflected some other trait which in turn affected CHD development. Several reasonable hypotheses seemed worthy of investigation: vital capacity affects CHD because of its relation to the following:

(1) Body height.
(2) Body weight.
(3) Presence of pulmonary disease.
(4) Cigarette smoking.
(5) Pre-existing heart disease.
(6) Level of physical activity.

Vital capacity decreased with age while CHD increased with age. However, this age-vital capacity relationship could not explain the association between vital ca-

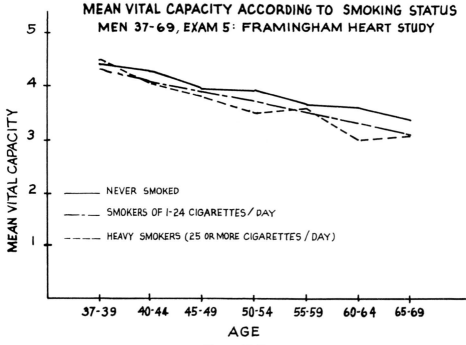

Figure 31–7.

pacity and disease development since the morbidity ratios (observed to expected cases) used to determine relative risk in the Framingham Study adjusted for the age composition of each vital capacity subgroup under consideration.

Vital Capacity and Height

Vital capacity was positively correlated with height which was also slightly related to the incidence of CHD. Since the relationship of vital capacity to disease was stronger than that of height, it seemed unlikely that height could explain the vital capacity effect. Also the effect of height was manifested primarily as an excess incidence of CHD in short women, whereas vital capacity was related to CHD in both sexes.

Vital Capacity and Obesity

Another factor which might possibly

explain the vital capacity-CHD relationship was that of obesity. Since overweight persons may have restricted vital capacity obesity might possibly explain the vital capacity-CHD relationship. However, observations in the Framingham Study have indicated that in men obesity was not related to myocardial infarction, but was related to angina pectoris, whereas vital capacity was somewhat more related to myocardial infarction than to angina pectoris (Fig. 31–6). Furthermore, when the study population was divided into two groups, those who were markedly obese and those who were not, the gradient of risk for vital capacity still held in each group. It did not appear that increase in weight could explain the effect of vital capacity on CHD development.

Vital Capacity and Pulmonary Disease

Neither the first-second volume, nor

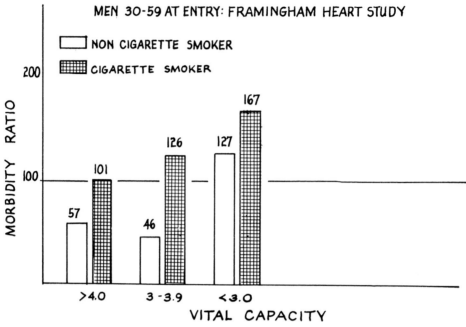

RISK OF DEVELOPING "HEART ATTACK" IN 10 YEARS
ACCORDING TO VITAL CAPACITY AND CIGARETTE SMOKING STATUS
MEN 30-59 AT ENTRY: FRAMINGHAM HEART STUDY

Figure 31–8.

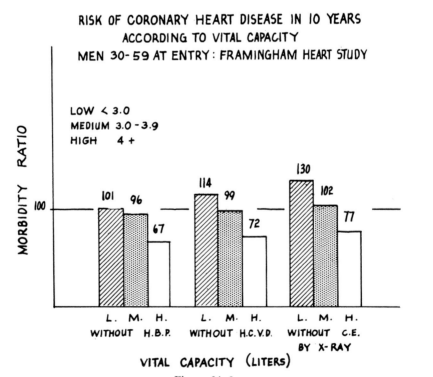

RISK OF CORONARY HEART DISEASE IN 10 YEARS
ACCORDING TO VITAL CAPACITY
MEN 30-59 AT ENTRY: FRAMINGHAM HEART STUDY

Figure 31–9.

the mid-expiratory flow rate were found to be related to the incidence of CHD. It is, therefore, unlikely that obstructive bronchopulmonary disease was responsible for the vital capacity-CHD relationship.

Vital Capacity and Cigarette Smoking

Cigarette smoking proved to be an important factor in increasing the risk of subsequent CHD development (Fig. 31–4). However, cigarette smokers had only a very slightly lowered vital capacity as compared to nonsmokers (Fig. 31–7). Thus, cigarette smoking did not appear to impair vital capacity sufficiently to explain the vital capacity-CHD relationship. In addition, the relationship of vital capacity to CHD held for nonsmokers as well as for smokers (Fig. 31–8).

Vital Capacity may Reflect the Presence of Heart Disease Already Developed.

It is conceivable that the vital capacity-CHD relationship might actually reflect the presence of existing heart disease (e. g., hypertensive heart disease), which carries a high risk of CHD development. In addition, the initial low vital capacity group might even have contained persons with CHD who had not yet developed clinical manifestations sufficient for diagnosis. Subjects with incipient congestive heart failure are believed to have decreased vital capacities. It is reasonable to suppose, therefore, that included in a group of persons with low vital capacities would be those individuals who have early congestive heart failure not otherwise manifest. The view that heart disease lowers the vital capacity, the degree depending on the clinical severity of the disease, has been supported in the

literature. The exact mechanism, whether because of increased blood volume in the lungs, decreased pulmonary compliance or some other factor, has been a matter of dispute. Peabody and Wentworth showed that cardiac patients who had dyspnea on moderate exertion without further evidence of decompensation had somewhat reduced vital capacities (6).

Thus it seemed worthwhile to study the risk of subsequent development of CHD according to vital capacity level comparing subjects with and without other evidence of myocardial impairment. This was accomplished by subdividing the population in three different ways according to whether or not (a) definite hypertension, (b) hypertensive heart disease or (c) cardiac enlargement by x ray was present on the initial examination. It is apparent that even when persons with these evidences of definite or possible heart disease were excluded, the gradient of risk according to vital capacity still held (Fig. 31-9).

Vital Capacity and Physical Activity

With failure to explain the relationship of vital capacity to CHD development on the above hypotheses the possibility that vital capacity might relate to life-long habits of physical activity which in turn might relate to subsequent CHD development was considered.

It has been frequently noted that physically active persons have higher vital capacities than inactive persons (7–9). However, it is not possible to determine whether the higher vital capacity was a trait helping to select the individual for athletics and vigorous occupations, or whether it was the result of such activity. There is conflicting evidence regarding the value of physical training in increasing the vital capacity (10, 11). If there is such an effect, it is probably small. The study of Gordon, Levine and Witmaers (12) showed that trained marathon runners had a "normal" range of vital capacities which could have been predicted on the basis of surface area, casting doubt on the ability of physical activity to increase vital capacity. However, this does not rule out the possibility that vital capacity in middle-aged persons might reflect long-term habits of physical activity especially during the years of body growth and development.

Investigation of the relationship between vital capacity and hand grip strength in the Framingham Study showed that these measurements were correlated with a coefficient of about +0.4 to +0.5 in the age groups studied. This correlation could reflect factors other than physical activity, such as body size and motivation.

The evidence relating physical activity to heart disease has been well reviewed by Montoye (13). Men in active occupations requiring greater exertion appear to have lower rates of fatal coronary disease than those in sedentary occupations (14–16). This argument is weakened by evidence of differences in body build which might have led to the selection of different occupations (17).

The possible mechanisms by which exercise is thought to exert this particular beneficial effect are multiple. There have been animal studies in which some protection against induced atheromatous lesions seems to have been provided by exercise (18, 19). Several studies have indicated that exercise may lower the serum cholesterol concentration, or may prevent the rise caused by overfeeding (20–22). Other animal experiments have indicated that exercise can improve the collateral circulation of the heart (23, 24). If this were also true in man, the occlusion of a coronary artery would be less likely to produce myocardial necrosis in persons who are accustomed to exercise vigorously. There is some suggestion that exercise decreases the tendency of blood to form a clot after a fatty meal (25, 26). It has also been suggested that regular exercise lowers the myocardial oxygen requirements by decreasing sympathetic activity (27).

For these reasons investigation of the relationship of physical activity to development of CHD and the relationship of vital capacity to physical activity were undertaken. It was hoped that there would be a sufficiently wide distribution of levels of physical activity reflecting biologically important variation in the Framingham population to permit the study of this factor in relation to subsequent disease. However, as may be expected in adults in a United States community, there was a relative shortage of subjects engaged in vigorous daily activity (Fig. 31–10).

A sufficient time has now elapsed to permit preliminary estimates of the subsequent rate of development of CHD in this population classified according to antecedent Physical Activity Index. There appeared to be an inverse relationship between physical activity level and subsequent CHD incidence (Fig. 31–11). In general, the risk was greater as the degree of usual physical activity lowered. It is important to recognize that these results are based on small numbers of cases accumulated since the fourth biennial examination, and may be altered as further experience accumulates. Fur-

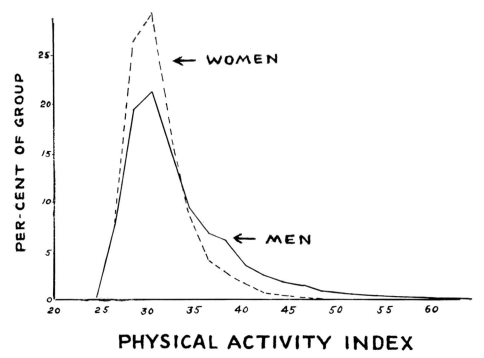

Figure 31-10. Distribution of levels of physical activity in group of 1,826 men and 2,214 women, aged 35 to 64 Framingham Study Group, Exam. IV.

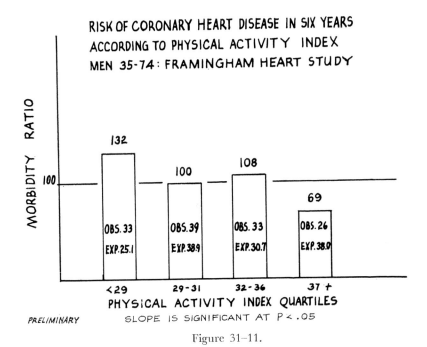

Figure 31–11.

thermore, this study has been carried out in a relatively sedentary population, If there had been greater variability in physical activity, a stronger relationship might have been demonstrable.

While low levels of vital capacity and the Physical Activity Index were both associated with excess risk of subsequent CHD development, the two measures were not correlated (correlation coefficient: $r = -.01$). It thus appears that the original purpose of this investigation, an attempt to explain the relationship of the vital capacity to subsequent CHD, still has not been achieved. The exploration of several different hypotheses has not resulted in any good explanation for the vital capacity effect and this still remains an area for further investigation. It is possible that each of the factors studied contributes slightly to the vital capacity-CHD relationship, but when studied individually the contributions were not evident. It is conceivable that the small contributions of all of these factors, taken together, produce the vital capacity-CHD relationship.

In any event, at this stage of our understanding it appears desirable to have a high vital capacity and do physical work. Exercise of a type requiring high energy expenditure, which can be continued over the years, seems highly desirable as a possible way to prevent premature CHD. If such activity improves the vital capacity, this also would appear to be beneficial.

SUMMARY

In a longitudinal study of 5,127 men and women aged 30 to 59, in Framingham, Massachusetts, several personal attributes have been demonstrated to relate to the risk of development of coronary (ischemic) heart disease (CHD). These have included age, sex, serum lipids, blood pressure, cigarette smoking, obesity, certain electrocardiographic abnormalities, and the vital capacity. Because the relationship of the vital capacity to the subsequent development of CHD failed to fit any hypotheses concerning the pathogenesis of CHD, several correlates of the vital capacity were studied in an effort to explain the observed relationship. Age, obesity, cigarette smoking, height, lung disease and other evidence of heart disease were all explored, but none could account for the vital capacity-CHD relationship. Habitual physical activity was also investigated because of a possible relationship of this characteristic to both the vital capacity and to CHD. In preliminary observations, persons with higher levels of energy expenditure did tend to show a lower incidence of CHD. However, the index used to measure activity did not correlate with vital capacity in the population studied. It would appear desirable on the basis of present information, to engage in regular vigorous physical activity as a possible means of preventing or delaying the onset of CHD.

REFERENCES

1. DAWBER, T. R., MEADORS, G. F., and MOORE, F. E.: Epidemiological approaches to heart disease: the Framingham study. *Amer J Public Health, 41:*279, 1951.

2. KANNEL, W. B., DAWBER, T. R., KAGAN, A., REVOTSKIE, N., and STOKES, J.: Factors of risk in the development of coronary heart disease—six year followup experience. *Ann Intern Med, 55:* 33, 1961.

3. DAWBER, T. R., and KANNEL, W. B.: Susceptibility to coronary heart disease. *Mod Conc Cardiov Dis, 30:*671, 1961.

4. KANNEL, W. B., DAWBER, T. R., FRIEDMAN, G. D., GLENNON, W. E., and McNAMARA, P. M.: Risk factors in coronary heart disease: an eval-

uation of several serum lipids as predictors of coronary heart disease. The Framingham study. *Ann Intern Med, 61:*888, 1964.

5. DOYLE, J. T., DAWBER, T. R., KANNEL, W. B., KINCH, S. H., and KAHN, H. A.: The relationship of cigarette smoking to coronary heart disease. *JAMA, 190:*108, 1964.

6. PEABODY, F. W., and WENTWORTH, J. A.: Clinical studies of respiration: IV. The vital capacity of the lungs and its relation to dyspnea. *Arch Intern Med, 20:*443, 1917.

7. DREYER, G.: The normal vital capacity in man and its relation to the size of the body. *Lancet, 2:*227, 1919.

8. HUTCHINSON, J.: On the capacity of the lungs. *Lancet, 1:*630, 1846.

9. FOSTER, J. H., and HSIEH, P. L.: The vital capacity of the Chinese: an occupational study. *Arch Intern Med, 32:*335, 1923.

10. STEINHAUS, A. H.: Chronic effects of exercise. *Physiol Rev, 13:*103, 1933.

11. ÅSTRAND, P. O.: Human physical fitness with special reference to sex and age. *Physiol Rev, 36:*307, 1956.

12. GORDON, B., LEVINE, S. A., and WITMAERS, A.: Observations on a group of marathon runners with special reference to the circulation. *Arch Intern Med, 33:*425, 1924.

13. MONTOYE, H. J.: Summary of research on the relationship of exercise to heart disease. *J Sport Med, 2:*35, 1962.

14. MORRIS, J. N., RAFFLE, P. A. B., ROBERTS, C. G., and PARKS, J. W.: Coronary heart disease and physical activity of work. *Lancet, 265:*1053, 1111, 1953.

15. MORRISON, S. L.: Occupational mortality in Scotland. *Brit J Industr Med, 14:*130, 1957.

16. KAHN, H. A.: The relationship of reported coronary heart disease mortality to physical activity of work. *Amer J Public Health, 53:*1058, 1963.

17. MORRIS, J. N., HEADY, J. A., and RAFFLE, P. A. B.: Physique of London busmen: epidemiology of uniforms. *Lancet, 271:*569, 1956.

18. WONG, H. Y. C., SIMMONS, R. L., and HAWTHORNE, E. W.: Effects of controlled exercise on experimental atherosclerosis in androgen-treated chicks. *Fed Proc, 15:*203, 1956.

19. KOBERNICK, S. O., NIWAYAMA, G., and ZUCKLEWSKI, A. C.: Effect of physical activity on cholesterol atherosclerosis in rabbits. *Proc Soc Exp Biol Med, 926:*623, 1957.

20. WONG, H. Y. C., ANDERSON, M. B., KIM, J. K., LIN, D. J., and HAWTHORNE, E. W.: Hypocholesterolizing effect of exercise on cholesterol-fed cockerels. *Fed Proc, 16:*138, 1957.

21. MYASNIKOV, A. L.: Influence of some factors on development of experimental cholesterol atherosclerosis. *Circulation, 17:*99, 1958.

22. MANN, G. V.: Importance of caloric disposition in cholesterol and lipoprotein metabolism of human subjects. *Fed Proc, 14:*442, 1955.

23. ECKSTEIN, R. W.: Effect of exercise and coronary arterial narrowing on growth of interarterial coronary anastomoses. *Fed Proc, 15:*54, 1956.

24. ECKSTEIN, R. W.: Effect of exercise and coronary artery narrowing on coronary collateral circulation. *Circ Res, 5:*230, 1957.

25. McDONALD, G. A., and FULLERTON, H. W.: Effect of physical activity on increased coagulability of blood after ingestion of high-fat meal. *Lancet, 2:*600, 1958.

26. WARNOCK, N. H., CLARKSON, T. B., and STEVENSON, R.: Effect of exercise on blood coagulation time and atherosclerosis of cholesterol-fed cockerels. *Circ Res, 5:*478, 1957.

27. RAAB, W.: The neurogenic metabolic factor in ischemic heart disease: pathogenesis and prevention. *Dis Chest, 46:*150, 1965.

Chapter XXXII

THE NATIONAL DIET-HEART STUDY: A STUDY IN ENVIRONMENTAL CHANGE

ROBERT B. McGANDY

(Boston, Massachusetts, U.S.A.)

EXTENSIVE epidemiological, clinical, pathological, and experimental evidence shows that multiple factors are associated with the development of coronary heart disease and the underlying atherosclerotic process. The relative importance of, and the interrelationships between, these several factors are well known to persons interested in preventive cardiology and will not be reviewed in this paper. Certain alterations in blood lipids (elevation of blood total cholesterol level has received the most attention) are undoubtedly associated with an increased risk of coronary heart disease. In the last 10 years or so, much has been learned about the dietary regulation of blood lipid levels; again, the emphasis has been on cholesterol response. Although diet alone cannot account for all variations in blood cholesterol, either between or within population groups, it is known with certainty that alterations in the kind and/or the amount of dietary fats and sterols can significantly lower circulating cholesterol levels in most individuals.

Thinking in terms of the primary prevention of coronary heart disease leads one to consider the feasibility of favorably altering the environmental and host factors known to be associated with an increased risk. Dietary reduction of blood cholesterol presently seems the one factor most amenable to a practical, large-scale approach to this major public health problem. At this moment, of course, there is little or no direct evidence that a reduction of blood cholesterol by diet (or by drugs or hormones for that matter) can significantly reduce risk. The possibility of a large-scale field trial to test this hypothesis led to the establishment in 1960 of an Executive Committee on Diet and Heart Disease. This committee was made up of leading medical, nutritional, and epidemiological scientists under the chairmanship of Dr. Irvine H. Page of Cleveland, Ohio.

For over 2 years this group explored the possibilities of carrying out this kind of study. It concluded that a well controlled, mass field trial involving middle-aged American men ought to test the dietary hypothesis without simultaneously altering other risk factors such as obesity, hypertension, and smoking habits. Analysis of the epidemiologic data relating cholesterol level to incidence suggests that a study population of middle-aged men with a cholesterol level 15 to 20 per cent less than the "average" range of 235 to 245 mg% has a coronary heart disease incidence some 30 to 40 per cent less than men in the "average" cholesterol range. This is, of course, the result of many years exposure to a lower cholesterol level. Assuming that only part of this benefit could be manifest during a 4 or 5 year study but also with the knowledge that a 15 per cent cholesterol reduction can be attained through dietary manipulation, one can calculate that about 100,000 research subjects would be required to detect, with reasonable certainty, a 20 per cent reduction in the incidence of myocardial infarction. Cholesterol reductions of 15 to 20 per cent have been achieved in smaller scale studies—ones using highly motivated persons or in secondary prevention studies. The committee concluded that a study of this magnitude was obviously a formidable undertaking and that many logistic problems needed to be resolved first. It was therefore decided to establish a small-scale "feasibility" study before making a decision on a large-scale effort.

In the spring of 1963, working under a common protocol, five groups of investigators in as many American cities (Baltimore, Boston, Chicago, Minneapolis, and Oakland) recruited a total of 1,500 men eligible for this undertaking. Eligible men between the age of 45 and 54, married and living at home, and free of manifest cardiovascular disease, diabetes, and other major systemic disease, were recruited. The eligible men were also limited in the amount of traveling and eating away from home.

Following a thorough clinical, radiological, electrocardiographic, biochemical, and nutritional evaluation during a base-line period, participants (with their wives present) received detailed and individualized dietary instructions which allowed for a pattern of food intake similar to those previously followed. A major feature facilitating these nutritional changes is that the participants purchase most of their fat-containing foods from a Diet-Heart Study warehouse in each city. Well-known food companies have prepared special fat-controlled foods including meats, dairy products, cooking fats, table spreads, and many baked goods for the study. These foods are modified in various degrees in the kind and amount of fat and sterols they contain.

Follow-up visits at monthly, and then bimonthly, intervals involve a physician and nutritionist as well as a blood sample for lipid analyses. Neither the participant nor the research personnel know what diet a participant is on or what his cholesterol response has been.

No results of this study will be announced until these feasibility studies have been terminated. It is still too early to speculate on the possibility of a large-scale definitive study. The fact that all is going well to date in a cooperative operation as complex at this one suggests that controlled mass field trials involving the manipulation of environmental factors in disease may indeed be feasible.

SUMMARY

The background, organization, and current status of the National Cooperative Diet and Heart Disease Study are presented. The immediate aim of these studies is to determine the feasibility of a large-scale study to assess whether or not a reduction of blood cholesterol by dietary means can significantly reduce the risk of coronary heart disease in healthy, middle-aged American men.

SECTION III

PREVENTIVE MEASURES

Chapter XXXIII

DIETARY FACTORS AND SERUM CHOLESTEROL IN MAN

FRANCISCO GRANDE

(Minneapolis, Minnesota, U.S.A.)

IT HAS been known for more than 50 years that atherosclerotic lesions can be produced in animals by feeding diets rich in fat and cholesterol (1, 2). The frequency of severe atherosclerosis and its complication of coronary heart disease among populations is closely related to the average serum cholesterol level of the population (3, 4, 5). Keys (5, 6, 7) has shown that the incidence rate of infarction is an exponential function of the "effective cholesterol level." About 70 per cent of the total risk is related to the serum cholesterol level.

These facts, without excluding other factors, indicate a close relationship between serum cholesterol level and the development of the atherosclerotic process and offer great promise for its prevention by reducing the serum cholesterol level.

Among the various factors known to influence serum cholesterol level, the diet deserves special consideration. It is our purpose to analyze the quantitative relationships between dietary changes and changes in serum cholesterol in man and its application to the prevention of the atherosclerotic process.

Dietary Fat and Serum Cholesterol Concentration in Man

Populations subsisting on diets high in saturated fat have higher serum cholesterol levels than comparable populations subsisting on low fat diets or on diets containing oils rich in polyunsaturated fatty acids (8, 9, 10). Controlled dietary experiments show that man's serum cholesterol concentration can be changed by changing the amount and kind of dietary fat (11, 12, 13, 14).

Other facts being constant, an increase in the proportion of dietary saturated fatty acid glycerides is associated with an increase in serum cholesterol concentration, whereas an increase in the proportion of polyunsaturated fatty acid glycerides causes a decrease of cholesterol. Monoene (= mono-unsaturated) fatty acids are indifferent, that is to say that when isocalorically substituted for carbohydrates, do not produce significant changes of serum cholesterol (15, 16).

The effect of the saturated fatty acids depends on their molecular size. Those with 10 or less carbon atoms have little or no influence on serum cholesterol (17, 18, 19, 20). The saturated fatty acid with

18 carbon atoms (stearic) seems to be devoid of cholesterol increasing effect (21). The cholesterol increasing effect of the common saturated fats, therefore, is due to that of the fatty acids with 12, 14 and 16 carbon atoms (lauric, myristic and palmitic). The effect of the polyunsaturated fatty acids does not increase with the degree of unsaturation (22, 23).

The unnatural trans isomers of monoene fatty acids produced during the partial hydrogenation of natural oils have shown a cholesterol raising effect, in contrast to the lack of effect of the natural cis isomers, and a tendency to elevate the serum triglycerides (24). The study of the effects of the trans isomers is far from completed, but these observations are important because of the significant amounts of hydrogenated fats consumed in many countries.

These effects refer to the human species. Animal experiments have shown (25, 26) significant differences in the responses of the serum lipids to dietary fat between man and animals.

The Influence of Other Dietary Factors

Other dietary factors also influence serum cholesterol concentration. Recent work has given valuable data concerning the effects of dietary cholesterol (17, 27–33, 40), the carbohydrates of the diet (35–38), and the unsaponifiable material of some vegetable oils (17, 39). Work from this laboratory (27, 28, 40, 41), and by others (30–33), has shown that up to a certain level of dietary cholesterol, changes of cholesterol intake cause corresponding changes of serum cholesterol concentration.

The total calorie intake influences serum cholesterol concentration. Serum cholesterol tends to increase during periods of positive calorie balance, and to decrease during periods of negative calorie balance.

The Fatty Acid Composition of the Diet and Serum Cholesterol

Natural fats are mixtures of glycerides containing various proportions of different fatty acids, and we have indicated that the different fatty acids have different effects on serum cholesterol concentration. The prediction of the serum cholesterol changes to be expected when the dietary fat is changed requires a knowledge of their quantitative relationships. The derivation of an equation for the prediction of the serum cholesterol changes from the changes in fatty acid composition of the diet was reported by Keys, Anderson and Grande in 1957 (42). A complete analysis of their results appeared in 1959 (43). The data used were obtained in middle-aged males, free of metabolic abnormalities, fed standard diets in which fats or fat mixtures of different composition, in terms of the various groups of fatty acids, were exchanged isocalorically for each other or for an isocaloric amount of carbohydrate. The changes of serum cholesterol were studied after 3 weeks of subsistence on the different diets. The data included 60 sets of dietary comparisons, each in groups of 12 to 27 individuals.

The basic hypothesis was that the effect of a given fat on serum cholesterol is the resultant of the effects of the various kinds of fatty acids and that each of the main groups of fatty acids has a specific effect independent of the effects of the others. We considered 3 main types of fatty acids: saturated, monoene (or monounsaturated) and polyene (or polyunsaturated).

Accordingly, the serum cholesterol concentration (mg/100 ml) on a given diet 1, (Chol.$_1$) can be represented by the equation:

1. Chol.$_1$ = a + bS$_1$ + cM$_1$ + dP$_1$

where a represents the part of the serum cholesterol independent of the dietary fat, that is to say the serum cholesterol level on a fat-free diet and b, c, and d are the coefficients expressing the effects of the saturated, monoene and polyene fatty acids, respectively. S, M, and P represent the proportions of the saturated, monoene and polyene fatty acids in the diet, as per cent of the total calorie intake.

On another dietary situation 2, the serum cholesterol concentration will be given by the equation:

2. Chol.$_2$ = a + bS$_2$ + cM$_2$ + dP$_2$

The change of serum cholesterol produced when changing from one diet to the other will be the following:

3. Chol.$_2$ − Chol.$_1$ = b (S$_2$ − S$_1$) + c (M$_2$ − M$_1$) + d (P$_2$ − P$_1$)

or, using Δ for the differences:

4. ΔChol. = b (Δ S) + c (Δ M) + d (Δ P)

The values of the coefficients b, c, and d were calculated by the least squares method. Coefficient b was positive, coefficient c was statistically not different from O, and coefficient d was negative. This indicates that changes in the monoene content of the diet, as already mentioned, are not associated with changes in serum cholesterol concentration. The prediction of serum cholesterol changes can be made by the following equation, which omits the term for the monoene fatty acids:

5. Δ Chol. = 2.68 Δ S − 1.23 Δ P

Where Δ Chol. represents the change of serum cholesterol concentration in mg/100 ml and Δ S and Δ P, respectively,

the changes in saturated and polyunsaturated glycerides (as per cent of the total calorie intake). This means that, other factors being constant, the serum cholesterol concentration increased by 2.68 mg/100 ml, when the intake of saturated fatty acids increased by 1 per cent of the total calories and that it decreased by 1.23 mg/100 ml, when the intake of polyunsaturated fatty acids increased by 1 per cent of the total calories.

Since the coefficient of Δ S in equation 5 is approximately twice that of Δ P, it follows that Δ Chol. is a linear function of 2 Δ S − ΔP.

Limitations of the Prediction Equation

The limitations of the prediction by equation 5 have been discussed in detail (42–44). The equation was derived from data obtained in groups of middle-aged men who had average serum cholesterol levels between 200 and 250 mg/100 ml when they were eating diets of the usual United States type of about 3,000 calories per day, with total fat providing 40 to 45 per cent of the total calories, cholesterol intake of the order of 600 mg/day, and in caloric equilibrium (that is to say that their body weights were kept constant throughout the experiments). No satisfactory prediction is expected when the equation is applied to data obtained from men who differ from these specifications. However, equation 5 has predicted with reasonable accuracy the serum cholesterol changes reported by other workers when applied to their data (11, 20, 44–48).

This may be considered as indication of its validity. A recent new analysis of 11 sets of dietary comparisons has given results in agreement with equation 5 (44).

The Iodine Value and the P:S Ratio as Indexes of the Effect of a Given Fat on Serum Cholesterol Concentration

Any index not including the proportion of fat calories will be only of limited predictive value. Iodine value has been suggested as an index of the effect of a given fat on serum cholesterol concentration (11, 48), but we have discussed the reasons why iodine value, alone or in combination with the amount of fat, is a poor predictor (16, 42–44).

The same applies to the so-called P:S ratio. It is obvious that highly unsaturated fats (with a high P:S ratio) will tend to produce lower serum cholesterol than fats lower in polyunsaturated and rich in saturated fatty acids (low P:S ratio), but the quantitative effect will depend also on the amount of fat which is used.

The Effect of Dietary Cholesterol

We reported (27, 40) that for cholesterol intakes between 50 and 1550 mg per day, serum cholesterol concentration is a function of the square root of the dietary cholesterol. More recently we have analyzed other results from the literature as well as our own experimental data (41). This analysis shows that, other things being equal, the change in serum cholesterol in mg/100 ml (Δ Chol.) caused by changing the cholesterol content of the diet is defined by the following equation.

6. $\Delta \text{Chol.} = 1.5 \ (Z_2^{\frac{1}{2}} - Z_1^{\frac{1}{2}})$

where Z_1 and Z_2 represent the cholesterol content of the diets expressed in mg per 1000 calories.

The effect of changing the cholesterol content of the diet can be illustrated by the following example. Assuming a cholesterol intake of 250 mg/1000 calories,

which is in the range of the cholesterol intake in the usual American diets, a reduction of 30 per cent in the cholesterol intake (to 175 mg/1000 calories) will produce a decrease of serum cholesterol concentration of only 4 mg/100 ml.

Prediction of Serum Cholesterol Changes from Changes of Dietary Fat and Dietary Cholesterol

Our observations (40) have shown that the effects on serum cholesterol concentration of changing the fatty acid composition and the cholesterol content of the diet are additive. Accordingly, it is possible to predict the serum cholesterol changes by combining equations 5 and 6. But the effect of the saturated fatty acids is limited to those of 12, 14 and 16 carbon atoms, and for this reason it is advisable to correct equation 5, taking into account the content of these fatty acids in place of the total saturated fatty acids. We have recalculated the data of 45 sets of dietary comparisons from our own experiments and those of 18 sets of comparisons from other workers (21). The serum cholesterol changes can be predicted by the following equation:

7. $\Delta \text{Chol.} = 1.2 \ (2 \ \Delta S' - \Delta P) + 1.5 \ \Delta Z$

where $\Delta S'$ represent the change in saturated fatty acids of more than 10 and less than 18 carbon atoms, (as per cent of the total calorie intake), P the change in polyunsaturated fatty acids, (as per cent of the total calorie intake) and ΔZ represents the difference between the square roots of the cholesterol content (in mg/100 calories) of the two diets. This term is equal then to the term $(Z_2^{\frac{1}{2}} - Z_1^{\frac{1}{2}})$ of equation 6.

The correlation coefficient between observed and predicted serum cholesterol differences is 0.95 for the 45 sets of experiments from this laboratory, and 0.93 when all the 63 sets of available data are included.

The Prediction of Serum Cholesterol Changes in Individuals

Men intrinsically hypercholesterolemic respond to a given dietary change with greater cholesterol changes than men intrinsically hypocholesterolemic. Keys, Anderson and Grande (43, 49) have shown that the response of an individual to a given dietary change can be predicted when his serum cholesterol (as per cent of the average serum cholesterol of the group) is known, by an equation of the type:

$$\Delta \% = a + b\ X\%$$

where $\Delta \%$ represents the serum cholesterol change of the individual as per cent of the average change of the group, and $X\%$ the serum cholesterol of the individaul as per cent of the average of the group on the standard diet.

Values for the coefficients a and b were obtained (49) using data from our experiments and from other laboratories, including 227 men in 10 sets of studies. Introducing these values, equation 8 can be written as follows:

8. $\Delta \% = 1.84\ X\% - 84$

This equation makes it possible to calculate the cholesterol change expected in a given individual belonging to a group, if his serum cholesterol and the average cholesterol of the group on a standard diet are known. Once $\Delta \%$ is computed from equation 9, this value applied to the prediction for the group, computed by the equations previously described, will give the expected value for the individual.

Diet and Prevention of Atherosclerotic Heart Disease

The data reported indicate that it is possible to modify serum cholesterol concentration in man by proper modification of the diet. Reduction of the amount of saturated fatty acids with an increase of polyunsaturated fatty acids will produce in most individuals a significant reduction of serum cholesterol concentration without increasing the total amount of fat in the diet. Limitation of cholesterol intake will also cause a reduction of serum cholesterol but, as indicated above, the reduction of dietary cholesterol necessary to produce significant changes in serum cholesterol concentration demands extreme changes in the diet. It is easy to avoid some cholesterol containing foods like eggs and butter, but it is difficult to prepare diets of very low cholesterol content unless animal foods are drastically limited.

With the information given, it is possible to predict the serum cholesterol changes expected for a given dietary change. Conversely, it is possible to determine the dietary change needed to obtain a given reduction of serum cholesterol concentration.

The practical application of our equations has been described in our recent papers (21, 34, 41, 44, 49). Dr. E.S. Fetcher from our laboratory has prepared a nomogram for the graphical computation of the data.*

The evidence available does not yet permit to evaluate the effect of a reduction of serum cholesterol concentration

---

*This nomogram will be sent upon request to the Laboratory of Physiological Hygiene, University of Minnesota, Stadium Gate 27, Minneapolis, Minnesota, 55455.

on the course of the atherosclerotic process in man. Much work has still to be done, but our present knowledge indicates that reduction of serum cholesterol concentration may be very effective in the prevention of atherosclerosis and of its consequences.

SUMMARY

The relationship between serum cholesterol concentration and development of atherosclerosis is supported by the results of animal experimentation and by epidemiological studies. This suggests that reduction of serum cholesterol concentration could result in a substantial degree of prevention or delay in the development of the atherosclerotic process.

It is possible to produce predictable changes of serum cholesterol concentration in man by changing the composition of the diet.

Equations relating the changes in the composition of the diet with the changes in serum cholesterol concentration are presented as a guide for planning the dietary control of serum cholesterol concentration in the prevention of atherosclerotic coronary heart disease.

REFERENCES

1. KATZ, L. N., and STAMLER, J.: *Experimental Atherosclerosis.* Springfield, Thomas, 1953.
2. KRITCHEWSKI, D.: Experimental atherosclerosis. In: *Lipid Pharmacology.* R. Paoletti, Ed. New York, Academic Press, 1964.
3. KEYS, A.: Epidemiological aspects of coronary artery disease. *J Chronic Dis, 6:*552, 1957.
4. KEYS, A.: Diet and coronary heart disease throughout the world. *Cardiol Prat, 13:*225, 1962.
5. KEYS, A.: Cholesterol and anticholesterol agents in regard to arteriosclerosis and its complications. *Mal Cardiov, 4:*93, 1963.
6. KEYS, A.: The risk of coronary heart disease. *Circulation, 23:*805, 1961.
7. KEYS, A., TAYLOR, H. L., BLACKBURN, H., ANDERSON, J. T., and SIMONSON, E.: Coronary heart disease in Minnesota business and professional men followed fifteen years. *Circulation, 28:*381, 1963.
8. KEYS, A.: Diet and the epidemiology of coronary heart disease. *JAMA, 164:*1912, 1957.
9. KEYS, A.: Role of the diet in human atherosclerosis and its complications. In: *Atherosclerosis and Its Origin.* M. Sandler and G. H. Bourne, Ed. New York, University Press, 1963.
10. KEYS, A., and GRANDE, F.: Diet and epidemiology of coronary heart disease. *Amer J Public Health, 47:*1520, 1957.
11. AHRENS, E. H., JR., HIRSCH, J., INSULL, W., TSALTES, T. T., BLOMSTRAND, R., and PETERSON, M. L.: The influence of dietary fat on serum lipid levels in man. *Lancet, 1:*943, 1957.
12. ANDERSON, J. T., KEYS, A., and GRANDE, F.: The effect of different food fats on serum cholesterol concentration in man. *J Nutr, 62:*421, 1957.
13. BEVERIDGE, J. M. R., CONNELL, W. F., MAYER, G. A., FIRSTBROOK, J. B., and DEWOLFE, M. S.: The effects of certain vegetable and animal fats on plasma lipids of humans. *J Nutr, 56:*311, 1955.
14. KINSELL, L. W., PARTRIDGE, J., BOLLING, L., MARGEN, S., and MICHAELS, G.: Dietary modification of serum cholesterol and phospholipid levels. *J Clin Endocr, 12:*909, 1952.
15. GRANDE, F., MATSUMOTO, Y., ANDERSON, J. T., and KEYS, A.: Effect of dietary rapeseed oil on man's serum lipids. *Circulation, 26:*653, 1962.
16. KEYS, A., ANDERSON, J. T., and GRANDE, F.: The effect on serum cholesterol in man of monoene fatty acid (oleic acid) in the diet. *Proc Soc Exp Biol Med, 98:*387, 1958.
17. BEVERIDGE, J. M. R., CONNELL, W. F., HAUST, H. L., and MAYER, G. A.: Dietary cholesterol and plasma cholesterol levels in man. *Canad J Biochem Physiol, 37:*575, 1959.
18. GRANDE, F.: Dog serum lipid responses to dietary fats differing in the chain length of the saturated fatty acids. *J Nutr, 76:*255, 1962.
19. GRANDE, F., ANDERSON, J. T., and KEYS, A.: The influence of chain length of the saturated fatty acids on their effect on serum cholesterol concentration in man. *J Nutr, 74:*420, 1961.
20. HASHIM, S. E., ARTEAGA, A., and VAN ITALLIE, T. B.: Effect of a saturated medium chain triglyceride on serum lipid in man. *Lancet, 1:*1105, 1960.
21. KEYS, A., ANDERSON, J. T., and GRANDE, F.: Serum cholesterol response to changes in the diet. IV. Particular saturated fatty acids in the diet. *Metabolism, 14:*776, 1965.
22. AHRENS, E. H., JR., INSULL, W., HIRSCH, J., STOFFEL, W., PETERSON, M. L., and FARQUHAR, J. W.: The effect on human serum lipids of a dietary fat highly unsaturated but poor in essential fatty acids. *Lancet, 1:*115, 1959.

23. GRANDE, F., ANDERSON, J. T., and KEYS, A.: A comparison of the effects of fish oil, poly-unsaturated fatty acids and of linoleic acid on man's serum lipids. *Amer J Clin Nutr, 12:*331, 1963.

24. ANDERSON, J. T., GRANDE, F., and KEYS, A.: Hydrogenated fats in the diet and lipids in the serum of man. *J Nutr, 75:*388, 1961.

25. GRANDE, F., AMATUZIO, D. W., and WADA, S.: The effect of dietary fat on serum cholesterol concentration in the dog. *Circulation, 22:*680, 1960.

26. GRUNBAUM, B. W., GEARY, J. R., GRANDE, F., ANDERSON, J. T., and GLICK, D.: Effect of dietary lipids on rat serum cholesterol and tissue mast cells. *Proc Soc Biol Med, 94:*613, 1957.

27. ANDERSON, J. T., GRANDE, F., CHLOUVERAKIS, C., PROJA, M., and KEYS, A.: Effect of dietary cho-lesterol on serum cholesterol level in man. *Fed Proc, 21:*100, 1962.

28. ANDERSON, J. T., GRANDE, F., and KEYS, A.: Interaction of dietary fat and cholesterol. *Fed Proc, 22:*268, 1963.

29. BEVERIDGE, J. M. R., CONNELL, W. F., MAYER, G. A., and HAUST, H. L.: The response of man to dietary cholesterol. *J Nutr, 71:*61, 1960.

30. CONNOR, W. H., HODGES, R. E., and BLEILER, R. E.: Effect of dietary cholesterol upon serum lipids in man. *J Lab Clin Med, 57:*331, 1961.

31. CONNOR, W. E., HODGES, R. E., and BLEILER, R. E.: The serum lipids in men receiving high cholesterol and cholesterol free diets. *J Clin Invest, 40:*894, 1961.

32. CONNOR, W. E., STONE, D. B., and HODGES, R. E.: The interrelated effect of dietary cholesterol and fat upon human serum lipid levels. *J Clin Invest, 43:*1691, 1964.

33. ERICKSON, B. A., COOTS, R. H., MATTSON, F. H., and KLIGMAN, A. M.: The effect of partial hydro-genation of dietary fat, of the ratio of poly-unsaturated to saturated fatty acids and of dietary cholesterol upon plasma lipids in man. *J Clin Invest, 34:*2017, 1964.

34. GRANDE, F., and ANDERSON, J. T.: Prediction of serum cholesterol changes caused by dietary fat in man. *Minnesota Med, 47:*645, 1964.

35. ANDERSON, J. T., GRANDE, F., MATSUMOTO, Y., and KEYS, A.: Glucose, sucrose and lactose in the diet and blood lipids in man. *J Nutr, 79:*349, 1963.

36. GRANDE, F., ANDERSON, J. T., and KEYS, A:. Effect of the carbohydrates of bread, potatoes and leguminous seeds on serum cholesterol con-centration in man. *J Nutr, 86:*313, 1965.

37. KEYS, A., ANDERSON, J. T., and GRANDE, F.: Diet-type (fat constant) and blood lipids in man. *J Nutr, 70:*257, 1960.

38. KEYS, A., GRANDE, F., and ANDERSON, J. T.: Fiber and pectin in the diet and serum choles-terol concentration in man. *Proc Soc Exp Biol Med, 106:*555, 1961.

39. GRANDE, F., ANDERSON, J. T., and KEYS, A.: Serum cholesterol in man and the unsaponifiable fraction of corn oil in the diet. *Proc Soc Exp Biol Med, 98:*436, 1958.

40. GRANDE, F., ANDERSON, J. T., CHLOUVERAKIS, C., PROJA, M., and KEYS, A.: The effect of dietary cholesterol on man's serum lipids. *J Nutr, 87:*52, 1965.

41. KEYS, A., ANDERSON, J. T., and GRANDE, F.: Serum cholesterol responses to changes in the diet. II. The effect of cholesterol in the diet. *Metabolism, 14:*759, 1965.

42. KEYS, A., ANDERSON, J. T., and GRANDE, F.: Prediction of serum cholesterol responses of man to changes of fats in the diet. *Lancet, 2:*959, 1957.

43. KEYS, A., ANDERSON, J. T., and GRANDE, F.: Serum cholesterol in man: diet fat and intrinsic responsiveness. *Circulation, 19:*201, 1959.

44. KEYS, A., ANDERSON, J. T., and GRANDE, F.: Serum cholesterol response to changes in the diet. I. Iodine value of dietary fat versus 2S–P. *Metabolism, 14:*747, 1965.

45. MALMROS, H., and WIGAND, G.: The effect on serum cholesterol of diets containing different fats. *Lancet, 2:*1, 1957.

46. TURPEINEN, O., ROINE, P., PEKKARINEN, M., KAROVONEN, M. J., RAUTANEN, Y., RUNEBERG, J., and ALIVIRTA, P.: Effect on serum cholesterol level of replacement of dietary milk fat by soy-bean oil. *Lancet, 1:*196, 1960.

47. GRANDE, F.: Prediction of serum cholesterol changes produced by dietary fat. *Amer J Clin Nutr, 13:*122, 1963.

48. KINSELL, L. W.: Some thoughts regarding the P:S ratio concept. *Amer J Clin Nutr, 12:*228, 1963.

49. KEYS, A., ANDERSON, J. T., and GRANDE, F.: Serum cholesterol response to changes in the diet. III. Differences among individuals. *Metab-olism, 14:*766, 1965.

Chapter XXXIV

THE ROLE OF DIET IN THE PREVENTION OF CORONARY HEART DISEASE

SEYMOUR H. RINZLER and GEORGE CHRISTAKIS

(New York, New York, U.S.A.)

THE rationale for a dietary approach to the prevention of coronary heart disease is based on the following major sequential advances of the past two decades:

1. International epidemiologic studies have indicated statistical associations between diet, the level of serum cholesterol in population groups, and the incidence of coronary disease (1).

2. The discovery of the serum cholesterol depressant effects of diets relatively rich in polyunsaturated fatty acids (2, 3, 4).

3. The identification of risk factors associated with the development of coronary heart disease in prospective studies (5), two of which could be modified by diet (serum cholesterol level and obesity).

4. The association between fat consumption and death rates for coronary heart disease in various countries of the world were made more significant when the death rates were compared with the consumption of saturated fats rather than total fat (6).

Since 1957, the "Anti-Coronary Club," the Diet and Coronary Heart Disease Study Project of the Bureau of Nutrition, Department of Health, City of New York, has been in progress (7–20). The overall objective was to investigate a dietary approach to the prevention of heart disease. This was done by developing practical diets for use by the general public, which were nutritionally adequate and palatable and which would lower the blood cholesterol level in most free-living subjects who modified their diets. The main objective was accomplished when it was determined that a favorable change in the blood level produced and maintained by diet was associated with a favorable change in morbidity from coronary heart disease in male subjects, aged 40 to 59 years.

The Anti-Coronary Club Study Diet ("The Prudent Diet")

The basic nutritional principle of the Prudent Diet was to provide approximately equal quantities of the 3 types of fats: saturated, polyunsaturated and monounsaturated. Beef, mutton or pork was limited to 4 meals per week, with the remaining meals comprised of poultry and fish, the latter consumed a minimum of 5 meals weekly. Eggs may not exceed 4 per week. Butter and hydrogenated shortenings were replaced by high P/S

TABLE 34–I
THE ANTI-CORONARY CLUB STUDY DIETS
FOR NORMAL WEIGHT AND OBESE SUBJECTS

Nutrient	"Prudent Diet" (2,000–2,700 Calories)		"Prudent Reducing Diet" (1,600 Calories)	
	g	Per cent of Calories	g	Per cent of Calories
Protein	130–150	23–26	140	35
Carbohydrate	225–280	42–45	180	45
Fatty acids	66–97	30–33	33.5	19.0
Saturated fatty acids	19–21	7–8	13.8	7.8
Oleic acid	25–26	8–9	11.4	8.5
Polyunsaturated fatty acids	20–33	9–11	8.3	4.7
P/S ratio	1.25–1.50		0.6	

ratio margarines and a minimum of 1 ounce of vegetable oil daily. Ice cream and hard cheeses were avoided. Overweight subjects were placed on a diet averaging 1600 calories and containing 19 per cent of the total calories as fat. When weight reduction was completed, this diet was changed to the standard study diet by the addition of 1 ounce of vegetable oil plus additional calories, when needed, from bread, nuts, fruits and vegetables. The constituents of this diet, available from food markets everywhere, are palatable, fulfill the nutrient requirements of the National Research Council, and are free of food fad characteristics. (See Appendix for example and recipes.)

The approximate composition of the Prudent Diet and the Prudent Reducing Diet is presented in Table 34–I. A typical Prudent reducing dietary prescription, adjusted as much as possible to the patient's cultural habits, appears in Table 34–II. It can be seen in Table 34–I that the proportion of calories from total fat is reduced from 30 to 33 per cent in the Prudent Diet and just under 20 per cent in the Prudent Reducing Diet. Saturated fatty acids (with no distinction made

between short, medium, and long-chain types) are reduced from 19 to 21 g in the Prudent Diet to 13.8 g in the Prudent Reducing Diet. On a relative basis, however, the saturated fatty acids as per cent of total calories in the two diets are the same. The monounsaturated fatty acids, chiefly oleic, are reduced from about 25 g in the Prudent Diet to 11.4 g in the Prudent Reducing Diet. The polyunsaturated fatty acids made up 9 to 11 per cent of total calories in the Prudent Diet, but only 4.7 per cent of total calories in the Prudent Reducing Diet. The P/S ratio of the Prudent Diet is 1.25 to 1.50 compared to 0.6 in the Prudent Reducing Diet.

Difficulties That May be Encountered While on the Anti-Coronary Club Study Diet

In over 7 years experience with more than 800 men in the Anti-Coronary Club Study Project, the following difficulties in adherence to the diet have been encountered:

1. The giving up of pastries made with highly saturated fat (such as Danish pastry, coffee cake, pound cake, "plain" cake, cookies, and pies) may constitute

TABLE 34–II

THE 1,600 CALORIE ANTI-CORONARY CLUB STUDY REDUCING DIET

	Calories	
Breakfast		
4 oz. citrus fruit or juice or 50 calories from tomato juice, strawberries or lemon in season	50	
1 egg* or 2 oz. cottage cheese	75	
1 slice bread (1 oz.)	75	
		200
Lunch or Supper		
4 oz. fish or seafood† or poultry or lean meat‡	200	
12½ calorie-value vegetable (all you want) ¶§	25	
2 slices bread	150	
1 serving fruit containing 75 calories	75	
		450
Dinner		
8 oz. fish** or poultry or meat††	150	
1 portion 25 calorie-value vegetable	25	
12½ calorie-value vegetable (all you want) ¶§	25	
1 slice bread	75	
1 serving fruit containing 75 calories	75	
		550
Between meals and at bedtime		
2 glasses skim milk††		
3 servings of fruit or fruit juice, 75 calories each	225	
Total		1,595

*No more than 4 eggs per week.
†At least three lunches (preferably more) per week should be of fish or seafood.
‡No more than one lunch per week should be from the leaner cuts of beef, lamb, or pork.
¶Cooked or raw.
§Vinegar, lemon juice, or a noncalorie dressing for salad portion.
**At least 2 dinners (preferably more) per week should be of fish.
††No more than 2 dinners per week should be from the leaner cuts of beef, lamb, pork or veal.

a real deprivation for many people, and causes the most frequent difficulty. These products need not be prohibited for the person whose wife is willing to make them with vegetable oil or a linoleate-rich margarine.

2. Limiting the portion size and frequency of serving of meats containing high proportions of saturated types of fats (such as beef, mutton, and pork) also is difficult. Many men in our affluent society have become accustomed to consuming 8, 10 or 12 ounce portions of meat per meal.

3. Prohibition of ice cream constitutes a sacrifice for some persons, although this ranks well below the first two complaints listed. Water ices, with an occasional sherbet, are the best substitutes.

4. Restaurant meals present difficulty for some of our subjects, but this is more apparent than real. No problem exists if a person can afford to eat in restaurants where the food is prepared to order. In restaurants and cafeterias where the food is prepared on a large scale, the problem is greater. In this instance, the entree should be boiled, broiled or baked fish, sea food or poultry. The dessert is limited to fruit. The unavailability of

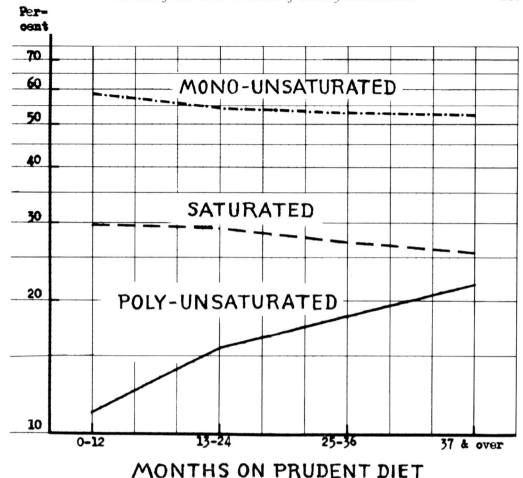

Figure 34–1. Change in composition of adipose tissue fatty acids with time on the Prudent Diet—78 males 50 to 59-years-old.

margarines with corn or safflower oil in restaurants is a definite disadvantage.

5. Hard cheeses of all varieties present a minor difficulty for a few of our study subjects. For those who must have hard cheese, 1 ounce may be substituted occasionally for half of the beef, mutton, or pork allowance; this entire allowance may be replaced by 2 ounces of cheese.

Metabolic Attributes of the Prudent Diet Studied on Anti-Coronary Club Members

The serum triglyceride level has also

TABLE 34–III

SERUM TRIGLYCERIDE LEVELS BY NUMBER OF MONTHS ON THE PRUDENT DIET

Months	Number	Serum Triglyceride mg per cent
0	53	122.0
1–12	25	144.7
13–24	22	96.5
25–36	11	100.6
37 & more	37	111.3
Total	148	

been implicated as a lipid factor of importance in coronary heart disease. Table 34–III shows the mean serum triglyceride

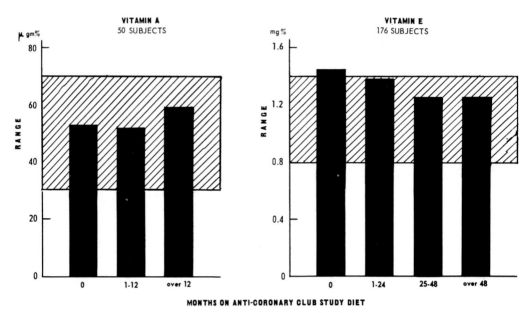

Figure 34–2. Serum levels of Vitamin A and E by months of adherence to the Anti-Coronary Club Study Diet.

levels of subjects consuming the study diet for a period up to 5 years. After an initial rise, the serum triglyceride level was maintained well within normal range (18).

In order to study certain metabolic aspects of the study diet and to provide an objective measurement of dietary adherence, the effect of the diet on depot fat consumption was also assessed (20). Figure 34–1 shows the progressive incorporation of linoleic acid in the adipose tissue of study subjects.

The relationship between Vitamin E requirements and serum cholesterol-lowering diets has invited considerable attention. Figure 34–2 shows the Vitamin E and A levels of a group of study subjects and indicates that normal levels were maintained after 4 years of adherence to the study diet.

The Effect of The Anti-Coronary Club Study Diet on Serum Cholesterol and Coronary Heart Disease Incidence

Figure 34–3 shows the trends in the level of serum cholesterol of the 40 to 59-year-old men still active in the experimental and control groups as of December 31, 1963 (21).

In the experimental group, a highly significant drop of about 30 mg per 100 ml serum from an average initial level of 260 mg per 100 ml was observed in the study after one year. Thereafter the concentration of serum cholesterol leveled off at about 225 mg per 100 ml. In the control group the serum cholesterol fell about 7 mg per 100 ml during the first two years, but rose thereafter so that by the end of the fourth year, the latest for which data are available, the average

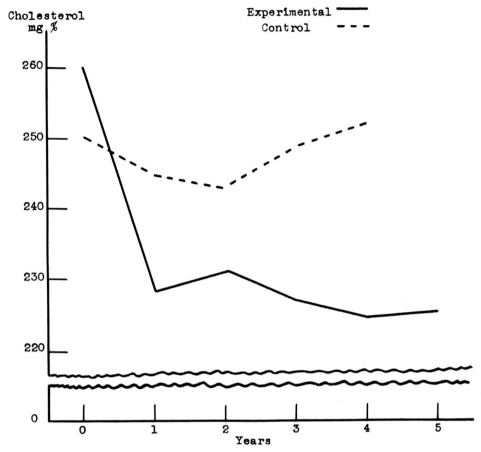

Figure 34–3. Trend of average serum cholesterol levels of men with no evidence of coronary heart disease on entry in active experimental and control groups by year of participation in study.

level had returned to its initial concentration.

During the 2,357 person-years of active experience accumulated by the 814 experimental subjects, 8 new coronary events occurred. This represents an overall incidence rate of 339 per 100,000 comprised of the age-specific rates of 196 and 379 per 100,000 for the 40 to 49 and 50 to 59-year-old men, respectively.

Similarly, the 463 men of the control group in comparable age catagories have accumulated 1,224 person-years of experience and 12 new coronary events, resulting in an overall incidence rate of 980 per 100,000 or 642 and 1,331 per 100,000 for the 40 to 49 and 50 to 59-year-old men, respectively.

The incidence rates in the control group were thus more than three times as high as the rates in the experimental group in each age category. It was desirable to test the statistical significance of the difference between the total active experimental and control groups rather than within the separate age groups because of the smaller sample sizes in the separate age groups. However, when doing so it was necessary to adjust the incidence rates observed in each total group for the difference in age distribution between the two groups. Therefore, age-adjusted numbers of "observed" new coronary disease events were calculated for the total experimental and control groups, and the difference between the two was found to be statistically significant.

Of the 8 new coronary events among active experimental subjects, 7 occurred during the 1353 person-years of experience accumulated during the first two years of each individual's participation in the study. This is not much below the expected number of 9 based on the experience of the control group. Only 1 of these 8 new events occurred among active experimental subjects during the 1,004 person-years of full participation accumulated subsequent to the first two years of an individual's participation when, presumably, the diet had a greater opportunity to exert its effect.

Of the 12 cases with new coronary disease events in the control group, all were still alive at the end of the observation period. This does appear somewhat unusual, although again the series is small. We have not been able to adequately evaluate this finding at this time and it will be analyzed further as follow up of the group continues.

Changes in Risk Factor Status Resulting from Study Participation

Since the experimental subjects experienced a significantly lower incidence of coronary heart disease during their period of Anti-Coronary Club participation than did the control group, it is of interest and importance to recognize the changes which took place in their status with respect to the three risk factors which have been considered in this study (obesity, elevated cholesterol and hypertension). An analysis was performed for the 332 subjects in the active experimental group and the 329 subjects in the control group who participated in the study for 4 years or more. This analysis compared their risk factor status at time of entry to the study and their status after 4 years of participation.

With regard to risk factors as seen in Figure 34–4, the experimental and control groups were quite comparable with respect to the proportion of subjects with initial hypercholesterolemia. However, the experimental group had a higher proportion with initial obesity and with hypertension than did the control group. From the aspects of demographic characteristics, and from risk factor status, the experimental group was not more biased toward an expected lower incidence of coronary heart disease than was the control group.

Figure 34–5 shows that, in the control group, the prevalence of initial risk factors and those calculated after 4 years have remained substantially the same. In the experimental group, as seen in Figure 34–6, four-year exposure to the Anti-Coronary Club program resulted in a definite decrease in risk factor prevalence. Thus, 59 per cent of the experimental group were free of all 3 risk factors after 4 years of study participation as compared to 35 per cent in the control.

Public Health Implications

The data from the Anti-Coronary Club have shown that the level of serum cholesterol can be effectively lowered over the course of a 5-year period

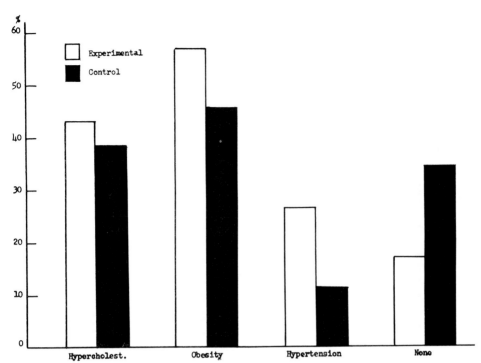

Figure 34–4. Prevalence of risk factors at time of enrollment in study—332 men in experimental group and 329 men in control group 40 to 59-years-old.

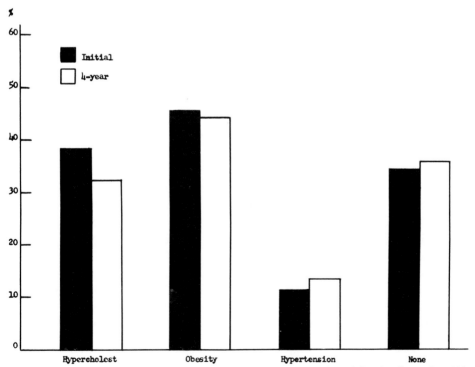

Figure 34–5. Change in prevalence of risk factors after 4 years of participation in study—329 men in control group 40 to 59-years-old.

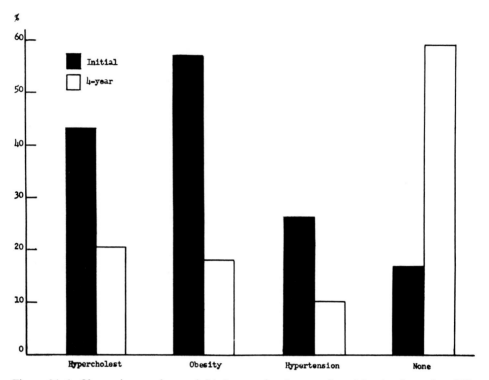

Figure 34–6. Change in prevalence of risk factors after 4 years of participation in study—332 men in experimental group 40 to 59-years-old.

without incurring a rebound. Moreover, such effective and prolonged lowering of serum cholesterol was associated with an incidence of coronary heart disease in subjects on the study diet which was significantly lower than that in our control group or in other populations under long-term observation consuming the usual American diet.

The public health significance of this salutory effect on coronary heart disease morbidity comes into proper perspective when it is realized that 30 to 40 per cent of all American males 40 to 59 years of age exhibit serum cholesterol levels above 260 mg% and are therefore exposed to six times the risk of developing coronary heart disease compared to populations whose serum cholesterol is 220 mg% or

below. It would also appear desirable to prevent the high levels of serum cholesterol observed in males age 40 to 59. The rapid increase in serum cholesterol observed in younger adult males (22) may be preventable by a dietary pattern similar to that of the study diet.

Over the course of the past 5 decades there has been an increase in beef and dairy product consumption and an increase in the daily caloric contribution by fat from approximately 30 to 33 per cent to 40 to 44 per cent of total calories. Two-thirds of this fat consumption is saturated. Though not the sole cause, this trend has almost certainly played a major role in causing what may be called "national dietary hypercholesterolemia."

A critical reappraisal of our nutritional

way of life would appear indicated. It is realized that a consideration of changes in our national diet pattern requires profound study and incurs great responsibility. While we have investigated certain effects of the study diet on serum triglyceride, serum vitamin levels and depot fat composition, not all the possible long-term metabolic effects of the Anti-Coronary Club study diet are now known.

However, the strong possibility exists that a diet pattern based on the principle of moderation in saturated fat consumption which provides a varied, nutritionally sound diet while lowering serum cholesterol may constitute a contribution to the development of a more physiologically optimal diet pattern for adults. We admonish, however, that a change in the diet pattern correcting the current over-consumption of saturated fats should not be misconstrued to mean a pattern in which polyunsaturated fats predominate, or in which any food group is over-emphasized to the exclusion of other foods supplying essential nutrients. It should also be emphasized that the apparently successful experience reported here involved a continuing program of supervised diet adherence and periodic medical examination.

If a consensus of medical and public health judgment concurs that dietary changes for the public are indicated, how are these to be implemented? Public health officials bear the responsibility of designing and operating nutrition education programs (23). The practicing physician must familarize himself with the meaning of the serum cholesterol level, the principles of the diet which can control it, and the difficulties likely to be encountered by his patient. Industry has

already shown that palatable fat-modified foods can be produced; such foods can effectively lower serum cholesterol under experimental conditions (24). It would be up to the government to develop suitable standards and labelling regulations enabling easier consumer identification of foods useful in a serum cholesterol-lowering regimen. It would also no longer appear prudent for governmental agencies to urge the public to increase consumption of products containing large quantities of saturated fat on the grounds that such products exist in surplus.

Many factors operate in the causality of coronary heart disease; however, the experience of the Anti-Coronary Club in lowering serum cholesterol and coronary heart disease incidence appears to have established a reasonable basis for public health action. Though the problems of program planning and implementation will be many and complex, there now appears to be real hope that effective programs for the control of coronary heart disease can be developed.

SUMMARY

After 7 years of observation, the Anti-Coronary Club Study of the Department of Health of New York City has indicated that men, aged 40 to 59 years, have a lower incidence of new coronary heart disease while on a prudent diet than the control group eating the usual American diet.

The principles of the Prudent Diet are as follows: |

1. It decreases the total dietary fats from 40 to 44 per cent of total daily calories to 30 to 33 per cent.

2. It reverses the predominance of saturated fatty acids found in the American diet by contributing approximately

isocaloric amounts of the three types of fat: saturated, polyunsaturated, and monounsaturated.

The Prudent Diet is able in most subjects to lower the serum cholesterol, while neither increasing the serum triglyceride level or decreasing the serum Vitamin E or A level.

REFERENCES

1. KEYS, A., and WHITE, P. D.: *World Trends in Cardiology. Vol. I. Cardiovascular Epidemiology.* New York, Paul B. Hoeber, Inc., 1956.
2. KINSELL, L. W., PARTRIDGE, J., BOLING, L., MORGEN, S., and MICHAELS, G.: Dietary modification of serum cholesterol and phospholipid levels. *J Clin Endocr,* 12:909, 1952.
3. AHRENS, E. H., TSALTAS, T. T., HIRSCH, J., and INSULL, W.: Effects of dietary fats on the serum lipids of human subjects. *J Clin Invest, 34:*918, 1955.
4. BEVERIDGE, J., CONNELL, W. F., MAYER, G. A., FIRSTBROOK, J. B., and DEWOLFE, M. D.: The effect of certain vegetable and animal fats on plasma lipids of humans. *J Nutr,* 56:311, 1955.
5. DAWBER, T. R., KANNELL, W. B., REVOTSKIE, N.: Factors associated with the development of coronary heart disease: six years' follow-up experience in the Framingham study. *Amer J Public Health,* 49:1349, 1959.
6. JOLLIFFE, N., and ARCHER, M.: Statistical associations between international coronary heart disease death rates and certain environmental factors. *J. Chronic Dis,* 9:636, 1959.
7. JOLLIFFE, N.: Fats, cholesterol and coronary heart disease. *New York J Med,* 57:2684, 1957.
8. JOLLIFFE, N.: Fats, cholesterol and coronary heart disease. A review of recent progress. *Circulation,* 20:109, 1959.
9. JOLLIFFE, N., RINZLER, S. H., and ARCHER, M.: The anti-coronary club: including a discussion of the effects of a prudent diet on the serum cholesterol level of middle-aged men. *Amer J Clin Nutr,* 7:451, 1951.
10. RINZLER, S. H., ARCHER, M., and JOLLIFFE, N.: Effect on serum cholesterol of a prudent-type reducing diet: study of 111 obese men 50 to 59 years of age. *Circulation,* 22:799, 1960.
11. RINZLER, S. H., ARCHER, M., MASLANSKY, E., and JOLLIFFE, N.: The anti-coronary club. The effect of diet on the control of serum cholesterol. *Health News,* 38:13, 1961.
12. JOLLIFFE, N., and RINZLER, S. H.: Practical dietary control of serum cholesterol in free-living American men aged 50 to 59 years. *Postgrad Med,* 29:569, 1961.
13. JOLLIFFE, N., RINZLER, S. H., and ARCHER, M.: Prudent reducing diet. Effects on serum cholesterol. *Arch Intern Med,* 109:566, 1962.
14. JOLLIFFE, N., RINZLER, S. H., ARCHER, M., MASLANSKY, E., RUDENSEY, F., SIMON, M., and FAULKNER, A.: Effect of a prudent reducing diet on the serum cholesterol of overweight middle aged men. *Amer J Clin Nutr,* 10:200, 1962.
15. RINZLER, S. H.: Lessons from the anti-coronary club. *Fed Proc,* 21:33, 1962.
16. RINZLER, S. H.: Nutrition in relation to heart disease. *Arch Environ Health,* 5:60, 1962.
17. JOLLIFFE, N., BAUMGARTNER, L., RINZLER, S. H., ARCHER, M., STEPHENSON, J. H., and CHRISTAKIS, G. J.: The anti-coronary club. The first four years. *New York J Med,* 63:69, 1963.
18. CHRISTAKIS, G. J., RINZLER, S. H., ARCHER, M. HASHIM, S. A., HILLMAN, R., VAN ITALLIE, T. B.: The effect of a cholesterol-lowering diet on the serum cholesterol, triglycerides, vitamin E and A levels, and fatty acid composition of subcutaneous fat in man. *Circulation,* 28:703, 1963.
19. RINZLER, S. H.: The relation of dietary fats to serum cholesterol and arteriosclerotic heart disease. *J Amer Geriat Soc,* 12:135, 1964.
20. CHRISTAKIS, G., RINZLER, S. H., ARCHER, M. S., HASHIM, S., VAN ITALLIE, T. B.: Effect of a serum cholesterol lowering diet on the depot fat composition of Man. *Amer J Clin Nutr,* 16:243, 1965.
21. CHRISTAKIS, G., RINZLER, S. H., ARCHER, M., WINSLOW, G., JAMPEL, S., STEPHENSON, J., FREEDMAN, G., FEIN, H., KRAUS, A. and JAMES, G.: The Anti-Coronary Club: a dietary approach to the prevention of coronary heart disease—a seven year report. *Am J Publ Health,* 56:299, 1966.
22. SCHILLING, F. J., CHRISTAKIS, G., COYLE, J. F., BENNETT, N.: An epidemiological and pathogenetic interpretation of the serum cholesterol levels of 4,244 New York City office personnel. *Amer J Public Health,* 54:461, 1964.
23. CHRISTAKIS, G.: Diet and coronary heart disease: a public health viewpoint. *Acad Med of New York Bull,* 10:262, 1964.
24. BIERENBAUM, M. L., GHERMAN, C. and EASTWOOD, G.: Fat-modified frozen food dietary pattern. Effect on blood cholesterol levels of young men with proved myocardial infarction. *J Am Med Assoc,* 182:296, 1962.

Chapter XXXV

APPROACHES OF THE CORONARY PREVENTION EVALUATION PROGRAM TO THE PRIMARY PREVENTION OF CLINICAL CORONARY HEART DISEASE IN MIDDLE-AGED AMERICAN MEN*

JEREMIAH STAMLER, H. A. LINDBERG, D. M. BERKSON, Y. HALL, W. A. MILLER, L. MOJONNIER, M. B. EPSTEIN, F. BURKEY, D. B. COHEN, M. LEVINSON and Q. D. YOUNG

(Chicago, Illinois, U.S.A.)

A VAILABLE knowledge concerning the etiology and pathogenesis of atherosclerotic coronary heart disease makes it possible to undertake the primary and secondary prevention of this disease on a rational and scientific basis (1). These advances may be summarized as follows:

1. Severe atherosclerosis is the underlying pathogenic process in most cases of clinical atherosclerotic ischemic heart disease.

2. A several-fold increase in cholesterol—particularly esterified cholesterol—is the biochemical hallmark of the atherosclerotic plaque.

3. The excess cholesterol in the plaque is derived from the cholesterol-bearing lipoproteins of the circulating plasma.

4. Sustained hypercholesterolemic hyperlipidemia is associated with frequent, premature, severe atherosclerotic coronary heart disease.

5. In groups of middle-aged patients with clinical CHD, higher mean serum cholesterol-lipid-β-lipoprotein levels are found than in matched control groups.

6. Sustained ingestion of diets containing increased quantities of cholesterol and fat is a virtual prerequisite for the production of significant atherosclerosis in a wide range of experimental animals.

7. In animals ingesting high-cholesterol, high-fat diets, other factors (e.g., hypertension, hypothyroidism, renal damage) may act synergistically to intensify atherogenesis, or to prevent or reverse the pathologic process (e.g., estrogens).

8. Marked contrasts exist among populations in different part of the world in habitual diets, levels of serum cholesterol-lipid-β-lipoprotein, and occurrence rates of premature atherosclerotic coronary heart disease; these three variables are generally correlated.

9. From data on social class differ-

*This study was aided by grants from the American Heart Association, the Chicago Heart Association, the National Dairy Council, the Wesson Foundation, the Corn Products Institute of Nutrition, and the National Heart Institute, National Institutes of Health, U.S. Public Health Service (H4197, HE 09426 and CH 00075); furthermore, by the cooperation of the Chicago Board of Health, Peoples Gas Light and Coke Company, the American Oil Company, Newspaper Division, Field Enterprises and the Department of Statistics and Biological Sciences Computation Center, University of Chicago.

ences, on the influences of migration, and on the effects of two world wars, it is evident that the marked international differences in occurrence rates of premature CHD are due to socioeconomic factors (i.e., differences in living habits, principally dietary habits), and not to racial, ethnic, climatic or geographic factors.

10. Where the mean serum cholesterol levels of populations are low, clinical CHD and severe coronary atherosclerosis at postmortem are rare, particularly in middle age.

11. High mean serum cholesterol levels in populations and high rates of middle-age clinical coronary heart disease occur only where the habitual diets are high in calories, total fat, saturated fat and cholesterol.

12. In populations studied prospectively, risk of premature atherosclerotic disease is increased in the presence of hypercholesterolemia-hyperlipidemia.

13. In populations with the nutritional-metabolic prerequisites for severe premature atherosclerotic disease, risk is also increased by hypertension, diabetes, overweight, cigarette smoking, and a positive family history of premature vascular disease. Physical inactivity (sedentary living habit) and psychological stress are in all likelihood additional significant risk factors.

14. Atherosclerosis is, at least in part, a reversible disease.

15. Serum cholesterol-lipid-β-lipoprotein levels are amenable to dietary influence, being responsive particularly to intake of cholesterol and saturated fat (less so to intake of calories, unsaturated and polyunsaturated fats, type of carbohydrate, meal-eating pattern, etc.).

16. The other major coronary risk factors—hypertension, diabetes, overweight, cigarette smoking, physical inactivity—are amenable to control and correction by nutritional-hygienic-pharmacologic means.

The foregoing phenomena have been massively documented, to an extent far exceeding most phenomena in medicine. They compel the conclusion that diet is of key importance among the multiple factors involved in the etiology and pathogenesis of atherosclerotic coronary heart disease (1, 2).

Based on these advances, the decisive preventive measures are nutritional and hygienic—the control and correction of those living habits (particularly eating, smoking and exercise habits) which are of central importance in the etiology and pathogenesis of the disease.

Since the late 1950s, several major research studies have accrued extensive experience in the utilization of such preventive measures in middle-aged men (1–21). At the present time, under the leadership of the American Heart Association, a major effort is being made to aid the medical and health professions and the public in the acquisition of the essential "know-how" of preventive approaches to controlling atherosclerotic coronary disease, particularly nutritional approaches (22, 23).

THE CORONARY PREVENTION EVALUATION PROGRAM

The Coronary Prevention Evaluation Program, in progress at the Chicago Board of Health for the last 7 years, is a research study aimed at assessing ability to achieve primary prevention of coronary heart disease by nutritional-hygienic means in higher-risk men of age 40 to 50. Volunteers have been accepted into

TABLE 35-I

CORONARY RISK FACTORS, HIGHER-RISK PARTICIPANTS IN THE
CORONARY PREVENTION EVALUATION PROGRAM, AS OF
APRIL 30, 1965

Coronary Risk Factors	No. of Participants	Rate/1000
Hypercholesterolemia (260–324) +overweight	42	201.9
Hypercholesterolemia (325 and >) +overweight	17	81.7
Hypercholesterolemia (260–324) +hypertension	3	14.4
Overweight +hypertension	21	101.0
Hypercholesterolemia (260–324) +overweight +smoking	41	197.1
Hypercholesterolemia (325 and >) +overweight +smoking	4	19.2
Hypercholesterolemia (260–324) +hypertension +smoking	2	9.6
Overweight +hypertension +smoking	12	57.7
Hypercholesterolemia (260–324) +overweight +ECG-STT abnormality	3	14.4
Hypercholesterolemia (325 and >) +overweight +ECG-STT abnormality	1	4.8
Overweight +hypertension +ECG-STT abnormality	6	28.8
Hypercholesterolemia (260–324) +overweight +hypertension	6	28.8
Hypercholesterolemia (260–324) +overweight +hypertension +smoking	14	67.3
Hypercholesterolemia (325 and >) +overweight +hypertension +smoking	2	9.6
Hypercholesterolemia (260–324) +overweight +hypertension +STT	1	4.8
Overweight +smoking +ECG-STT abnormality	5	24.0
Hypertension +smoking +ECG-STT abnormality	1	4.8
Hypercholesterolemia (260–324) +overweight +smoking +ECG-STT abnormality	2	9.6
Hypercholesterolemia +hypertension +smoking +ECG-STT abnormality	2	9.6
Overweight +hypertension +smoking +ECG-STT abnormality	2	9.6
Hypercholesterolemia 325 and >	1	4.8
Hypercholesterolemia 325 and > +smoking	2	9.6
ECG-STT abnormality +overweight	18	86.5
All hypercholesterolemia (260–324)	116	557.7
All hypercholesterolemia (325 and >)	27	129.8
All overweight	197	947.1
All hypertension	72	346.2
All cigarette smoking	89	427.9
All ECG-STT abnormality		197.1

the program only after thorough medical examination has demonstrated them to be free of clinical coronary heart disease and other major systemic diseases, and has revealed the presence of significant coronary risk factors (Table 35–I).

The program works closely with the volunteer participants and their wives in the effort to control and correct key coronary risk factors and faulty living habits—hypercholesterolemia, hypertension, overweight, cigarette smoking, and lack of exercise. A detailed description of the medical and nutritional methodology

has been presented previously (1, 3). Overweight is controlled utilizing moderate caloric restriction with individually prescribed diets of mixed ordinary foodstuffs high in nutrients and low in calories. Hypercholesterolemia is controlled by structuring these diets so that they are moderate in total calories, moderate in total fat (approximately 30 per cent of total calories), low in saturated fat (less than 9 per cent of calories), and low in cholesterol (less than 300 mg per day).

Husband and wife are indoctrinated

in detail as to the foods to eat, menus, recipes, cookbooks, and "eating out" suggestions so that the stated objectives can be achieved while enjoying the pleasures of good eating (1, 3, 24–30).

The participant is also advised concerning other habit patterns, such as sedentary living—lack of physical activity. In one of the early visits, a full discussion is had concerning the possibility of his getting regular, frequent, moderate exercise, with particular attention paid to his previous experiences, and details are reviewed at each visit.

For obese participants with hypertension, no recommendations with respect to pharmacologic treatment are made in the initial months of the program, unless the hypertension is very severe (e.g., fixed diastolic pressures of 110 mm Hg or more). In accordance with longstanding knowledge, the experience has been that a significant per cent of hypertensives do respond well to the nutritional-hygienic approach. For those who do not after 3 to 6 months, consultation proceeds with private physicians in regard to appropriate pharmacologic treatment (1, 31).

A similar approach is taken to control of abnormalities of carbohydrate metabolism in the absence of clinical symptoms or signs of diabetes. Nutritional-hygienic management with weight reduction results in the rectification of abnormal glucose tolerance in a significant per cent of obese persons with so-called mild maturity onset diabetes. For those whose glucose tolerance curves remain abnormal, consultation proceeds with private physicians in relation to possible therapy with oral antidiabetic drugs or insulin.

Correction of the cigarette smoking habit is one of the major efforts of the Coronary Prevention Evaluation Program. For most of the higher-risk men, no effort is made simultaneously to alter several habit patterns (e.g., diet, exercise, smoking) since diet control is particularly in jeopardy when the effort is being made to stop cigarette smoking. In general, the first effort is to achieve effective institution of the new dietary pattern for purposes of correction of obesity and hyperlipidemia. The effort to control cigarette smoking is postponed until the participant has "gotten over the hump" in dietary alteration. Usually, therefore, definite action on smoking is deferred until 3, or often 6, months after the nutritional recommendation is made with particular attention to appropriate steps for avoidance of marked weight gain during the initial weeks off cigarettes. Where indicated, medications (e.g., sedatives or tranquilizers) are prescribed short term.

The fundamental approach is one of maintaining "friendly persuasion" and "firm steady pressure" on the matter of smoking without "bugging" the participant in a long-term program, which includes frequent repeat visits to the research center.

Obviously, all of the above listed recommendations are at least as meaningful and as practicable for secondary prevention (i.e., for the effort to prevent recurrent clinical attacks and prolong life in persons already victimized by the disease).

RESULTS

Long-term Participation. As of April 30, 1965, a total of 208 higher-risk men of age 40 to 59 had become long-term participants in the Chicago Coronary Prevention Evaluation Program. Of this group, 130 men have been in the study 3 years or longer. A recent life table

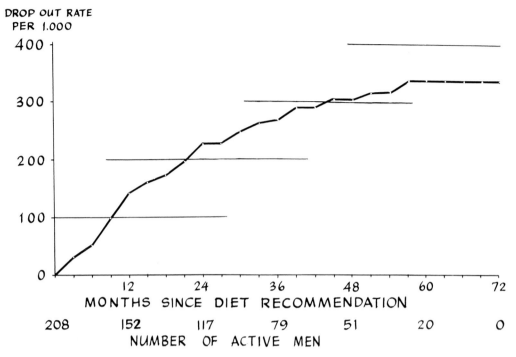

Figure 35–1. Drop out rate in the 208 coronary-prone men age 40 to 59 participating in the Coronary Prevention Evaluation Program. Data from life table analysis of the findings as of April 30, 1965.

analysis revealed the six-year drop-out rate to be 34.6 per cent. Most of the drop-outs occur during the first 24 to 30 months. Thereafter, the drop-out rate is low (Figure 35–1). The study has been in progress for 7 years. Therefore, it has become clear that it is possible to retain a majority of such men in such a program long term. A New York study has had a similar experience (6–8).

Nutritional Alterations. Men in the Coronary Prevention Evaluation Program keep a one week food record four times a year. Development of a computer program has made possible detailed interval analyses of the nutritional data (4). These tabulations incidentally serve an additional purpose: they are excellent teaching and motivational tools for use in reviewing their status with partici-

pants. The overall changes in daily foodstuff and nutrient intake for the first 99 men—given their diet recommendations 3 or more years ago (before April, 1962)—are presented in Figures 35–2 A, B, C and 35–3 A, B, C (4). The data indicate that during the early months of the study the diets of the men, in accordance with the recommendations made to most of them (94.7 per cent were evaluated as obese—Table 35–I), were moderate in total calories (about 1700 per day on the average), with an estimated caloric deficit of about 500 to 800 calories, calculated to effect weight loss at a rate of about 1.0 to 1.5 pounds per week. They were moderate in carbohydrate and total fat (about 30 per cent of total calories, rather than the usual American 40 per cent or more), low in saturated fatty

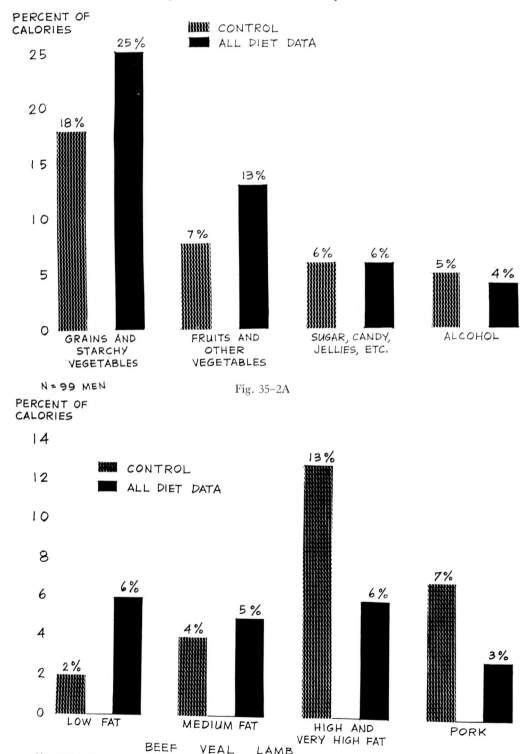

Fig. 35–2A

Fig. 35–2B

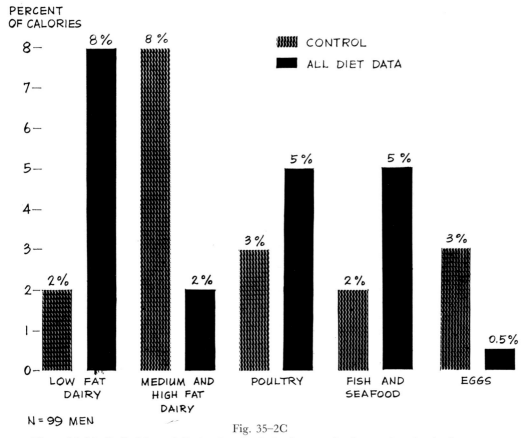

Fig. 35–2C

Figure 35–2A, B, C. Mean daily intake of calories from each of several major food groups as obtained from food records kept by the first 99 participants in the Coronary Prevention Evaluation Program. Data are expressed as per cent of total calories from each food group during the control period and the period on diet.

acids (less than 20 g per day, 10 per cent or less of total calories, rather than the usual 45 or more g per day, 17 per cent or more of total calories), low in cholesterol (300 mg per day or less, rather than the usual 600 mg or more) and moderate in unsaturated and poly-unsaturated fatty acids. The diets were ample in all essential nutrients, proteins, amino acids, vitamins, minerals, despite caloric restriction.

As shown by correlated t-tests, the major changes effected in intake of the critical food groups and nutrients were highly significant statistically (4).

The nutritional patterns of the men in the Coronary Prevention Evaluation Program closely resembled those of the men in the New York Anti-Coronary Club (6–8). They were also similar in several critical respects, (e.g., low saturated fat and low cholesterol intakes) to those of other related studies, with the difference that these latter gave strong emphasis to high levels of unsaturated and polyunsaturated oils in the diet, resulting also in high total fat intakes (40 per cent of total calories) (9–12, 18, 19). Our group believes that the approach of the Coronary Prevention Eval-

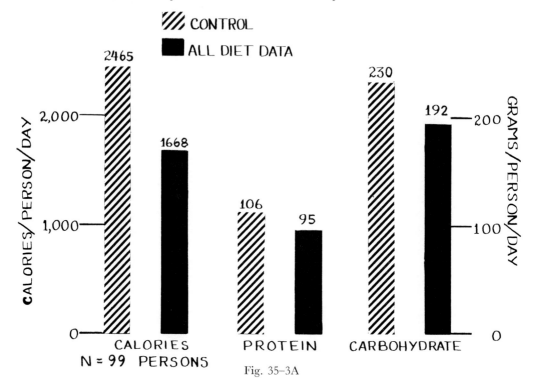

Fig. 35-3A

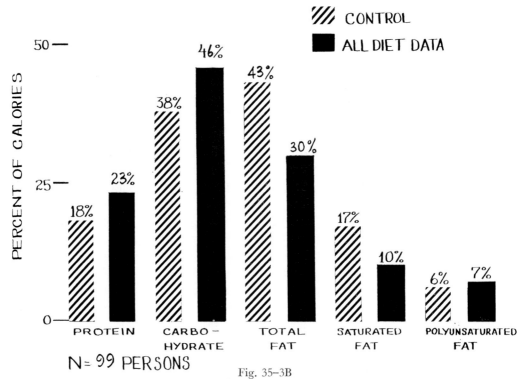

Fig. 35-3B

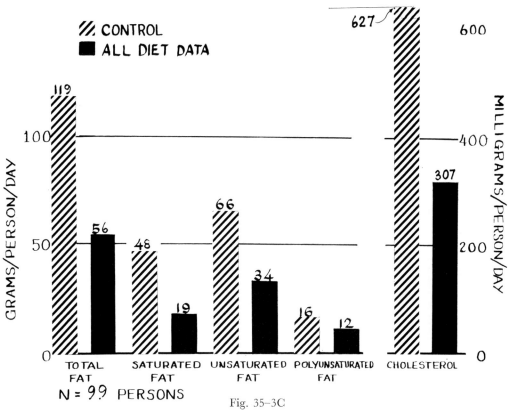

Fig. 35–3C

Figure 35–3A, B, C. Mean daily intake of nutrients by the first 99 participants in the Coronary Prevention Evaluation Program during the control and experimental (on diet) periods.

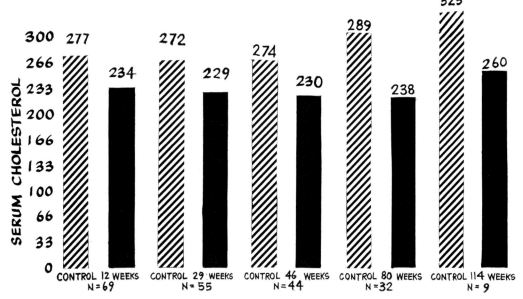

Figure 35–4. Serial mean serum cholesterol levels of the participants in the Coronary Prevention Evaluation Program. Since the number of men yielding data for each time period differs, 2 sets of bars at each time period are presented, with matching control and experimental (on diet) data for the given number of participants.

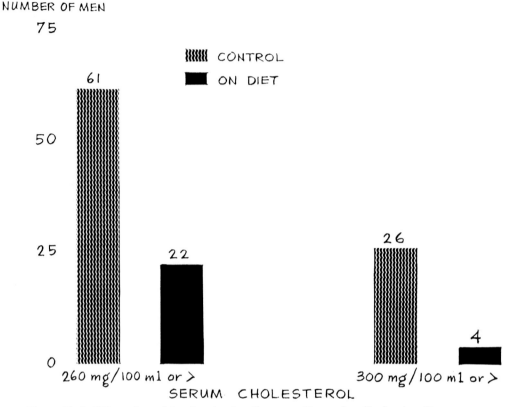

Figure 35–5. Effect of participation in the Coronary Prevention Evaluation Program on status with respect to frank hypercholesterolemia.

uation Program and the Anti-Coronary Club in this area is preferable.

Changes in Serum Cholesterol. The men in the Coronary Prevention Evaluation Program experienced a highly significant overall decline in serum cholesterol concentration (Fig. 35–4) without utilizing jiggers of oil, special oil allotments or fat-modified foods. Ordinary foodstuffs sufficed, particularly since the main emphasis was not on achieving a high intake of unsaturated oils. Rather, it was on assuring a low-saturated fat, low-cholesterol intake, with consumption of oils adjusted in a flexible, discretionary and permissive fashion, depending on need for caloric restriction and on individual's food preference.

Weight and Blood Pressure also were significantly reduced (4). Decline in weight tended to be greatest during the first 3 months on diet. For some men, correction of gross obesity was critically related to curtailment or cessation of intake of beer and other alcoholic beverages. In a sizeable number of men, the reductions resulted in their attaining levels of serum cholesterol, weight and blood pressure below those set as criteria for the high-risk designation (Figs. 35–5–7). Thus, among the 61 men who were originally hypercholesterolemic, the levels in 39 fell below 260 mg/100 ml with treatment. Of the 84 men designated as obese, 38 had a sufficient decline in the ratio of observed weight to desirable

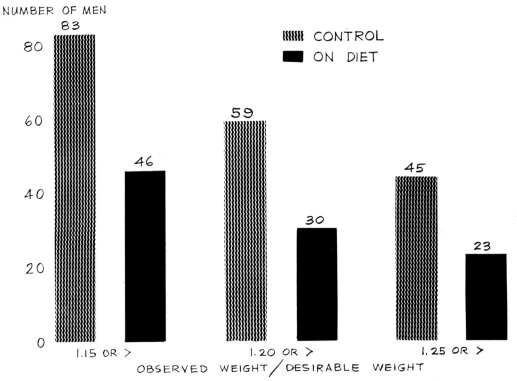

Figure 35–6. Effect of participation in the Coronary Prevention Evaluation Program on status with respect to frank overweight.

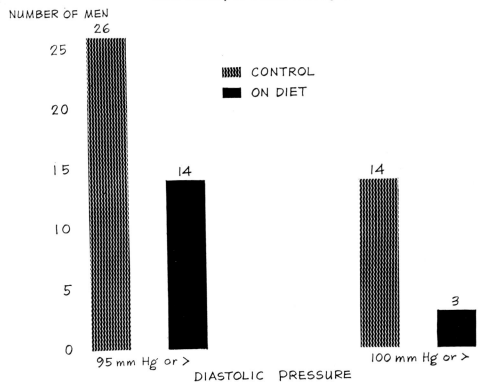

Figure 35–7. Effect of participation in the Coronary Prevention Evaluation Program on status with respect to frank hypertension.

TABLE 35–II

LONG TERM EFFECTS OF THE CORONARY
PREVENTION EVALUATION PROGRAM ON
WEIGHT AND SERUM CHOLESTEROL

54 Higher Risk Men Participating for over Four Years

Time on Diet	Weight Pounds	Serum Cholesterol mg/100 ml
Control	189.2 ±4.4*	274.9 ±7.3
One Year	175.0 ±3.8	231.0 ±4.9
Two years	173.8 ±3.9	234.9 ±5.0
Three years	174.9 ±3.7	237.5 ±5.9
Four years	176.8 ±3.8	246.4 ±6.2
Years 1–4	175.1 ±3.8	237.4 ±5.5

*Standard error of the mean.

weight so that it fell below 1.15. Of the 26 hypertensive men, 12 experienced a fall in diastolic blood pressure to levels below 95 mm Hg. These changes were effected within the first 12 weeks, and persisted thereafter with continued adherence to the recommended nutritional pattern (4).

The range of percentage decreases in serum cholesterol was wide. Among the 99 men, the levels in 61 fell 10 per cent or more; in 43, 15 per cent or more; in 27, 20 per cent or more; in 13, 25 per cent or more. In part, this variability of response may be attributed to the differing control serum cholesterol levels, since percentage decline was a function of control concentration (4). The levels in those with control values of 300 mg/100 ml or greater declined the most, 22.9 per cent on the average (a mean absolute fall of 77.8 mg/100 ml).

However, the initial level is not the sole factor involved. Thus, in the 26 men with control serum cholesterol of 300 mg/100 ml or greater, response to recommended diet also varied considerably. While the mean fall for this group was 22.9 per cent, serum cholesterol declined less than 10 per cent in three men,

10 to 19.9 per cent in nine men, 20 to 29.9 per cent in nine men, and 30 per cent or more in 5 men. Two men experienced falls of 47.1 per cent and 47.9 per cent, respectively. Of the three men showing no significant decline, nutritional data revealed poor adherence to recommended diet in one. The other two poor responders had dietary data indicative of better adherence.

In addition to the foregoing analyses, our group recently reviewed data on 54 men in the Coronary Prevention Evaluation Program for over 3 years, on active status throughout (i.e., all nondrop-outs) (Table 35–II). The data unequivocally confirm that with long-term nutritional change, reduction in both serum cholesterol and body weight persists throughout. The slight tendency to "rebound" undoubtedly reflects "back-sliding" in terms of adherence to the diet. For the total 4-year time period, the mean serum cholesterol fall of these 54 men was 13.6 per cent (from 274.9 mg/100 ml before diet recommendation to a mean value of 237.4 overall). The per cent decreases for years 1, 2, 3 and 4 were 15.9, 14.5, 13.6 and 10.4, respectively.

Serum triglyceride levels also declined in hypertriglyceridemic participants.

Changes in Smoking and Exercise Patterns. Of 94 cigarette smokers in the Chicago study long term, 15 have stopped smoking entirely, 12 have switched to pipe or cigars in moderation (i.e., 28.7 per cent have abandoned the cigarette smoking habit). Of the 15 men who quit smoking altogether, 5 did so during the first 6 months in the program, 4 during the next 6 months, 2 during the second year, 2 during the third year, and 2 thereafter.

Valid assessment of change in exercise

habit is difficult in a free-living population unless a supervised exercise program is developed. From the information obtained by interview at each visit, it is our impression that a significant per cent of men in the Coronary Prevention Evaluation Program have made a transition from sedentary habits to light regular exercise, principally in the form of walking and household chores. This aspect of the approach to prevention needs further intensive research effort, particularly on the methodology, feasibility and utility of supervised exercise programs. †

Effects on CHD Incidence. The fundamental end-point in all investigations of this type is information with respect to long-term incidence of clinical coronary heart disease. For purposes of comparison, the Coronary Prevention Evaluation Program has access to data on three other groups of higher-risk men age 40 to 59, being followed in long-term prospective epidemiologic studies involving no systematic intervention (32-34). At the present juncture both the size of the experimental group and the duration of the follow-up period are too small to warrant any definitive statement on incidence of clinical coronary disease.

Based on available data from prospective epidemiologic studies, it is possible to estimate hypothetically what might be accomplished by changes in serum cholesterol, weight, blood pressure, cigarette smoking and exercise status. For example, leaving aside any possible concomitant effects of altered nutritional patterns on other risk factors (e.g., obesity and hypertension), a 15 to 20 per cent reduction in mean serum cholesterol levels alone might be associated with a 25 to 50 per cent reduction in coronary

disease incidence rates in middle-aged men (35).

The hypothetical effects of simultaneous correction of hypercholesterolemia and two or more other risk factors (hypertension, obesity, cigarette smoking, physical inactivity) can also be estimated, and reductions in CHD incidence considerably greater than 20 to 50 per cent might be anticipated.

Lest there be any tendency to minimize the significance of these figures, a few additional statistics are worth reiterating. In 1962, atherosclerotic coronary heart disease caused the death of 528,000 Americans (1, 36). Of these, 151,000 occurred in persons less than 65 years of age. A reduction in CHD mortality of as little as 10 per cent would save the lives of 15,000 persons in their prime of middle life. A 25 per cent reduction would save the lives of 38,000 middle-aged persons. A 50 per cent reduction in CHD mortality would save the lives of 76,000 middle-aged persons.

Of course, the validity of these estimates remains to be ascertained. Nevertheless, the likelihood that these projections are meaningful, and not mere wild speculations, is underscored by data on special population groups in the United States with exceptional eating and smoking habits, lower serum cholesterol levels and lower CHD incidence rates (e.g., Seventh Day Adventists) (37). In addition, the New York Anti-Coronary Club recently presented data indicating a sizeably lower mortality incidence in the active participants in that study (8).

Hopefully data on incidence will be forthcoming from other long-term studies currently in progress in this country and abroad, and appropriate national cooperative mass field trials will be under-

_____
† See Chapters 15, 16, 29, 30, 31, 36-51 of this book.

taken, based on the experiences and find-ings of several studies, including the National Diet-Heart Study. Such studies are sorely needed, it should be empha-sized, not only with regard to the effects of dietary change, but also of cessation of cigarette smoking and of sedentary living habits. Only limited attention and energy have this far been devoted to developing mass field trials in these latter two areas. Serious efforts are in order to rectify this situation as soon as possible, especially since the practical problems of mass field trials are complex, and the time requirements lengthy.

Based on the experiences and findings to date, every reason exists to encourage wider efforts to realize the possibilities inherent in the new approaches to the primary prevention of premature athero-sclerotic disease of the coronary arteries and associated ischemic heart disease.

SUMMARY

The Coronary Prevention Evaluation Program is a long-term research study on the ability to correct and control coronary risk factors (hypercholesterol-emia, overweight, hypertension, cigarette smoking, physical inactivity) and thereby to prevent first heart attacks in higher-risk men of age 40 to 59.

The main forms of management are nutritional and hygienic. Experience since 1958 in over 200 men demonstrates that the preventive program is feasible, i.e., that long-term cooperation can be obtained from a majority of such men, with resultant significant improvements in risk factor status. Longer follow-up of larger numbers of men is necessary to assess effects of the program on incidence and mortality from atherosclerotic heart disease.

REFERENCES

1. STAMLER, J.: *Lectures on Preventive Cardiology*. New York, Grune and Stratton, in press.
2. KATZ, L. N., STAMLER, J., and PICK, R.: *Nutrition and Atherosclerosis*. Philadelphia, Lea and Febiger, 1958.
3. STAMLER, J.: Current status of the dietary pre-vention and treatment of atherosclerotic coronary heart disease. *Progr Cardiov Dis, 3:*56, 1960.
4. STAMLER, J., BERKSON, D. M., YOUNG, Q. D., LINDBERG, H. A., HALL, Y., MOJONNIER, L., and ANDELMAN, S. L.: Diet and serum lipids in atherosclerotic coronary heart disease—etiologic and preventive considerations. In: Rickets, H., Ed., *Medical Clinics of North America*. Philadelphia, W. B. Saunders, January, 1963, p. 3.
5. KEYS, A.: The role of the diet in human athero-sclerosis and its complications. In: Sandler, M., and Bourne, G. H., Eds., *Atherosclerosis and Its Origin*. New York, Academic Press, 1963, p. 263.
6. JOLLIFFE, N., RINZLER, S. H., and ARCHER, M.: Prudent reducing diet: effect on serum choles-terol. *Arch Intern Med, 109:*566, 1962.
7. JOLLIFFE, N., BAUMGARTNER, L., RINZLER, S. H., ARCHER, M., STEPHENSON, J. H., and CHRIS-TAKIS, G. H.: The Anti-Coronary Club: the first four years. *New York J Med, 63:*69, 1963.
8. CHRISTAKIS, G. H., RINZLER, S. H., ARCHER, M., WINSLOW, G., JAMPEL, S., STEPHENSON, J., FRIEDMAN, G., FEIN, H., KRAUS, A., and JAMES, G.: The Anti-Coronary Club: a dietary approach to the prevention of coronary heart disease. A seven year report, presented to the Annual Meeting of the Amer. Public Health Assn., Oct., 1964.
9. DAYTON, S., PEARCE, M. L., HASHIMOTO, B. S., FAKLER, L. J., HISCOCK, E., and DIXON, W. J.: A controlled clinical trial of a diet high in un-saturated fat—preliminary observations. *New Eng J Med, 266:*1017, 1962.
10. BROWN, H. B., and PAGE, I. H.: Lowering blood lipid levels by changing food patterns. *JAMA, 168:*1989, 1958.
11. GREEN, J. G., BROWN, H. B., MEREDITH, A. P., and PAGE, I.: Use of fat-modified foods for serum cholesterol reduction. *JAMA, 183:*5, 1963.
12. BIERENBAUM, M. L., GHERMAN, C., and EAST-WOOD, G.: Fat-modified frozen food dietary pat-tern: effect on blood cholesterol levels of young men with proved myocardial infarction. *JAMA, 182:*296, 1962.
13. PILKINGTON, T. R. E., STAFFORD, J. L., HANKIN, V. S., SIMMONDS, F. M., and KOERSELMAN, H. B.: Practical diets for lowering serum lipids—a long-term study on out-patients with ischemic heart disease. *Brit Med J, 1:*23, 1960.
14. OLLENDORF, P., GEILL, P., ASTRUP, T., and LUND, E.: The influence of diets containing cer-

tain animal and vegetable fats on the initiation of blood coagulation. *Acta Med Scand, 170:*351, 1961.

15. HANSEN, P. F., GEILL, T., and LUND, E.: Dietary fats and thrombosis. *Lancet,* 2:1193, 1962.

16. TURPEINEN, O., ROINE, P., PEKKARINEN, M., KARVONEN, M. J., RAUTANEN, Y., RUNEBERG, J., and ALIVIRTA, P.: Effect on serum-cholesterol level of replacement of dietary milk fat by soybean oil. *Lancet,* 1:196, 1960.

17. BUZINA, R., KARVONEN, M. J., ROINE, P., and TURPEINEN, O.: Effect of changes in dietary fat on whole-blood coagulation-time in man. *Lancet,* 2:287, 1961.

18. ROSE, G. A., THOMSON, W. B., and WILLIAMS, R. T.: Corn oil in treatment of ischemic heart disease. *Brit Med J,* 1:1531, 1965.

19. WATSON, W. C.: Long-term administration of corn oil in management of patients after myocardial infarction. A four-year study. *Brit Med J,* 2:1366, 1963.

20. TOOR, M.: Personal communication.

21. BAKER, B. M., FRANTZ, I. D., JR., KEYS, A., KINSELL, L. W., PAGE, I. H., STAMLER, J., and STARE, F. J.: The National Diet-Heart Study: An initial report. *JAMA, 185:*105, 1963.

22. American Heart Association: Dietary fat and its relation to heart attacks and strokes. *Circulation, 33:*133, 1961.

23. American Heart Association: *Diet and Heart Disease.* New York, American Heart Association, 1965.

24. BLAKESLEE, A., and STAMLER, J.: *Your Heart Has Nine Lives—Nine Steps to Heart Health.* New Jersey, Prentice-Hall, 1963.

25. JOLLIFFE, N.: *Reduce and Stay Reduced on the Prudent Diet.* New York, Simon and Schuster, 1963.

26. KEYS, A., and KEYS, M.: *Eat Well and Stay Well.* New York, Doubleday, 1963.

27. ROSENTHAL, S.: *Live High on Low Fat.* Philadelphia, J. B. Lippincott, 1962.

28. WALDO, M.: *Cooking For Your Heart and Health.* New York, Pocket Books, 1962.

29. ZUGIBE, F. T.: *Eat, Drink and Lower Your Cholesterol.* New York, McGraw-Hill, 1964.

30. BELINKIE, H.: *The Low-Fat Cookbook for Gourmets.* New York, David McKay, 1964.

31. BERKSON, D. M., and STAMLER, J.: The therapy of hypertension. *Worldwide Abstr Gen Med, 8:*8, 1965.

32. STAMLER, J.: Atherosclerotic coronary heart disease—the major challenge to contemporary public health and preventive medicine. *Conn Med, 28:*9, 1964.

33. PAUL, O., LEPPER, M. H., PHELAN, W. H., DUPERTUIS, G. W., MACMILLAN, A., MCKEAN, H., and PARK, H.: A longitudinal study of coronary heart disease. *Circulation, 28:*20, 1963.

34. TAYLOR, H., KLEPETAR, E., KEYS, A., PARLIN W., BLACKBURN, H., and PUCHNER, T.: Death rates among physically active and sedentary employees of the railroad industry. *Amer J Public Health,* 52:1697, 1962.

35. STAMLER, J.: The problem of elevated blood cholesterol. *Amer J Public Health, 50:* Part II, 14, 1960.

36. Cardiovascular Diseases in the United States—Facts and Figures. The American Heart Association, in Cooperation with the National Heart Institute and the Heart Disease Control Program, Public Health Service, U.S. Dept. of Health, Education and Welfare, New York, 1965.

37. WALDEN, R. T., SCHAEFER, L. E., LEMON, F. R., SUNSHINE, A., and WYNDER, E. L.: Effect of environment on the serum cholesterol-triglyceride distribution among Seventh-Day Adventists. *Amer J Med, 36:*269, 1964.

Chapter XXXVI

PREVENTIVE ASPECTS OF PHYSICAL FITNESS*

HANS KRAUS

(New York, New York, U.S.A.)

WHEN physical fitness is discussed, the question arises, "Fit for what?" It is evident that people who do heavy labor and people who have a sedentary occupation require different levels of fitness. However, they all have one need in common: the need for the minimum fitness compatible with healthful living. It is this minimum physical fitness which becomes the concern of the physician, and which is the topic of this presentation.

As long as man had to use his muscles to provide for his daily needs and as long as he lived in primitive surroundings, this minimum fitness was automatically guaranteed by his way of life. This condition has changed, and in our mechanized, over-stimulated and sedentary society, life does not provide enough exercise to keep muscles strong and flexible and keep the cardiovascular system sufficiently exercised to maintain that minimum physical fitness.

STRESS AND UNDEREXERCISE

While the lack of physical activity weakens the heart and muscles by disuse, the overstimulation which is inherent in urbanized living keeps man in almost constant alert reaction to which there is

hardly ever a direct or even vicarious outlet. This imbalance in our lives, namely excessive stimulation, which per se can be the cause of emotional disturbance, combined with underexercise, which in itself produces disuse states, is built into our mechanized society. Therefore, we all live in a potentially pathogenic environment.

Besides causing disturbance in itself, underexercise and overstimulation are combined in a constant suppression of "fight and flight" response (1, 2). This constant suppression of an otherwise normal reaction is an additional source of stress (3) and, therefore, in the long run, of disease (Fig. 36–1) (4).

To add insult to injury, this source of stress is compounded by conditioned responses which make mere signals of irritation stressful (5).

We all experience the irritations of the telephone. Those who have many irritating calls have frequently felt like throwing the telephone at someone or running away from it. Neither is done, and we have to accept this daily repeated occurrence of a stressful interruption of our defense response. After some time, the mere ringing of the telephone becomes an alert reaction as irritating as the actual call.

What are the effects of this pathogenic

---

*This article is reprinted with permission of the New York State Journal of Medicine where it had been published in Volume 64, No. 10, May 15, 1964.

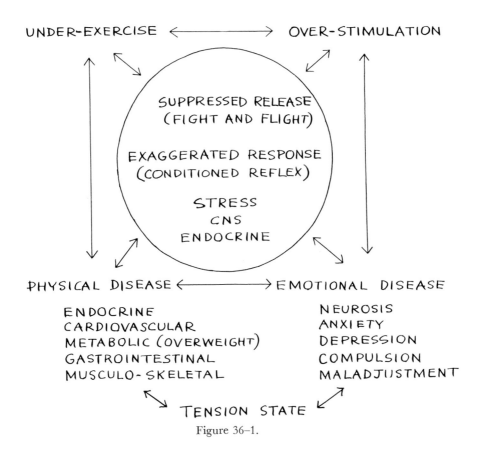

MECHANIZED, URBANIZED, UNBALANCED INDIVIDUAL :

OVER-RESTED, OVERFED, OVER-STIMULATED, OVER-PROTECTED, UNDER-EXERCISED, UNDER-RELEASED, UNDER-DISCIPLINED

UNDER-EXERCISE ⟵⟶ OVER-STIMULATION

SUPPRESSED RELEASE (FIGHT AND FLIGHT)

EXAGGERATED RESPONSE (CONDITIONED REFLEX)

STRESS
CNS
ENDOCRINE

PHYSICAL DISEASE ⟵⟶ EMOTIONAL DISEASE

ENDOCRINE
CARDIOVASCULAR
METABOLIC (OVERWEIGHT)
GASTROINTESTINAL
MUSCULO-SKELETAL

NEUROSIS
ANXIETY
DEPRESSION
COMPULSION
MALADJUSTMENT

TENSION STATE

Figure 36–1.

milieu? Muscle tension together with weakness of essential posture muscles combine to produce the ubiquitous back pain (6), the "tension neck," the "tension headaches," and other pain in almost any part of the musculoskeletal system (4, 7–10). Lack of exercise makes the limitation of caloric intake mandatory to avoid overweight (11–13). Lack of exercise combined with tensions is an important factor in producing degenerative heart disease (Fig. 36–2), duodenal ulcer, and diabetes (14–17). The emotional disturbance of the underexercised and over-

irritated person is well known (18). Much literature has been accumulated in the paet 2 decades illustrating the role of unsderexercise and stress in production of disease. Prevention of chronic degenerative disease, be it musculoskeletal or cardiovascular, overweight, nervousness, or tension syndrome, has been discussed in many speciality meetings, ranging from orthopedic and cardiovascular to occupational and physical medicine.

PREVENTIVE MEASURES
Only recently, Selye in his book, Pluri-

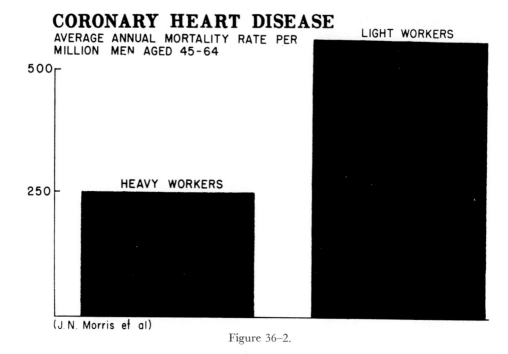

CORONARY HEART DISEASE

AVERAGE ANNUAL MORTALITY RATE PER MILLION MEN AGED 45-64

LIGHT WORKERS

500

HEAVY WORKERS

250

(J. N. Morris et al)

Figure 36-2.

causal Cardiopathies (19), has demonstrated that exposure to cold and exercise are the best and most easily accessible means of preventing stress disease. We now have scientific evidence, based on many years of research and animal experimentation, that the idea of "toughening up" and of exercising regularly may be old but is still valid. Preventive medicine has yet to be practiced on a national basis from that point of view, and while we have nearly perfected our prevention of contagious diseases, we still have not started in the prevention of "hypokinetic disease" (4) (underexercise disease) or "imbalance disease." Other countries have gone a long way in the last decades to establish preventive institutions where "pre-sick" people (20), that is, people who are underexercised and overstressed, can spend sufficient time (4 to 6 weeks minimum) to rest and get reconditioned by exercise and an appropriate diet (Fig. 36-3 †) (21). These same countries have strict physical training programs in their schools and have developed excellent facilities for physical training at every age level.

Where do we stand in this immensely important preventive job? What have we done? A Council for Youth Fitness was established under President Eisenhower, and President Kennedy reinforced this council and changed its scope from youth fitness to physical fitness, to include all age groups. His administration attempted to support the idea of regular physical exercise for all age groups, and on a compulsory basis for children and adolescents. Unfortunately, the actual effect of these councils has not gone beyond sparking a few pilot programs and beyond public relations efforts. The ac-

†W. Raab, Queen City Printers, Burlington, Vermont, 1962

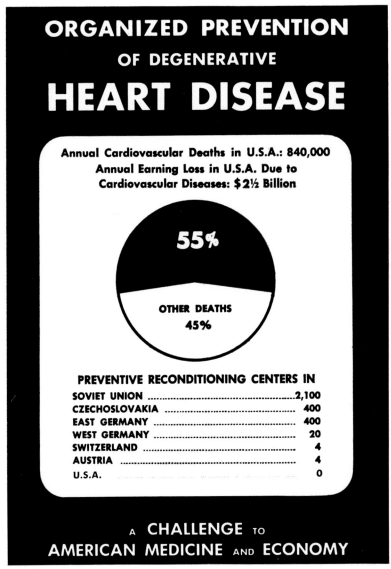

Figure 36-3.

tual need is to establish an intense program of daily basic exercise and basic physical activities (not games) for all school children and to provide opportunities for adult physical workouts.

For overstressed and underexercised persons there should be institutions, such as are found abroad, where they can really receive systematic reconditioning under expert guidance. Much suffering, much working time, and much money can be saved by prevention. Our specialty of physical medicine and rehabilitation should be familiar with the elements of exercise and reconditioning. We are the specialty best equipped to organize and conduct this essential part of disease prevention.

SUMMARY

Mechanized society deprives man of movement. He cannot react to stimuli but is forced to suppress the defense responses which are elicited by irritations. He lives in chronic imbalance. Underexercise and overstimulation produce stress disease, tension syndrome, overweight, orthopedic disability (painful backs, necks, and so forth), cardiovascular disease and endocrine and emotional imbalance.

Exercise from cradle to grave, designed to substitute for previously normal everyday activity and serving as a vicarious outlet for tensions, is the simplest preventive measure.

Specialists in physical medicine and rehabilitation should take the lead in establishing such preventive programs as exist abroad.

REFERENCES

1. CANNON, W. B.: The mechanism of emotional disturbance of bodily functions. *New Eng J Med, 198:877, 1928.*
2. CANNON, W. B.: *Bodily Changes in Pain, Hunger, Fear and Rage.* 2nd Ed. New York, Appleton Co., 1929.
3. SELYE, H.: *The Physiology and Pathology of Exposure to Stress.* Montreal, Acta, Inc., 1950.
4. KRAUS, H., and RAAB, W.: *Hypokinetic Disease—Diseases Produced by Lack of Exercise.* Springfield, Thomas, 1961.
5. PAVLOV, I. P.: *Conditioned Reflexes: An Investigation of the Physiological Activity of the Cerebral Cortex.* London, Oxford University Press, 1927.
6. KRAUS, H.: Diagnosis and treatment of low back pain. *GP, 5:55, 1952.*
7. KRAUS, H., and HIRSCHLAND, R. P.: Muscular fitness and orthopedic disability. *New York S J Med, 54:212, 1954.*
8. STIMSON, B. B.: The low back problem. *Psychosom. Med, 9:210, 1947.*
9. THOMPSON, W. A.: Keeping the patient with low back pain employable. *Industr Med, 22:318, 1952.*
10. SAINSBURY, P., and GIBSON, J. G.: Symptoms of anxiety and tension and the accompanying physiological changes in the muscular system. *J Neurol Neurosurg Psychiat, 17:216, 1954.*
11. MAYER, J.: Genetic, traumatic and environmental factors in the etiology of obesity. *Physiol Rev, 33:472, 1953.*
12. MAYER, J.: Mechanism of regulation of food intake and multiple aetiology of obesity. *Voeding, 16:62, 1955.*
13. MAYER, J., ROY, P., and MITRA, K. P.: Relation between caloric intake, body weight, and physical work: studies in an industrial male population in West Bengal. *Amer J Clin Nutrition, 4:169, 1956.*
14. MORRIS, J. N.: A social-medical reconnaissance of coronary disease. From: *Needed Research in Health and Medical Care—A Bio-social Approach,* Chapel Hill, University of North Carolina Press. 1954.
15. MORRIS, J. N., and BARLEY, R. G.: Coronary heart disease in medical practitioners. *Brit Med J, 1:503, 1952.*
16. MORRIS, J. N., and HEADY, J. A.: Mortality in relation to the physical activity of work: a preliminary note on experience in middle age. *Brit J Industr Med, 10:245, 1953.*
17. MORRIS, J. N., and RAFFLE, P. A.: Coronary heart disease in transport workers; a progress report. *Brit J Industr Med, 11:260, 1954.*
18. APPLETON, L.: Study on fitness or performance of West Point cadets, in press.
19. SELYE, H.: *Pluricausal Cardiopathies.* Springfield, Thomas, 1961.
20. RAAB, W.: Metabolic protection and reconditioning of the heart muscle through habitual physical exercise. *Ann Intern Med, 53:87, 1960.*
21. RAAB, W.: Prevention of degenerative heart disease by neurovegetative reconditioning. *Public Health Rep, 78:317, 1963.*

Chapter XXXVII

THE EFFECT OF TRAINING ON HEART AND CIRCULATION AND ITS IMPORTANCE IN PREVENTIVE CARDIOLOGY

HARALD MELLEROWICZ

(Berlin, Germany)

THE biological principle of Roux (1), that all organs are maintained and developed by function also applies to the heart of man. Lack of function and movement leads to atrophy and disease, especially hypokinetic disease.

So far all progress made in modern medicine has not been able to prevent a steady increase in heart and circulation diseases. In our days we expect everything from the remedies made available to us in excessive numbers, but training surpasses by its efficiency-increasing effect on heart and circulation the effect of all other drugs. A certain amount of training is the best way to keep heart and circulation efficient and healthy.

As a result of training, the muscle fibers of the heart and the whole heart grow with retention of their natural proportions (2). Such large hearts reach a considerable weight (up to 500 g) and large volume (up to 1400 cc). This physiological increase in the size of the heart makes possible an economical O_2-saving volume output of the heart, and an augmentation of the cardial and general physical power reserves. On the other hand, the small "civilization heart" is continually forced to carry out an uneconomical frequency work with a large O_2-consumption. Accordingly, the coronary reserves are more or less reduced and coronary insufficiency is more likely to occur.

The coronary arteries are also extended roughly in proportion to the growth of the muscular system of the heart. An extension of the ventricles of the heart and auricles causes a lengthening of the whole cardiac capillary network and an increase in its total internal area. According to the investigations of Petrén, Sjöstrand and Sylvén (3), the capillarization of the trained heart muscle is increased.

The investigations of Eckstein (4) show that the new growth of collaterals after blocking a coronary artery in untrained dogs was considerably smaller than in trained dogs. Accordingly, signs of coronary hypoxia and heart infarction do not occur in persons with trained hearts, except for very rare instances. By contrast, persons with small "office hearts" suffer often from coronary insufficiency and angina pectoris. Just as these persons become short of breath even after small physiological efforts, in a similar way their hearts are also inclined to "shortness of oxygen."

Through physical training, the num-

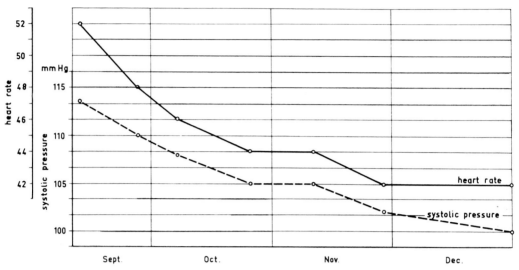

Figure 37–1. Reduction of heart rate and systolic pressure by one training period of 4 months
in one typical case (16).

ber of heart beats per minute at rest and
during performance can be decreased to
approximately 50 per cent of the initial
rate (Fig. 37–1). It is not uncommon for
highly-trained persons to have 30 to 40
heart beats per minute. With bradycardia, the O_2-consumption of the heart
muscle is more economical while the
same work of the heart, with a higher
pulse rate, requires a larger cardiac
O_2-consumption, and the coronary O_2-
reserve is reduced. This applies especially
to the small "civilization hearts." They
have to work with a higher frequency to
expel the same volume per minute with
a relatively small stroke volume per beat.

Training, by reducing the cardiac
sympathetic tone, leads to a considerable
lengthening of the isometric period and
of the ejection period (5, 6). This alteration in cardiac work results in a saving
of energy and O_2 according to Burger
(7), Wezler and Böger (8), and Frick
et al. (27). A slow pace of the systole
also increases the degree of effectiveness

of the contraction phase according to
Bohnenkamp (9). Reduction of training
on the other hand, brings about a reduction of cardiac efficiency and an increase
in the cardiac O_2-consumption.

The lengthening of the diastole by
training is of great importance for the
nutritive condition of the myocardium,
in particular of the aging myocardium.
The longer the diastole, the longer is the
time available for optimal O_2 supply of
the heart muscle. A progressive shortening of the diastole due to lack of training
automatically leads to a deterioration of
the prerequisites for optimal O_2 supply
to the myocardium.

The minute volume (cardiac output)
at rest and with the same effort is very
much smaller in trained persons than in
untrained ones. Our investigations and
those by other authors using different
methods have all shown that minute-
volumes of 3 liters are by no means rare
in highly-trained persons. By comparison,
the circulation of untrained persons works

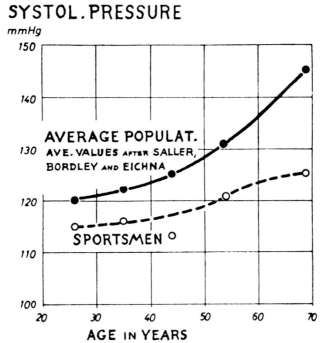

Figure 37–2. Systolic blood pressure in an average population as compared with that of 107 well-trained sportsmen (5). (Courtesy of Dr. D. Steinkopff, Darmstadt, 1956.)

uneconomically with relatively high volumes per minute and a lowered coronary reserve. The small volume per minute of the trained circulation with a low O_2 consumption by the heart is associated with a richer capillarization in the periphery and with an increased arteriovenous difference. Lack of training can cause a deficiency in capillarization in the periphery with a relatively low arteriovenous difference, a large volume per minute, and an increased wear and tear on the circulation.

Training over long periods often leads to a lowering of the systolic pressure (Fig. 37–1) and, with a concomitant slight rise of the diastolic pressure, to a reduction of the arterial mean pressure. This can be observed during every training period. With reduced pressure work of the heart, the cardiac O_2-consumption

also diminishes and the coronary reserve is increased. The rise in the systolic pressure with age is much slower in persons who engage in sports regularly and sufficiently, as our comparative investigations have shown (Fig. 37–2).

Due to the lower cardiac pressure and volume work in the trained person, the work of the heart is greatly reduced, even after only one hour's training per day (Fig. 37–3). With a heart work of 10,000 to 15,000 mg (at rest), the cardiac O^2 consumption per minute is approximately 25 to 40 cc in office workers. On the other hand, hearts of trained persons need only 15 to 25 cc O_2 per minute for a considerably lower daily heart work (at rest), amounting to 5,000 to 10,000 mg.

According to the investigations of Raab (10), the increased liberation of adrenalin

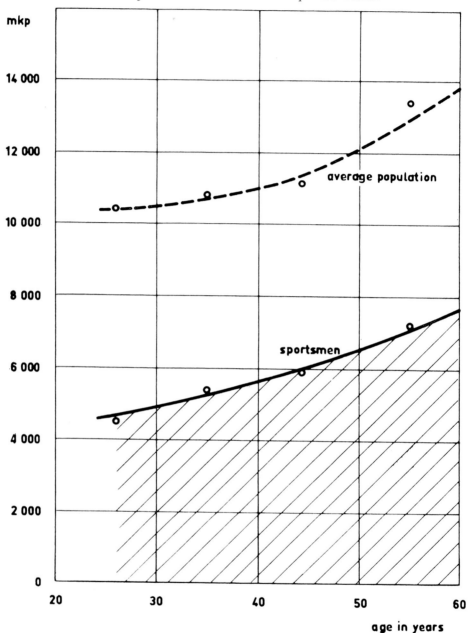

Figure 37–3. Daily cardiac work of 20 to 70-year-old trained persons is only 5000 to 10,000 mkp. at rest, while in untrained people it reaches 10,000 to 15,000 m/kg (5).

and noradrenalin in sympathicotonic untrained persons can endanger the O_2 economy of the myocardium and elicit a hypoxia-producing discrepancy between vascular O_2 supply and myocardial O_2 consumption, especially in the presence of coronary atherosclerosis, whereas the cardiac sympathetic tone is reduced and the vagal tone augmented by training.

In a thorough statistical study on a

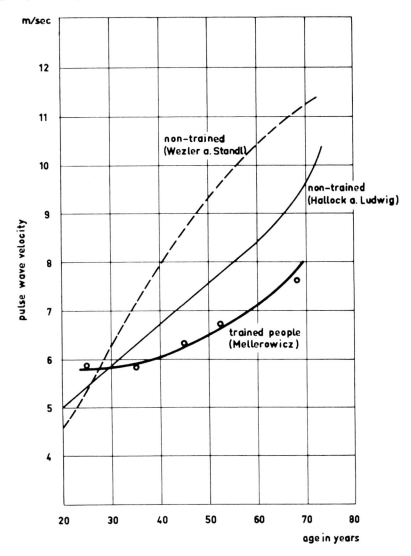

Figure 37–4. Rise of pulse wave velocity with age is much lower in 107 trained people (17) in comparison with untrained persons (18-20).

large group of persons, Morris demonstrated an inverse proportionality between the amount of occupational physical work and the mortality from coronary disease. Occupations associated with heavy bodily work had the lowest coronary mortality. The incidence of death due to coronary disease was 3 to 4 times higher in sedentary workers. Similar observations have been made by Luongo (4), and many others. It is not training and hard physical work which leads to coronary insufficiency, but the lack of it.

Sedentary living causes a reduction of maximal O_2 intake and performance ability of the whole organism, together with a lowering of the coronary reserve and increased danger of myocardial hypoxia. Owing to lack of movement, physical work and exercise in our mechanized civilization, coronary insufficiency has become one of the most common diseases of our age, while persons who regularly engage in physical exercise very rarely suffer from it, according to the experience of the Sportärzliche Hauptberatungsstelle Berlin over a period of 12 years.

Various investigations have shown that prolonged hard physical training reduces the lipid level of the blood. The serum cholesterol level was found significantly lower in Finnish long-distance ski runners compared with the rest of the Finnish population (12).

Keys (13) and others observed that the rise of the serum cholesterol level after rich meals can be reduced by physical exercise.

A lowering of the lipid level through physical work and exercise is believed by some investigators to have an inhibitive effect against atherosclerotic changes. This seems to be supported by observations of Myasnikov (14) and others, who found the development of experimental atherosclerosis less marked in trained animals than in untrained controls.

As our own comparative studies have shown (Fig. 37–4), the age increase of the pulse wave velocity occurs in trained persons to a lesser degree than in untrained ones, suggesting a longer preservation of vascular elasticity.

Everyone should exercise for the benefit of his circulation at least 3 minutes daily, with heart rates reaching 30 to 60 beats above the resting level (15).

SUMMARY

Physical training of the endurance type reduces heart rate and systolic pressure. It promotes a more economical frequency, volume and pressure work of the heart, and thereby a considerable reduction in the daily energy expenditure of the heart muscle.

Training improves the economy effect of dynamic and metabolic regulatory mechanisms in the cardiovascular system.

Prolonged training lowers the lipid level of the blood and may possibly play an important part in the prevention of atherosclerotic vascular lesions.

Animal experiments have shown that training favors the formation of collaterals and capillaries in the coronary vascular system. Persons with trained hearts rarely suffer from myocardial infarction.

By physical training, the oxygen consumption of the heart muscle is reduced and the coronary reserve increased due to diminution of oxygen-wasting sympathetic overactivity and to augmentation of the parasympathetic tone and sympathoinhibitory counter-regulation. Lack of training produces the opposite effect with its potentially pathogenic consequences.

Even though training can be considered as only one among several preventive factors, it is a very important one.

REFERENCES

1. Roux, W.: Gesammelte Abhandlungen über Entwicklungs-mechanik der Organismen. Bd. I, *Funktionelle Anpassung*, Leipzig, 1895.
2. Linzbach, A. J.: (a) Das ökonomische Prinzip in der Sauerstoffversorgung der Nieren, des Herzens und des Stützgewebes. *Z Ges Inn Med*, 2:144, 1947. (b) Die Muskelfaserkonstante und das Wachstumsgesetz der menschlichen Herzkammern. *Virchow Arch Path Anat*, 318:575, 1950.
3. Petrén, T., Sylvén, B., and Sjöstrand, T.: (3) Der Einfluss des Trainings auf die Häufigkeit der Kapillaren in Herz- und Skeletmuskulatur. *Arb Physiol*, 9:376, 1936.
4. Eckstein, R. W.: Effect of exercise and coronary artrey narrowing on coronary collateral circulation. *Circ Res*, 5:230, 1957.

5. MELLEROWICZ, H.: Vergleichende Untersuchungen über das Oekonomieprinzip in Arbei- und Leistung des trainierten Kreislaufs und seine Bedeutung für die pärventive und rehabilitative Medizin. *Arch Kreislaufforsch, 24:*70, 1956.

6. EMMRICH, J., KLEPZIG, H., and REINDELL, H.: Zur Frage der klinischen Bedeutung einer Unterteilung der Anspannungszeit des linken Ventrikels in Umformungszeit und Druckanstiegszeit. *Arch Kreislaufforsch, 24:*177, 1956.

7. BÜRGER, M.: *Altern und Krankheit.* Leipzig, Thieme, 1957.

8. WEZLER, K., and BÖGER A.: Abhängigkeit der Arterienelastizität von Alter und Zustand der Wandmuskulatur. *Z Kreislaufforsch, 27:*721, 1935.

9. BOHNENKAMP, H.: Der Stoffwechsel des Herzens und seine Leistungsgrenzen. *Verh Deutsch Ges Verdauungskr,* Leipzig, 1937.

10. RAAB, W.: *Adrenergic—cholinergic control of cardiac metabolism and function.* In: Advances in Cardiology, Karger, S., New York, Basel, 1956.

11. LUONGO, E. P.: Health habits and heart disease. Challenge in preventive medicine. *JAMA, 162:*1021, 1956.

12. KARVONEN, M. J., *et al.*: Herzgrösse bei Skimeistern. *Ann Med Intern Fenn, 46:*169, 1957.

13. KEYS, A., LARSON, PH., and MANN, G. V.: Exercise in the disposition of dietary calories. Regulation of serum lipoprotein and cholesterol levels in human subjects. *New Eng J Med, 253:*349, 1955.

14. MYASNIKOV, A. E., (quoted by Reindell, H.): Sport- und Schreibtischherz. *Die Aerztl Fortbildg, 9:*168, 1959.

15. MAIDORN, K., and MELLEROWICZ, H.: Vergleichende Untersuchungen über Leistungssteigerung durch Intervalltraining bei unterschiedlicher Intervallzahl. *Int Z Angew Physiol, 19:*27, 1961.

16. PROKOP, L.: Die Wirkung des sportlichen Trainings auf den menschlichen Organismus. Habilitation Thesis, Univ. of Vienna, 1952.

17. MELLEROWICZ, H.: *Präventive Cardiologie.* Berlin, Medicus-Verlag, 1961.

18. WEZLER, K., and STANDL, R.: Die normalen Alterskurven der Pulswellengeschwindigkeit in elastischen und muskulären Arterien des Menschen. *Z Biol, 97:*265, 1936.

19. HALLOCK, PH.: Arterial elasticity in man in relation to age as evaluated by the pulse wave velocity method. *Arch Intern Med, 54:*770, 1934.

20. LUDWIG, H.: Die Pulswellengeschwindigkeit bei Gesunden und Kranken. *Schweiz. Med Wschr, 99:*352, 1936.

21. FRICK, M. H., KONTINEN, A., and SARAJAS, H. S. S.: Effects of physical training on circulation at rest and during exercise. *Amer J Cardiol, 12:*142, 1963.

Chapter XXXVIII

PREVENTIVE SIGNIFICANCE OF EXERCISE TRAINING IN ELDERLY ADULTS*

SERAFIM P. LETUNOV and RAKHIL' E. MOTYLYANSKAYA

(Moscow, U.S.S.R.)

WE CARRIED out investigations concerning the mechanism of the influence exerted by a regime of systematic physical exercise on the state of health and on the working capacity of adults in advanced age categories.

Health groups are organized by many sports installations in various cities of the Soviet Union. One of these is located in Moscow in the Central Stadium, named after V. I. Lenin. Exercise periods are arranged two to three times weekly, lasting 1½ hours and offering specific exercise programs, including gymnastics, elementary light athletics, swimming, lively games, skiing and skating.

We endeavored to evaluate the work capacity of the body and the range of its adaptability to muscular activity under conditions of physiological aging as well as in the presence of certain abnormalities connected with the pathology of old age.

Multiple parameters were recorded by means of electrocardiography, ballistocardiography, arterial oscillography, blood oximetry, gasometry, electroencephalography, including tele- and radiotelemetry during exercise, chemical determination of lipids, ketobodies and proteins in the blood and the assay of adrenal steroids in the urine.

In 82 per cent of older sportsmen we found that the usual age-induced bodily changes were present only to a relatively minor extent and those individuals were classified as "healthy." Eighteen per cent of this group displayed pathological alterations, especially of the circulatory system, such as manifest atherosclerosis of the aorta and coronary vessels and arterial hypertension.

By contrast, persons who had not started on a specifically organized regime of physical training before the age of 50 to 65 showed, in 30 per cent of the instances, certain age-induced abnormalities of the circulatory, respiratory and nervous systems. Clinical manifestations of myocardial ischemic were demonstrable in 45 per cent, hypertensive disease in 10 per cent and metabolic abnormalities (lipids, electrolytes) in 15 per cent of the cases. Thus, the incidence of clinical derangements was substantially lower among the sportsmen than in the untrained group.

In persons in whom physical exercise training was initiated at an advanced age, a distinct improvement of their general well-being and self-confidence was usually noticeable 3 to 6 months after the beginning of regular exercise. In 90 per cent of the cases an increase of

---

*Translated by W. Raab.

stamina and diminished fatigability was reported. This was accompanied by a regression or disappearance of angiospastic phenomena, headaches and precordial pain, which had only poorly responded to medication in 83 per cent, by improved sleep in 54 per cent and also by better digestion and bodily motility.

Under the *influence of physical training* the heart rate at rest was diminished, diastole and isometric period of the ventricular systole as well as the period of ventricular relaxation were prolonged, the maximal, minimal and mean blood pressure were more or less lowered, the pulse wave velocity in blood vessels of both the elastic and muscular type was diminished, and the peripheral resistance was decreased.

Comparative analysis of numerous *electrocardiograms* from sportsmen of different ages revealed certain differences between older and younger subjects. The former displayed a greater stability, sometimes even "rigidity" of the cardiac sinus rhythm, in some instances a lower amplitude of QRS and T in the standard and chest leads, in 12 to 16 per cent of the cases a tendency toward lengthening of the PQ interval and in 33 per cent of the QRS complex, however, remaining within normal limits. In 8 per cent there was a prolongation of the relative QT interval and in 50 per cent a horizontal or left deviation of the electrical axis of the heart. A horizontal or semihorizontal position of the heart itself was seen in the majority of instances.

The ratio of the amplitudes of R and T in the second chest lead of young sportsmen was on an average 1.53, and in the fifth chest lead 3.07. In older sportsmen the corresponding ratios were 1.09 and 2.11, respectively. In the electrocardiographic standard leads the angle between the vectors of QRS and T did, as a rule, not exceed 45°; thus it remained within the normal range of variations.

In persons who had not engaged in sports activities, abnormal electrocardiograms were quite frequently observed, such as arrhythmias, low voltage of QRS and T in standard and chest leads, prolonged PQ in the range of 0.20 to 0.22 seconds (in 24 per cent of the cases), widening of the P wave (in 35 per cent), augmentation of its amplitude and deformation of its shape (in 22 per cent). Discordant directions of the beginning and end of the ventricular complex, a wide angle between vectograms of QRS and T (60° and above) indicated a true left preponderance of the ECG. Trophic changes of the myocardium of atherosclerotic origin were suggested by other electrocardiographic signs, such as deformation of the QRS complex, conduction disturbances in chest and standard leads and prolongation of the intrinsic deflection in $V_5 - V_6$.

In a group of 159 subjects who started training at an advanced age, 2 to 5 years of physical activity were associated with the development of the following modifications of the electrocardiogram: slowing of the heart rate (in 59 per cent), shortening of the PQ interval in 7.2 per cent, of the QRS interval in 2 per cent, and of QT in 22 per cent; increase of the voltage of R in 36 per cent, and of T_1 and T^2 in 33 per cent; reduction of the angle between the QRS and T vectors in 30 per cent and elevation of the ST interval in 5 per cent of the cases.

The influence of muscular training on *myocardial contractility* and on the tonus of the larger vessels were expressed by ballistocardiographic observations. In older sportsmen changes of the ballistocardiogram of the third degree were found in 26 per cent and of the fourth degree in 8 per cent, whereas in persons of comparable age who had previously not been trained, such changes were seen in 32 per cent and 30 per cent, respectively. After periods of systematic training of this latter group, the ballistocardiographic trainings suggested a diminution of resistance on the part of the large vessels, and an improvement of myocardial contractility.

Indications of a definite influence of physical training upon the *fat and lipid levels* in the blood are of special interest. The cholesterol concentration in the blood of older sportsmen was found to be much lower than that of persons who had not started their training program at the same age. After 6 to 18 months of systematic physical activity, a marked and more or less stable lowering of the blood cholesterol level was observed in these latter subjects, accompanied by a tendency toward normalization of the ratio between serum proteins and lipids (diminution of β-globulins and β-lipoproteins, augmentation of albumins and α-proteins with a corresponding increase of the albumin-globulin coefficient). This was paralleled also by a normalization of the previously elevated level of neutral fats and reduction of ketobodies in the blood (1, 2, 3).

Indirect evidence concerning a positive effect of prolonged training on the age-induced alterations of *metabolism* was supplied by the relation between body length and weight. In old sportsmen the average values were 170 ± 1.2 cm and 74.3 ± 1.19 kg and in untrained persons 168 ± 1.8 cm and 78.8 ± 1.2 kg. The untrained group included a number of obese individuals. During the first year of training, the weight was reduced from 2 to 8 kg in 50 to 60 per cent of the subjects in this group.

The *vital capacity of the lungs* in older sportsmen was on an average 4600 ± 127 ml; in beginners of a sports regime it was 3650 ± 200 ml. However, in the older sportsmen this so-called vital sign could be assessed as being even significantly higher in consideration of their lower body weight. Within 1½ to 2 years of systematic training, the vital capacity of the lungs increased 200 to more than 1000 ml.

Measurement of the *oxygen saturation* of the blood in a large number of older subjects revealed variations between 87 and 96 per cent. Independently of age, the degree of oxygenation of the blood after 2 years of training proved higher than in those who were just beginning their program of regular exercise. The blood oxygenation in 20 of 37 subjects of this latter group increased an average 3 per cent within a few months of training (4).

An augmented resistance against hypoxia in old sportsmen was suggested by the following data: during breath holding tests the duration of apnea amounted to an average 143.3 ± 1.89 seconds, while the arterial oxygen saturation fell an average 15.5 ± 1.62 per cent. In physically inactive persons the apnea lasted 70.6 ± 3.8 seconds while the oxygen saturation fell 6.2 ± 0.83 per cent. The respective durations of "resistance" (section A-B of the oxyhemogram) were 55 ± 3.89 and 44.4 ± 2.4 seconds.

Older sportsmen displayed a remarkable capability of performing *strenuous physical feats*. For example, 5 and 10 km runs, skating races of 500 to 3000 m, and ski races of 5 to 10 km were carried out in excellent form and without signs of undue fatigue.

Even if physical training is started only in middle or advanced age, an increased adaptability of the organism can be achieved. After 2 to 3 years of training, we observed in 53 per cent of the trainees the following improved reactions to standard exercises (step test). A lesser cardiac acceleration, and improvements of the ballistocardiogram and electrocardiogram; a decreased elevation of the maximal, minimal and mean blood pressures, and a shortening of the blood pressure recovery period. However, in 30 per cent significant improvements of this latter kind were not noticed, and in 17 per cent a tendency toward higher rises of the blood pressure appeared.

Our observations seem to explain the fact that after 3 to 4 years of training the physical work capacity of older subjects is markedly increased. While at the outset of the training program most of the trainees could not continue the two-step test for more than 3 minutes, they were able after completion of 2 to 3 years of systematic training to do this for an average 26 minutes, in some instances even for one hour or more.

From all this the conclusion appears justified that a regime of active physical motion in middle and advanced age is of great value for the maintenance of health. Functional changes in the condition of vital organ systems of the body are being directed toward an improved economy of blood circulation, respiration, general metabolism, blood supply and contractility function of the myocardium; furthermore toward normalization of the peripheral blood flow and toward a distinct augmentation of the adaptability

of the organism. We interpret these phenomena in terms of the reflex theory by ascribing them to a perfection of unconditioned and development of manifold conditioned reflex processes, connecting the nervous centers which govern the functions of internal organs on the one hand with the muscular motor apparatus on the other. We attach an outstanding significance to the motor-visceral reflex mechanisms (especially to vasodilator proprioceptive impulses on the coronary arteries), originating in the widely distributed proprioceptive areas of the skeletal muscular system.

An important role is played by the *augmentation of the vagal tone* in the cardiovascular system such as evidenced by slowing of the cardiac rhythm and reduction of the blood pressure. These features suggest an economizing effect upon the function of the heart. Modern concepts of cardiology attribute to an excess of adrenergic substances a major role in the origin of degenerative diseases of the heart muscle. (5, 6, 7). On this basis we feel entitled to consider the augmentation of cholinergic and sympathoinhibitory mechanisms which results from physical training as an essential factor involved in the pathogenically-oriented approach to therapy.

A stimulating influence of muscular exercises upon the activity of the adrenal cortex was revealed by determinations of the basal urinary excretion level of 17-oxycorticosteroids. In older sportsmen it was found higher than in untrained persons. After 1 year of physical training the basal excretion was augmented and the response to administered ACTH was increased (8).

Among the measures intended for the prevention of premature aging and for the elimination of diseases of old age, the universal application of active physical exercise regimes appears as a primary obligation of modern medicine.

SUMMARY

Sports installations in many cities of the Soviet Union are organizing systematic exercise training programs for middle-aged and elderly people.

Comparative studies were carried out on older, perennially trained sportsmen (age 50 to 65) and on previously untrained persons of comparable age. The results revealed in the sportsmen a lower incidence of electrocardiographic and ballistocardiographic abnormalities, lower blood cholesterol and lipid levels, a greater pulmonary vital capacity and breath-holding ability, lower body weight, greater physical work capacity and a higher degree of adrenal cortical activity.

Within training periods of 2 to 5 years, the corresponding parameters of previously physically inactive subjects showed a progressive improvement and approach to the characteristics of older sportsmen.

These favorable changes are attributed to a shift in central nervous system-mediated motor-visceral reflexes, especially to an increase of cardiovascular cholinergic and sympathoinhibitory mechanisms, resulting from regular physical training. Universal prophylactic application of the latter appears as one of the foremost tasks of modern medicine.

REFERENCES

1. BABARIN, P. M., and MOTYLYANSKAYA, R. E.: Theory and practice of physical culture. ——, 23: 673, 1960.
2. BABARIN, P. M., and ROMANOVA, L. S.: Proceedings of the Summarizing Scientific Session of the Central Scientific Institute of Physical Culture and Research, Moscow, 1964, p. 178.
3. ROMANOVA, L. S., and BABARIN, P. M.: *Kardiologiia*, No. 6, 1961, p. 36.
4. BUKREYEVA, D. C., and TISHLER, V. A.: *Conference on Problems of Gerontology and Geriatrics.* Thesis of lectures, Kiev, 1961, p. 125.
5. RAAB, W.: Adrenergic-cholinergic regulation of metabolism and function of the heart. In: *Dostizheniya Kardiologii.* Moscow, Medgiz, 1959.
6. MYASNIKOV, A. L.: Pathogenesis of myocardial infarction. *Kardiologyia*, No. 4, 1963, p. 3.
7. SOFIYEVA, I. E.: Significance of the catecholamines for the pathogenesis of coronary insufficiency. *Ter Arkh, 34*:3, 1962.
8. EREZ, V. P.: *Ukr Biokhim Zh*, No. 1, 1963, p. 58.

Chapter XXXIX

THE RELATIVE VALUE OF VARIOUS EXERCISE PROGRAMS TO PROTECT ADULT HUMAN SUBJECTS FROM DEGENERATIVE HEART DISEASE

THOMAS K. CURETON

(Champaign, Illinois, U.S.A.)

ASSESSMENT OF IMPROVEMENTS OR RETROGRESSION.

SINCE 1941 programs have been under way in the College of Physical Education, University of Illinois, Urbana, Illinois, to assess the value of various activity programs to improve cardiovascular functioning and to prevent heart disease. This effort has involved (a) evaluating improvements in terms of the Schneider Index and the Harvard 5-Minute Step Test; (b) blood pressure changes, especially post-exercise blood pressures; (c) improving the angle of the wave front, the amplitude and area under the brachial pulse wave (sphygmogram); (d) improvement in the gross oxygen intake capacity and all-out treadmill run, or similarly on the ergometer bicycle; (e) changes in the newly developed velocity and acceleration (1st and 2nd derivative) waves, taken with high frequency electronic pick-up, a pulse wave divider, a differentiator and 5-channel simultaneous recording, permitting the assessment of the latent period preceding contraction of the ventricles, and (f) using derived calculations of peripheral resistance in terms of formulae (Wiggers 1, 2). (See Fig.

39–1.) More recently we have added the 5-channel records of ECG, BCG and heartograph (3 channels) with high-frequency electronic pick-up (Fig. 39–2, Table I).

Middle-aged persons with relatively high cardiovascular measurements in the terms described above do not have as much heart disease as those with poor scores on these same tests; in fact, those with the highest scores are relatively immune within the range of our observations. Therefore, attention should be paid to the types of programs which will improve these scores. My method of low, middle and high gear progression was introduced in 1955 into the Cleveland YMCA and became generally used by Cumler, Meadow, Morris, Hellerstein and others in that project, as has been described by Waxman (3). Ten types of experiments were conducted at our research station in which the validity of various exercise methods was probed and the results reported (4) (Table II.)

We test individuals first in the quiet state, as we take basal metabolism, ECG, BCG, heartograph and Schneider Index. Then we use the 5-Step Progressive Pulse Ratio Test, developed at our own station.

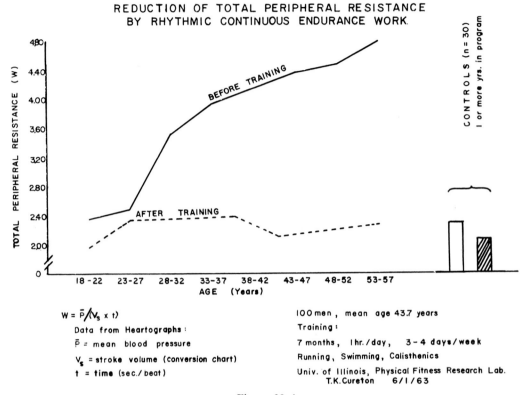

REDUCTION OF TOTAL PERIPHERAL RESISTANCE
BY RHYTHMIC CONTINUOUS ENDURANCE WORK.

$W = \bar{P}/(V_s \times t)$

Data from Heartographs:

$\bar{P}$ = mean blood pressure

V_s = stroke volume (conversion chart)

t = time (sec./beat)

100 men, mean age 43.7 years

Training:

7 months, 1 hr./day, 3 – 4 days/week

Running, Swimming, Calisthenics

Univ. of Illinois, Physical Fitness Research Lab.
T.K. Cureton 6/1/63

Figure 39–1.

We have noted that a sharp break in the progressive pulse ratio line follows very closely the oxygen debt as experimentally determined for the 12, 18, 24, 30 and 36 per minute rates of stepping.

THE AMOUNT AND NATURE OF EXERCISE

There is no easy way. It takes 2 to 3 months to induce an out-of-condition adult into such condition that he can take 300 to 500 calories per hour of physical work and live with it 5 to 6 days per week for several months at least. Over the 25-year period we have succeeded in getting about 8,000 men to do this and we have kept a varying sort of laboratory record upon them. Gradually the controls have become tighter in fear that we would hurt someone, but none has had a heart attack or has been "knocked out," as far as we know. The low rate of heart attacks in this group over such a long period seems much lower than among the sedentary adults around us in the University and the Champaign-Urbana population, where there is a relatively high incidence of coronary infarction. Certain individuals who called the exercise method "rubbish" suffered heart attacks themselves. Heart attacks occurred in over 60 of my sedentary acquaintances.

In a program of 5 to 6 hours of swimming and land exercises per day, including walking and running a mile for each cigarette smoked, the trainees at the U.S. Navy Underwater Swimmer's School, as

TABLE 39–I

RESULTS OF PROGRESSIVE PHYSICAL TRAINING FOR ADULT MEN (SWIMMING)

(15 men, 26 to 60 years—Six weeks)

(Raw scores are converted to SS (standard scores) by table)

Fitness Test Items	Units	June, 1950 T' Mean	August, 1950 T_2 Mean	Improvement (D)	σ Diff.	D/σ Diff.
Cardiovascular:						
1. Heartograph area	sq cm	43.71 SS	67.43 SS	24 SS	10.18	2.33
2. Systolic pulse wave amplitude	cm	57.43 SS	76.00 SS	19 SS	11.64	1.60
3. Diastolic pulse wave amplitude	cm	52.58 SS	72.28 SS	20 SS	10.53	1.90
4. Sitting pulse rate	beats ——— min.	54.57 SS	68.57 SS	14 SS	5.77	2.47
5. Schneider index	units	56.00 SS	64.00 SS	8 SS	8.78	.92
6. 5-Min. Step Test (Brouha)	beats	32.62 SS	54.50 SS	22 SS	7.94	2.76
7. Barach index	units	180.88 SS	141.10 SS	19 SS	19.97	1.99
8. Standing pulse rate	beats ———	50.30 SS	71.40 SS	21 SS	5.42	3.56
Respiratory:						
9. Basal metabolic rate	Cal/Hr /Sq m	−21.9%	−14.2%	7%	3.82	2.02
10. Breath holding after 2 min step-up 30/min	sec	14.9 SS	15.3 SS	4.0 SS	2.31	.173
11. Normal breath holding	sec	72.9 SS	80.9 SS	8.0 SS	8.90	.90
12–18 Eliminated						
Physique:						
19. Total fat (sum of 6)	mm	154.3 SS	145.2 SS	5.0 SS	3.78	2.42
20. Weighted fat index	lbs	231.6 SS	216.9 SS	5.0 SS	4.47	3.28

Note: Forty-two other items were dropped because of low significance. These included the blood pressure items, the separate strength items, vital capacity, the ECG vertical deflections, the skeletal index, and the muscular girth index.

measured by us in 1955 (5), improved a great deal in cardiovascular fitness, endurance in the mile run, and in many other kinds of fitness tests. From years of experience with swimming, I would say that endurance swimming and the associated land drills, such as those in the Bob Kiphuth System, are extraordinarily good for developing cardiovascular endurance (6, 7). Reports from our laboratory on middle-aged men have featured a progressive walking, jogging program (8, 9).

We have developed a progressive system of exercising which has been effective with middle-aged and older adults for over 20 years at Urbana, and we have spread its use to many YMCA's through men who have come to be trained for this special type of exercise and learn the testing procedures which are used for evaluation (10, 11). Our studies have shown the progressive improvement of the triglycerides, serum cholesterol, working capacity and the force in the BCG record (12, 13, 14). We have demonstrated significant improvements in the brachial pulse wave and in its velocity and acceleration components (15, 16, 17). We also have found good correlation

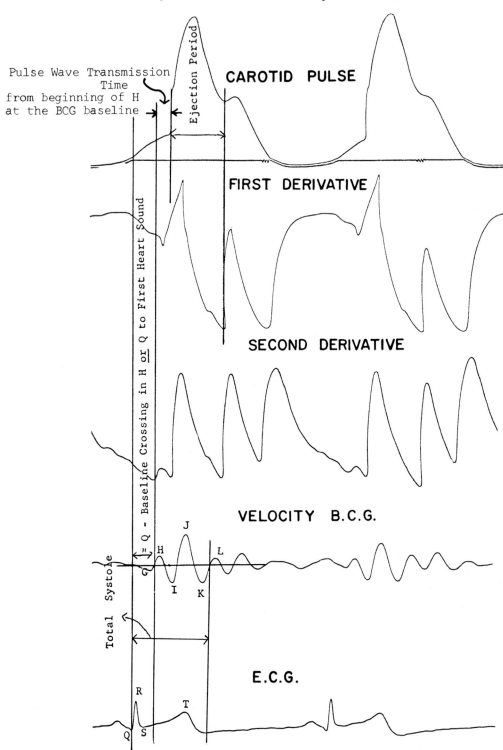

Figure 39–2.

TABLE 39–II

IMPROVEMENT OF A MIDDLE-AGED SUBJECT
BY RHYTHMIC RUNNING AND SWIMMING

Subject: R. L. (*No. 61*) Test Items	Units	Age 49-6 T'		Age 50 T_2		Ht. 71.0 Gain
Treadmill run	min and					
5 Mi/Hr	sec	2:07	(37)	4:00	(53)	16
Vital capacity residual	cu in	6	(58)	41	(75)	17
Breath Holding after						
1' exercise	sec	14	(45)	16	(47)	2
After 2' exercise	sec	13	(22)	25	(39)	17
Cardiovascular Tests:						
Brachial pulse wave/SA		.219	(65)	.363	(105)	40
Standing sys. BP	mm Hg	118	(55)	112	(63)	8
Standing dias. BP	mm Hg	100	(21)	80	(54)	2
Heartograph sys. amp.	cm	1.50	(59)	2.37	(125)	66
Pulse rate (sitting)	beats/min	64.6	(67)	62.8	(73)	6
Schneider index	score	12	(55)	15	(68)	13
5' Step test	beats	176	(28)	140	(89)	61
Barach index	score	191.8	(22)	181	(39)	17
Gale BMR	%	−1.0	(44)	+11	(56)	12
BMR (basal O_2	%	−18.8	(35)	−11.04	(43)	8
Av. P P ratio	score	2.47	(42)	2.14	(65)	23
Area brachial pulse wave	sq cm	2.50		4.96		
Area frontal x-ray	sq cm	180		141.1		
ECG (T_{IV-V} wave)	mm	9.9		11.6		
Total O_2 in jog	L	10.29	(38)	12.13	(46)	8
Post-Ex BP	mm/Hg	207/86		170/78		
Physique Tests:						
Fat	mm	179	(32)	139.5	(58)	26
Vital capacity residual	cu in	+6	(58)	+41	(75)	17
Chest expansion	in	4.5	(85)	5.5	(112)	27
Exp. chest girth—ab. girth	in	6.0	(61)	9.6	(87)	26
Heart size	%	5.5	(58)	−2.56	(43)	−15
Weight	lbs	183.8	(74)	170.8	(65)	9

Note: Figures in parentheses are standard score values, based upon 6 sigma spread; these are necessary to compare the relative gain on the tests.

between the Arbeit direct body ballistocardiographic IJ wave and the Ballistocor ultra low-frequency IJ wave, a rank-order correlation of 0.80 between the two methods (14). By computing the total peripheral resistance

$$\left(= \frac{\text{Mean Blood Pressure}}{\text{Stroke Output X Time per Beat}} \right)$$

in 100 men from our files with stroke output data taken from the heartograph (Cameron), we found that a striking reduction of total peripheral resistance had occurred in our training course of 6 to 7 months (Fig. 39–1). This course involves an hour of exercise 4 to 5 times per week and a long walk once per week, or a swim, run, row, treadmill climb, comparable to 300 to 600 calories per workout period. In our basic chart of exercises (8), the first month all-around series of rhythmic muscular endurance exercises totals about 100 calories; the second month 200, and the third month 300 or more. Some of our men have done as much as 600 calories of work on one day, working two hours.

STUDIES ON EXERCISE PROGRAMS AND SPORTS

Various studies completed by our graduate students on volleyball, golf, casual walking and weight lifting show much lower calorie cost and almost no circulatory-respiratory improvements. Badminton and tennis 3 times per week were a little better. The Canadian 5-BX Program was shown to be relatively ineffective in two studies. Only insignificant cardiovascular changes accrue as a result, except when running is added. Compared to the work our subjects have done, as in Skinner's study (12), I have said that "Golf is a good way to spoil a good walk," thinking of the restricted breathing, the waiting to play, the long time spent on the greens, and the sudden explosive efforts, not to mention the anxiety created by betting per hole, the drinking and smoking between rounds. It just isn't effective physical training for the cardiovascular-respiratory mechanisms, even if played fairly regularly. Getchell's (20) recent energy-cost study of golf verifies this. We saw in one study that weekend activity did not improve individuals over and above those who took almost no exercise at all (21). It has been our rule to work out a full hour 3 to 5 times per week, and in addition walk, hike or swim on weekends.

We have many men from 50 to 75 who do a whole hour of rhythmic endurance exercises in our program. We try to motivate them and to get their interest in our program by interviewing each man, requiring a medical examination, and by giving out some papers to read.

MANY TYPES OF EXERCISE DO NOT SUFFICE

The USA is afflicted by many schemes which are advertised, but do not work, such as use of gadgets; isometric 6-seconds per day routines; trifling 10 minutes per day exercises for muscle tone and posture. Most of these are too short to even induce a good circulatory respiratory warm-up and do not induce new capillary development or improved vital capacity residual, nor better breath-holding after exercise (1 minute at 30 per minute on a 17 inch bench), nor more velocity or acceleration in the heart stroke. There are slip-rods, bend-rods, elastics, vibrating tables, electric rockers, motor-driven bicycles and dozens of other gadgets now advertised. Our research work has shown that there is nothing better than free exercise to improve the circulation and respiration, and it may be made into the highest calorie-cost work by gradually working both harder and longer. Several 10 to 12 minute programs examined by us averaged 40 to 100 calories per workout. The rhythmic free exercise work, done mainly in the interval training style, averaged 300 to 500 calories for an hour's work, as done by men 26 to 75 years of age after their introductory 3-month period. Swimming is relatively high calorie work if done on a continuous basis. Running is the best for calorie cost (Fig. 39–1).

THE PROBLEM OF COMMUNICATION BETWEEN SPECIALTIES

The study of the relative effectiveness of various exercise programs is an old field of work in physical education but there has been a problem of communication between the several groups of professional health workers. The evidence which has accumulated within the physical education field (and adult fitness) in the past 20 years is still not too well known in certain medical specialties. The physical education approach has been one which aims to develop endurance, mainly with aerobic, moderate, rhythmic endurance exercises continued for a relatively long time (an hour or more).

Sudden, spurty, high intensity weight lifting or tensing (isometric) exercises may cause a depressed circulation and inotropic effect, possibly reflecting an oxygen deficiency in the heart muscle, as evidenced by (a) a shortened interval between Q and the very beginning of ventricular contraction, taken from the 1st sound or the beginning of H in the direct body BCG (where G to H crosses the baseline in the velocity tracing), (b) a general oxygen deficit; (c) depression of the ST segment of the ECG; (d) a shift in the fibrinogen curve, and (e) breathlessness which such exercise induces.

By contrast, a walk which very gradually is increased in pace, along with forced ventilation, then built up to walking and jogging, and finally jogging and interval training, does not induce such distressful symptoms. After 20 to 30 minutes of warm-up with very easy exercise, men can do more of the harder exercise than they ever thought they could do, and still feel good. Such graduated adjustment of the circulation, respiration, and body heat is essential if men are to make good psychological and physiological adjustments to an exercise program. It is also important to taper off for 10 to 15 minutes with stretching, deep breathing and rhythmic movement, balancing, upside down posture, and self-massage. Total calorie cost should be 300 to 500 or more per day.

There is good agreement now that the working capacity is adjusted to by (a) increasing the stroke volume; (b) dilating the muscle capillary beds and the lung capillary beds; (c) increasing the total circulatory turnover per minute; (d) using ballistical (relaxed) movements rather than tensed movements, and (e) by alternating the muscle groups or distributing the load so that no one muscle is overloaded too severely. All of this is facilitated by adequate warm-up. An important point is that after hard work one should rest enough. Soreness comes from overworked and overtensed muscles. The rhythmical endurance work at moderate levels of intensity is least offensive. Frequent stretching is indicated as is also deep breathing.

If people with poor circulatory capacity and poor respiratory reserve are kept away from the type of progressive exercise program we have described, then good circulation will seldom, if ever, develop.

The fundamental problem of method is one of training men to bear stress by a very gradual method of progression and slow adaptation. We have termed this progressive exercise, not primarily designed to improve strength but to induce better circulatory, respiratory and nervous features of physical fitness.

By alternating walking, jogging, and doing muscular endurance exercises (such as push-ups, sit-ups, leg-raisings, flutter kicks, side leg-raisings, hops, squat jumps, stepping up and down on a bench) the work can be made adequate if continued for 30 minutes or more. In the government outline, *Adult Physical Fitness*, we eliminated the 10 to 12-minute idea because of its inadequate calorie cost (23).

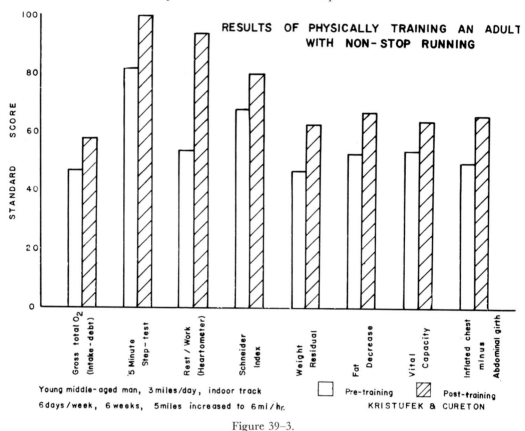

Figure 39–3.

In all of our standard tests the improvement of our subjects is very good. Reference may be made to Figure 39–3, a study which used most of these tests. We also see that if the training is hard enough and long enough, the post-exercise diastolic blood pressure will drop rather than rise, as in poorly conditioned subjects. In a 20-week program carried out on Marine underwater demolition trainees at Little Creek, Virginia, impressive changes were noted (5). Holloszy (13, 15) and Naughton (24) have made medical evaluations of our work with middle-aged men, as have Morris and Hellerstein, in Cleveland (2).

In a few subjects with heart disease, referred by their doctors, we have noticed a sluggish heart stroke and low Ft or Mv (28) and, in particular, we saw a loss of the fast deceleration following the heart ejection stroke. The unfit, not-yet classified medical case, who has poor circulation and relatively high peripheral resistance shows the same sluggishness of heart stroke, poor respiratory reserve, and low tolerance of exertion of the step-up and step-down type. We have noted consistent improvement in all of these measures in over 15 years of observations.

Improvements in the amplitude of the precordial R and T waves, in the amplitude of the brachial pulse wave and in the amplitude of the IJ wave of the ultra-low frequency BCG, are all positively correlated in the same direction.

Reduction of fat, cholesterol and trigly-cerides are in the opposite direction. Better time in the mile run is paralleled by greater amplitude, velocity and ac-celeration of the deflections which are due to heart contraction. Vigor can be trained into the heart, and it persists in what is called "physical fitness" (26, 30, 31, 33). It is reflected in the brachial and carotid pulse waves.

SUMMARY

Since 1941 testing programs have been under way in the College of Physical Education of the University of Illinois to assess the relative value of various types of physical activity with regard to improvement of cardiovascular function and, thereby, prevention of degenerative heart disease.

A progressive program, consisting mainly of rhythmic endurance exercises, with an adequate breathing technique, proved most effective.

Golf, handball, volleyball, and similar social sports of an intermittent nature are much less effective. Weight lifting and tensing (isometric) exercises are of least value. Many programs are too short, too low in calorie cost, too intermittent, and not sufficiently progressive.

The Canadian 5-BX program proved less valuable for cardiovascular training than expected.

Programs such as the "6-seconds per day" "fitness without movement" are practically useless.

Rhythmic activities during 30 to 60 minutes per day, 5 or 6 times per week, combined with emphasis on adequate breathing, are most useful. They include swimming, walking, jogging, running, skating and skiing. Campbell (35) found cholesterol reduction to be significant with running cross-country, but not in weight training or games.

REFERENCES

1. WIGGERS, C. J.: *Circulatory Dynamics.* New York, Grune and Stratton, 1952, p. 107.
2. CURETON, T. K., JR.: Anatomical, physiological and psychological changes induced by exercise programs (exercises, sports, games) in adults. In: *Exercise and Fitness.* Chicago, The Athletic Institute, University of Illinois Colloquium Report, 1960, p. 152.
3. STALEY, S. C., CURETON, T. K., HUELSTER, L. J., and BARRY, A. J.: *Exercise and Fitness.* Chicago, 1960, p. 183.
4. STALEY, S. C., CURETON, T. K., HUELSTER, L. J., and BARRY, A. J.: *Ibid.,* p. 152.
5. CURETON, T. K., JR.: Improvements resulting from a U.S. Navy underwater swimming training program, with and without dietary supplements. *Res Quart, 34:*440, 1963.
6. KIPHUTH, R. J. H.: *How to be Fit.* (2nd Ed.) New Haven, Yale University Press, 1963, p. 205.
7. KIPHUTH, R. J. H.: *Swimming.* London, Nicholas Kaye, 1950, p. 116. (Amer. Ed.: New York, A. S. Barnes and Co., 1942, p. 110.
8. CURETON, T. K., JR., with White, W. H.: Exercises to keep fit. *Sports Illustrated, 2:*63, 1955.
9. CURETON, T. K., JR.: *Physical Fitness and Dynamic Health.* New York, Dial Press, 1965, p. 200.
10. CURETON, T. K., JR.: *Physical Fitness Appraisal and Guidance.* St. Louis, C. V. Mosby and Co., 1947, p. 566.
11. CURETON, T. K., JR.: *Physical Fitness of Champion Athletes.* Urbana, University of Illinois Press, 1951, p. 458.
12. SKINNER, J. S., HOLLOSZY, J. O., and CURETON, T. K., JR.: Effects of a program of endurance exercises on physical work. *Amer J Cardiol, 14:* 747, 1964.
13. HOLLOSZY, J. O., SKINNER, J. S., TORO, G., and CURETON, T. K., JR.: Effects of a six-month program of endurance exercises on the serum lipids of middle-aged men. *Amer J Cardiol, 14:*753, 1964.
14. HOLLOSZY, J. O., SKINNER, J. S., BARRY, A. J., and CURETON, T. K., JR.: Effect of physical conditioning on cardiovascular function. *Amer J Cardiol, 14:*761, 1964.
15. BANISTER, E.: Cardiovascular parameters including the time derivatives of the brachial pulse wave in the assessment of physical condition and the efficiency of a training program. Urbana, Unpublished PhD thesis, University of Illinois, 1965, p. 92.
16. CURETON, T. K., JR.: Improvement of physical

fitness in a middle-aged man. *Res Quart, 23:*149, 1952.

17. CURETON, T. K., JR.: The hearts of athletes. *Illinois Med J, 99:*143, 1951; and *Sci News Letter, 66:*10, 1954.

18. HOLLOSZY, *et al.*: see reference 14.

19. MICHAEL, E. D., and CURETON, T. K., JR.: Effects upon the cardiac output at ground level and at 15,000 feet simulated altitude. *Res Quart, 24:*446, 1953.

20. GETCHELL, L. H.: A comparative study of the effects of a season of golf on cardiovascular, respiratory, metabolic and muscular endurance tests of middle-aged men, and the calorific cost of golf. Unpublished PhD thesis, University of Illinois, 1965, p. 130.

21. FARHI, A.: Physical fitness of the officers, U.S. Air Force Defense Command. MSc Thesis, Physical Education, University of Illinois, 1962, p. 143.

22. CURETON, T. K., JR.: Physical fitness work with normal aging adults. *J Ass Phys Ment Rehab, 11:*145, 1957.

23. President's Council on Physical Fitness. Adult Physical Fitness, Washington, Government Printing Office, Nov., 1963, p. 64.

24. NAUGHTON, J., and NAGLE, F.: Peak oxygen intake during physical fitness program for middle-aged men. *JAMA, 110:*899, 1965.

25. CURETON, T. K., JR.: The case for physical fitness. *Think*, Sept., 1958.

26. CURETON, T. K., JR.: The nature of cardiovascular conditioning and protection by exercise fitness programs. *J Phys Educ, 61:*30, 1963.

27. CURETON, T. K., JR.: Shrinkage in heart size resulting from the progressive physical training of three middle-aged adults. *J Ass Phys Ment Rehab, 10:*75, 1956.

28. CURETON, T. K., JR.: The analysis of physical education and athletic activities and the effects produced by such programs. 59th Annual Proc Coll Phys Educ Assn, Urbana, Illinois, 1955.

29. CURETON, T. K., JR.: Effects of physical education and athletics upon college men. Urbana, Illinois, Coll. Phys Educ Assoc, 1955, p. 79.

30. CURETON, T. K., JR., and POHNDORF, R. H.: Influence of wheat germ oil as a dietary supplement in a program of conditioning exercises for middle-aged men. *Res Quart, 26:*391, 1955.

31. CURETON, T. K., JR.: Results of moderate physical training on middle-aged men. Fed Int d' Education Physique, Lund, Sweden, *1:*58, 1955.

32. CURETON, T. K., JR.: The effect of physical training sports and exercises on weight, fat and tissue proportions. Washington, D.C. *Proc Acad Phys Educ*, Professional Contribution No. 6, 1956, p. 24.

33. CURETON, T. K., JR., and PHILLIPS, E. E.: Physical fitness changes in middle-aged men attributable to equal eight-weeks of training. *J Sport Med, 4*, June, 1964.

34. RUSHMER, R. F.: Initial ventricular impulse, a, potential key to cardiac evaluation. *Circulation 29:*268, 1964.

35. CAMPBELL, D. E.: Influence of several physical activities on serum cholesterol concentrations in young men. *J Lipid Res, 6:*478, 1965.

Chapter XL

A PRIMARY AND SECONDARY CORONARY PREVENTION PROGRAM—IN-PROGRESS REPORT

H. K. HELLERSTEIN

(Cleveland, Ohio, U.S.A.)

THIS report summarizes three years' experience in a projected ten-year prospective study of the effects of enhanced physical fitness on the development and course of primary coronary artery disease.

Beside the capacity for muscular work, other somatic biochemical and psychological factors and living habits were evaluated, including 48 hours of continued ECG monitoring. Subjects were classified into (a) coronary-stricken (myocardial infarcts), and (b) normals with low or high coronary proneness.

The subjects are middle-class sedentary men. The program emphasizes physical fitness and includes medical care, nutritional counseling, abstinence from tobacco, and informal group psychotherapy. The individualized training program includes 3 to 5 hours per week of supervised graduated exercises, home calisthenics, walking, and stair-climbing.

To date 300 subjects have entered into the program with 80 per cent adherence rate. Pretraining physical fitness of normal subjects was similar to that of normotensive coronary subjects without congestive heart failure; their "Physical Work Capacity 150" (steady state work load to elicit a heart rate of 150 per minute) was 603 and 608 kgm/min, respectively, compared to 925 kgm/min for trained normals.

Ninety per cent of both groups experienced definite subjective improvement. Over 75 per cent improved their vital and work capacities, heart rate, and blood pressure responses to exercise. After reconditioning, the ECG response to the same muscular effect normalized in 40 per cent of subjects with initial abnormal ECG responses.

It has been demonstrated that coronary subjects as well as normals can engage in a physical training program without untoward effects. The former are rehabilitated (restored to near-normal levels) and the latter habilitated (improved to a normal level previously unattained).

CARDIOPULMONARY RESPONSES DURING PHYSICAL TRAINING IN PATIENTS WHO HAVE RECOVERED FROM MYOCARDIAL INFARCTION*

JOHN NAUGHTON

(Oklahoma City, Oklahoma, U.S.A.)

THE association of a physically active life with a reduced incidence of clinically manifest coronary heart disease has been established by several retrospective epidemiological studies (1–4). Whether this seemingly preventive role can be converted into therapeutic usefulness in the care of patients who have recovered from myocardial infarction needs widespread investigation. The rationale for this latter approach stems from previous investigations which have shown that patients with healed myocardial infarction have physiological adaptations to work similar to those of noncardiac subjects (5, 6). The minor differences in response that occur during work between these two groups of individuals may be accounted for by a variation in the level of daily physical activity rather than solely by the fact that one group has underlying myocardial disease. It seems, therefore, that such patients should have the same response to physical conditioning as that observed in presumably healthy individuals. If the quality of response were simi-

lar, it might then be fair to speculate that regular vigorous physical activity has a dual role in the care of cardiac patients; one, therapeutic, directed toward the restoration of physical work capacity lost through illness, and the other, preventive, aimed at the promotion of increased coronary arterial collateral circulation (7) with a concomitant decrease of sympathetic inotropic and increase of parasympathetic, chronotropic tone (8).

To initiate the testing of this hypothesis a group of patients with healed myocardial infarcts participated in a physical training program. It is the purpose of this report to present various observations recorded on these individuals before and during the course of training.

MATERIALS AND METHODS

Ten white men with well-documented episodes of myocardial infarction volunteered for study. Their initial examination included a physiological evaluation with a modified work capacity test (9). In this test each subject begins walking on a motor-driven treadmill at a pace of 2.0 mph on a 0 per cent grade. The speed is held constant and the grade is

*This study was supported, in part, by U.S. Public Health Service Grants No. HTS 54-06 and HE 06286-04.

elevated 3.5 per cent every 3 minutes. Each level of energy expenditure represents an additional multiple of the resting metabolic state (i.e., 2, 3, 4) times the energy expenditure of rest. Blood pressure, pulse rate and the oblique lead electrocardiogram (10) are recorded during rest, the last half of each minute of work, and during each of the first 10 minutes of recovery. Respiratory gas exchange is recorded during every third minute of work. The test is terminated either at an energy expenditure not greater than seven times that of the resting metabolic state or at a lower energy demand if the patient develops fatigue, chest pain or claudication. A venous blood specimen for determination of the serum cholesterol concentration is drawn during rest and immediately after work (11).

The program was started with interval training on a treadmill. The energy demand was individualized daily so that a subject's physiological limitations were not exceeded. The intensity and duration of the work was increased as the patient's condition permitted. After the first month of training he was introduced into a more active daily program of simple, competitive games (12). These did not demand special skills, yet were capable of producing the work intensities needed to obtain a training effect. Eventually, each day's activity period lasted from 45 to 60 minutes with each patient utilizing about 300 kilocalorie per session.

The patients were retested in the above manner 6 weeks and 4 months after entering the program.

RESULTS

The men ranged in age from 37 to 62 years, with a mean age of 47 years. Eight patients entered the study from 2 to 7 months post-infarct; the other 2 subjects had myocardial infarcts 3 to 5 years prior to the program. The group's mean weight was 76.7 ± 13.3 kg.

Hypertension, excessive weight, a history of heavy smoking and an elevated serum cholesterol concentration were common findings. Two or more of these factors were present in each individual. Six patients stopped smoking and 2 lost weight during the training program. Five others gained weight so that there was no mean change in weight in the group.

The mean performance time for the initial work capacity evaluation was 12 minutes at an energy expenditure of 17.5 ml O_2/kg/min. This level of oxygen intake is about five times that of the resting state. Reasons for terminating the first evaluation varied from subjective signs of fatigue to moderately severe dyspnea. None of the patients experienced angina pectoris or developed electrocardiographic evidence of subendocardial ischemia. All were able to perform the entire test without difficulty after 6 weeks of physical training.

Systolic and diastolic blood pressures were slightly lower at rest and during standing following training (Fig. 41–1). Both parameters remained lower at comparable levels of energy expenditure. The degree of elevation of systolic pressure above the resting value was almost equal during work in both states of physical condition. Following training the diastolic pressure decreased slightly with each new level of work, a response similiar to that usually observed in healthy, vigorously active individuals.

The mean pulse rate at the termination of the pretraining evaluation was 131/

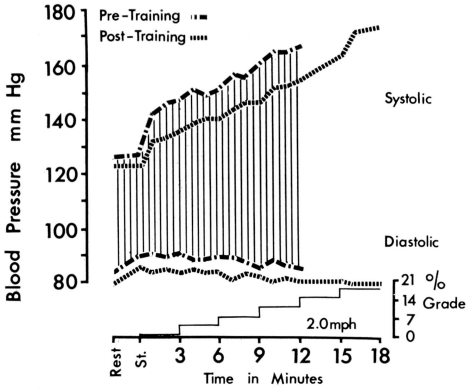

Figure 41–1. Lower values for the systolic and diastolic blood pressures were found during rest, standing and various levels of energy expenditure in the 10 patients 4 months after the initiation of physical training. The subjects were able to complete the post-training evaluation in contrast to performances which averaged 12 minutes before the initiation of the physical conditioning. (All values represent the mean determinations for 10 men.)

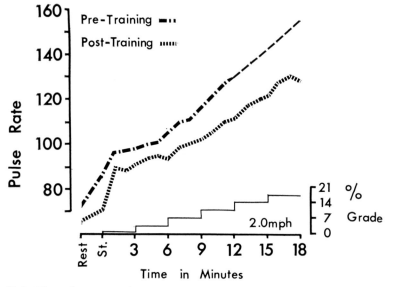

Figure 41–2. The pulse rate was lower at all comparable levels of energy expenditure following 4 months of physical conditioning (see text). (Values represent mean determinations for 10 men.)

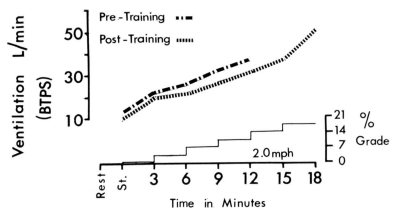

Figure 41–3. The minute ventilation was slightly decreased in the men during comparable physiological conditions after training. This indicates that there was an increased ventilatory efficiency with training. (Values represent mean determinations for 10 men.)

min (Fig. 41–2). If this curve is extrapolated to the usual end-point of the test, that is, to an oxygen intake approximating 7 times that of the resting metabolic state, the final pulse rate would have approached 156/min, a value comparable to that usually recorded with this test in presumably healthy, sedentary men (6). Training was accompanied by a lower resting and standing pulse rate and by a more gradual elevation during work. The final pulse rate, recorded at the greater energy demands during testing after 4 months of training, was identical to the value recorded at the lower levels of energy expenditure before training. The lowered pulse rate at various levels of metabolic activity reflects an increased cardiovascular efficiency which can be expressed as an increased oxygen pulse.

Improved respiratory efficiency was reflected by a slightly lowered minute ventilation during standing and comparable levels of energy expenditure (Fig. 41–3). The final value of 50 liters/min (BTPS) is far below the levels recorded

in subjects as they near their maximum aerobic capacity with other types of testing, and slightly below the values obtained in healthy, sedentary individuals at this level of energy expenditure.

The serum cholesterol concentration was investigated as a possible metabolic indicator of the training response (Fig. 41–4). Even though the group's mean weight remained unchanged and the quality of the caloric intake was not altered, the concentration of serum cholesterol decreased from 236 ± 44.9 to 212 ± 20.0 mg/100 ml. The 2 subjects who lost weight showed no greater decrease in cholesterol than did others who gained slightly. This difference was significant at the .05 level. Both work tests were accompanied by a transitory elevation in the serum cholesterol concentration.

Upon entering the study most subjects were tense and somewhat fearful of exercising in view of the prevailing popular opinion that "cardiacs" should restrict activity. Two subjects had typical angina pectoris prior to training but neither

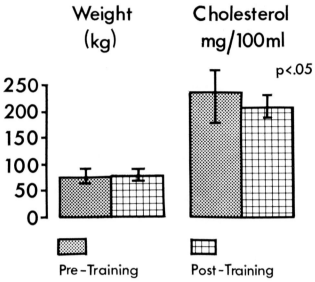

Figure 41–4. There was a reduction of the serum cholesterol concentration in the men even though there was no appreciable alteration of their weight during the period of observation.

developed any episodes of chest pain or electrocardiographic changes while under observation. All of them developed an intense desire to compete and to win. The number of somatic complaints decreased as a patient's ability to compete improved.

One subject terminated training after 4 months when he moved out of town, Another who dropped out for 2 months. gained 4.0 kg; his serum cholesterol concentration had increased from 198 to 300 mg/100 ml, and his exercise electrocardiogram revealed recurrent ventricular extrasystoles. Four weeks after resuming training he had lost the added weight, cholesterol had fallen to 212 mg/100 ml and only an occasional ventricular extrasystole was recorded during recovery from exercise. A third patient has been rehospitalized 3 times; twice for an acute anxiety reaction and once for chest pain which was not associated with electrocardiogram changes and did not have the characteristics of angina.

DISCUSSION

These data indicate that the patient with an uncomplicated, healed myocardial infarction can return to levels of physical performance which are comparable to, and in some instances may exceed, the performance of presumably healthy, sedentary individuals. The mechanisms used to adapt to work in the trained cardiac appear to be the same as those employed by healthy individuals.

A physical training program involving cardiac patients must be multifaceted. The initial phase should provide ample psychological reassurance to each patient and should avoid having him perform beyond his physiological limitations. When a patient's capacity for work increases he can be permitted to participate in more strenuous group games where competition provides a large portion of the training stimulus. If a patient develops a maximum training effect from group games his program may be individualized so that a continuing training effect can be induced by ever-increasing work demands.

Whether such a program should be a part of the therapeutic regimen of the cardiac patient is not yet definitely known. Only after a large group of patients have trained regularly over a period of several years will we know whether the course of events has been affected, favorably or unfavorably. It seems fair to speculate, however, that physical conditioning might induce increased coronary arterial collateralization which could be beneficial to the cardiac patient. In addition, the increased cardiopulmonary efficiency developed through vigorous physical activity might aid these patients in coping with environmental stresses more effectively, thus providing a protective influence.

SUMMARY

Ten middle-aged men who had recovered from well-documented episodes of myocardial infarction participated in a physical conditioning program. Their physiological response to work was evaluated before and after 4 months of training. Conditioning was accompanied by a reduction in the levels of systolic and diastolic blood pressure, pulse rate, minute ventilation and serum cholesterol concentration at rest. Their work capacity increased and they used the same physiological mechanisms to adapt to the stresses of work and of training as

have been found in healthy individuals. Somatic complaints decreased as the training effect increased.

REFERENCES

1. MORRIS, J. N., HEADY, J. A., RAFFLE, P. A. B., ROBERTS, C. G., and PARKS, S. W.: Coronary heart disease and physical activity of work. *Lancet*, 2:1053, 1953.
2. MORRIS, J. N., and CRAWFORD, M. C.: Coronary heart disease and physical activity of work. *Brit Med J*, 2:1485, 1958.
3. MORRIS, J. N.: Health and social class. *Lancet*, 1:303, 1959.
4. TAYLOR, H. L., KLEPETER, E., KEYS, A., PARLIN, W., BLACKBURN, H., and PUCHNER, T. C.: Death rates among physically active and sedentary employees of the railway industry. *Circulation*, 22: 822, 1960.
5. CHAPMAN, C. B., and FRASER, R. S.: III. Cardiovascular responses to exercise in patients with healed myocardial infarction. *Circulation*, 9:347, 1954.
6. NAUGHTON, J., BALKE, B., and POARCH, A.: Modified work capacity studies in individuals with and without coronary artery disease. *J Sport Med*, in press.
7. ECKSTEIN, R. W.: Effect of exercise and coronary narrowing on collateral circulation. *Circ Res, 5:* 230, 1957.
8. RAAB, W.: The neurogenic metabolic factor in ischemic heart disease. Pathogenesis and prevention. *Dis Chest, 46:*150, 1964.
9. NAUGHTON, J., SEVELIUS, G., and BALKE, B.: Physiological responses of normal and pathological responses to a modified work capacity test. *J Sport Med*, 3:201, 1963.
10. LINDEMAN, R., KYRIAKOPOULOS, J., and CONRAD, L.: Evaluation of a new oblique chest lead for the detection of electrocardiographic abnormalities. *Amer Heart J*, 64:24, 1962.
11. ZAK, B., DICKERMAN, R. C., WHITE, E. G., BURNETT, H., and CHERNEY, P. I.: Rapid estimation of free and total cholesterol. *Amer J Clin Path, 24:*1307, 1954.
12. EDMONDSON, J.: *Games and Activities.* Isaac Pitman and Sons, 1952, pp. 124–126.

Chapter XLII

STRENUOUS SPORTS AS TREATMENT FOR DEGENERATIVE HEART DISEASE

VIKTOR GOTTHEINER

(Tel-Aviv, Israel)

ADVANTAGES OF STRENUOUS SPORTS FOR CARDIAC HEALTH

IN OUR industrial civilization the sedentary person drifts into a state of increasing physical unfitness due both to a primary lack of desire for physical motion and to a self-perpetuating and aggravating loss of ability to move vigorously. His limbs are becoming stiff and unwieldy, his breath short, his heart beat unduly fast and pounding. Early fatigue and discomfort generate a feeling of insecurity and fear, and serve as an excuse for further immobilization (1).

In order to conquer these shortcomings and renew his confidence in his potential physical capacity and enjoyment of life, the contemporary victim of sedentary degeneration must undergo a thorough physical reconditioning (2). It is imperative, however, that this be done in a systematic, carefully graded fashion because an overdosage as well as an underdosage would defeat the purpose (3, 4, 5).

Some of the fundamental principles to be observed in reconditioning and rehabilitation programs are the following:

1. The exercises performed must be of a strenuous character in keeping with the individual's increasing maximal exercise tolerance.

2. Exercises must be carried out daily for a lifetime.

3. The control of exercise tolerance, and prescription of exercise dosage should be entrusted to a sports physician (6).

4. Apart from training under periodic supervision, unsupervised, independent training must be systematically continued according to instructions received.

5. Tobacco smoking should be avoided.

6. The diet should be kept within the limitations which active sportsmen impose upon themselves to avoid weight gain.

A variety of gentle motion treatments, without and with the aid of gadgets which have been recommended for acutely and chronically severely disabled persons, are without value for the restoration of optimal cardiovascular function and fitness. Many physicians who lead a conspicuously sedentary life themselves confine their advice to the lukewarm admonition that the patient should do "some" walking, gardening, golf playing or "some" home gymnastics, without recommending any systematic dosage or control. Such forms of "exercise therapy" may occasionally be more harmful than useful if they lull the patient into a false sense of security and induce him to sporadic bouts of unwise overexertion which may lead to disastrous consequences. Foreseeable and avoidable cardiac accidents of this kind have been misinterpreted and indiscriminately adduced to condemn the principle of strenuous exercising in middle-aged and elderly people and in cardiacs altogether.

In reality, the widely disregarded general benefits to the cardiovascular system, accruing from strenuous physical training, are the following:

1. Improved energetic and oxygen economy of the heart muscle due to a reduction of exaggerated oxygen-wasting sympathetic activity, and development of a more effective parasympathetic and sympathoinhibitory counterbalance; slower heart rate at rest and lesser cardiac acceleration during effort, faster deceleration after exertion, reduction of peripheral resistance due to dilatation of muscular blood vessels, increased residual volume in the heart which facilitates the transition from rest to work, and slowing of circulation with a resulting better utilization of oxygen by the tissues.

2. Improved coronary blood flow due to augmented collateral capillarization of the heart muscle; prolongation of the diastole (during which coronary flow is optimal), and diminished hemodynamic compression of subendocardial coronary ramifications.

3. Prolongation of coagulation time and lowering of the serum cholesterol level.

4. Improved emotional equanimity and augmented self-reliance with their beneficial hypothalamic neurohormonal implications (7).

Among the different ways in which adult fitness can be attained, a change of occupation from sedentary work to heavy strenuous labor is the least practical for obvious socioeconomic reasons and because an abrupt alteration of physical habits entails considerable risks.

Systematic physical training in reconditioning centers like those in the eastern European countries, West Germany (8), Switzerland, etc. is associated with additional environmental and emotional benefits, but is limited in time. Its lasting effectiveness depends decisively on the individual's willingness and motivation for continued maintenance of indoctrinated and acquired health habits.

Regular, properly guided and supervised sports activities (after a preliminary basic fitness training) offer superior physical as well as psychological advantages to those whose geographic location and occupational time schedule permit their regular active participation. It is evident that the initiation and systematic conduction of such programs must be carried out by competent sports physicians who, over and above their professional knowledge, must be capable of supporting their trainees' enduring motivation by a psychologically effective approach and by their personal active example.

Unfortunately, these prerequisites for a successful preventive and rehabilitative sports training are only rarely available.

Most practicing physicians are unfamiliar with the physiological principles and practical results of exercise therapy and, therefore, reluctant to make the necessary emphatic recommendations to their patients.

As a specific point concerning the training of persons with anginal symptoms on exertion, we would like to mention that, contrary to common practice, we do not necessarily prohibit physical activity in such cases. On the contrary, we have found that, with proper en-couragement, such persons can often overcome the painful sensation by slow-ing down but not altogether interrupting their effort. The situation can be com-pared to the "crisis before the second wind" among athletes who often pass through a phase of "choking" discomfort before reaching the level of maximal performance. In no instance did we see any complications arising in patients who succeeded in continuing their exercises through and beyond the stage of what we like to describe as "pain of adapta-tion."

CHOICE OF SPORTS FOR CARDIAC RECONDITIONING

Both acute exertion and prolonged training exert powerful influences on the autonomic nervous system and, thereby, on the metabolism and function of the heart muscle.

Whereas muscular effort as such is associated with a transient strong stimu-lation of the sympathetic system, its fre-quent repetition as in regular sports ac-tivities pays long-range dividends. These consist in a gradual and sustained reduc-tion of the exaggerated and unnecessary, oxygen-wasting sympathetic overexcit-ability which characterizes the sedentary individual, plus an augmentation of the oxygen-preserving parasympathetic tone.

The potentially hypoxiating cardio-metabolic disadvantages of the inevitable exercise-induced acute sympathetic stim-ulation in persons with coronary athero-sclerosis seem to be largely compensated by the associated favorable hemodynamic reactions to effort (decreased peripheral resistance, augmented coronary perfusion pressure, decreased compression of sub-endocardial coronary branches.)

Emotional excitements, connected with certain sports, are superimposed stimu-lants to the hypothalamo-sympathetic system. Hence it is advisable to exclude from the physical training of pre-cardiacs and cardiacs all types of sports which, by their very nature or by competitive application, elicit emotional tension or fear.

From this point of view, preference is given to sports which involve endurance in rhythmical locomotion over distances, such as walking, running, swimming, cycling, and rowing. By contrast, body contact games, such as boxing, wrestling, and judo, are unsuitable. Tennis de-mands too much constant preparedness to cope with the moves of an opponent. The combat character of team ball games (soccer, rugby, football, and hockey) makes them likewise objectionable. Volley ball is the most useful among ball sports games.

The individual choice among the gen-erally recommended sports should be flexible according to the trainee's psycho-logical attitude and inclinations, degree of fitness and body build.

PATTERNS OF TRAINING

In our program (1), actual sports ac-tivities are preceded by exercises which promote flexibility and strength as a "warm-up" preparation, lasting 10 to 20 minutes and carried out, in part, with dumbells (½ to 3 kg) in each hand (Figs. 42–1–3).

Strength training (45 minutes) is added twice or three times per week and consists of 5 kg weight one-armed, and 10 kg weight both-armed exercises. This may be increased according to dynamometer tests.

The "warming-up" exercises are car-

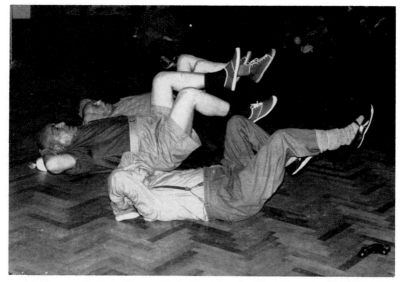

Figure 42–1. Exercises in Class I.

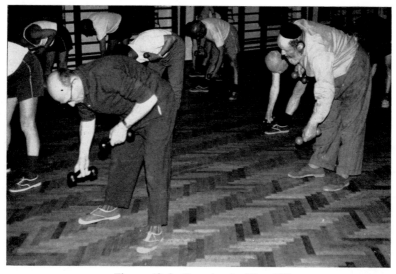

Figure 42–2. Exercises in Class III.

ried out at home in the morning, followed by step-climbing (see below) and a cold and hot shower.

Our *specific cardiac endurance training* in the afternoons is implemented in 3 ways, namely (a) climbing steps; (b) out-of-door distance endurance effort, and (c) team games.

Step-climbing serves mainly as a substitute for distance effort when either weather conditions or the time factor are incompatible with the latter. Applying the interval method, step-climbing is practiced by sprints (30 seconds each) alternating with intervals of 60 seconds. The speed of the sprints is being set at

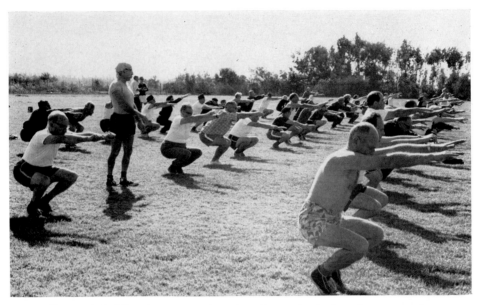

Figure 42–3. Warming-up exercises of cardiacs at beginning of sports meeting.

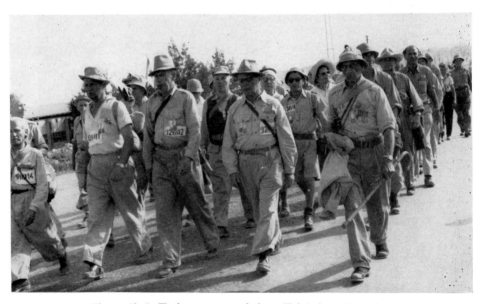

Figure 42–4. Trainees on march from Tel Aviv to Jerusalem.

80 per cent, and that of the intervals at 40 per cent of the maximal speed, determined by the step test (Table 42–I). The number of repetitions depends on the previously measured exercise tolerance of the trainee (9).

Distance sports are begun with walking (Fig. 42–4), cycling or rowing, all of which are feasible in small doses, even by the least trained individuals. Swimming and running are started in more advanced stages of training a few months

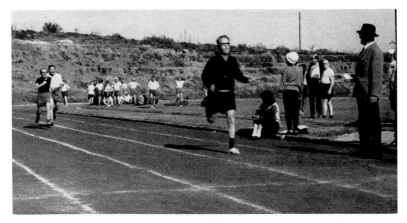

Figure 42–5. Trainee C. J.; employee; 59-years-old. Myocardial infarctions 10 and 2 years ago. No previous physical training. At beginning of training: intensive anginal symptoms when walking on level ground; Class I.—Present status: 3-times weekly running and 3-times strength training with 20 kg; Class V.—Walks 25 km in 5 hours, runs 60 meters in 10.2 sec, jumps 3.0 meter, throws 5 kg ball 5.90 meter. Recipient of Israel Sports Medal. Optimal performance before training: 90 watt; now 130 watt; O_2 pulse at maximal steady state performance rose from 8.5 to 11.2.

TABLE 42–I

DOSAGE OF ENDURANCE TRAINING IN RELATION TO THE STEP TEST

Class	Maximum Perform- ance in Watt	Maximum O_2 Consumption per Minute	Walking (Plain) m/min	km/hr	Running (Plain) m/min	km/hr	Swimming (Breast Stroke) m/min	km/hr	Cycling (Race Bicycle) m/min	km/hr	Rowing (Skiff) m/min	km/hr
II	40	600	46	2,8					100	6,0	59	3,5
II	50	750	72	4,3					133	8,0	68	4,1
II	60	900	90	5,4					167	10,0	74	4,5
III	70	1050	97	5,8					200	12,0	80	4,8
III	80	1200	106	6,4					233	14,0	86	5,2
III	90	1350	112	6,7					265	16,0	92	5,5
IV	100	1500			112	6,7	35	2,1	285	17,0	98	5,9
IV	110	1650			123	7,5	38	2,3	300	18,0	108	6,5
IV	120	1800			134	8,1	41	2,4	320	19,0	118	7,1
V	130	1950			145	8,7	44	2,6	345	20,6	128	7,7
V	140	2100			172	10,3	47	2,8	370	22,2	138	8,3
V	150	2250			200	12,0	50	3,0	395	23,8	148	8,9
VI	160	2400			220	13,2	53	3,2	425	25,4	158	9,5
VI	170	2550			240	14,5	56	3,4	450	27,0	168	10,1
VI	180	2700			254	15,2	59	3,5	475	28,6	178	10,7
VII	190	2850			268	16,2	62	3,7	500	30,2	188	11,3
VII	200	3000			282	17,0	65	3,9	525	31,8	198	11,9
VII	210	3150			295	17,5	68	4,1	550	33,0	208	12,5

later, unless bodily defects or peripheral arterial disease make this impossible. All nonhandicapped trainees are schooled in at least 2 sports, one of which is always swimming. Games of volley ball are inserted once a week to avoid monotony.

Distance training is subdivided in 3 stages: sprints (Fig. 42–5) with intervals

TABLE 42–II

DISTANCE SPORTS

Type of Sport	Sprint	Middle Distance	Long Distance
Walking	40–80 m	100–200 m	5–10 km
Running	60–120 m	300–400 m	2–10 km
Swimming	25–50 m	75–200 m	400–2000 m
Cycling	100–200 m	300–600 m	15–45 km
Rowing	80–160 m	300–400 m	4–10 km

TABLE 42–III

REPETITION PROGRAM

Type of Sport	Sprint	Middle Distance
Walking	8–12 times	3–6 times
Running	8–15 times	4–10 times
Swimming	6–15 times	4–10 times
Cycling	10–30 times	6–15 times
Rowing	8–15 times	3–6 times

Note: The interval between individual efforts is twice as long as the effort periods.

(the latter lasting twice as long as the sprint and consisting of a slowing but not cessation of movement); medium distances with intervals as above, and long distances. We aim at 80 per cent of the maximum speed in the sprints, 60 per cent in runs over medium distances, and 50 per cent over long distances (Table 42–II). The number of phase repetitions is increased every other week (Table 42–III).

The general time arrangement of the training programs is represented in Table 42–IV.

ORGANIZATION OF GRADED CLASSES

Our trainees are divided in 7 classes, 3 of which are designated as preparatory classes, while the 4 following ones are sports classes. The lowest class comprises full invalids. Some of these had been bedridden for long periods but a large section of this group has regained a certain measure of activity and joy of life. Some have even reached degrees of fitness surpassing that of healthy individuals of their age category. The initial exercise therapy of such patients excludes all attempts at step-climbing, "warming-up," strength and distance training. It begins with simple breathing exercises, followed by slow walking (about 20 minutes twice a day). If a thorough medical examination permits it, promotion into

TABLE 42–IV

INDIVIDUAL WEEKLY PLAN

	Sun.	Mon.	Tues.	Wed.	Thurs.	Fri.	Sat.
Preparatory Groups Activities							
"Warming up"	+	+	+	+	+	+	
Step climbing	+	+	+	+	+	+	
Hot-cold shower	+	+	+	+	+	+	+
Walking	+	+	+	+	+	+	
Sports Groups Activities							
"Warming up"	+	+	+	+	+	+	
Step climbing	+	+	+	+	+	+	
Hot-cold shower	+	+	+	+	+	+	+
Strength training*	+				+		
Distance sports*		+		+		+	

*Every other week the order is reversed; 3-times strength training and 2-times distance sports. In the afternoon of the once weekly group gymnastics there is no individual training.

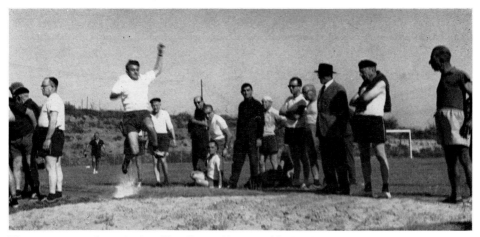

Figure 42–6. Trainee S. S.; Chauffeur; 43-years-old. Healed myocardial infarction. Had been 3 years in military service. No further previous training. At the beginning of training: intensive anginal pain on walking slowly; Class I.—Present status: trained in running, swimming, strength (with 25 kg); Class VI.—Throws 5 kg ball 8.14 meters. Recipient of Israel Sports Medal. Optimal performance before training: 120 watt; now 170 watt; O_2 pulse at maximal steady state performance rose from 10.0 to 13.8.

TABLE 42–V

Sex	Types of Cases	Number of Cases	Age Groups (years) and Numbers of Cases per Groups with Ischemic Heart Disease				
			30-39	40-49	50-59	60-69	70 and over
Male	Ischemic Heart Disease						
	(a) With infarction	650	32	186	214	187	31
	(b) Without infarction	520	56	114	185	121	44
	Other (rheumatic, hypertensive, etc.)	390					
	"Normal" (prevention)	780					
Female	Ischemic Heart Disease						
	(a) With infarction	99	—	—	69	30	—
	(b) Without infarction	192	—	32	90	58	12
	Other (rheumatic, hypertensive, etc.)	239					
	"Normal" (prevention)	130					

The last 3,000 subjects who have passed through the training program (2,340 men and 660 women), subdivided in morbidity and age groups. Of the 1462 cases with ischemic heart disease, the following numbers are still under observation: (a) with infarction, 505 males; 43 females; (b) without infarction, 395 males; 160 females.

a higher class takes place within a few months.

Admission of sufficiently pretrained persons into the lowest sports class is usually possible after 9 months. From then on, progress is slower. Graduates of the top class are equal in fitness to well-trained sportsmen of their age group (Fig. 42–6). They are organized in teams which compete with each other. Some continue their training individually or join other sports clubs. Many take part in the periodical community evening gymnastics sessions of our association.

TABLE 42–VI

TIME INTERVALS BETWEEN BEGINNING OF TRAINING AND DEATH

Trainees with Ischemic Heart Disease (Remaining Under Observation)	Men		Women	
	Total Number	Number of Deaths	Total Number	Number of Deaths
With Infarction	505	27	43	3
Without Infarction	395	5	160	1

Numbers of Deaths Within Time Intervals After Beginning of Training Program

	Men	Women
0– 3 months	10	0
3– 6 "	2	0
6– 9 "	1	0
9–12 "	0	1
12–24 "	11	2
24–36 "	4	0
36–48 "	1	1
over 48 "	3	0

Number of deaths, subdivided by heart disease categories and time intervals after beginning of training program. No death occurred during the physical activities of training. Nine of the 36 deaths were due to noncardiac causes: cerebral thromboses, brain tumor, perforated ulcer, prostatectomy, automobile accident.

Practically all trainees remain under our permanent control. Even those who have dropped out remain influenced by our programs in that they have changed their way of life at least to some extent.

Our sports organization for cardiacs and precardiacs has more than 3,000 organized members and nonorganized participants (2,340 men and 660 women) and is located in 5 cities of Israel with the center in Tel Aviv. Coronary infarction has been diagnosed in 749 of the trainees, coronary insufficiency in 712, nonischemic heart diseases (rheumatic valvular and hypertensive) in 629. In the remaining 910 no definite cardio vascular diagnosis was made (Table 42–V).

A total of 36 trainees (mostly men with sedentary occupations) have died since inception of our program. The time intervals between beginning of training and death are given in Table 42–VI. The number of deaths in relation to the train-

ing classes attained was the following: First class, 11; second class, 15; third class, 4; fourth class, 1; fifth class, 2; sixth class, 1; seventh class, 2. One of the latter two had been a complete invalid after an anterior wall infarction. He reached the highest fitness category and died 8 years after joining our organization at age 58 from a perforated ulcer.

The organization is self-supporting and covers all expenses for training staff, equipment, space rent, and a monthly bulletin from membership fees ($4 per month).

SUMMARY

Over the past 10 years a sports organization for the rehabilitation of cardiacs (for the most part patients with past myocardial infarctions, coronary insufficiency, and hypertensive heart disease) and for the reconditioning of sedentary precardiacs has been developed in Israel.

According to their initial condition, the trainees are assigned to 7 classes, beginning with minimal breathing exercises and walking, and progressing to intensive strenuous sports activities under periodic medical supervision.

Preparatory daily training for flexibility and strength is followed by regular endurance activities (step-climbing and distance training, such as running, swimming and rowing), volley ball, and finally strenuous team games. Contact and combat sports are avoided.

Out of more than 3,000 trainees, 36 have died up to date, 9 of these from noncardiac causes.

The risk of carefully graded physical training for cardiac patients is usually much overrated. Its rehabilitative and reconditioning value deserves wide and systematic application under the guidance of competent sports physicians.

REFERENCES

1. KRAUS, H. and RAAB, W.: *Hypokinetic Disease.* Charles C Thomas, Springfield, Ill., 1961.
2. GOTTHEINER, V.: Die Renaissance des Zivilisationskranken und die Wiederherstellung des Herz-Gefäss-Leidenden durch maximale körperliche Uebung. *Die Rehabilitation, 3:*172, 1964.
3. GOTTHEINER, V. and KOST, R.: Heart stroke volume during effort, XIV Internat'l. Physiol. Congr., Rome, 1932 in: Herxheimer, H.: *Grundriss der Sportmedizin.* G. Thieme Verlag, Leipzig, 1933.
4. GOTTHEINER, V.: Myocardial infarction and sport. *Sympos. on Sports Medicine,* XVII. Olympic Games, Rome 1960.
5. GOTTHEINER, V.: Richtlinien zur Beurteilung des Herzkranken und zur Dosierung seines Trainings, XXI. *Deutscher Sportärzte-Kongress,* Münster, 1963.
6. GOTTHEINER, V.: Improvement of physical fitness—the task of the sports physician. *Hygiene and Health,* Jerusalem, 3:15, 1943.
7. RAAB, W.: The adrenergic-cholinergic control of cardiac metabolism and function. *Advances of Cardiology, 1:*65. S. Karger, Basel–New York, 1956.
8. BECKMANN, P.: Gesundheitserziehung als Krankenbehandlung. *Innternat. Rundschau f. Physikal. Med., 11:*1, 1958.
9. GOTTHEINER, V.: Der Stufentest, ein einfaches Mittel zur Schätzung der Kreislaufökonomie. *Der Sportarzt,* No. 6, 1961.

Chapter XLIII

THE EFFECT OF GRADED WORK EXERCISE IN 100 PATIENTS WITH ISCHEMIC HEART DISEASE: TWO YEAR FOLLOW-UP

MENDEL WASSERMIL and MORDECAI TOOR

(Petah Tikva, Israel)

INTRODUCTION

A NUMBER of recently published papers have shown that judicious use of graded exercise may improve the well-being and the circulatory status of patients suffering from ischemic heart disease (1–3). The exact way graded exercise may help these patients is not known. Some investigators suggest that exercise may open preexisting intercapillary anastomoses and thus improve the coronary circulation (4).

The purpose of this paper is to evaluate the effect of graded exercise performed during 2 years in 100 cardiac patients.

MATERIALS AND METHODS

The subjects were 100 male patients who suffered from ischemic heart disease. Patients with congestive heart failure, cardiomegaly or systemic hypertension were excluded.

The mean age was 55.5 years, ranging from 37 to 65 years.

Ninety-two patients had a history of myocardial infarction 6 months to 3 years prior to this study and their electrocardiogram indicated prior myocardial infarction. The remaining 8 patients had angina of effort with a normal ECG at rest.

All patients were subjected to a preliminary physical examination which included also the determination of blood cholesterol, chest x ray, electrocardiogram and erythrocyte sedimentation rate. The initial load of the graded exercise was established by means of an ergometric study performed on a bicycle ergometer (5).

The work load was submaximal, but sufficient to obtain a pulse rate of 150 beats per minute. The work capacity was expressed in terms of calories per minute, based on actual oxygen consumption during the ergometric test. Each subject performed this test for a period of 6 minutes at different work loads with a 4-minute rest period between tests, until pulse rates returned to control levels. Testing was begun with 300 kilopondmeter per minute and this load was increased according to the patient's reaction in terms of anginal pain, pulse rate and ECG changes. The minute ventilation and expired air samples were obtained during the test through the use of the Wolff IMP masks.*

The expired air samples were analyzed

---

*Integrating Motor Pneumograph (Wolff "IMP"), J. Langham Thompson, Ltd., Bushey Heath, England.

for oxygen content on a Beckman oxygen electrode. †

The ergometric studies were repeated at 6-month intervals to help assess the patient's physical status and progress.

According to the results of the ergometric studies, the subjects were divided into 3 groups; each group was given a specially prepared course of calisthenics of Swedish-type exercises. The energy expenditures of these exercises were known, ranging from 3.0 calorie/min for the lowest group to 6.0 calorie/min for the most advanced group.

All patients were trained under medical supervision twice weekly for 3 minutes in a gymnasium and, in addition, they were urged to perform these exercises daily at home before breakfast.

RESULTS

Adverse Effects. Four patients were removed from this study after 3 months of training because of adverse effects of exercise, as evidenced by increased ischemic changes in the ECG in 1 patient, and increased severity and frequency of angina on effort in the remaining 3 patients. Two patients died suddenly at home under circumstances not related to exercise training.

Beneficial Effects. In the remaining 94 patients who continued to participate in this study, improvement was noted in several parameters.

Angina of Effort. Thirty-eight patients noted less anginal pain on exertion. They were able to perform more strenuous tasks without chest pain, while prior to participation lesser tasks had caused anginal pain. Ten patients claimed lesser use of nitrates and 5 patients discontinued this medication completely.

---

†Beckman Physiological Gas Analyser Model 160, Spinco Division, Beckman Instruments, Inc., Stanford Industrial Park, Palo Alto, California.

Physical Tolerance. Physical tolerance was increased in 57 patients. On close questioning they stated that they were able to walk longer distances and perform arduous physical tasks without tiring. All 94 patients claimed a sense of well-being and stated that they were no longer apprehensive of their heart disease.

Objective Improvement. The control physical fitness was a mean of 3.6 calorie/min; after two years of training the physical fitness rose to 4.2 calorie/min.

ECG Changes. The electrocardiogram was remarkably stable. In 88 patients it did not show any appreciable changes as compared to the control tracing. In 6 patients, however, the ECG showed marked improvement with return of the tracing to normal limits. It should be stated, however, that spontaneous ECG improvement in the course of years can be seen without the use of graded exercise.

DISCUSSION

Ischemic heart disease is the major cause of morbidity and mortality in modern sedentary society.

Among other causes of ischemic heart disease, it is natural to inquire into the connection between physical activity and the frequency of its occurrence. Many authors who have studied the influence of hard physical work on the development of ischemic heart disease concluded that exercise has a beneficial effect and prevents, to some extent, against its development (6–9). Eckstein, in an ingenious experimental study on dogs, confirmed that physical activity favors the development of coronary anastomoses (10). As a direct corollary to this beneficial effect of exercise on the coronary circulation, it was postulated that graded exercise training may be used clinically. The use of graded exercise in patients with ischemic heart disease in order to improve their physical fitness and cardiac status is relatively new and most clinicians are not yet ready to accept it into the therapeutic armamentarium until there is more evidence that graded exercise training really helps these patients and actually improves their physical status without causing any harm in the long run.

It must be recognized, however, that the graded exercise must be used persistently in the form of prolonged training, advancing the patient from one group of calisthenics to a harder one according to the results of careful physical examination and ergometric studies.

As we noted in our results, the most significant achievement was the psychological improvement. All patients who participated stressed a remarkable sense of well-being. It was most probably related to the relief of anxiety and fear of the disease.

Several conclusions may be drawn from this study. The cardiac patients with previous infarction or with anginal syndrome can perform physical work and can safely participate in graded exercise training.

Further work is required to clarify whether the use of such training programs actually improves the cardiac output, the coronary flow, and the metabolism of the heart muscle, and thus prolongs life expectancy, or if improvement of physical fitness is due only to relief of anxiety and other psychological causes.

SUMMARY

One hundred patients with ischemic heart disease participated for a period of two years in a training program utilizing graded work levels, consisting of specially prepared series of calisthenics. Only 4 patients showed adverse effects and were excluded from the study. Two patients died at home. The remaining 94 patients who followed the prescribed training improved significantly. The physical fitness rose from 3.6 calorie/min. to 4.2 calorie/min. The severity of anginal pain diminished. The physical tolerance of 57 patients improved subjectively and they were able to participate in long and arduous hikes. The ECG in 88 patients was stable while in 6 patients it reverted to within normal limits.

It is concluded that graded exercise training programs are safe for selected patients with ischemic heart disease.

REFERENCES

1. HELLERSTEIN, H. K., HIRSCH, E. Z., CUMLER, W., ALLEN, L., POLSTER, S., and ZUCKER, N.: Reconditioning of the coronary patient; a preliminary report. *Coronary Heart Disease.* Likoff, W., and Moyer, J. H., Ed. New York, Grune and Stratton, Inc., 1963, p. 448.
2. HELLERSTEIN, H. K.: Assessment of work capacity of cardiovascular patients. Scientific approach to the training of patients with cardiovascular disease for work. *WHO Expert Committee on the Rehabilitation of Patients with Cardiovascular Disease,* Agenda item No. III, 3a and c, July, 1963.
3. HELLERSTEIN, H. K., and FORD, A. B.: Comprehensive care of the coronary patient. *Circulation,* 22:1160, 1960.
4. LAURIE, W., and WOODS, J. D.: Coronary interarterial anastomoses. *Amer Heart J,* 65:579, 1963.
5. DOBELN, W. VON: A simple bicycle ergometer. *J Appl Physiol,* 7:222, 1954.
6. MORRIS, J. N., and CRAWFORD, M.: Coronary heart disease and physical activity of work. *Brit Med J,* 2:1485, 1958.
7. MORRIS, J. N., HEADY, J., and RAFFLE, P.: Physique of London busmen. *Lancet,* 2:569, 1956.
8. BRUNNER, D., and MANELIS, G.: Myocardial infarction among members of communal settlements in Israel. *Lancet,* 2:1049, 1960.
9. SKINNER, J. S., HOLLOSZY, J. O., and CURETON, T. K.: Effects of a program of endurance exercises on physical work capacity and anthropometric measurements of fifteen middle-aged men. *Amer J Cardiol,* 14:747, 1964.
10. ECKSTEIN, R.: Effect of exercise and coronary artery narrowing on coronary collateral circulation. *Circ Res,* 5:230, 1957.

Chapter XLIV

INTERVAL TRAINING IN CARDIOVASCULAR DISEASES

VOJIN SMODLAKA

(New York, New York, U.S.A.)

IN THE last decade the spotlight has been turned on the rehabilitation of cardiac patients and the preventive reconditioning of prepatients. After Oertel's pioneering work (1), various reconditioning techniques have been employed, mostly consisting of continuous exercise, such as walking on different levels and inclines, calisthenics, cycling and swimming.

About 20 years ago, Zatopek, the famed Czech endurance runner, developed the method of interval training by alternating short periods of running and resting (2, 3, 4).

Interval training for patients was introduced only several years ago (5, 6, 7, 8) with good results achieved in convalescents from cardiac surgery, cases of neurocirculatory asthenia, healed myocardiac infarction, arteriosclerotic heart disease, and juvenile hypertension.

EFFECT ON HEART RATE

Karrasch (9) was the first to study the behavior of the heart rate during interval exercise in normal subjects. Figure 44–1 shows three tests performed by a subject working on a bicycle ergometer at the rate of 20 kgm/sec for 5 minutes during which the heart rate rose to 140 beats per minute. After 7.5 minutes rest he worked for another 6 minutes and the heart rate rose to 165. After this (a total of 11-minutes work, amounting to 12,000 kgm), the subject was exhausted.

During a second session he did a total of 28,800 kgm of work, divided into 12 two-minute periods of exercise, with rest periods of 3 minutes each inbetween. Following the last working period the heart rate was 160 beats per minute and the subject was again exhausted.

In the third session the same amount of work was performed as in the second, but it was divided into 48 working periods of 30 seconds each, with 48 seconds rest periods inbetween. This time, again after a total of 28,800 kgm the heart rate remained below 100 and the subject was not exhausted.

Similar reactions were observed by us (10) (e.g., in a subject who worked on a bicycle ergometer for one-half minute periods with one minute resting inbetween). He started with 3.5 kgm/sec the first day and gradually increased his work load until a maximum of 20 kgm/sec was reached. His heart rate increased depending on the work load, but the peaks remained at a steady state and always on a relatively low level, with the maximal heart rates on 7 successive days being 125, 110, 106, 106, 96, 92, and 92.

Another example concerns an elderly

man with a healed myocardial infarction and a history of arteriosclerotic gangrene. During 25 exercise periods of 1 minute each and one-half minute resting periods each at 2 kgm/sec to a total load of 3,100 kgm and work time of 25 minutes, his rate remained below 98 beats per minute. On the next day he exercised continuously with the same load per second and was exhausted after only 8 minutes at a peak heart rate of 122 (10).

Thus it is possible by the interval training method to perform large amounts of work with minimum exertion and at a relatively low heart rate.

OXYGEN INTAKE AND CARBON DIOXIDE OUTPUT

The oxygen intake and carbon dioxide output of normal young adults during interval training was found increased during short but lengthening work periods, and gradually rose also somewhat during the equally long resting intervals (11, 12). Maximum oxygen intake during work was reached when the exercise periods exceeded one minute. This made work periods of less than 60 seconds appear more rational.

STROKE VOLUME, HEART VOLUME, AND OXYGEN PULSE

Nöcker et al. (19) concluded from the ballistocardiogram that the stroke volume was greatest at termination of work periods and during the beginning of the subsequent rest periods. Reindell et al. (4), using the Flack principle, and Schneider et al. (20), using a similar method, found maximal stroke volumes during rest periods only when the working heart rates had reached 120 to 140 in normal adults. This phenomenon is ascribed to

a work-induced temporary lowering of the peripheral resistance.

Hollmann (21) recommends limitation of the individual work periods to 1½ minutes because of the occurrence of capillary constriction in the muscles after 3 to 4 minutes of exercise.

According to Reindell et al. (4), an augmented stroke volume represents the main stimulus for an enlargement of the systolic capacity of the heart and the increases of the stroke volume during the resting intervals appeared to serve as a factor contributing to enlargement of the heart as manifested by myocardial hypertrophy. An increase of the heart volume takes place both during conventional and interval training (4, 8).

The oxygen pulse (oxygen uptake per heart beat) was found to be highest during the first 30 to 40 seconds of the resting intervals owing to the augmented stroke volume of that phase.

WORK LOAD, DURATION AND NUMBER OF INTERVALS

During work periods the load was kept submaximal, not exceeding 80 per cent of the subjects' maximal work capacity. Mellerowicz et al. (23) have shown that 25 per cent of the latter suffices in normal young people to attain the same level of training as exercising with maximal work loads, although it requires longer periods of time. An augmentation of muscular strength can be achieved by isometric exercises with less than 30 per cent of maximal work capacity (24, 25).

Paul D. White points out the need for investigations concerning the work capacity of cardiacs (26). While in normal adults the duration of intervals is usually kept between ½ and 1½ minutes (4, 5, 21, 22), we used in cardiacs work

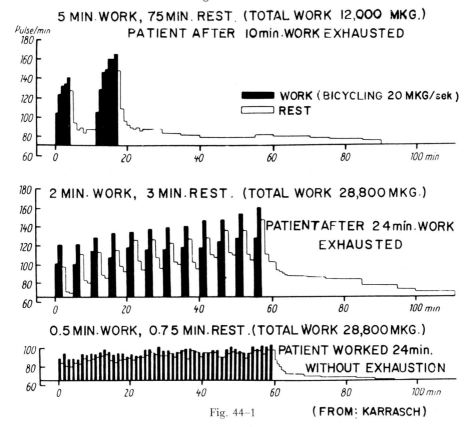

Fig. 44–1 (FROM: KARRASCH)

periods of ½ to 1 minute and longer resting intervals (5, 7).

Depending on the physical condition of the subject, training programs are begun with small numbers of work-rest cycles (e.g., 5 to 10), which are then increased by one or two at each session. For healthy athletes the full training sessions were extended to one or two hours. For elderly persons and cardiacs their length was limited to a maximum of 45 minutes (4, 6).

LENGTH OF RECONDITIONING PERIODS

In normal individuals it is possible to double the work capacity within 20 weeks of daily training. After 40 weeks of training the gains in work capacity proved more stable and could be main-

tained at a 75 per cent level up to 70 weeks following discontinuation of training (22).

In cardiac patients, the training has to be carried out at a slower pace. With training sessions only three times a week and with work loads of only one-third or one-half of maximal working capacity, adequate results may, in our experience (4, 6, 7), be expected within 3 months. This question is being further investigated.

Studies of strength development by isometric exercises have revealed a drop of strength gains from a maximum of 100 per cent to 80, 60 and 40 per cent, respectively, when the number of training sessions per week was reduced from 6 to 3, 2 and 1 (24, 25).

In athletic training it has been observed that short exercise periods with heavy loads and long resting intervals favor primarily the building-up of strength, whereas long exercise periods with low work loads and short resting intervals are more apt to develop endurance.

Hettinger (24, 25) has emphasized that the degree to which an individual may forseeably be trained cannot be predicted until at least 4 to 6 weeks of daily training have elapsed. This rule requires, however, certain modifications in the case of cardiacs and precardiacs.

PRETESTING OF CARDIACS BEFORE TRAINING

The patient works in recumbent position using a bicycle ergometer, starting with a work load of 0.5 kgm/sec during 30 seconds, followed by 60 seconds of rest. After each work-rest cycle the load is augmented by 0.5 kgm/sec until the patient displays a high heart rate and feels exhausted. Heart rate and electrocardiogram are recorded by means of telemetry at the end of exercise and rest periods.

On this basis increasing loads of muscular work can be safely imposed on the patient without unduly over-straining the cardiovascular and respiratory systems (27). The fact that older workers, despite a reduced capacity for oxygen intake, often remain active in physically strenuous jobs, such as forestry and farming, seems to be due to their instinctive choice of alternating timing of work and rest (18).

RECONDITIONING PROGRAMS FOR CARDIACS

After clinical examination and performance of the above-described introduc-

tory test (plus spirometry), each patient is subjected to standard spiroergometric test procedures preceding and following training periods. The patient lying in supine position is provided with a breathing mask and connected with a basal metabolism tester*, RQ Meter†, and telemetric electrocardiograph.‡ After 3 minutes rest, he pedals continuously for 5 or 6 minutes on the bicycle ergometer, then rests again for 6 minutes. Throughout the test, the ventilation per minute, oxygen and carbon dioxide in the expired air, and heart rate are recorded for each minute. From these data the oxygen uptake and carbon dioxide production in cc/min, the respiratory quotient, the ventilatory equivalent, and the oxygen pulse are calculated.

Using one of several types of ergometers,¶ the patient starts with 0.5, 1, 2 or 3 kgm/sec of work, depending on heart rate, and the load is slowly increased to higher levels. Initially 3 to 6 short exercise periods are carried out and their number is increased by 1 or 2 periods in each training session. Ordinarily the optimal number of 25 to 30 work-rest cycles per training session is reached within 10 to 12 sessions.

Ten patients with neurocirculatory asthenia exercised 3 times a week for 6 weeks. The first interval training session started with 3 work periods of ½ minute each and 1 minute rest. The number of work periods was gradually increased to 30 per session. Like in normal subjects,

---

*Hartmann-Braun, A.G., Frankfurt/Main.

†Instrumentation Association, Inc., New York, New York.

‡Telemedics, Southampton, Pennsylvania. Medical System Corporation, Great Neck, Long Island.

¶Dargatz, Hamburg; Richard Lauckner, Berlin Tempelhof; Joseph B. Wolffe, Norristown, Pennsylvania; Lode, Groningen.

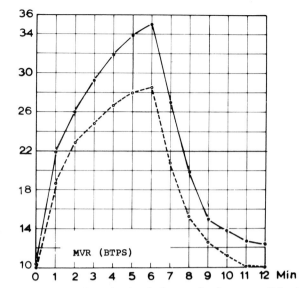

Figure 44–2 Minute volume of respiration before and after reconditioning of a group of of young subjects with neurocirculatory asthenia. (*Before—solid line; after—dotted line.*)

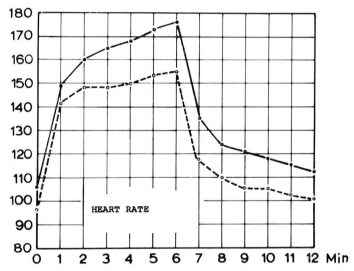

Figure 44–3. Heart rate of a group of subjects with neurocirculatory asthenia before and after reconditioning by interval training. (*Before—solid line; after—dotted line.*)

the respiratory minute volume (Fig. 44–2), the heart rate per minute (Fig. 44–3) and the ventilatory equivalent (Fig. 44–4) decreased significantly.

A group of patients who had undergone cardiac surgery (5, 6, 7) (Fig. 44–5) and a group of patients with healed myocardial infarctions (unpublished) reacted in the same fashion.

Mellerowicz (23) has summarized from the literature the character of work done by sportsmen at different types of sports activity (Table 44–I), as expressed in ergometer work equivalents. From these

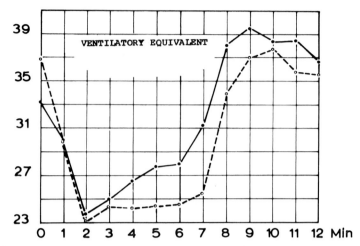

Figure 44–4. Ventilatory equivalent in a group of young subjects with neurocirculatory asthenia before and after reconditioning by interval training. (*Before—solid line; after—dotted line.*)

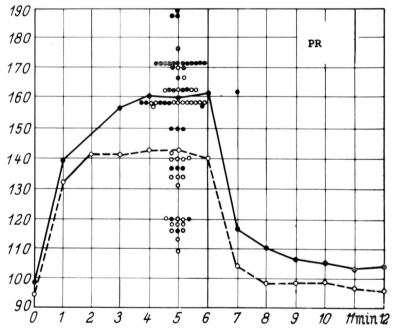

Figure 44–5. Heart rate of a group of patients after cardiac surgery before and after reconditioning by interval training. (*Before—solid line and black discs; after—dotted line and white discs.*)

data it appears possible to substitute various athletic disciplines for ergometer work and to use short periods of sports activities with appropriate interruptions in practical reconditioning programs, such as walking, running, and swimming.

Contraindications against physical training in cardiovascular patients in-

TABLE 44-I

Type of Movement	Speed		O_2 Consumption in cc kg and m	O_2 Consumption in cc 70 kg/min	Watt Equivalent Ergometer	MVR Liters
	m/min	km/h				
Walking	70	4.2	0.104	510	25–30	15
Liljestrand and Stenstrom	90	5.4	0.123	778	40	20
	115	6.9	0.162	1340	90–110	33
Running	150	9.0	0.191	2000	180–210	40
Liljestrand and Stenstrom	200	12.0	0.161	2250	200–240	48
	250	15.0	0.148	2630	250–280	70
Skiing	120	7.2	0.191	1600	130–150	30
Liljestrand and Stenstrom	150	9.0	0.183	1900	160–190	36
	250	12.0	0.175	2450	230–260	65
Bicycling	150	9.0	0.058	620	30	19
Zuntz	250	15.0	0.061	1060	60–80	25
	350	21.0	0.076	1860	150–180	38
Swimming	20	1.2	0.584	825	50	18
Liljestrand and Stenstrom	30	1.8	0.602	1290	80–100	27
	50	3.0	0.652	2290	210–240	46
Rowing with Fixed Seat	50	3.0	0.177	625	30	15
Liljestrand and Stenstrom	70	4.2	0.244	1250	70–90	25
	90	5.4	0.328	2060	180–210	52
Rowing with Moving Seat	50	3.0	0.123	430	20–30	14
Ewig	75	4.5	0.158	835	50	27
	100	6.0	0.219	1540	130–150	43
Kayak	75	4.5	0.062	360	20	14
Wohlfeil	125	7.5	0.198	1640	130–150	64

clude the following: Congestive heart failure or borderline cardiac decompensation; angina pectoris at rest; fresh myocardial infarction; uncontrolled arrhythmias and attacks of tachycardia; extrasystoles, bundle branch block, paroxysmal tachycardia, and auricular fibrillation occurring during exercise; S-T changes of the electrocardiogram or accentuations of preexisting S-T displacements occurring during exercise; bacterial endocarditis; excessive cardiac acceleration (130 to 170) during exercise; recent pulmonary embolism; fatigue, shortness of breath, cyanosis and fainting.

SUMMARY

Interval training is indicated in the physical reconditioning of prepatients and in patients with cardiovascular diseases (except for certain contraindications). It produces demonstrable beneficial effects on the cardiovascular and respiratory systems and increases work capacity.

At the outset, the baseline condition of reconditioning candidates must be evaluated by means of a spiroergometric test.

The recommended duration of individual work periods is one-half to one minute each with interpolated rest periods of about equal length.

The number of work periods per session (in 2 to 6 sessions per week) is gradually increased from 3 to 30 with a total training period of several months.

The work load is gradually increased from 0.5 to 10 kgm/sec and more for each individual work period.

The heart rate at termination of each work period is a practical, simple and adequate criterion of the training effects achieved and of the indication for or counterindication against further work augmentations.

REFERENCES

1. OERTEL, quoted by Atzler, E.: *Körper und Arbeit*. Leipzig, Thieme Verlag, 1927.
2. KOZIK, F.: *Der Marathonsieger Emil Zatopek*. Prague, Artia Verlag, 1953.
3. NETT, T.: *Die Entwicklung der Trainingsmethoden im Mittel-und Langstreckenlauf*. IV. International Congress, Track and Field Coaches Assn., (ITFCA.) Duisburg, Germany, March, 1964.
4. REINDELL, H., ROSKAMM, H., and GERSCHLER, W.: *Das Intervalltraining*. Munich, Johann Ambrosius Barth, 1962.
5. SMODLAKA, V.: *Untersuchungen uber das ergometrisch dosierte Intervalltraining nach Herzoperationen*. Doctor's Thesis, Berlin, Freie Universitat, 1960.
6. SMODLAKA, V.: Interval training in heart disease. *J Sport Med*, 3:93, 1963.
7. SMODLAKA, V., JANKOVIC, M., MELLEROWICZ, H., NEUHAS, G., PAEPER, H., and SCHMUTZLER, H.: Das ergometrisch dosierte Intervalltraining nach Herzoperationen. *Z Kreislaufforsch*, 51:152, 1962.
8. REINDELL, H., *et al.*: *Herz, Kreislaufkrankheiten und Sport*. Munich, Johann Ambrosius Barth, 1960.
9. KARRASCH, K.: Grundriss der Biologie der Leibesübungen, quoted by Nöcker, J., ed. Sportverlag, Berlin, 1959.
10. SMODLAKA, V., TRAINOR, F., SOKOLOW, J., and DACSO, M.: Interval training in rehabilitation of the amputee. Amer. Congress of Phys. Med. and Rehab., 43rd Annual Session, Philadelphia, August 22–27, 1965.
11. v. GOOR, H., and MOSTERD, W. L.: Gas exchange during and after muscular work. *Kon Ned Akad Wetensch, Amsterdam*, 64:96, 1961.
12. v. GOOR, H., and MOSTERD, W. L.: Gas exchange during interval training. *Kon Ned Akad Wetensch, Amsterdam*, 64:15, 1961.
13. CHRISTENSEN, E. H.: Zum Problem: Pause-Erholung, Sportliche Dauerleistung und Intervalltraining. Verhandlgn. 18. *Deutsch Sportärztekongr*, Hamburg, 1957, Frankfurt a/M, 1957.
14. CHRISTENSEN, E. H.: Intervallarbeit und Intervalltraining. *Int Z Angew Physiol*, 18:345, 1960.
15. CHRISTENSEN, E. H., HEDMAN, R., and HOLMDAHL, I.: The influence of rest pauses on mechanical efficiency. *Acta Physiol Scand*, 48:443, 1960.
16. CHRISTENSEN, E. H., HEDMAN, R., and SALTIN, B.: Intermittent and continuous running. (A further contribution to the physiology of intermittent work.) *Acta Physiol Scand*, 50:269, 1960.
17. ROSSKAMM, H., REINDELL, H., and KEUL, J.: Zur Frage der Pausenwirkung des Intervalltrainings. *Sportarzt*, 12:170, 1960.
18. ÅSTRAND, I., ÅSTRAND, P. O., CHRISTENSEN, E. H., and HEDMANN, R.: Intermittent muscular work. *Acta Physiol Scand*, 48:448, 1960.
19. NÖCKER, J., *et al.*: Der Sauerstoffpuls in Abhängigkeit vom Lebensalter. *Ver Deutsch Ges Kreislaufforsch*, 24:225, 1958.
20. SCHNEIDER, K. W., and GATTENLÖHNER, W.: Hämodynamischer Beitrag zu den physiologischen Grundlagen des Intervalltrainings. *Arch Kreislaufforsch*, 46:114, 1965.
21. HOLLMANN, W., VALENTIN, H., and VENRATH, H.: Ueber wissenschaftliche Grundlagen des Intervalltrainings. *Sportmed*, 8:204, 1958.
22. NÖCKER, J.: Grundriss der Biologie der Körperübungen. *Sportverlag*, Berlin, 1959.
23. MELLEROWICZ, H., MELLER, W., and MÜLLER, J.: Vergleichende Untersuchungen über Leistungssteigerung durch Intervalltraining und Dauertraining (bei gleicher Trainingsarbeit). *Int Z Angew Physiol*, 18:376, 1961.
24. HETTINGER, T.: Zur Physiologie des Muskeltrainings. *Sportmed*, 7:237, 1956.
25. HETTINGER, T.: *Physiology of Strength*. Springfield, Thomas.
26. WHITE, P. D., RUSK, H., WILLIAMS, B., and LEE, P.: *Cardiovascular Rehabilitation*. New York, McGraw-Hill Book Co., 1957.
27. CHRISTENSEN, H.: Neue Forschungsresultate auf dem Gebiet der Sportmedizin. Intervallarbeit. *Sportarzt*, 6:147, 1961.

Chapter XLV

THE HYPOTENSIVE EFFECT OF PHYSICAL ACTIVITY IN HYPERTENSIVE SUBJECTS

JIŘÍ A. KRÁL, JOSEF CHRÁSTEK, and JIŘINA ADAMÍROVÁ

(Prague, Czechoslovakia)

PHYSICAL activity is in general accompanied by a "catabolic" phase, followed by an "anabolic" phase. This rule applies also to the blood pressure. The present study concerns its behavior in hypertensive, as compared with normotensive, individuals.

A fall of the systolic blood pressure (1) and, to a lesser extent and less regularly, also of the diastolic pressure has often been observed after short, as well as prolonged physical exercise (2), both in the upper and lower extremities (3). This phenomenon is ascribed to a more or less protracted reduction in peripheral vascular resistance (4), induced by muscular exercise.

In men and women, physical training has also been found to lower the blood pressure (1, 5). Unusually low blood pressure levels (below 100/60 mm Hg) occur relatively frequently in athletes (6, 7). In top athletes they are more common than in sportsmen of lower performance (7). The average blood pressure levels recorded in 107 well-trained German sportsmen were lower than in comparable groups of the general population (8). Particularly low readings were obtained in gymnasts, basketball players and swimmers (6).

In hypertensive subjects, the post-exercise fall of the blood pressure is usually more marked than in normal ones. This is equally true for individuals with labile and with fixed hypertension (2, 9–21). Here, too, a diminution of the total peripheral resistance seems to be responsible (18).

In juvenile vascular hyperreactors, the pressor reaction to a 3-minute run was found reduced after a 7-day ski training (22).

Remedial exercises, combined with physio- and climatotherapy seem to counteract the hypertensive state through their influence on the central nervous system (6, 10, 16, 23) and, thus, to exert their apparent preventive effect (9).

SUBJECT MATERIAL

Our subject material consisted of (a) juvenile labile hypertensives (24) (age 19 to 29 years, with pressure readings from 150 mm systolic and/or from 80 mm diastolic pressure up), including cases of the first stage, according to the classification of Vančura (25); (b) patients with essential hypertension (age 50 to 60 years, with pressure readings from 180mm systolic and/or 110 mm diastolic pressure up, having persisted for at least 10 years). All medications were discontinued before testing.

TABLE 45–I

MEAN SYSTOLIC AND DIASTOLIC BLOOD PRESSURE AND PULSE RATE
AFTER 20 KNEE-BENDS WITHIN 30 SECONDS IN 15 SUBJECTS WITH
JUVENILE HYPERTENSION

Number of Subjects 15	*Systolic Pressure*		*Diastolic Pressure*		*Pulse Rate*		
	$\bar{x}$	σ	$\bar{x}$	σ	$\bar{x}/10\ sec$	σ	$\bar{x}/1\ min$
Before	145	11,6	88	6,5	13	5,2	(78)
After:Immediate	180	13,5	88	9,6	21	6,8	(126)
1′	158	10,2	84	6,0	15	6,2	(90)
2′	149	7,6	84	5,5	14	7,2	(84)
3′	145	7,4	83	6,2	13	6,1	(78)
4′	139	8,5	83	5,1	13	4,7	(78)
5′	138	8,0	85	4,1	13	5,8	(78)
6′	133	3,0	83	5,8	13	2,5	(78)
7′	136	7,8	81	5,5	13	6,8	(78)
Difference of BP before and after exercise	−12		−7				

TABLE 45–II

MEAN SYSTOLIC AND DIASTOLIC BLOOD PRESSURE AND PULSE RATE
AFTER 3-MINUTE RUN IN 21 SUBJECTS WITH JUVENILE HYPERTENSION

No. of Subjects 21	*Systolic Pressure*		*Diastolic Pressure*		*Pulse Rate*		
	$\bar{x}$	σ	$\bar{x}$	σ	$\bar{x}/10\ sec$	σ	$\bar{x}/1\ min$
Before	143	14,0	90	7,7	14	5,8	(84)
After:Immediate	196	20,1	86	9,9	26	6,5	(156)
1′	169	15,5	81	19,6	20	10,3	(120)
3′	154	14,6	84	15,6	18	8,3	(108)
4′	147	13,3	85	12,2	17	8,0	(102)
5′	136	12,1	85	8,8	16	7,1	(96)
7′	133	12,8	86	8,9	16	6,8	(96)
10′	130	11,6	87	7,1	16	6,6	(96)
Difference of BP before and after exercise	−13		−3				

TESTS IN LABORATORY AND GYMNASIUM

Pachon - Martinet's Test: 20 Knee Bends Within 30 Seconds. Fifteen juvenile subjects with labile hypertension (Table 45–I). The mean resting systolic pressure (145±11.6 mm) decreased after effort by 12 mm; the mean resting diastolic pressure (88 ± 6.5 mm) decreased by 7 mm.

Three-Minute Run In Place (180 Steps Per Minute). Twenty-one juvenile hypertensives (Table 45–II). The mean resting systolic pressure (143 ± 14 mm)

decreased after effort by 13 mm, the mean resting diastolic pressure (90 ± 7.7 mm) by 3 mm Hg.

Step Test (5 Minutes, 6112.5 KPM). In a 42-year-old man with second stage hypertension of more than 10 years standing, with normal body weight and in excellent physical training, the step test was followed by a significant drop of the systolic and diastolic blood pressure (Fig. 45–1).

Standing Up and Sitting Down. Some older patients with arthritic conditions and unable to carry out the pre-

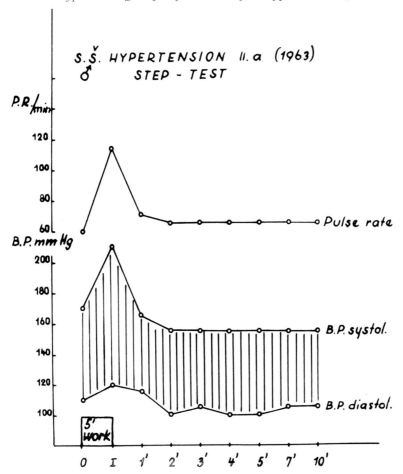

Figure 45–1. Changes of blood pressure and pulse rate after the Harvard step-up test in a patient with hypertension of stage II^a.

TABLE 45–III

No. of Subjects 12	Systolic Pressure $\bar{x}$	σ	Diastolic Pressure $\bar{x}$	σ	Pulse Rate $\bar{x}$	σ
Before	168,7	28,89	100,8	11,27	68,5	7,48
Immediately	205,8	27,03	100,4	9,43	130,5	16,40
After: 1'	184,5	24,21	97,5	9,89	91,00	13,52
2'	171,0	19,42	97,5	10,09	79,0	9,27
3'	158,7	12,61	98,3	9,38	76,1	8,49
Difference of BP before and after the effort	−10,0		−2,5			

viously mentioned exercises were subjected to a test devised by us (17) which consisted in standing up from and sitting down on a chair (45 cm high) once every 2 seconds during a total of 5 minutes.

Figure 45–2 shows the reaction of a 54-year-old patient with fixed hypertension (II^b stage) who also complained of anginal symptoms in cold weather.
The entire group of 12 subjects with

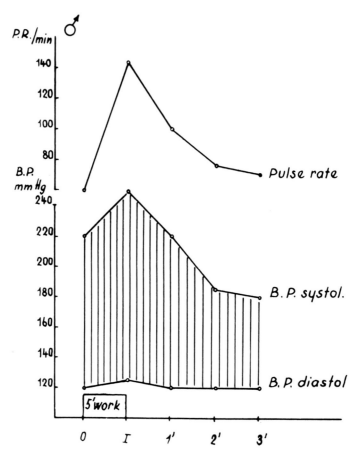

Figure 45–2. Changes of blood pressure and pulse rate after 5 minutes standing-up and sitting-down test in a patient with hypertension of stage II[a].

a mean resting pressure of 168.7 ± 28.9 mm systolic and 100.8 ± 11.27 mm diastolic, showed after effort a mean pressure fall of 10.0 mm systolic and 2.5 mm diastolic (Table 45–III).

Exercises in the Gymnasium. Nine juvenile hypertensives and 12 comparable control subjects carried out an intermittent and increasingly strenuous exercise program in a gymnasium (total: 25 minutes of actual effort) consisting of exercises (a) on rings, (b) on parallel bars, and (c) running over obstacles. Figure 45–3

shows the results. Fifteen minutes after termination of the various types of exercise, the systolic pressure was lowered considerably more in the hypertensives than in the control subjects. Changes of the diastolic pressure were less regular and of a minor degree.

TESTS IN A CHANGED ENVIRONMENT

In order to study the effect on the blood pressure of exercises more resembling those of recreational physical ac-

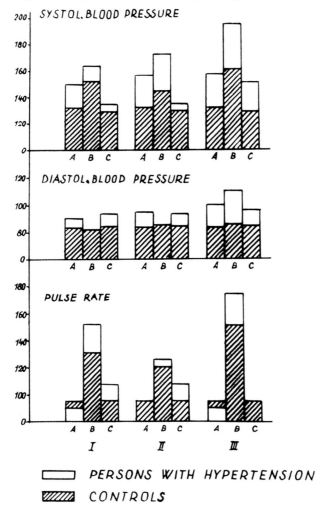

Figure 45–3. Blood pressure and pulse rate before (A), immediately (B), and 15 minutes (C) after three types of exercises (rings, parallel bars, run over obstacles) in 9 juvenile hypertensive and 12 control subjects.

tivities, tests were carried out in hypertensive subjects before, during, and after swimming, winter touring in the mountains, and ski training.

Swimming. During swimming, the horizontal position of the body, as well as the temperature factor, modify the circulatory reactions. Contact of the skin with the cool water increases the peripheral vascular resistance of hypertensive individuals, as observed in cold tests (26, 27).

Twenty-eight students (age 18 to 25 years) with labile hypertension swam for 55 minutes in a pool (water temperature, 22 to 25 °C; air temperature, 24 to 28 °C). Ten normal students of the same age group served as controls.

As shown in Table 45–IV, the systolic pressure, 15 to 20 minutes after swimming, was lowered more distinctly in the hypertensives than in the normotensive subjects. The diastolic pressure

TABLE 45–IV

CHANGES OF SYSTOLIC AND DIASTOLIC BLOOD PRESSURE AND
OF PULSE RATE AFTER A 55-MINUTE SWIM-TRAINING

| | Juvenile Hypertension (n = 28) | | | | | | Control Group (n = 10) | | | | | |
| | Systolic Pressure | | Diastolic Pressure | | Pulse Rate | | Systolic Pressure | | Diastolic Pressure | | Pulse Rate | |
	$\bar{x}$	σ	$\bar{x}$	σ	$\bar{x}$	σ	$\bar{x}$	σ	$\bar{x}$	σ	$\bar{x}$	σ
Before swimming	158,3	10,05	96,0	10,90	80,0	8,36	125,0	11,20	70,50	12,30	86,0	7,60
Immediately after	167,4	11,09	101,0	11,80	102,0	6,32	138,0	10,60	86,50	12,60	98,0	11,70
15–20′ later	148,0	12,49	90,0	10,67	89,0	13,03	122,5	12,60	82,50	11,40	77,0	7,30
Difference of BP	−10,3		−6,0				−2,5		+12,0			

TABLE 45–V

SYSTOLIC AND DIASTOLIC PRESSURE AND PULSE RATE IN 14 SUBJECTS WITH
JUVENILE HYPERTENSION DURING A 7-DAYS SKI-TRAINING IN THE MOUNTAINS

| Number of Subjects 14 | Prague | | 1st Day | | Significance of the Difference | 7th Day | | Significance of the Difference |
	$\bar{x}$	σ	$\bar{x}$	σ		$\bar{x}$	σ	
Systolic pressure	156	±6,9	144	±11	p>0,01	126	+11	p>0,01
Diastolic pressure	96	+5,0	95	±7	0	89	±4	p>0,05
Pulse rate	83	±9,4	77	±16	0	69	±13	0

was also decreased in the hypertensives but remained elevated in the controls.

Winter Touring and Skiing of Juvenile Hypertensives.

Observations were made on 50 students in 4 separate groups, at an altitude of 1000 meters (3,279 ft) during 7-day periods.

The exercise program consisted of 3 hours walking and/or ski training in the forenoon, and 2½ hours in the afternoon. Blood pressure measurements were taken (a) early in the morning; (b) 10 to 20 minutes after return from the forenoon occupation; (c) following the early afternoon rest period; (d) 10 to 20 minutes after return from the afternoon occupation, and (e) between 9:30 and 10:00 pm. We were aware of the fact that under the conditions of these tests, both the element of physical exertion per se, and psychological-environmental factors had to be taken into account in the interpretation of the results.

As shown in Table 45–V, which represents one group of 14 subjects, a reduction of systolic and diastolic blood pressure was noticeable already on the first day in the mountains, as compared with the readings previously obtained in Prague. This initial change was obviously due to the environmental differences. However, on the seventh day, a further, statistically significant decline of the above-mentioned parameters was noted in which the elements of environment and training were presumably jointly involved. Similar results were recorded in the other groups.

Details of Figure 45–4 appear of interest insofar as by contrast with the preceding days of training, on the fourth day, which was entirely devoted to rest, the evening blood pressure levels were higher than those observed in the morning. Similarly, on the fifth day, the pressure levels were lowered after the forenoon training, but during the afternoon, which was again spent in the hotel, there was a renewed rise.

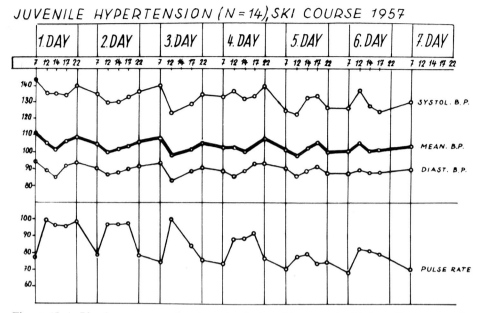

Figure 45–4. Blood pressure and pulse rate during ski course in 14 juvenile hypertensive subjects.

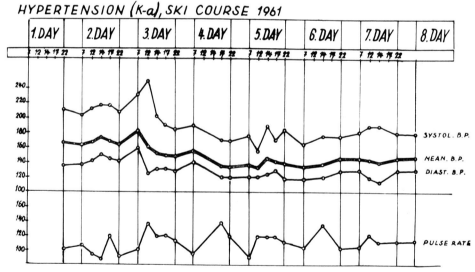

Figure 45–5. Blood pressure and pulse rate of one hypertensive patient who joined a ski course on the third day of his stay in the mountains.

Winter Touring and Skiing of Grade II^a Hypertensives. Twenty-four patients with more advanced hypertensive disease were exposed during wintertime to a similar, although less strenuous, exercise program in the mountains as the preceding group. Measurements were taken in the same sequence. All antihypertensive medication was discontinued 2 weeks before beginning of the experiment.

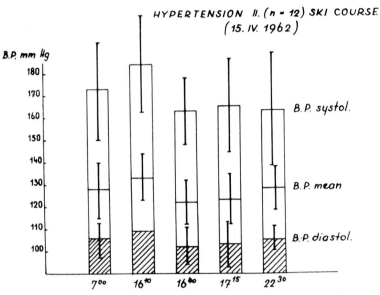

Figure 45–6. Blood pressure changes in a group of 12 hypertensive subjects (stage II) during a day of ski training.

Although a diminution of the blood pressure level did occur in 15 instances, the average end result was statistically not significantly different. However, some importance may be attached to the fact that, despite the abstinence from antihypertensive drugs, not one patient showed an elevation of the blood pressure at termination of the experimental period.

The vasodepressor effect which was noticeable in part of the patients may be exemplified by the case of one man, represented in Figure 45–5. This patient did not participate in the training during the first 2 days, but on the third day he joined the rest of the group. From that day on, a steady reduction of his systolic, diastolic, and mean blood pressure was clearly demonstrable.

A fall of blood pressure occurred also in 13 advanced hypertensives following one 6-hour walking excursion in the snow with two resting pauses, covering 14 km and including an ascent and descent of

400 meters each. The excursion elicited pulse rates of 120 to 140 beats per minute in these older patients (50 to 60 years) while the corresponding heart rates during the same walk were 100 to 130 beats per minute in untrained, and 100 to 120 beats per minute in well-trained controls.

Figure 45–6 shows the blood pressure measurement of 12 hypertensive patients before, during, and after a walk and ascent in the snow. Both systolic and diastolic pressure were lowered.

Another group of 13 fixed hypertensives (stage II-a) was subjected to a more prolonged training program at a lower sea level (Františkovy Lázně), consisting of 5 to 6-hour daily walks during 18 days (again without antihypertensive premedication for 2 weeks). In 9 of these cases (Fig. 45–7), both blood pressure levels were diminished immediately upon arrival at the spa due to environmental influences, and were further reduced during the entire stay (b, c), only to

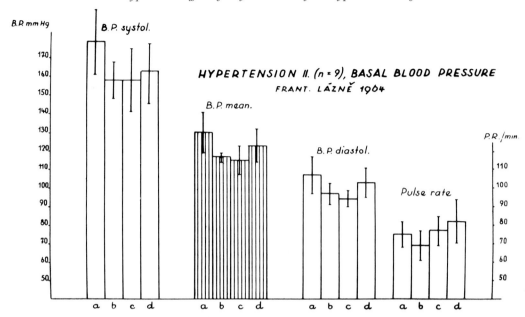

Figure 45–7. The basal (morning) systolic, mean, and diastolic blood pressure and pulse rate of 9 hypertensive subjects (stage II), taken (a) before departure from Prague, (b) on the first day at a spa (Františkovy Lázně), (c) on the last (18th) day at the spa, and (d) on the second day after return to the city.

TABLE 45–VI

BLOOD PRESSURE AND PULSE RATE DURING AND AFTER A 95-MINUTE TENNIS
GAME BETWEEN A HYPERTENSIVE SUBJECT (II-a) AND A HEALTHY CONTROL

	Hypertensive Subject			Control		
	Blood Pressure		Heart	Blood Pressure		Heart
	Systolic	Diastolic	Rate	Systolic	Diastolic	Rate
Before	220	140	72	125	75	78
During the game highest values	235	130	144	160	85	144
After the end:				ǀ		
0′	210	130	198	140	70	174
1′	185	130	126	120	80	144
2′	180	135	120	120	80	114
3′	170	125	114	125	80	96
4′	175	120	114	120	80	108
5′	170	120	108	110	80	90
10′	155	130	96	120	90	108
20′	145	115	90	110	90	90
40′	160	120	102	115	85	90
Difference of BP before and after exercise	−75	−25		−15	+5	

return to near pretraining levels after return to the city (Prague) (d). In the 4 remaining cases, no change of the blood pressure was observed.

COMPETITIVE SPORT

The influence of a competitive sport performance on the blood pressure was tested in a 42-year-old trained sportsman

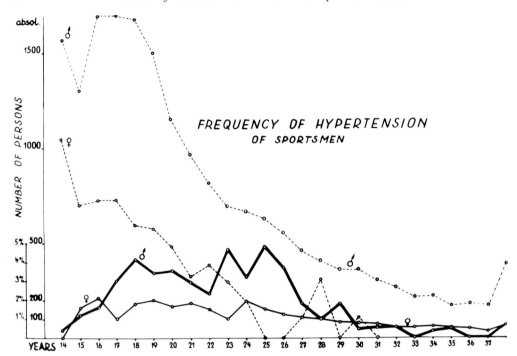

Figure 45–8. The percentual incidence of blood pressure levels higher than 160/100 mm Hg in 27,578 sportsmen (over a period of 30 years), observed in the evening consulting room. (*Dotted lines: absolute numbers of men and women; drawn-out lines: per cent hypertensives per age group.*)

with grade II-a hypertension, who played a game of tennis (95 minutes) against a 37-year-old, equally well-trained normotensive sportsman as control.

Blood pressure and heart rate were determined at 5-minute intervals during the game, and until 40 minutes after its conclusion (Table 45–VI). After the game, the systolic pressure fell in the hypertensive player 75 mm, in the normotensive one only 15 mm. The average diastolic pressure fell 25 mm in the hypertensive, and rose 5 mm (after a transient fall) in the normotensive player.

PREVENTION OF HYPERTENSIVE DISEASE BY REGULAR EXERCISE

As previously reported (23), we found in 31 subjects who had, over at least 30 years, regularly engaged in gymnastics 3 times per week, and whose average age was 62 ± 3.05 years, systolic blood pressure levels ranging from 95 to 190 mm Hg (mean: 141.3 ± 25.7 mm), and diastolic levels only in 3 instances higher than 100 mm Hg (mean: 85.3 ± 13.86 mm).

An overall review of 27,578 sportsmen and sportswomen, studied in our institute over the last 30 years, revealed the fact that, based on the WHO criteria of hypertension (160/100 mm Hg), only 0.884 per cent cases of hypertension were present among sportsmen, and only 0.416 per cent among sportswomen.

Figure 45–8 shows by dotted lines the absolute numbers of sportsmen and sportswomen of rising age categories who were examined. The drawn-out lines represent the incidence of hypertensive individuals in the respective age groups as per cent of the corresponding absolute numbers examined. The percentage declines markedly in the advancing age categories. This may be due, in part, to an increasing withdrawal of hypertensive individuals from sports activities, either upon advice of their physicians or because of ill health. Nevertheless, the trend does at least suggest the possibility that regular physical activity may exert a certain protective influence against the gradual development of hypertensive disease which tends to occur on the basis of a labile hypertension in younger years (7, 28, 29).

DISCUSSION

Hypertension, according to one hypothesis, is being interpreted as a derangement in the vascular adaptation to muscular activity (4, 30).

Under conditions of physical exercise, the peripheral vascular resistance in the skeletal musculature decreases, while that in the splanchnic area, and often in the skin, and possibly also that in the central nervous system, rises.

Simultaneous emotional tension accentuates the pressor effect of physical effort. This is manifested by the higher elevations of the blood pressure during competitive muscular exertions (e.g., competitive running over obstacles as in Fig. 45–3/III).

An acute lowering of the systolic and, to a lesser extent, of the diastolic blood pressure within 15 to 20 minutes after physical exercise was seen in most of our acute exercise tests with a variety of exercises and under different environmental conditions. Interferences of the central nervous system (hypothalamus) (37) were probably involved in these reactions.

The vasodepressor effect of acute physical exertion appeared more pronounced in individuals with juvenile, labile and advanced fixed hypertension than in normotensives.

Prolonged and regularly repeated physical exercise, especially if combined with favorable environmental influences, seems to contribute to a more sustained reduction of the blood pressure levels and, thus, to constitute a valuable factor in the prevention or retardation of hypertensive disease which otherwise often develops on the basis of juvenile, labile hypertension.

As far as cardiac function is concerned, it seems worthy of note that the post-exercise cardiac deceleration within 15 to 20 minutes was much slower and less complete in the hypertensives than in the normotensive groups.

SUMMARY

Acute physical exertion elicits a transient rise of blood pressure (especially the systolic pressure) which is followed by a fall during 15 to 20 minutes. This hypotensive reaction is more pronounced in subjects with juvenile, labile, as well as in those with more advanced, fixed hypertension than in normotensives. It is manifested more distinctly in the systolic than in the diastolic pressure.

The degree of post-exercise hypotension is approximately proportionate to the intensity of the preceding physical effort.

The hypotensive phenomenon was studied under a variety of types and durations of exercise, and in combination with different environmental influences.

Prolonged regular physical activity of hypertensive city dwellers in a changed, mountainous and rural environment, evoked after several days a longer sustained lowering of the blood pressure level. This occurred more regularly in juvenile, labile than in advanced, fixed hypertensives.

All of these observations, as well as the relatively low incidence of hypertensive disease in sportsmen and sportswomen of older age groups, suggest that regular vigorous physical exercise serves as a protective agent against the development and progression of hypertensive disease.

REFERENCES

1. HERXHEIMER, H.: *Grundriss der Sportmedizin.* Leipzig, Thieme, 1933.
2. KOHLRAUSCH, W., and TEIRICH-LEUBE, H.: *Lehrbuch der Krankengymnastik bei inneren Erkrankungen.* Fischer, Jena, 1954.
3. CHRÁSTEK, J., ADAMÍROVÁ, J., and KOPŠÍK, J.: Experiences with juvenile hypertensives in special physical education. *Tělových Sborník,* 6:243, 1961, (Czech).
4. BROD, J.: Hemodynamic basis of acute pressure reaction and hypertension. *Brit Heart J,* 25:227, 1963.
5. KRÁL, J., JONÁŠ, V., and STŘÍTESKÝ, J.: Les relations de l'hypotension artérielle et de la réserve alcaline. *Rev Méd de l'Est,* 57:117, 1929.
6. VOLKOV, N. I.: About the arterial blood pressure level of sportsmen. *Ter Arkh,* 30:65, 1958, (Russian).
7. VOLKOV, N. I.: *The Arterial Pressure of Sportsmen.* Dissertation, Leningrad, 1959, (Russian).
8. MELLEROWICZ H.: *Ueber Wirkungen der Leibesübungen auf denmen schlichen Organismus und ihre Bedeutung für die präventive Medizin.* Training, Leistung, Gesundheit, Berlin, 1958.
9. ADAMÍROVÁ, J., CHRÁSTEK, J., and KOPŠÍK, J.: The influence of winter training courses on students with hypertensive disease. *Telových Sborník,* 4:309, 1959.
10. ANDREYEVA, V.: Modification de l'état fonctionel du système nerveux central des malades d'hypertension sous l'action de la gymnastique médicale. XII. Congress Sports Med., Moscow, 1958, p. 366.
11. HENSEL, J., and KOCINGER, A.: The influence of the remedial exercises on hypertensive disease. *Fysiatr Věstník,* 36:1, 1958.
12. ISRAEL, S.: Das Senkungsphänomen des arteriellen Blutdruckes nach körperlicher Belastung. *Das Deutsche Gesundheitswesen,* 14:75, 1959.
13. KHYTRIK, I.: La gymnastique médicale dans le complexe du traîtement de l'hypertension combinée avec les bains d'hydrogène sulphuré artificiels. XII. International Sports Med. Congress, Moscow, 1958.
14. MYASNIKOV, A. L.: *Gipertoneecheskaya Bolyezn'.* Medgiz, Moscow, 1951.
15. MOGA, A., OBRASCO, C., DOBO, S., TOMAS, A., BLENDEA, O., CHETIANU, O., MACAVI, E., MAZILU, A., and POP, V.: Le traîtement de la maladie hypertonique par la culture physique médicale. XII. International Sports Med. Congress, Moscow, 1958, p. 377.
16. MOSHKOV, V. N.: Lječebná tělovýchova pri vnútorných chorobách. *Slov Akad Vied.* Bratislava, 1955, (Slovak).
17. POCHOPOVÁ, K., PATOCKOVÁ, M., POCHOPOVÁ, V., and NEMCOVÁ, Z.: The influence upon the impaired regulation of the blood pressure by means of physical exercise. *Telových Sborník,* 3: 301, 1957.
18. SANNERSTAEDT, R., and VARNAUSKAS, E.: Total peripheral resistance during muscular exercise in arterial hypertension. Cardiol. Congress, Prague, 1964, p. 289.
19. SOROKINA, Z.: L'application de la gymnastique médicale et de la marche dosée dans le traîtement des malades atteints d'hypertension dans l'ensemble du traîtement thermal et climatique, XII. International Sports Med. Congress, Moscow, 1958.
20. VICH, J.: Psychothérapie et gymnastique médicale comme traîtement de l'hypertension. XII. International Sports Med. Congress, Moscow, 1958.
21. WALKO, K.: Die Herzarbeit bei jugendlichen Hypertonikern beim Sport. Congress International d'Education Physique et de Sport, Amsterdam, 1928, p. 125.
22. FEJFAR, Z., FEJFAROVÁ, M., LINHART, J., MALÁ, V., PŘEROVSKÝ, J., WIDIMSKÝ, J., and MATOUŠKOVÁ, M.: Contribution to the study of juvenile hypertension. *Hypertensní Nemoc SAV,* Bratislava, 1955, (Czech).
23. KRÁL, J.: L'équilibre acido-basique des vieux sportifs hypotendus. XX. Congrès Français de Médecine, Montpellier, 1929, p. 139.
24. WIDIMSKÝ, J., FEJFAROVÁ, M., EXNEROVÁ, M., DEJDAR, R., and PIRK, F.: *Juvenilní Hypertense.* Prague, STN, 1957, (Czech).
25. VANČURA, A.: *Vysoký Krevní Tlak.* Prague, 1942.
26. BROD, J., FENCL, V., GEROVÁ, M., HEJL, Z., JIRKA, J., KOTANOVÁ, E., PRAT, V., SEIDLOVÁ, P., and ZAJÍC, F.: Attempt at judgement of

regulatory mechanisms of blood pressure by the method of dynamic cold test. *Hypertensní Nemoc, SAV*, Bratislava, 1955, p. 71.

27. BROD, J., *et al.*: Changes of skin temperature and finger plethysmogram of normotonic and hypertensive subjects during the cold test. *Hypertensní Nemoc, SAV*, Bratislava, 1955, p. 72.

28. ROBINSON, S. C., and BRUCER, M.: Range of normal blood pressure. A statistical and clinical study of 11,383 persons. *Arch Intern Med, 64:*429, 1939.

29. VANČURA, A.: On transient hypertension in young subjects. *Cardiologia, 16;*124, 1950.

30. BROD, J.: Hemodynamic changes in hypertensive disease and their relation to the pathogenesis of the illness. *Vnitřní Lék, 5:*940, 1959.

31. LANG, A. F.: *The Hypertensive Disease.* Leningrad, 1950, (Russian).

Chapter XLVI

PREVENTION OF HYPERTENSIVE DISEASE AND OF ISCHEMIC HEART DISEASE IN THE SOVIET UNION

ALEKSANDR L. MYASNIKOV*

(Moscow, U.S.S.R.)

THE prevention of a disease should be based on the current concept of its etiology and pathogenesis. According to Soviet authors, hypertensive disease, in its initial stages, is a neurosis conditioned by damage and overstrain of the higher nervous system. At the same time, an important role is played by hereditary predisposition and by aging factors. Functional disorders of the endocrine glands and changes in the kidneys also promote its appearance.

Atherosclerosis too is regarded as the result of a long-term disorder in the nervous regulation of the lipoid, and particularly the cholesterol metabolism, in connection with certain alimentary conditions. Changes in the vascular walls have a predisposing influence and neuro-hormonal as well as endocrine factors, partly connected with social conditions, play an important role in the pathogenesis of the disease (1). (Fig. 46–1).

Disorders of the coronary circulation appear against a background of atherosclerotic lesions of the coronary vessels, together with such factors as spasm of the coronary vessels, changes in the coagulating and anticoagulating system of the blood, metabolic overstrain of the myocardium and, lastly, collateral circulation (2).

The close interrelations between hypertensive disease and coronary insufficiency (etiological, pathogenic and clinical) are explained by the fact that both diseases are essentially central nervous disorders in the functioning of the arterial system with involvement in the pathological process of the vasomotor centers (in hypertensive disease), and of the trophic centers (in atherosclerosis) (3).

With regard to the prevalence of symptomless forms of hypertensive disease and disorders of the coronary circulation, primary importance must be given to their early recognition. In detecting the initial preclinical stages, the possibility of hypertension beginning during youth and coronary atherosclerosis in the thirties must be taken into account.

For the purpose of differentiating hypertensive disease from symptomatic hypertonia it is important to use special examination methods to detect anomalies in the renal and other vessels, disorders of the endocrine glands, and chronic pyelonephritic hypertonia (3).

Mass screening, carried out in recent

---

*Deceased, Nov. 19, 1965.

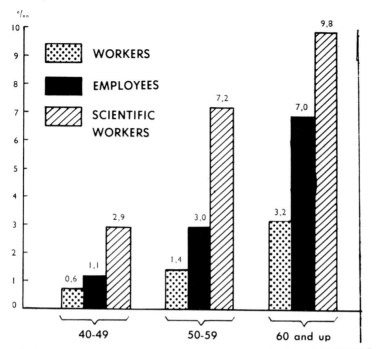

MYOCARDIAL INFARCTIONS IN SOCIAL GROUPS

(A. L. MYASNIKOV, Cardiologia Pratica
13: 71, 1962)

Figure 46–1. Data obtained from the City of Moscow. The incidence of myocardial infarction is highest among mentally stressed, sedentary scientific workers; lowest in physically active manual workers.

years in the Soviet Union, has shown an increased rate of hypertensive disease and disorders of the coronary circulation in persons engaged in work involving mental and nervous strain. It is in these groups that preventive measures should be taken in the first place. Speaking of factories and workshops, the improvement of technical processes and abatement of noise and vibration are undoubtedly of preventive importance as is the provision of hygienic equipment in workshops. For those already suffering from hypertensive disease and coronary atherosclerosis, a change of occupation and special measures to relieve their workload are desirable.

In our experience, it is essential at large industrial plants to organize *day and night preventoria*, i.e., in-patient clinics to which workers and employees in early stages of cardiovascular diseases can be admitted without discontinuing their employment, and where they can follow a healthy regime with proper diet and physiotherapy· One-and-one-half to two months stay in these preventoria has proved effective in improving the subsequent condition of patients for a considerable period (4).

Nutritional factors, of course, play an important role in the pathogenesis of atherosclerosis. We cannot, however, agree with the present widely-advocated theory that the intake of animal fats should be severely restricted in preventing or treating atherosclerosis. The first essential is to work out differentiated dietetic recommendations for different population groups in the light of health status and energy expenditure. To solve the problem of prevention, we believe it is most important that further long-term mass studies and experimental work should be undertaken.

Since a moderate amount of physical activity improves the metabolic processes, thereby inhibiting the development of atherosclerosis, great importance is being attached to *physical culture* (5) in all forms, for the young, the elderly, and those in the milder stages of cardiovascular disease. Big campaigns to promote various forms of physical exercise and walking daily, during free time and on Sundays, and to organize special training groups for the elderly and enfeebled persons, are run by the health authorities and by the trade unions.

The tremendous value of *sufficiently long and deep sleep* at night as a means of prevention and treatment is well known. The *campaign against smoking* and alcoholism is an important factor in preventing hypertensive disease and coronary heart disease.

The *elimination of the different factors that disturb the central nervous system* and maintain chronic excitation and stress is of great significance in prevention and treatment. Here relationships between people at work, in their families, and in the community, are of decisive importance. Proper upbringing from childhood on in diligence, honesty, politeness, mutual respect and comradeship, and development of the right reaction to criticism and comments from older people in the family and at work to a great extent forestall situations of conflict and the associated neurovascular reactions. The same is true of promoting a sense of responsibility and of the need to maintain working discipline. Naturally, the fulfillment of all these conditions largely depends on social structure and community relationships.

Candidates for and patients with hypertensive disease and coronary insufficiency receive *preventive care and treatment* conforming to a systematic, appropriately adapted program, including suitable preventive medication at their factory or office (antihypertensive therapy, vascular-dilating agents, anticoagulants, lipotropics, sedatives, and other preparations) and the control of corpulence due to physical inactivity.

Active observance of the above measures calls for a strong sense of health consciousness on the part of the population as a whole. *Popular lectures* on the nature of hypertensive disease and coronary atherosclerosis, their prevention and treatment are, therefore, one of the main issues in preventive work.

Successful accomplishment of the measures described depends largely on the organization of a *dispensary service* for patients and persons with so-called premorbid conditions. Among the latter are to be included, for reasons already mentioned, persons with heightened neurovascular reactivity, excess weight, and a high serum cholesterol content as well as those with a family history of such conditions.

The prevalence of hypertensive disease and disorders of the coronary circulation urgently calls for a *special cardiological service* with departments in hospitals and policlinics and, in large cities, special cardiological hospitals (with therapeutic, neurological, surgical and urological departments, angiocardiography and radio isotope diagnostic facilities, completed by biochemical and hormonal laboratories).

As part of the *network of sanatoria and spas*, special attention should be paid to local sanatoria and out-of-town hospitals for expanding the treatment of patients. An appropriate use of the Sunday rest is of great importance. For this purpose, all possible means should be used to increase facilities for *out-of-town rest periods*, giving priority to patients with hypertensive disease and coronary insufficiency (6).

At *sports centers, physical culture grounds, and swimming baths*, special groups should be organized for elderly people and for patients with cardiovascular derangements.

Doctors need to improve their qualifications in angiocardiography. This could contribute greatly to the prevention of hypertensive disease and coronary insufficiency. Systematic *postgraduate training for doctors*, from the local doctors to the chief physician of the *oblast* (region) or republic, should be run on a planned basis in regional medical clinics, institutes for the postgraduate training of doctors, and special cardiological institutes.

To assure success on all fronts in the campaign against cardiovascular diseases, the work must be given a definite form. The following structure (already partly accepted and put into practice in the Soviet Union) is tentatively put forward: in the rayon (district) policlinic, there is a cardio- and rheumatological consulting room which advises local doctors and gives them organizational and technical assistance in the control of cardiovascular diseases; in addition, in large towns and *oblasts, cardiology centers* (or dispensaries) have been set up to coordinate and direct the work of the *rayon* consulting room.

Communal amenities play an important role in the prevention of cardiovascular diseases. The planting of trees in towns, noise abatement, dust and air-pollution control, water supply and sewerage, convenient urban transport and, above all, healthy accommodations are essential elements. Details like the provision of ground floor flats, isolated from the noise of the town, for patients with cardiovascular disorders must also be solved.

The problem of diseases of the cardiovascular system can be solved by the joint efforts not only of medical workers, but of other state and voluntary organizations. It is, therefore, advisable to prepare a *national plan for the control of cardiovascular diseases, with legal status*, and in which all the relevant authorities play their part.

SUMMARY

The active, organized prevention of functional and degenerative diseases of the cardiovascular system occupies a prominent place in Soviet medicine.

Early diagnosis of a predisposition to hypertensive disease and to ischemic heart disease is made possible by mass screening in dispensaries and regional cardiology centers.

In consideration of the central nervous factors involved in the pathogenesis of cardiovascular diseases, measures are being taken to reduce the harmful influences of social tensions, physical inactivity, noise, and inadequate sleep, and to offer relief from them in spas, rural sanatoria, preventoria at industrial plants, and in sports centers also for the middle-aged and elderly.

Popular educational talks and propaganda campaigns for physical culture and against smoking help to activate the large-scale programs for the maintenance of cardiovascular health.

REFERENCES

1. MYASNIKOV, A. L.: *Atherosclerosis (Origin, Clinical Forms, Treatment)*. Medgiz, Moscow, 1960, (Russian).
2. MYASNIKOV, A. L.: Myocardial necroses of coronary and non-coronary genesis. *Amer J Cardiol, 13;*435, 1964.
3. MYASNIKOV, A. L.: Diagnostic and pathogenic borderlines between hypertensive disease and atherosclerosis. *Amer J Cardiol, 5;*692, 1960.
4. KURASHOV, S. V.: *The Organization of the Control of Cardiovascular Diseases*. Translation: Office of Technical Services, U.S. Dept. of Commerce, Washington 25, D.C., 1961.
5. LETUNOV, S. P., and MOTYLYANSKAYA, R. E.: Prophylactic significance of a regimen of physical activity in advanced age. *Klin Med, 11;*115, 1964, (Russian).
6. GOL'DFAYL, L. G.: *A Guide for Physicians Concerning the Sanatorium and Kurorty System*. Medgiz, Moscow, 1963, (Russian).

Chapter XLVII

PROPHYLAXIS OF CARDIOVASCULAR DISEASES IN THE SOVIET UNION

DMITRI D. VENEDIKTOV

(Moscow, U.S.S.R.)

THE prophylactic approach to major diseases is one of the dominant principles of medicine in the Soviet Union. Cardiovascular diseases, especially, atherosclerosis and its complications and hypertension provide a good example of the practical application of this principle.

Prophylaxis of cardiovascular diseases is necessary because in the USSR, like elsewhere, these diseases threaten national health and are the leading cause of deaths. The average span of life in the USSR is 70 years. The number of citizens over 100-years-old is the highest in the world (21,000 centenarians or 10 per 100,000 of population). With a birth rate of 19.7:1000 and total mortality of 7.0:1000, the annual increase of the USSR population is about 3.5 million and the age structure of the nation is gradually changing.

The percentage of people above 40 and 50 years of age is increasing and it is among them that degenerative cardiovascular diseases take the heaviest toll.

In 1962 the share of cardiovascular diseases among all causes of death was 38.7 per cent (30.8 percent for males and 46.3 per cent for females), and various forms of atherosclerosis and hypertension accounted for 85 per cent of all cardiovascular deaths. These diseases account for 72 to 80 disability days for every 100 workers and employees, and for more than one-fifth of all cases of permanent invalidity.

Modern scientific knowledge of the nature and pathogenic mechanisms of cardiovascular diseases is still limited, and there are still no means to reverse the pathological process. In terms of national health, the belated, curative approach is a very costly and relatively inefficient way of dealing with the problem.

Obviously, one cannot wait until "the last button" of the medical and scientific gown will be fixed. However, our present knowledge on the relations of degenerative cardiovascular processes to various environmental, emotional, nutritional, physical and occupational factors, although imperfect, does permit the systematic planning and carrying out of various measures, aimed at prevention of these pathological processes.

Experiences in the USSR, as well as studies of many scientists of other nations, demonstrate beyond any doubt that a prophylactic approach to cardiovascular disease is not only feasible, but also effective.

In developing broad prophylactic measures against these diseases one must, however, bear in mind the following:

1. Since it is impossible to say at which point the degenerative changes in the heart and in the blood vessels begin and from when they might elicit serious complications, prophylactic measures should be started early in life and embrace all age groups.

2. There are no specific methods to prevent atherosclerosis, but various internal, central nervous and environmental factors are known which contribute significantly to the development of ischemic and degenerative cardiovascular disease. Prophylactic measures should be directed primarily and as systematically as possible towards these factors.

3. Many of the prophylactic methods available now are of such a nature that participation of the State is needed in their implementation and in organized efforts toward large-scale national measures. In the USSR, considerable progress has been made in coordinating individual, public and governmental actions for prevention of cardiovascular diseases, whereby the main responsibility rests with the Central Soviet Government, the individual republican Ministries of Health and their various branches and institutions.

This is in full compliance with Articles 119 and 120 of the USSR Constitution, which not only proclaim "the right of the citizens of the USSR for rest and leisure. . .for the maintenance in old age and in case of sickness and disability . . .," but also state that these rights ". . .are ensured by extensive development of social insurance of industrial, office and professional workers at state expense, free medical service for the working people, and the provision of a wide network of health resorts for the use of the working people."

GENERAL LIVING CONDITIONS

Conditions of life can profoundly influence general health. Therefore, an improvement of living conditions of the population constitutes one of the most important prophylactic measures. The solution of this problem was not (and still is not) easy for the Soviet Union with its growth of the urban population, and with 1,710 cities and almost 70,000 villages ruined during the last war.

All available resources have been called upon by the Soviet Government and people, resulting in the highest rate of housing construction programs in the world. During the last 7 years alone (1958–1964), 84.3 million people (more than one-third of the total population) moved into new apartments, all of which are under the surveillance of health and other authorities. The rent does not exceed 4 to 5 per cent of the family's income. More than 5,000 epidemiologic sanitation stations supervise all planning or construction of new city sections and industrial plants.

WORKING CONDITIONS

Special attention in prophylaxis is being paid to conditions of work and to measures which can be carried out directly at the industrial installations and offices. Studies of the Institute of Labor, Hygiene and Occupational Diseases have clearly demonstrated variations in cardiovascular morbidity, not only in different branches of industry, but also in different groups of workers and employees at the

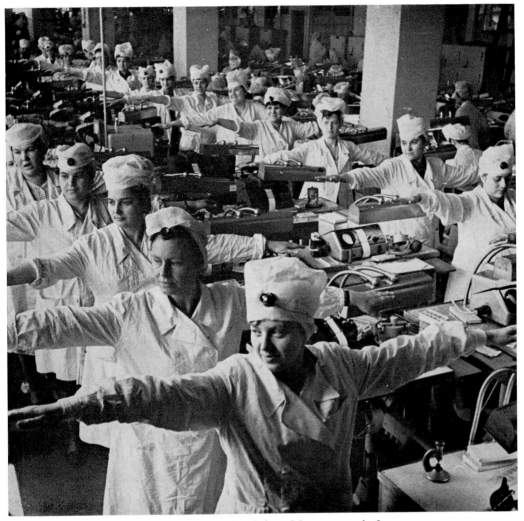

Figure 47–1. Exercise break in a Moscow watch factory.

same plant or enterprise. Loud noise and vibrations can derange neuroreflex mechanisms and cause unfavorable cardiovascular reactions, and chemical agents (lead, benzole, beryllium) affect muscular elements of the blood vessel walls and myocardium.

Therefore, continuous control over working conditions is carried out at all factories and enterprises either by a general network of epidemiologic sanitation stations or by special medical sanitation units and departments. The structure of these departments includes, in addition to central hospital and outpatient clinics, an assignment of special physicians to every workshop (one workshop physician for 2,000 workers in general industry or 1,000 workers in coal, oil and chemical industry).

Among the important functions of physicians and other medical personnel at the industrial enterprises are health education lectures and demonstrations to

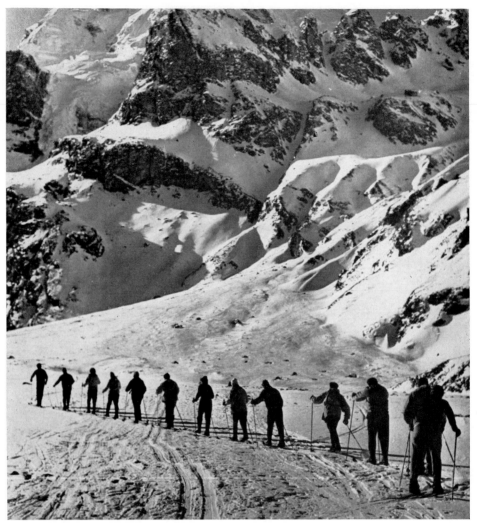

Figure 47–2. Trade union sports club "Labor" at training camp Ullu Tau in the Caucasus.

workers, aimed at explaining to them the principles of hygiene and of a rational regime, and medical supervision of the physical exercise breaks (3 to 5 minutes every few hours) during the working day (Fig. 47–1).

NUTRITION AND HEALTH EDUCATION

Derangements of lipid metabolism play an important role in the pathogenesis of atherosclerosis and related conditions. Therefore, the average diet should not only be sufficient in quantity and quality, but should also be balanced in relation to energy requirements and other biological factors. A decrease of animal fats in the nutrition is considered desirable and the increased consumption of plant oils, fish and other sea food is recommended. Also sufficient amounts of methyl-containing compounds (choline,

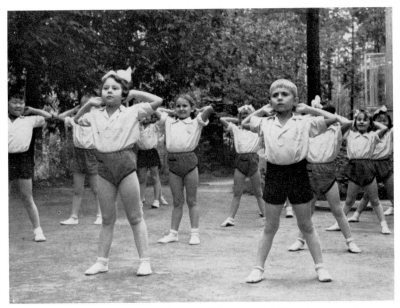

Figure 47–3. Morning exercises at Malachovka children's sanatorium.

methionine, choline-phosphates), and of vitamins of the C, P and B groups are important.

Health education of the population in relation to nutrition, and nonsmoking is widely carried out by all medical establishments in the USSR and by more than 370 special institutes and houses of health education established in all republics and in the major cities by Red Cross societies and by educational and cultural organizations, using books and brochures, films, slides, TV programs and lectures.

In recent years, more than 1,000 People's Health Universities were organized in urban and rural areas to disseminate medical knowledge about prophylaxis and treatment, and to promote desirable health habits by people at home and at work. The duration of the course is 2 years, with a 3-months interval during the summer. Tuition is free. Two-hour "after work" class sessions are conducted twice a month by the staffs of medical and research institutes and by doctors from local medico-prophylactic establishments.

In addition, it has been estimated that every month about 150 million Soviet people watch television features or listen to radio broadcasts on subjects of health protection.

PHYSICAL ACTIVITY AND SPORTS

In the USSR physical activity and sports have long been considered as very effective means of raising the general level of health of the population. There are about 187,000 sport clubs and societies (Fig. 47–2) in the Soviet Union with nearly 33 million members, who have more than 2000 stadiums, 18,000 sport grounds, and many other facilities at their disposal. From the point of view of health preservation, it is important to note that numerous sports festivals and competitions in the USSR are carried

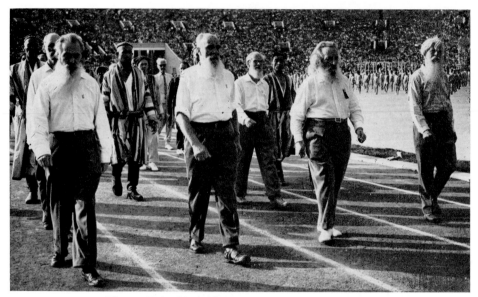

Figure 47–4. Old athletes at Moscow sports meeting.

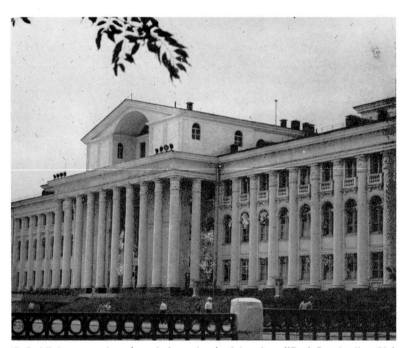

Figure 47–5. Night sanatorium (prophylactorium) of the plant "Red October" at Volgograd.

out with an endeavor to involve as many people as possible in active participation and not merely as spectators. The Spartakiad of the USSR peoples in 1963, for instance, drew more than 66 million contestants.

Sports are widely cultivated during vacations, in summer camps, holiday homes, etc. The propaganda of sports is started early in life (in school or even kindergarten) (Fig. 47–3), and continues into adult and elderly age (Fig. 47–4).

Special emphasis on sports is being aimed at people above 30 or 40 years, at which age many of those previously active in sport gradually give it up, and at intellectuals whose work does not provide them with vigorous physical activity, but keeps them instead under constant intensive emotional and mental tension and stress.

EARLY RECOGNITION AND PROPHYLACTIC TREATMENT OF CARDIOVASCULAR DISEASES

Various approaches to an early recognition of degenerative cardiovascular diseases are used in the USSR. All persons visiting one of the local policlinics for the first time, irrespective of the cause of the visit, are submitted to a thorough physical examination. If any abnormalities are detected, the patient is examined in more detail, and appropriate further examinations are recommended.

Beyond this, periodic prophylactic examinations of the healthy population are being carried out in the USSR on a very large scale. Organizational patterns of such examinations may be different. Very large groups may be examined by teams of medical specialists for some particular diseases; in 1963, for instance, more than 80 million people were examined for tuberculosis, more than 45 million for cancer, and many millions for cardiovascular diseases.

Groups of the population (preschool and school children, students, industrial workers, employees) and people suffering from cardiovascular and other definite diseases are placed under "dispensary care," that is, they are taken under active supervision and treatment by special medicoprophylactic establishments, the so-called dispensaries. (In 1963 there were more than 3,000 special dispensaries of different types in the USSR.)

Dispensary care means thorough periodical examinations (once or twice a year), including consultations with various specialists, x-ray studies, and laboratory tests. If any abnormalities are noted, the patients are referred to local physicians or clinical institutions and treatment is initiated.

All the above named methods are effective in discovering early forms of degenerative cardiovascular diseases and in determining the proper preventive therapy.

Treatment might be given in the local policlinic or medical unit at the factory, including drug and physical therapy, changes in the working regime and temporary transfer of the worker to a lighter job without loss in wages.

Many industrial plants have special "prophylactoria" or "night sanatoria" (more than 1,000 of such institutions were operated in the USSR in 1963) (Fig. 47–5) where patients can stay after their working day for rest and medical treatment without interrupting their usual work, and without forfeiting their rights for a paid holiday. Treatment in these "prophylactoria" is free and the cost of maintenance is paid by the worker only in part, or covered completely by labor union funds.

A 24-day course of treatment in such establishments helps to bring the elevated blood pressure down to normal limits for up to 5 to 8 months in a majority of patients with the first stage of the dis-

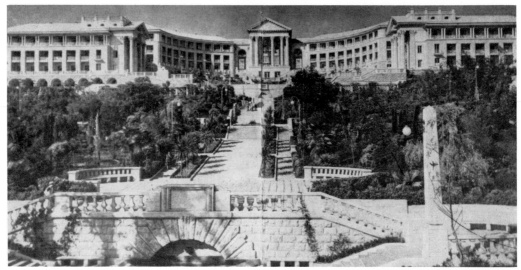

Figure 47–6. Sanatorium "Metallurg" for metal workers at Sochi on the Black Sea Coast.

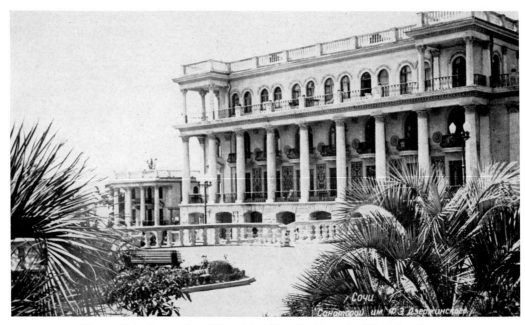

Figure 47–7. Sanatorium "Dzershinski" at Sochi on the Black Sea Coast.

ease, and up to 2 to 3 months in the second stage. The treatment can be repeated whenever necessary.

During vacations, many people obtain additional prophylactic treatment at special sanatoria and health resorts or reconditioning centers. These have been developed since 1919 all over the country in areas where natural conditions favor undisturbed rest and offer environmental advantages.

In 1963 there were over 3,000 recon-

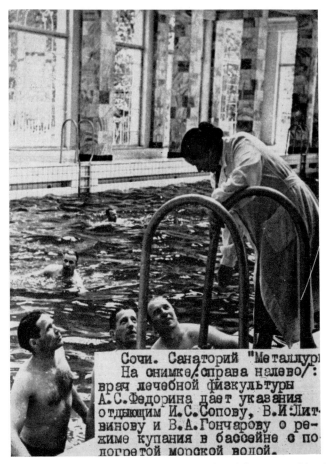

Сочи. Санаторий "Металлур;
На онимке/справа налево/:
врач лечебной физкультуры
А.С.Федорина дает указания
отдыющим И.С.Сопову, В.И.Лит-
винову и В.А.Гончарову о ре-
жиме купания в бассейне с по-
логретой морской водой.

Figure 47–8. Indoor seawater swimming pool with ultraviolet-penetrable glass ceiling.

ditioning centers in the USSR with accommodations for 547,000 people. Many of the centers are located along the coast of the Black Sea, in the Caucasus, on the Riga Seashore, and in other scenic areas (Figs. 47–6–8). More than 6 million workers, employees and members of their families per year spend their vacations in these establishments. Approximately 3.5 million of them receive accommodations and treatment free of charge or at a 70 per cent discount at the expense of social insurance funds, paid by the labor unions and by the State.

Local doctors and policlinics examine each person before referring him to a particular center, e.g., at the Black Sea or in the woods of Central Russia. Since the reconditioning centers are predominantly intended for prophylaxis and periodic preventive treatment of people with mild and chronic forms of cardiovascular diseases, the indications for admission are rather liberal. It is generally considered unwise to wait until a person develops advanced ischemic heart disease or hypertension before sending him to a health resort instead of doing so while he is still relatively well. Counterindications on the other hand are more

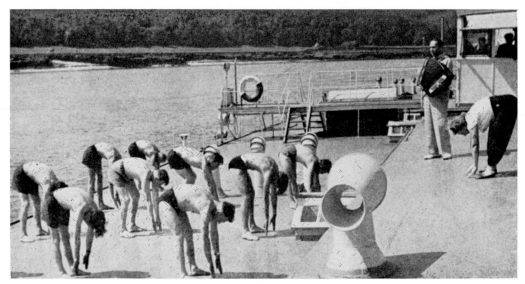

Figure 47–9. Calisthenics aboard a Russian floating reconditioning center on the Don river.

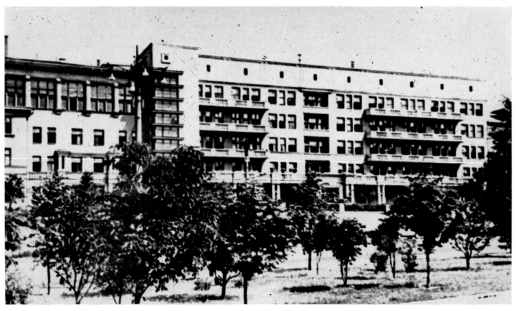

Figure 47–10. Central Research Institute of Kurortology and Physiotherapy in Moscow.

strictly defined since the stay in hot and humid climates, or else in the mountains, or taking sulfur baths, may do some patients more harm than good.

After arriving at a health resort, the person is seen by a special staff physician of the center who examines his medical record and arranges for his individual regime, such as regular physical activity, sea-swimming, physiotherapy, and sun bathing, all under constant medical supervision (Fig. 47–9). The stay in a sanatorium usually lasts 28 days.

The effectiveness of prophylactic treatments at the sanatoria of the USSR has been convincingly confirmed by many physicians, and especially by the staffs of 12 Health Resort and Physiotherapy Research Institutes in various areas of the USSR, whose main task is the evaluation of various forms of physiotherapy, exercise therapy, and climatotherapy, and the follow-up of late results after such treatments (Fig. 47–10).

Despite all these extensive prevention programs, Soviet physicians are far from considering the present achievements in this field as completely satisfactory and they are looking for all possible improvements of today's methods. In May, 1965, the Academy of Medical Sciences of the USSR—the highest scientific body in Soviet Medicine—has devoted its entire annual session to a comprehensive and multidirectional discussion of the problem "Prophylaxis of Cardiovascular Diseases." (The Proceedings of this session are to be published soon.)

Forty-seven years of prophylactic Soviet medicine and public health services demonstrate quite clearly that it is within the possibilities of modern society to organize large-scale, effective programs for the at least partial prevention of degenerative cardiovascular diseases. Soviet specialists are eager to share their experience in the fight against cardiovascular diseases with that of other countries and to join forces with them in the pursuance of that vital common goal.

SUMMARY

Many problems of etiology and pathogenesis of degenerative processes in the heart and blood vessels are still unsolved. Nevertheless, our present state of knowledge in these fields makes it possible to carry out various prophylactic measures, embracing all age groups, and directed toward different contributing pathogenic factors.

Effective implementation of these measures demands close cooperation of the public, the medical profession, and governments.

The main features of cardiovascular prophylaxis, as practiced in the USSR in accordance with the constitutional rights of the Soviet citizens, are the following:

(a) Improvement of the living standard; (b) social security of the individual; (c) hygienic control of working conditions; (d) balanced nutrition; (e) intensive and incessant health education of the population; (f) encouragement of regular vigorous physical activities and sports; (g) early diagnostic recognition and a system of comprehensive care of the mild preclinical forms of cardiovascular diseases, and (h) an extensive network of People's Health Universities, sports facilities, policlinics, dispensaries, prophylactoria, night sanatoria, holiday homes, and reconditioning centers on the seashore or in the mountains.

Further determined efforts toward the development of even more effective large-scale prevention programs for the control of degenerative cardiovascular diseases are urgently needed in all nations.

Chapter XLVIII

PREVENTIVE MEASURES AGAINST CARDIOVASCULAR DISEASES IN CZECHOSLOVAKIA*

JAN BADAL

(Františkovy Lázně, Czechslovakia)

THE growing incidence of cardiovascular diseases constitutes a grave problem of public health in Czechoslovakia. They occupy the first place in mortality statistics.

Mortality per 100,000 inhabitants rose from 248 in 1937 to 321 in 1963 (1, 2). In 1962, 26.9 per cent of these deaths were due to arteriosclerosis, degenerative cardiovascular diseases and arterial hypertension.

Morbidity is rather prolonged and often leads to permanent invalidism. The average duration of incapacity for work, caused by cardiovascular disease, was 38.4 days in 1961 and 36.2 days in 1963 (3).

The Public Health Administration in Czechoslovakia, therefore, is intent on initiating prophylactic measures as early as possible in order to reduce these detriments to popular health and to national economy.

The following discussion will be focused on the prophylaxis against ischemic heart disease and hypertension, with particular emphasis on those measures which are being organized on a large scale (i.e., reconditioning treatment in spas, "dispensaire" methods in "night sanatoria," recreation programs and some others).

In Czechoslovakia a number of spas (or reconditioning centers) are dedicated to the special requirements of cardiological indications with primary attention paid to the prevention and medical care of ischemic heart disease and hypertension. According to legislation of 1951, spa treatment is an integral part of prophylaxis and therapy in Czechoslovakia.

The spa system is intended to serve the welfare of the working population and the healthy development of the young generation. Cure participants are selected on the basis of standardized indications which concern particularly the initial and early phases of disease, when it is still possible to achieve a postponement of impaired working capacity, or an improvement of existing disease, or the restoration of full working capacity, respectively.

Spa treatments are provided for workers and their dependents by the organization of the revolutionary labor unions and the corresponding agricultural unions, and for pensioners by the social

---

*Translated by W. Raab.

security administration. The state spas are operated directly by the Ministry of Health. With some exceptions, the cure participants contribute a small fee.

The spa treatment is characterized by its complex synthesis of diverse therapeutic measures which are adapted to individual needs. It includes balneological treatment (e.g., natural CO_2 baths), exercise therapy, physiotherapy and hydrotherapy, dietary therapy and, when necessary, medicinal treatment. The sojourn at the spas ordinarily lasts 25 days. In 1963, 40,000 cardiac patients and prepatients were treated in spas. (4). Half of these had ischemic heart disease or hypertension.

CO_2 baths primarily affect the peripheral vascular system. They lower the blood pressure, stimulate capillary blood flow, augment muscular tone and improve venous circulation and cardiac efficiency. Coronary circulation seems to be increased unless vascular lesions have reached an advanced stage (5). Bartussek (6) and Herkel (7) have observed a prolonged isometric period and longer duration of systole in diseased hearts under the influence of CO_2 baths. Venous return into the right ventricle is increased and the minute volume rises slightly. Due to the reduced blood pressure and slower heart rate, the heart muscle functions more economically and with a better blood supply.

Exercise therapy in the Czechoslovak spas is composed of gymnastics and the so-called "terrain" cure (hiking and hill climbing). The latter figures particularly prominently in reconditioning centers with terrain conditions suitable for graded, increasing efforts.

Gymnastic exercises serve the maintenance and improvement of physio-logical circulatory functions both concerning the peripheral vascular system and the economy of cardiac work. This form of treatment is particularly effective in an environment which provides freedom from the emotional and sensory burdens of everyday life.

It is necessary to explain to the cure participants the importance of prophylactic and therapeutic exercising in order to obtain their cooperation and for the purpose to exert an educational influence on them. Thus, efforts are made to build up their willingness to permanently continue exercise practices after their return home as a means of sustained prophylaxis, especially against ischemic heart disease and hypertension.

Exercise therapy is being conducted in agreement with the concept of those investigators who attribute its value to a reduction of sympathetic adrenergic activity in the heart (8, 9) which seems to be initiated by training-induced metabolic adjustments in the skeletal musculature (10). Myasnikov (11) and others assume a direct connection between lack of physical activity and the development of degenerative heart disease. Nevrayev (12) ascribes to the physical training in reconditioning centers an equilibration of stimulating and inhibiting processes in the central nervous system, and Morris and Crawford (13) provided evidence for an increased vulnerability of the myocardium resulting from sedentary living habits.

It should be mentioned here that preventive exercise therapy is being carried out in all Czechoslovak spas regardless of their various special areas of indication. Thus, the entire mass of people who spend cure periods in these places are included in the general preventive programs. This means approximately 300,-000 persons per year. Among these there are patients suffering from neurocirculatory asthenia, which seems to be a condition predisposing for the later development of degenerative heart disease.

The environmental emotional impact of the stay in reconditioning centers deserves particular emphasis. In a surrounding of quiet, serene natural beauty, the cure participant is relieved from disadvantageous domestic circumstances which not infrequently entail considerable nervous tensions. The scenic attractiveness of the location, undisturbed walks in the woods and frequent outdoor concerts contribute jointly to relaxation and subjective well-being. Pleasant living quarters and the solicitous, friendly attitude of physicians and personnel make the sojourn at the spas enjoyable and psychologically beneficial.

The educational value of the spa system rests in the fact that the cure participant learns to understand his condition, to live with it and to control it. He is thus being offered an extraordinarily favorable opportunity to acquire needed health habits. This psychologically motivational element constitutes one of the most important positive features of the complex reconditioning center treatment. It is considered of paramount importance for the early prevention and alleviation of the so-called diseases of civilization, notably ischemic heart disease and hypertension.

Several Czechoslovak spas are staffed and equipped primarily for specialized cardiological treatment (e.g., Františkovy Lázně, Poděbrady and Sliac). In 1960, Czechoslovakia operated 16 cardiological spa sanatoria with 3,153 beds for adults, and 5 children's sanatoria with 509 beds.

Since then, an additional sanatorium for teenagers and students has been established for prophylactic purposes.

Prevention is intimately connected with early diagnosis. The so-called "dispensaire" system is specifically directed toward this goal. It is aimed at the early detection of circulatory abnormalities, mainly of arterial hypertension, and of proneness to heart disease. On the basis of early registration and periodic follow-ups, appropriate preventive measures are being initiated with meticulous consideration of individual working conditions and living habits. This system is applied first of all for the benefit of workers in strenuous occupations and in jobs involving health hazards; furthermore for the protection of responsible leaders in industry, science and administration and of young individuals. This diagnostic system forms a part of the daily obligations of district and plant physicians who cooperate with specialized medical institutions, industrial administrations, labor unions and commissions for labor safety. Full documentation of the individual cases is thus guaranteed.

The value of the dispensaire system was demonstrated by the fact that during 1954, the first year of its existence, 50,000 cases of subclinical or fully developed hypertension were discovered, most of them at an early stage and, therefore, optimally amenable to prophylactic treatment.

Recreational programs are being conducted as an additional feature of the overall prevention system. These programs have been organized in Czechoslovakia since 1945 by the revolutionary labor movement and labor unions in recreation centers at scenic locations in order to provide for the workers a change of environment for periods of 2 weeks during the summer season, and of 7 to 10 days in the winter. These recreation periods are available to workers and employees and their families for a modest fee. The number of participants increases from year to year and has reached a total of 1,300,000 in 1964 (14).

The recreation programs are of a social rather than systematically preventive nature and are being granted largely as a reward for meritorious services. Nevertheless, the factor of physical activity in fresh air and the temporary escape from unfavorable environmental conditions do fit into the general aims of prevention in that they help to equilibrate the autonomic nervous regulation of cardiac metabolism and function. Raab (15) has shown that sedentary living causes a deficiency of vagal and sympathoinhibitory antiadrenergic counterregulation against an undue, oxygen-wasting and efficiency-impairing sympathetic preponderance in myocardial metabolism. Physical activity at the recreation centers is also of psychological value by inducing the participants to abandon the popular misconception of the benefits of total physical rest and to overcome the fear of bodily motion.

In approximately one-third of the Czechoslovak factories, "physminutes" (exercise breaks) are inserted in the working hours (i.e., short periods of about 5 minutes), which are used for group calisthenics.

In the so-called "night sanatoria," which are located on the precincts of the industrial plants, workers with coronary sclerosis and/or hypertension, who are in need of prophylactic treatment, are subjected to an appropriate regimen after working hours. They spend the nights at the sanatorium for 4 consecutive weeks without interrupting their regular working schedule at the plant.

Each spring a hiking venture, designated as the "100 spring kilometers," is organized for a change of scenery, combined with physical effort, both in the interest of prevention.

Public educational campaigns are emphatically concentrating on the subjects of atherosclerosis, ischemic heart disease and hypertension, and people are instructed with regard to the necessities of prevention, such as regular physical activity, abstinence from smoking, sensible living habits, fat-poor diet, reconditioning periods. Recently, a number of "reducing camps" have been established where, during the summer, 2 weeks are being spent for instruction in gymnastics and dietary rules.

A significant regression of rheumatic cardiac complications (valvular lesions) by means of antibiotics has been achieved as a demonstrable result of successful prevention in this particular area of cardiac pathology. By contrast, no unequivocal statistics are yet available concerning the effectiveness of current prophylactic measures against ischemic heart disease and hypertension.

One reason for this is the fact that large parts of the population have not yet carried out prophylactic practices with sufficient perseverance, which precludes an accurate statistical evaluation of results. In an attempt to obtain more objective data, some of the reconditioning centers have now introduced the systematic measurement of special cardiovascular functional parameters before and after reconditioning periods.

We are convinced, however, from general experience that the above-described prophylactic principles are rational and well-founded, and we hold them against the outdated opinion that only medicinal interference can be prophylactically helpful. Wide application of physical activity appears as a primary task of prophylaxis against ischemic heart disease and hypertension and is an important factor in the correction of the detriments inherent in our technical civilization.

SUMMARY

Large-scale preventive measures organized in Czechoslovalia against ischemic heart disease and hypertension are the following:

1. Treatment in spas (reconditioning centers) which consists of the influence of a quiet, pleasant environment; therapeutic exercises; CO_2 baths; physiotherapy, and an appropriate diet, in suitable combinations. More than 40,000 cardiac patients and prepatients avail themselves annually of such programs. Results are equilibration of autonomic nervous dysregulation, lowering of blood pressure, improved coronary circulation, psychotherapeutic and educational effects. Duration is 25 days.

2. The "dispensaire" system for early detection of hypertension, elimination of causative factors and early application of therapy.

3. Recreation centers and programs as supplements to reconditioning treatment, offering beneficial, relaxing change of environment and opportunities for physical activity. Duration in summer is 14 days; in winter, 7 to 10 days.

4. Exercise breaks and group calisthenics (once or twice daily for 5 minutes), given in about one-third of the factories.

5. Night sanatoria for the conducting of prophylactic regimens after working hours and overnight stays in special installations at industrial plants. Duration is 4 weeks.

6. Extensive periodic campaigns and incidental programs of public education toward preventive living habits.

REFERENCES

1. Statistická ročenka ČSSR, pp. 108, 112, 1964.
2. 15 let nového československého zdravotnictví, p. 71, 1960.
3. Statistická ročenka ČSSR, p. 450, 1964.
4. Lázeňská statistika minist. zdravotnictví, 1963.
5. MLÁDEK: Choroby koronarních tepen a jejich léčba, p. 263, 1940. Ed.: Čs. kardiologická společnost.
6. BARTUSSEK: *Balneologe, 5;*8, 1938, (quoted by Mládek, l.c.
7. HERKEL: *Balneologe, 5;*549, 1938, quoted by Mládek, l.c.
8. RAAB, W.: The nonvascular metabolic myocardial vulnerability factor in coronary heart disease. *Amer Heart J, 66;*685, 1963.
9. SELYE, H.: The prevention of adrenaline edema by the alarm reaction. *Amer J Physiol, 122;*347, 1938.
10. STEGEMANN, J.: Zum Mechanismus der Pulsefrequenz-Einstellung durch den Stoffwechsel. *Arch ges Physiol, 276;*480, 1963.
11. MYASNIKOV, A. L.: On epidemiology of atherosclerosis of heart coronary vessels in Soviet Union. *Cardiol Prat, 13;*72, 1962.
12. NEVRAYEV: Quoted by Paul E. Schennetten, F.: Einführung in die kardiologische Dispensairebetreuung als Grundlage zur Rehabilitation, p. 119. Ed.: VEB: Volk und Gesundheit, Berlin, 1959.
13. MORRIS, J. N., and CRAWFORD, M. D.: Coronary heart disease and physical activity of work, evidence of a national necropsy survey. *Brit Med J, 2;*1485, 1958.
14. Statistická ročenka ČSSR: p. 462-463, 1964.
15. RAAB, W., dePAULA e SILVA, P., MARCHET, H., KIMURA, E., and STARCHESKA, Y. K.: Cardiac adrenergic overactivity due to lack of physical exercise and its pathogenic implications. *Amer J Cardiol, 5;*300, 1960.
16. 15 let nového československého zdravotnictví, p. 185, 1960.

Further information to be found in "Československé zdravotnictví, IX, 1961, a survey of material presented by the Ministers of Health of the socialist countries at the V. Conference on the Prophylaxis and Treatment of Cardiovascular Diseases and Rheumatism in Moscow in September, 1960.

Chapter XLIX

COMBINED ENVIRONMENTAL-EMOTIONAL AND PHYSICAL CARDIAC PREVENTION PROGRAMS IN THE WEST GERMAN RECONDITIONING CENTERS*

PETER BECKMANN

(Ohlstadt, Germany)

Attempts at optimally influencing the predisposition to multifactorial myocardial degeneration and infarction demand a broader, more complex approach than a mere increase of physical activity within the accustomed daily environment of high-pressure urban living.

Common experience has shown that the emotional tensions, frustrations and anxieties, as well as the sensory annoyances of today's competitive life constitute a heavy burden on man's nervous system with all of its cardiovascular pathogenic implications.

The principle of at least temporary "getting-away-from-it-all" is basically sound but our contemporary style of vacationing usually provides only the replacement of one category of artificial overstimulation by another equally hectic one. Reasonably planned physical activity and the relaxing contact with a natural environment remain at a minimum.

Under the impact of rapidly rising cardiac mortality in prosperous postwar Germany, several far-sighted social insurance organizations and industries initiated in 1955 an organized system of active empirical prophylaxis against ischemic heart disease by sponsoring the development of reconditioning centers, primarily for infarction-prone executives, workers and employees, in scenically beautiful rural regions.

At present, West Germany has 20 such centers, representing an investment of about 10 million dollars, and accommodating some 20,000 persons per year. The first of these centers was established at Ohlstadt in the Bavarian Alps (1) (Fig. 49–1), where about 15,000 patients or "trainees" have been admitted over the last 9 years for periods of at least 4 weeks each, free of charge, and without curtailment of their regular vacation time.

Selection for admission is made by insurance or private physicians on the grounds of symptoms, which Delius has designated by the collective term of "tense exhaustion." They encompass a variety of complaints, such as fatigue which remains unrelieved by sleep, general nervous irritability, insomnia, decrease of initiative and work efficiency, feelings of frustration and despondency, abnormally elevated or abnormally low blood pressure, extrasystoles, angina-like

*Translated by W. Raab.

393

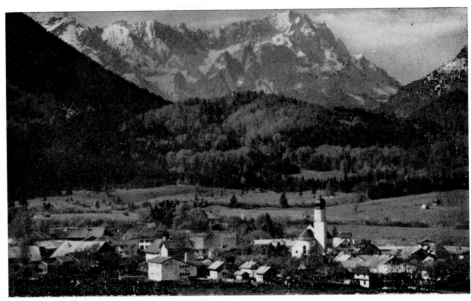

Figure 49–1. Ohlstadt in the Bavarian Alps, site of the first West German Reconditioning Center for Cardiovascular Diseases. (120 trainees live in private homes.) Operated by the Regional Insurance Administration, Unterfranken.

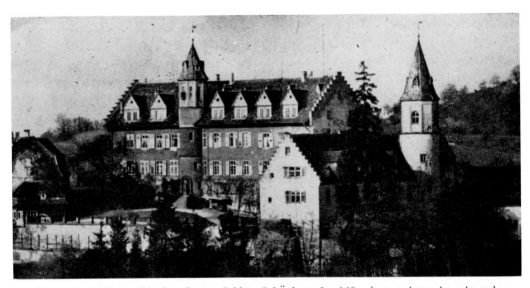

Figure 49–2. Reconditioning Center Schloss Schönberg for 140 mine workers. An adapted mediaeval castle. Operated by the Ruhr Mining Industry.

chest sensations, shortness of breath, and muscular weakness. Overweight is a frequent additional feature.

The admitted reconditioning trainees are accommodated either in private homes of the villagers, as for example at Ohlstadt, or in former castles, such as Schloss Schönberg (Fig. 49–2), or in former hotels. Some of the newer centers in Germany, Switzerland and Austria

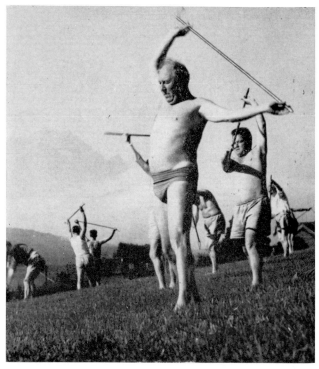

Figure 49–3. Outdoor exercises near Reconditioning Center, Ohlstadt.

were specially constructed for the purpose.

Certain important fundamental differences distinguish the programs at the reconditioning centers from the stay at spas or ordinary vacation spots (2): all admittances are subjected to a graded and progressing physical training program. The latter occupies 5 to 6 hours per day and consists of outdoor calisthenics, relaxation and breathing exercises, games, a great deal of hiking and mountain climbing, complemented by skinbrushing, cold water applications, and sauna baths.

Nearly all of this takes place in the open air, regardless of weather conditions, and in closest possible contact with the natural alpine environment (Figs. 49–3–6).

Systematically organized, so-called "terrain cures" had been introduced into official medicine by Oertel in 1880 and have retained their prophylactic as well as therapeutic significance ever since. Despite the differences in location and character of landscape, a certain degree of quantitative standardization of effort is possible. Groups of trainees are assigned, in accordance with their general condition and stage of training, to specified, marked footpaths with different degrees of steepness, and leading to goals at different distances and altitudes.

The personal satisfaction of having reached a certain height or mountain peak with a panoramic view, together with the esthetic reward of such achievements, are powerful factors in restoring the trainee's confidence in his physical

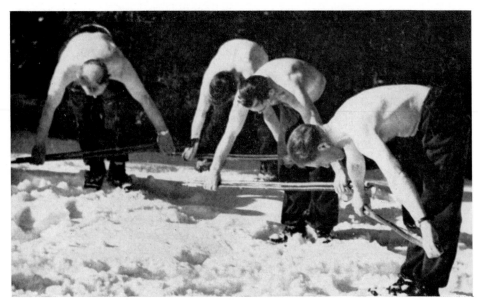

Figure 49–4. Winter exercises at Reconditioning Center, Ohlstadt.

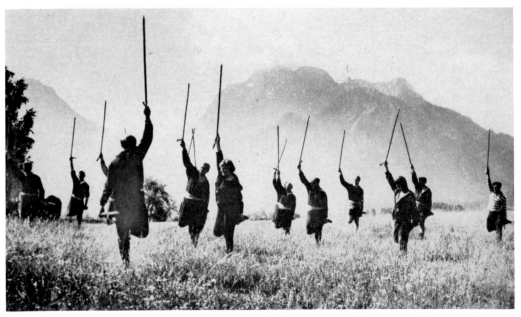

Figure 49–5. Morning exercises near Reconditioning Center, Schwangau. (Courtesy Dr. Chr. de Werth.)

abilities, and in motivating his continued interest in and ambition for lifelong active health maintenance. They go far beyond the effect of mere physical train-ing in a city gymnasium from which the trainee steps out directly into the usual harassment of noisy traffic and the de-pressing daily routine.

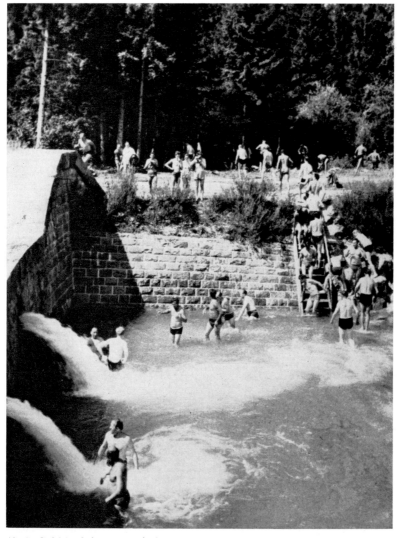

Figure 49–6. Cold bath in mountain brook at Reconditioning Center, Schwangau. (Courtesy Dr. Chr. de Werth.)

Competitive efforts and any semblance of drill are carefully avoided in the reconditioning centers. The training is conducted jointly by physical educators and physicians. The physicians participate personally in the greater part of the outdoor activities, gymnastics, and hikes. This enables them to observe deficiencies, reactions, and gradual gains of the trainees, and is of inestimable value in re-

enforcing the psychological element of the latters' growing self-confidence, as well as in preventing over-ambitious hazardous escapades.

The emotional effectiveness of the environmentally refreshing sojourns in the reconditioning centers (Fig. 49–7) is further accentuated in some of them by the so-called "autogenic training" (i.e., periods of repose in semi-darkness with soft music, eyes closed and deliberate concentration on soothing images of idyllic landscapes and the like). On free afternoons and evenings, hobby instructions are given in various handicrafts (Fig. 49–8). Weekends are used for excursions to nearby historic sites and art monuments.

Much emphasis is being placed on the educational opportunities available at the centers, with the aim in mind to make the best possible use of the trainees' gradually changing attitude toward themselves and toward their place in society. The powerful psychological influence of an entirely new and greatly appealing rural environment makes the originally tense and sometimes distrustful trainees increasingly amenable to a thorough indoctrination of basic health rules concerning diet, nonsmoking, and a meaningful utilization of leisure time.

The personal experience of an unexpected feeling of "rejuvenation" at the centers, combined with popular explanations of the medical principles involved, bolsters the trainees willingness to continue the active practice of newly acquired living habits when they return home. Such habits include the avoidance of elevators whenever possible, walking at least part of the way to work, home calisthenics, cold showers, hiking on Sundays and holidays, using the sports facilities which are in an increasingly large measure made available by prevention-minded industries and communities, non-smoking, and dietary restrictions.

It has been said that it would be difficult to popularize such a philosophy in other countries of the West because of differences in social and economic structure and in individual motivation. However that may be, there cannot be any doubt that without determined, systematically organized guidance by responsible health agencies, and without an enlightened active personal cooperation of the millions of prospective heart disease victims in highly industrialized soft-living nations, no reduction of premature mass mortality from the detriments of misused prosperity and over-civilization can be expected.

The reconditioning center at Ohlstadt, after which most of the other centers are patterned, accommodates 120 persons at a time. The staff consists of the medical director, 3 physicians, 3 physical educators, 2 medical substitutes, 2 laboratory technicians, 2 secretaries, 1 nurse, and other service personnel. Despite the expense involved in this organization, its economic profitableness has been demonstrated by a marked reduction of absenteeism. In 1,500 workers, followed over 2 years before and over 2 years after a reconditioning and indoctrination period, the average amount of lost working time was diminished by nearly 70 per cent (3). Furthermore, it has been estimated that the cost of one reconditioning period of 4 weeks is compensated by a 6 months postponement of invalidism and pension payments.

Subjective improvement is reported by about 90 per cent of the trainees at termination of the reconditioning periods. Objective studies of various cardiovascular parameters in several centers have shown an objective improvement of cardiac function, characterized chiefly be a diminution of cardiac sympathetic over-activity, and a partial normalization of both elevated and abnormally low blood pressure levels (4, 5).

These objective gains, aside from a prolonged improvement of subjective well-

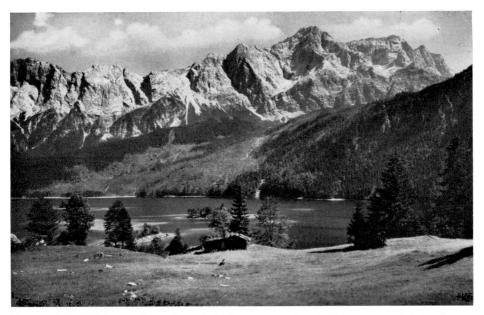

Figure 49–7. "All frets and worries and chafings sank to sleep in the presence of the benignant serenity of the Alps; the Great Spirit of the Mountains breathed his own peace upon their hurt minds and sore hearts and healed them."

MARK TWAIN

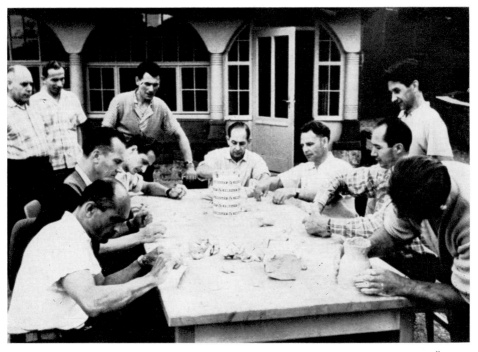

Figure 49–8. Instruction in clay modeling at Reconditioning Center, Schloss Schönberg. (Courtesy Dr. W. Schauwecker.)

being, were found to persist for more than a year, on an average. They depend largely on the degree of continued adherence to the health instructions given at the centers. Long-range morbidity and mortality statistics are not yet available, but follow-up data are now being collected over a 5-year period concerning 5,000 former trainees from several centers for comparison with corresponding non-reconditioned controls.

Research laboratories for the more detailed systematic study of immediate and long-range cardiovascular reconditioning effects were recently established at Ohlstadt by insurance groups, and an extensive research program is now being conducted here by several scientists under the sponsorship of the German Federal Air Force (5).

In 1963 thirteen representatives of the United States Public Health Service, the American College of Preventive Medicine, the American Heart Association, the National Health Council, and other American organizations spent 4 weeks in Germany as the guests of the German Federal Government to acquaint themselves with the German preventive heart reconditioning system (6, 7, 8). The expected establishment of similar centers in the United States and in other industrialized, prosperous countries will unquestionably help to reduce the staggering number of today's premature deaths from heart disease as a major effort toward urgently needed, organized, active prevention.

SUMMARY

In the German Federal Republic 20 reconditioning centers are operated by industries and insurance organizations for the early prevention and rehabilitation of chronic degenerative diseases of civilization, especially ischemic heart disease.

These centers are located in scenically beautiful, mostly mountainous areas. They combine the preventive principles of environmental-emotional relaxation, physical training under careful medical supervision, and a thorough indoctrination for lifelong adherence to acquired health habits.

Recently established scientific institutes at some of the centers have provided objective evidence for a clearly favorable influence of reconditioning periods on cardiovascular function.

Statistical morbidity and mortality studies on a large number of reconditioned subjects are in progress.

REFERENCES

1. BECKMANN, P., WALINSKI, W., and DeWERTH, CHR.: *Internistische Uebungsbehandlung.* Stuttgart, Hippokrates Verlag, 1961.
2. RAAB, W.: *Organized Prevention of Heart Disease.* Vermont, Queen City Printers, 1962.
3. BRUSIS, O.: Ueber die Indikation von Frühheilverfahren mit Terrainkuren bei Sozialversicherten mit Kreislaufschäden und über die Prüfung des Kurerfolges. Inaugural Dissertation, University of Munich, Munich, 1961.
4. NESSWETHA, W., and NATHUSIUS, W.v.: Untersuchungen über die prophylaktische und therapeutische Bedeutung der Terrainkur bei Regulationsstörungen des Kreislaufes der Industriearbeiter. *Int J Prophyl Med, 4;*No. 6, 1960.
5. KIRCHHOFF, H. W.: Cardiovascular function before and after "terrain cures" in the Alps. (See Chapter 50.)
6. American Medical Association: Postwar prosperity, cardiovascular disease, and reconditioning centers. *JAMA, 185;*49, 1963.
7. HELLERSTEIN, H. K.: Reconditioning and the prevention of heart disease. *Mod Med,* May 11, 1964, p. 266.
8. RAAB, W., and GILMAN, L. B.: Insurance-sponsored preventive cardiac reconditioning centers in West Germany. *Amer J Cardiol, 13;*670, 1964.

Chapter L

CARDIOVASCULAR FUNCTION BEFORE AND AFTER RECONDITIONING PERIODS IN A MOUNTAINOUS TERRAIN*
(Preliminary Studies)

(Fürstenfeldbruck, Germany)

So-called "Terrain-Kuren" of at least 4-weeks duration for the prevention and alleviation of cardiovascular disturbances are being carried out in Alpine reconditioning centers as described by Beckmann (1, 2). The basic principles of this type of preventive and rehabilitative treatment consist of combined physical training (hiking, mountain climbing, calisthenics, and breathing exercises) and environmental-emotional relaxation.

In the following, a description of techniques for the objective evaluation of functional results obtained at such centers will be presented (3). These techniques were developed both for the early detection of cardiovascular functional abnormalities and for the purpose of obtaining evidence of their response to reconditioning procedures. At the Reconditioning Center Ohlstadt and at the Medical Research Institute of the Federal German Air Force at Fürstenfeldbruck in the Bavarian Alps, 250 persons between 22 and 50 years of age were submitted to the following types of testing: (a) ergometric determination of heart rate and blood pressure; (b) determination of orthostatic tolerance by means of a tilting table (heart rate,

*Translated by W. Raab.

blood pressure, ECG); (c) low oxygen breathing, and exercise test in a low pressure chamber (ECG), and (d) combined examination of circulatory and respiratory parameters (spiroergometry).

HEART RATE AND BLOOD PRESSURE UNDER GRADED WORK LOADS

Indication. These tests were carried out in order to evaluate the individual effectiveness of circulatory regulation systems and its influence on the range of circulatory performance during physical exertion.

Procedure. With the aid of an ergometer, a photoelectric cardiotachometer and graphic registration of the blood pressure, measurements were taken each minute for at least 10 minutes of exercise in sitting or recumbent position at a work load of 50, 75 or 100 watt, and during the subsequent 5 minutes of recovery.

Comment. Under normal conditions heart rate and blood pressure rise during a constant work load (in a certain proportion to its magnitude) to a rather constantly maintained maximum level (steady state). If the workload exceeds the subject's adaptability, the heart rate

TABLE 50–I

AVERAGE HEART RATE AND BLOOD PRESSURE READINGS
AT REST AND UNDER DEFINED WORK LOADS
IN SUBJECTS OF AVERAGE FITNESS

Work Loads	Heart Rate (Per Minute)	Systolic Blood Pressure (mm Hg)	Diastolic Blood Pressure (mm Hg)
Resting state	50–70	120–140	70–85
50 watt	80–100	130–150	80–90
75 watt	100–120	140–160	80–95
100 watt	110–130	150–170	85–100
125 watt	120–140	160–180	85–100
150 watt	130–150	170–190	90–110

TABLE 50–II

INFLUENCE OF RECONDITIONING THERAPY UPON HEART RATE AND
BLOOD PRESSURE REACTIONS UNDER EFFORT

		Number of Reconditioning Subjects Displaying:				
Total Number of Test Subjects	Change from "Tachycardia of Exhaustion" to Steady State Values	Reduction of the Heart Rate Under Effort by Number of Beats per Min:		Shortening of the Time of Ascent of Heart Rate to Steady State Values:		
		1–10 beats	11–20 beats	1–2 min	3–4 min	
125	20	35	16	33	17	
	(16.0%)	(28.0%)	(12.8%)	(24.4%)	(13.6%)	
	Change from Constantly Rising Blood Pressure to Steady State Values	Lowering of the Systolic Blood Pressure by mm Hg		Lowering of the Diastolic Blood Pressure by mm Hg		
		10 mm	20 mm	10 mm	20 mm	
125	22	38	12	46	11	
	(17.6%)	(30.4%)	(9.6%)	(36.8%)	(8.8%)	

continues to rise until the exertion is stopped ("tachycardia of exhaustion"). The systolic blood pressure behaves in a similar fashion, whereas the diastolic pressure participates in the exercise-induced elevations only to a minor extent (usually 5 to 10 mm Hg) or it may even fall below the resting level. Accordingly, the amplitude of the blood pressure is increased during exertion primarily due to augmentation of the systolic pressure.

Deviations from normal reactions can be recognized by comparison with the ranges obtained by us on normal subjects and shown in Table 50–1.

A favorable condition of the circulatory regulation can be concluded from a rapid ascent of the heart rate to a relatively low steady state level, and a rapid deceleration during recovery. By contrast, a retarded ascent of the heart rate to a high steady state level or a progression of acceleration to a "tachycardia of exhaustion," and slow deceleration are to be regarded as criteria of an uneconomic functioning of the circulatory system. Similar principles apply to the interpretation of blood pressure reactions, whereby a particular significance is to be attributed to abnormally high elevations of the diastolic blood pressure.

Results. As shown in Table 50–II and in Figures 50–1 and 2, a modification of the above-mentioned criteria in the

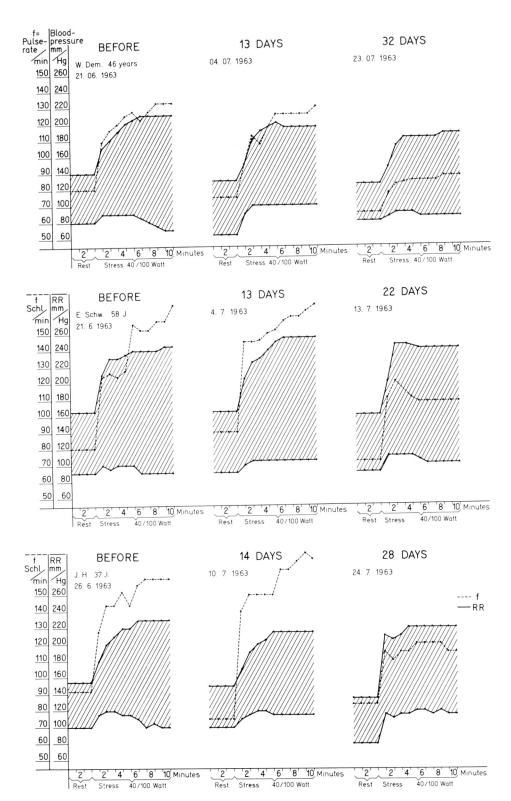

INFLUENCE OF RECONDITIONING THERAPY UPON HEART RATE AND BLOOD PRESSURE

H. W. Kirchhoff, Fürstenfeldbruck - Ohlstadt

Figure 50–1.

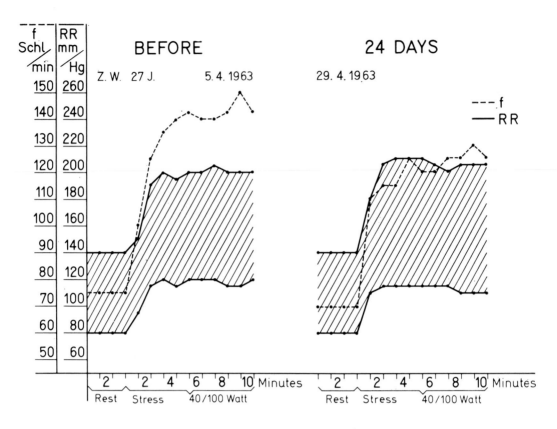

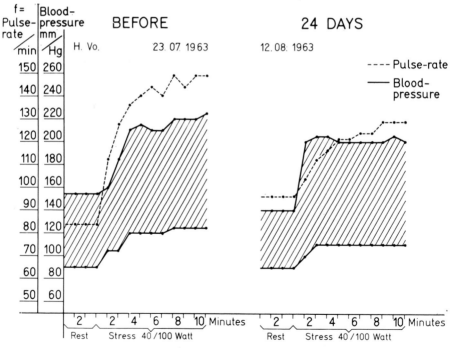

INFLUENCE OF RECONDITIONING THERAPY
UPON HEART RATE AND BLOOD PRESSURE

H. W. Kirchhoff, Fürstenfeldbruck–Ohlstadt

Figure 50–2.

sense of an improved circulatory regulation was observed in a substantial percentage of persons who had undergone 4 weeks of physical and environmental reconditioning in a mountainous terrain.

A reduction of cardiac acceleration during exercise was particularly conspicuous.

Exaggerated systolic pressure peaks are, as a rule, reduced first during the "Terrain-Kur." This is often followed by a lowering of the systolic steady state level. Diastolic pressure reductions appear latest, if at all. Other favorable effects on blood pressure regulation consist in some cases of a faster stabilization on a steady state level and of an acceleration of the post-exercise pressure decline. Hiking and mountain climbing toward the end of the reconditioning period seemed particularly effective in lowering the diastolic blood pressure.

ORTHOSTATIC TOLERANCE

Indication. Testing for orthostatic tolerance is indicated in subjects who complain of abnormal dizziness, fatigue, inclination to blackouts and fainting, suggestive of disturbances of circulatory regulation.

Procedure. The test subjects are fastened with a belt to a tilting table in a relaxed, recumbent position. Electrodes are attached with adhesive paste. After stabilization of heart rate and blood pressure, the table is raised to vertical position and measurements of heart rate, blood pressure and ECG are recorded each minute for 10 minutes, unless the patient is approaching collapse.

Comment. Normally the heart rate increases only slightly and the pulse pressure remains within adequate limits after upward tilting. "Orthostatic lability" is characterized by irregular fluctuations of the heart rate which may reach 110 to 130 beats per minute. The blood pressure may also vary considerably, and the pulse pressure may become narrowed down to as little as 10 mm Hg due to a systolic depression which not infrequently coincides with an elevation of the diastolic pressure level. If the pulse pressure shrinks to below 10 mm, if tachycardia becomes extreme, and if collapse occurs, the term "orthostatic insufficiency" is being used.

Results. In 36 subjects who had displayed the signs of orthostatic lability or insufficiency, the "Terrain-Kur" was followed by a stabilization and normalization of the respective circulatory parameters (Fig. 50-3), and initially observed abnormalities of T and ST were reduced or disappeared.

HYPOXIA TEST WITHOUT AND WITH EXERCISE

Indication. Low oxygen breathing tests and exercise tests under conditions of low oxygen pressure were carried out in order to bring to light a subclinical predisposition to coronary insufficiency.

Comment. In the conventional exercise tests and low oxygen breathing tests, two factors, indicative of the available coronary reserve, are being evaluated separately by either augmenting myocardial oxygen consumption (exercise) or by diminishing exogenous oxygen supply (low O_2 breathing). The combination of both techniques permits an earlier detection of a tendency toward myocardial ischemia (of either vascular or metabolic origin or both) than either procedure by itself alone.

Procedure. (a) Plain hypoxia tests

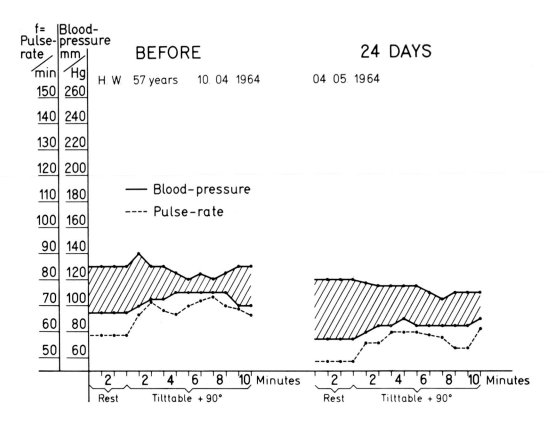

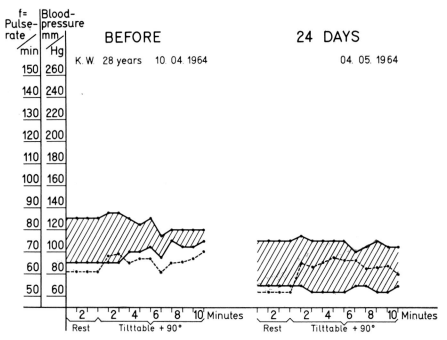

INFLUENCE OF RECONDITIONING THERAPY UPON REACTION
OF BLOOD PRESSURE AND HEART RATE TO TILTING

H. W. Kirchhoff, Fürstenfeldbruck–Ohlstadt

Figure 50–3.

were applied by breathing successively oxygen concentrations of 21 per cent, 14 per cent, 12 per cent and 10 per cent. With each concentration, standard and chest lead ECG's were recorded after 5 and 10 minutes.

(b) In a large low-pressure chamber, 12 ECG leads were taken first at atmospheric pressure, whereupon the subject had to repeat the double Master step test at a simulated altitude of 12,000 ft. Electrocardiograms were taken immediately, and 2 and 4 minutes after termination of effort.

Hypoxic changes of the T wave and depressions of ST were used as criteria of myocardial ischemia.

Results. In all of 26 subjects whose ECGs had shown hypoxic ST reactions in the low oxygen tests, the ECG was partly or completely normalized after completion of a "Terrain-Kur."

SPIROERGOMETRY

Indication. The parameters measured by spiroergometry are useful in assessing a subject's actual work capacity. They can be determined under a maximum tolerated work load (*vita maxima*) as well as during the steady state attained under a certain known amount of exertion.

Procedure. The following circulatory and respiratory data were recorded simultaneously: (a) O_2 uptake; (b) CO_2 exhalation; (c) respiratory quotient; (d) respiratory volume; (e) respiratory equivalent, and (f) oxygen pulse.

Comment. In principle, determinations of oxygen uptake during physical exertion can be considered as a criterion of total cardiocirculatory effectiveness in providing the active peripheral tissues with a maximum of oxygen as a direct result of maximal cardiac output. In physically unfit individuals, the oxygen uptake during exertion is reduced both under *vita maxima* and under steady state conditions. However, since the ideal "normal" values for a given individual are difficult to assess, it is preferable to determine simultaneously other parameters which offer additional information regarding cardiocirculatory efficiency. This applies particularly to work loads below the *vita maxima* level.

The respiratory quotient under minor and medium work loads ranges ordinarily between 0.8 and 0.9. When it rises to between 0.95 and 1.0, this indicates that the subject is approaching the limits of his work capacity.

Determination of the respiratory equivalent (relation between respiratory volume and oxygen uptake per minute) provides information concerning respiratory economy. A high quotient indicates that a relatively large respiratory volume is required to effectuate the uptake of a certain amount of oxygen, and vice versa. The range of variations of respiratory equivalents during exertion is narrower than at rest. Therefore, their informative value is greater under conditions of effort. High quotients are found in subjects with abnormalities of respiratory surface, diffusibility and regulation. Such factors are apt to interfere with work capacity.

The so-called "oxygen pulse" represents the calculated amount of oxygen taken up by the body per heart beat. This parameter serves as a criterion of circulatory economy in that any increase of the oxygen pulse reveals an augmentation of cardiovascular work capacity.

Results. Tables 50–III and IV show improvements of some coordinated parameters following reconditioning periods.

TABLE 50–III

RESPIRATORY AND CIRCULATORY PARAMETERS BEFORE AND AFTER
RECONDITIONING (UNDER STEADY STATE WORK LOAD 100 WATT

Number of Test Subjects 22	Oxygen Uptake in ml		Respiratory Volume in 1/min		Heart Rate Beats/min		Blood Pressure mm Hg	
	Before	After	Before	After	Before	After	Before	After
Average	1610	1560	44	41.5	144	126	195/100	175/95
SD	±106	±88	±6	±5	+11	±10	±12/±5	±8/±4
Certainty	80–95%		80–95%		>99.9%		>99.9%	

TABLE 50–IV

RESPIRATORY AND CIRCULATORY PARAMETERS BEFORE AND AFTER
RECONDITIONING (UNDER *VITA MAXIMA* WORK LOAD)

Number of Test Subjects 12	Oxygen Uptake in ml		Respiratory Volume in 1/min		Oxygen Pulse	
	Before	After	Before	After	Before	After
Average	2250	2940	88	112	11.4	15.6
SD	±168	±212	±12	±18	±2.4	±3.2
Certainty	>99.9		>99.9		>99.9	

SUMMARY

Preliminary studies of several cardiovascular and respiratory parameters were carried out in 250 test subjects.

Measurements in subjects with premorbid disturbances of cardiovascular regulation were made before and after reconditioning periods ("Terrain-Kuren") of at least 4 weeks duration at reconditioning centers in the Alps) and compared. In a substantial number of instances they suggest a definite improvement of cardiovascular regulation and respiratory efficiency.

There occurred a lowering of the heart rate and blood pressure at rest and during exercise, an improvement of orthostatic tolerance, normalization of exercise-induced hypoxic electrocardiographic changes at low oxygen pressure, and an increase of oxygen uptake, respiratory volume and oxygen pulse during physical effort.

These data seem to corroborate the concept of a preventive and rehabilitative value (for the autonomic nervous and cardiovascular systems) of physical and environmental-emotional reconditioning programs in appropriate rural centers.

REFERENCES

1. BECKMANN, P., WALINSKI, W., and DeWERTH, CHR.: *Internistische Uebungsbehandlung.* Stuttgart, Hippokrates Verlag, 1961.
2. BECKMANN, P.: Combined environmental-emotional and physical cardiac prevention programs in the West German reconditioning centers. (See Chapter 49.)
3. KIRCHHOFF, H. W.: *Praktische Funktionsdiagnostik des Herzens und Kreislaufs.* Munich, Johann Ambrosius Barth, 1965.

Chapter LI

OBJECTIVE RESULTS OF PHYSICAL TRAINING THERAPY AT RURAL RECONDITIONING CENTERS

MARIA BLOHMKE

(Heidelberg, Germany)

IN THE German Federal Republic, 700,000 "kuren"* are conducted yearly at the suggestion of referring doctors and at the expense of the State Insurance. The financial costs of the kuren are considerable and amount yearly to 250 million American dollars. "Kur" therapies have a long tradition in Germany and in Central Europe. Even the Romans reported the therapeutic action of the German spas, and a large part of the life of the social elite of Germany was spent at spa resorts in the past, as pointed out by Goethe.

In those days, one could afford a kur when one had time and money at ones disposal. In other words, it was a privilege of a very marginal social class. At the beginning of the thirties, the social insurance companies began to take over the costs of the kur therapy for their insured (in case of illness). In 1957 a law was passed establishing the possibility of kuren for the preservation, improvement and rehabilitation of the individual's working capacity. The doctor concerned can prescribe a kur for a patient purely as a matter of precaution when the patient does not yet show any manifest organic disease, but only reports subjective complaints and functional disturbances.

After passage of this law, the medical and pension insurance representatives of the coal mines (the Miner's Union) decided to introduce preventive kuren and thus bought for this purpose 3 kur-houses, one in the Black Forest in Hundseck, one in the Odenwald, Schloss Schönberg, and one on the North Sea at Borkum. In these 3 homes, 4,000 kuren are conducted per year. All 3 houses are situated in places having an extremely favorable climate. Miners who have worked underground for at least 10 to 15 years in the mines come to these kur-centers (reconditioning centers). Ninety-one per cent of the miners report functional complaints, while the rest are free from complaints. Ill persons are not admitted to these reconditioning centers. The cost of the 4 weeks kuren is borne completely by the respective insurance

---

*The term "kur" (pronounced "koor") with the plural "kuren" ("kooren") differs in meaning from the Enligh "cure." In contrast to the latter, it does not necessarily imply a successful course of treatment but rather a prolonged period of therapeutic procedures as such, regardless of the outcome. Specifically, the term "kur" is used for a period of time spent in a spa or reconditioning center.

agency. The only way in which the miner participates in this expenditure is by giving up 10 days of his yearly vacation, the length of which varies between 18 and 28 days.

In the 3 union homes the kuren are conducted as originally recommended by Beckmann (1). They consist of exercises such as gymnastics and hiking, in winter, also skiing, combined cold water applications according to the Kneipp method, and Sauna treatment. During every kur group lectures are held on various topics based on the theme: Health is teachable and learnable. Films are shown, painting and handicrafts are being taught. In short, an effort is made to help the trainee relax generally, and give him an interest in worthwhile leisure time recreational activities. The supervising doctors are always available for personal talks. "Autogenic training" (i.e., periods of complete physical and mental relaxation in a quiet, darkened room with soft music) is given 3 times a week to groups selected by the physicians.

It appeared to be of interest to investigate the objective functional effects of such kuren. For this purpose, the union-homes seemed to be especially suitable, as we could choose our subjects from about 100 kur trainees during each kur period. Thus healthy persons of similar ages and similar work capacities were selected for our tentative pilot study. With our methods we can obtain data concerning the level of physical fitness at the outset, and observe the eventual improvement of the fitness level of the muscles, the heart and circulatory system. Psychological tests have also been employed but are not yet sufficient for statistical evaluation.

We examined 40 trainees in the kur-home Schloss Schönberg and 60 in the kur-home Hundseck, the latter of which is located at an altitude of 2,500 feet in the Black Forest.

The following symptoms were reported by our subjects: sensations near the heart, such as stabbing, burning, feelings of pressure or palpitations (by 37 per cent), headaches (by 37 per cent), insomnia (by 27 per cent), dizziness (by 26 per cent), stomach complaints (by 22 per cent), cold hands and feet (by 21 per cent) and loss of weight (by 21 per cent). All in all, 91 per cent of our subjects had various complaints.

METHODS

Examinations took place within the first and last 3 days of a kur period. At the beginning of the kur, we first tested the work capacity of the individual subjects by means of an ergometer. The subsequent tests took place only in the morning, each subject being tested at the same hour of the day on the following 2 days. At the beginning the patient had to lie quietly for 30 minutes on a bed in an isolated room. After that, his pulse rate at rest, his blood pressure and breathing frequency were recorded. The patient was then taken into another room where an electrocardiogram was made. After this, with the chest electrodes and blood pressure cuff in place, the subject sat quietly for another 3 minutes on the ergometer. After exercising for 6 minutes, the subject lay down, his pulse rate being measured continuously. In the second minute after termination of exercise, an ECG was again recorded and the test was concluded 5 minutes after the end of exertion.

For estimation of the individual effort we used the acceleration of the pulse rate. In the first and second kur we made the subjects exert themselves to a mean pulse rate of 130 beats per minute and also regulated the watt-value at the end of the kur period. In the next kur groups (III, IV, V) the pulse rate was adjusted to a frequency of 145 beats per minute and the watt-value was not regulated at the end of the kur period. Since for technical reasons it was not possible to measure the oxygen uptake directly, we calculated the maximal oxygen uptake using Åstrand's (2) "nomogram for calculation of aerobic work capacity from submaximal pulse rate and work load." This value was then multiplied by the factor 0.87, which is an age correction factor for our 35-year-old subjects.

Furthermore, we recorded the pulse rate at rest, the pulse rate during the sixth minute of exercise, the total heart beats from the fourth to sixth minute of exercise, and the recovery pulse sum.

The blood pressure was measured at rest after 30 minutes of lying quietly, in the third minute of rest while sitting on the ergometer, and in the second, fourth and sixth minutes of exercise; also in the first, third and fifth minute of recovery. Hemoglobin values and erythrocyte counts were determined at the beginning and at the end of the kur.

RESULTS

Pulse Rate. Mean pulse rates showed a clear reduction at the end of the kuren. Before the kur, the mean pulse rate at rest was 71 beats per minute, after the kur it was 68 beats per minute. The mean difference was significant at $p = 0.05$ level.

Next we calculated the total pulse accelerations for the fourth to sixth minute of effort by adding the pulse rate

values for these 3 minutes and subtracting the resting pulse rates from this total.

The following values were thus obtained. The pulse total was reduced by 10 beats per minute, the mean difference being significant at the $p = 0.01$ level. The pulse total of the 5 minutes of recovery was calculated against the pulse rate at rest before the effort. The recovery pulse rate at the beginning of the kur was 67 beats per minute, at the end of the kur it was 57 beats per minute, but the difference was not statistically significant.

Maximal Oxygen Uptake. From the values of the maximal oxygen uptake at the beginning of the kur, one can conclude that the general bodily condition of the miners was relatively good, owing to the fact that their work is physically hard. The mean capacity of the subjects was 1.9 watts per kg or 0.83 watts per cm of body height. The maximal oxygen uptake per kg of body weight was 39.0 ml/kg/min at the end of the kur.

The means of the maximal oxygen uptake which we estimated from Åstrand's nomogram showed an increase of approximately 0.2 to 0.7 liters of oxygen. The mean values before and after the kur were 2.96 versus 3.27 liters/min, respectively. The difference was significant at the 0.001 p-level.

Blood Pressure. No regular reduction of either the systolic or diastolic blood pressure was observed and the mean blood pressure did not change distinctly. It must be noted here, however, that the first values recorded on each subject were all within normal limits (i.e., the systolic values were lower than 150 mm Hg, and the diastolic values were not higher than 95 mm Hg). In general, the latter were around 80 mm Hg.

In 36 per cent of the subjects an increase of blood pressure of 200 to 270 mm Hg was measured during effort. This abnormal increase in blood pressure we cannot, as yet, explain. The high blood pressure values were not dependent either on the height of the pulse frequency on effort, nor on the blood pressure level at rest, nor on the work load itself. These abnormally high blood pressure elevations did not show any definite reduction during the kur.

The hemoglobin values and erythrocyte counts rose in all cases. The differences of both values between the beginning and end of the kur were highly significant (p = less than 0.001).

Furthermore, we were interested in the correlations between the individual measured and calculated parameters. The mass correlations for all relevant combinations were calculated. They showed large differences for the various parameters.

Levels of Significance. A highly negative correlation of -0.71 † was obtained between the pulse frequency at rest and the sum of the pulse rates, from the fourth to sixth minute of effort. There was a highly positive correlation of 0.58 † between the fourth and sixth minute pulse total on effort and the recovery pulse total. It thus appears that a direct relation exists between the total pulse on effort and the recovery pulse total, because the latter starts to rise when the work load is well above the normal capacity level. On the other hand, the correlation coefficient between the pulse frequency at rest and the recovery pulse total was negative and very low at 0.26. The correlation coefficient between the pulse rate at rest and the oxygen uptake was highly negative (-0.84†). Between the heart rate at rest and the erythrocyte counts it was also negative (-0.67†).

The relatively high correlation coefficient between the pulse rate during the sixth minute on effort and the pulse total on effort for the fourth to sixth minute may be explained by the fact that the pulse rate of the sixth minute on effort is included in the calculation of the total pulse on effort.

CONCLUSIONS

It appears that, apart from the total recovery pulse, all of the parameters used are suitable to evaluate the influence of the kur on the individual level of physical fitness. The pulse during the sixth minute of effort was reduced in 68 per cent, the pulse total on effort in 70.4 per cent, and recovery pulse in 57.4 per cent of the 54 subjects. The pulse rate at rest was reduced in 62 per cent and the maximum oxygen uptake was increased in 70.8 per cent of the 100 subjects.

Out of the 54 subjects who were tested on all parameters, 10 showed an improvement in each of the 5 variables; 28 subjects improved in 4 parameters; 38 subjects in 3, and 46 in 2 parameters. Forty-nine subjects improved in only 1 parameter, 5 subjects did not improve in any of the parameters. At the present time we cannot give any particular reason for these irregularities of the results. It is more than likely that they are due to a variety of as yet unidentified factors. We assume that neuroses, depressions, hereditary and social influences affect the variables measured, but such factors were evident only in 2 of the cases. Currently applied psychological tests may help to elucidate these disturbing influences.

---

†Highly significant, significant, probably significant.

It ought to be kept in mind that in general the physical condition of our subjects was too good to be much improved. It is probable, therefore, that normalizing effects of kur periods as measured by our methods would be more impressive in persons doing sedentary work. A control group of vacationing miners not participating in any physical exercise program will be examined next.

SUMMARY

In 100 miners, who over a period of 4 weeks had participated in a physical exercise program in a German kur home (reconditioning center), a study was conducted in order to investigate the objective functional effects of such kuren, which lasted 4 weeks. Examinations took place within the first and last 3 days of a kur period.

The criteria measured at rest and after exercise were pulse rate, blood pressure and electrocardiogram. During the exercise, which lasted for 6 minutes, the pulse rate was registered continuously, and the blood pressure was measured every other minute.

The mean pulse rates showed a clear reduction at the end of the kuren. The mean values of the oxygen uptake, estimated from Åstrand's nomogram, showed a clear increase. No regular reduction of either the systolic or diastolic blood pressure was observed.

REFERENCES

1. BECKMANN, P.: Körperliche Ertüchtigung während der Kur. *Aerztl Prax, 13:*1295, 1961.
2. ÅSTRAND, I.: Aerobic work capacity in men and women with special reference to age. *Acta Physiol Scand, 49:* Suppl. 169, 1960.

Chapter LII

INFLUENCE OF HIGH ALTITUDES ON CARDIOVASCULAR AUTONOMIC NERVOUS AND HORMONAL REGULATION

MAX J. HALHUBER

(Innsbruck, Austria)

CLIMATIC conditions and altitude are of theoretical and practical interest for preventive cardiology in general, and especially with regard to sojourns in reconditioning centers in mountainous areas.

What are the reactions of the autonomic nervous system when one uses a chairlift in a skiing area or stays for 4 weeks near the top of Mt. Mansfield (4000 feet) in the Green Mountains of Vermont?

Some of the studies reported here were carried out during the last 10 years in the Austrian Alps at the University of Innsbruck in cooperation with Drs. H. Jungmann, F. Gabl, E. Haus, and others.

Acute changes of altitude precipitate phasic changes in the circulatory system. Immediately after arrival at a high altitude, bradycardia appears as a feature of the first phase, accompanied by a reduction of the pulse pressure and reduction of the cardiac output (Fig. 52–1).

After 1 to 2 hours, the initial parasympathicotonia gives way to the second phase with cardiac acceleration and an increase in the cardiac output. At an altitude of 6,500 feet, the increase in the pulse rate in the supine position is at least 10 percent; at 12,000 feet, more than 18 per cent, and at 15,000 feet more than 50 per cent. The pulse wave velocity, expressing arterial tonus, showed an upward trend in this phase, and a temporary increase of the blood pressure was observed.

As a result of an acute change in altitude up to 6,500 feet, the ECG showed no typical alterations in our studies. At 15,000 feet, Penaloza (1) found rather frequent ST variations at rest, developing after the first to the fourth day, and characterized by ST elevation and negative T waves over the right ventricle. The duration of the second phase depends both on the altitude and on the degree of preadaptation. At 6,500 feet, it lasts hours to days; at 10,000 feet about 3 days, and at 12,000 feet, 5 to 10 days.

The second phase is followed by further hemodynamic alterations. The initially increased pulse wave velocity drops markedly and reaches a minimum in about the third week; the cardiac output returns to the initial value. In the course of the third week, intensified reactions of the circulatory system occur under the influence of physical activity. Disturbances of the cardiac rhythm were observed in predisposed individuals, such as atrioventricular rhythm and extra-

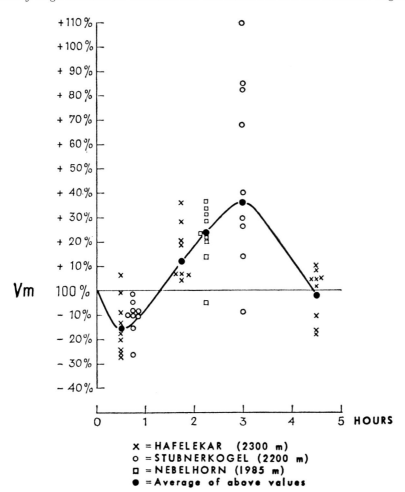

Figure 52–1. Two-phase alterations of cardiac output (Vm) after ascent to altitudes between 6,300 and 7,600 feet, expressed as percentage of the initial value at lower levels (2000 to 3000 feet).

systoles. Individual differences in cardio-vascular reactions are considerable, depending upon constitution and the degree of training.

Nearly all of the cardiovascular alterations caused by acute changes of altitude disappear when acclimatization is completed; the pulse rate at rest is then normal or decreased. Hartmann and von Muralt (2) regard the disappearance of tachycardia in higher altitudes as the most important sign of acclimatization.

The blood pressure becomes relatively low at rest as well as during effort; cardiac output is reduced; the initially increased pulse wave velocity is markedly diminished during the third week at altitude, and later seems to return to normal. The sensitivity to atropine and sympathomimetics is decreased alongside with an increased sensitivity to acetylcholine (3).

At an altitude of 6,500 feet, the vital capacity decreases during the first days,

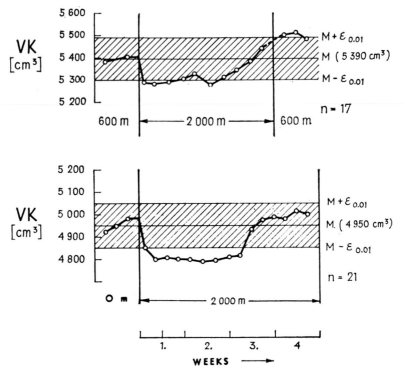

Figure 52–2. Average decrease of vital capacity at high altitude in 38 health students; values outside the shaded area are highly significant.

and even more so at a greater altitude difference, as shown in Figure 52–2. The lower vapor pressure of the air at high altitudes tends to dry and cool the respiratory mucosa. This is most noticeable during the first few days, especially under physical exertion, and predisposes to tracheitis and bronchitis. This factor probably explains the slowing of the maximum expiration rate (Tiffeneau test) during the first days.

Figure 52–3 shows the changes in the 17-hydroxy-corticosteroid excretion in the urine in 5 subjects who stayed 4 weeks at the highest European village, Obergurgl (20,000 feet). These changes suggest increases and decreases in adrenocortical activity during this period. We know from other investigations that the

transition from low to high altitudes causes a stimulation of the ardenal cortex (4).

The 17-hydroxy-corticosteroid excretion at sea level was about 3 mg/12 hr. During the first week at a high altitude the values were significantly increased to 4 and 4.5 mg/12 hr.

During the second week the average values fell to the range of those obtained at sea level with relatively narrow individual differences. During the third week there were pronounced discrepancies between the individual values, some of which were extremely high. During the fourth week, the results again resembled the initial values in Hamburg. In the last period, the differences between the individual values again were small (5),

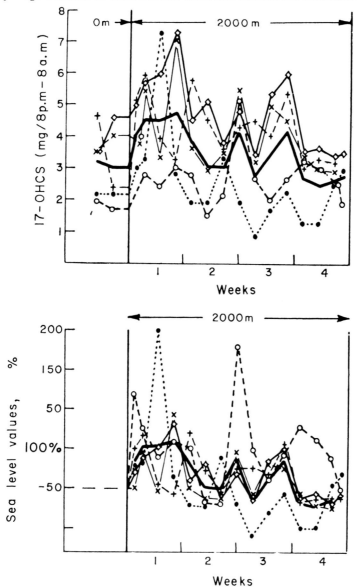

Figure 52–3. 17-hydroxy-corticosteroid (17-OHCS) excretion in the urine during 4 weeks at 6600 feet altitude. Single plottings of 5 test persons. (Mean value curve = heavy line) *Upper curves*: 12/hr 17-OHCS excretion in mg. The first 2 plottings stand for the initial Hamburg values. *Lower curves*: 17-OHCS excretion in Obergurgl (6600 feet) represented in percent of the initial values (mean value of the two initial Hamburg results).

SUMMARY

Acclimatization (i.e., adaptation to an unaccustomed altitude, e.g., in reconditioning centers in mountainous areas) is not a simple linear process. It involves cardiovascular manifestations indicating neural and hormonal instability during the first hours and days. These are followed by contrasting phases after the elapse of 2 to 3 weeks.

The concurrent alterations of heart rate, cardiac output, pulse wave velocity, blood pressure and ECG may be easily mistaken for symptoms of cardiovascular disease. They should be considered when functional effects of reconditioning periods in mountainous areas are evaluated.

REFERENCES

1. PENALOZA, R., MARTICORENA, E., ECCHEVARRIA, M., DYER, J., and GUTIERREZ, E.: Influence of high altitudes on the electrical activity of the heart. *Amer. Heart J, 61:*101, 1961.

2. HARTMANN, H., and VON MURALT, A.: Pulsfrequenz und Höhenanpassung. Untersuchungen der deutschen Himalaya-Expedition 1931 und in der Unterdruckkammer in Zürich. *Acta Aerophysiol, 1:*38, 1934.

3. JUNGMANN, H., and HALHUBER, M. J.: The physiology of high altitudes. In: *Medical Climatology.* New Haven, Sidney Licht, 1964.

4. KOLLER, F., SCHWARZ, E., and MARTI, M.: Ueber die Reaktion der Nebennierenrinde beim Aufstieg ins Hochgebirge. *Acta Endocr, 16:*118, 1954.

5. HALHUBER, M. J., and GABL, F.: Symposium on the effects of high altitude. Interlaken, Sept., 1962; Pergamon Press; Oxford, London, New York, Paris, 1963.

Chapter LIII

ENVIRONMENTAL RECONDITIONING TREATMENT OF PATIENTS WITH ISCHEMIC HEART DISEASE ON THE CRIMEAN COAST*

M. N. PERTSOVSKY

(Yalta, U.S.S.R.)

ON THE Southern coast of the Crimean Peninsula, a large number of patients with atherosclerotic ischemic heart disease are being accommodated and treated each year.

Personal investigations of Professor S. P. Tatyevosov have revealed in the majority of these patients both a subjective and an objective improvement, whereby the latter was manifested chiefly by electrocardiographic criteria. Drs. V. N. Lukyanov and A. S. Ukraynets observed a lowering of the serum cholesterol level in these cases.

Our own observations were obtained on 50 patients (44 men and 6 women). Four of these were between 40 and 50-years-old, 36 between 51 and 60 years and 10 over 60 years.

Forty-three of the patients suffered from myocardial ischemia of the first degree (according to the criteria of Lang). Seven did not show any signs of disturbed coronary circulation. Twenty-five were diagnosed as chronic coronary insufficiency on the basis of their clinical history and electrocardiogram. Six had sustained a myocardial infarction.

For evaluation of the functional state of the myocardium, we used the electro- and ballistocardiogram; for study of biochemical parameters we applied the Engelhardt-Smirnov method for serum cholesterol, the Bloor method for lecithin, the Hagedorn-Jensen method for blood sugar, and the Bogomolov method for determination of the prothrombin index. All of these tests were carried out within the first 2 to 3 days after admission and within the last 2 to 3 days prior to discharge.

The therapeutic program made extensive use of the climatic elements prevailing on the coast of the Black Sea. During the warm season (April to September) it consisted of exposure to open air and sunlight, bathing in the sea, sleeping nights on the beach, and hiking; during the cool season (October to March) baths were taken in indoor seawater pools. The patients slept on verandas and walked along the beach. These climatic-environmental measures were prescribed in individual dosages and applied under medical supervision.

No drugs were administered except validol in the case of acute anginal attacks. The sojourn at the reconditioning center lasted 26 days.

*Translated by W. Raab.

At the time of discharge, 4 patients reported a marked subjective improvement, 42 a considerable improvement, 3 no change, and 1 a worsening.

On admission, most of the patients complained of oppressing or painful sensations in the precordial area with or without characteristic irradiations, shortness of breath and palpitations. Objectively the majority showed an enlargement of the heart, notably of the left ventricle, muffled heart sounds, a systolic murmur near the apex, and an accentuation of the second aortic sound.

At termination of treatments, the precordial pain had disappeared in 76 per cent of the patients; shortness of breath had ceased in 27 per cent and was diminished in 68 per cent.

The electrocardiogram showed several definite changes. At the time of discharge a sinus rhythm with a normal heart rate was found in 40 cases, as compared with 33 on admission. Two patients had extrasystoles and a partial atrioventricular block, respectively. These phenomena did not subside.

Retarded intraatrial conduction was observed on admission in 2 cases, an atrioventricular conduction defect in 6, and a disturbed intraventricular conduction in 23. During the therapy period, intraatrial conduction was improved in one case, atrioventricular conduction in 3, and intraventricular conduction in 14 cases. In 3 patients the latter was worsened.

A shortening and normalization of the electrical systole after treatment was observed in 13 out of 26 patients; in 4 cases the duration of the systole became increased.

A normal position of the electrical axis was seen on admission in 17 cases, a left axis deviation in 29 and a right axis deviation in 4. These findings remained unchanged until discharge.

An augmentation of the voltage of R in 3 standard leads occurred under treatment in 26 instances, a decrease of the voltage of R in 12.

On admission, 23 patients presented a diphasic (positive-negative) or inverted T wave; 17 of these were in the third lead. At the time of discharge, this feature had disappeared in 5 cases; in 3 instances, an inversion of T became apparent in the third lead.

Under the influence of treatment, 52 per cent of the patients with coronary insufficiency showed a normalization of the position of the ST interval.

In the others, the electrocardiographic abnormalities were fixed. Furthermore, some patients with chronic coronary insufficiency of an advanced degree reacted to changing meteorological conditions (temperature, atmospheric pressure) with an appearance or aggravation of anginal symptoms and shortness of breath.

Ballistocardiograms were recorded by means of Dock's electromagnetic system. In order to establish the time relation of the ballistocardiographic deflections with the phases of cardiac activity, the ballistocardiogram was registered with simultaneous superimposition of the R wave of the second lead.

In analyzing the ballistocardiograms, the time lag between the electrical and the hemodynamic systole was determined (R-H interval); also the length of the mechanical systole (R-K) and the ventricular ejection period (H-K). The ballistic index was calculated.

Besides, the entire ballistocardiogram was studied according to the classification of Brown for evaluation of myocardial contractility (Table 53–I).

TABLE 53–I

Ballistocardiographic Parameters	Number of Cases	
	On Admission	On Discharge
R–H = 0.06–0.09 sec. (normal range)	21	29
R–H = >0.09 sec. (prolonged)	29	21
R–K = 0.26–0.36 sec. (normal range)	38	46
R–K = >0.36 sec. (prolonged)	12	4
Ballistic index 0.4–1.0 (normal range)	27	41
Ballistic index <0.4 (diminished)	23	9
"Early" or "late" M	26	22

At termination of the treatments, the contractile function of the heart was improved in a sizeable number of patients, as manifested by an augmented effectiveness of ventricular contraction. At the same time, the number of ballistocardiograms with abnormalities of the degrees O and I had become larger, and those with abnormalities of degrees III and IV were decreased.

Quite frequently, repeated ballistocardiographic tests revealed a reduction of deformed deflections, an augmentation of voltage and, in 4 instances, the disappearance of M-shaped deformations.

Clinical improvement was not always accompanied by a lowering of the serum cholesterol level or an increase of the concentration of lecithin. Hypercholesterolemia (above 200 mg%) was found only in half of the patients. This may be explained by the fact that in cases of coronary sclerosis of the third degree of the second period, according to Myasnikov's classification, vascular sclerotic processes attain prevalence over biochemical factors.

Average values at the start and termination of treatment periods, respec-

tively, were the following: cholesterol: 199.2 mg% versus 190.9 mg%; lecithin: 215.8 mg% versus 227.0 mg%; blood glucose 110 mg% versus 105 mg%; prothrombin index 90.4% versus 88.6%.

A post-treatment diminution of the serum cholesterol concentration was observed chiefly in patients who had had hypercholesterolemic levels from the beginning. There was a distinct tendency toward augmentation of lecithin in the blood. The ratio lecithin:cholesterol increased due to a simultaneous diminution of cholesterol. It varied within the range of 0.64 to 1.45. At the conclusion of the treatments, the ratio was increased in 31 cases; in 7 it was decreased.

At the beginning, the prothrombin index exceeded 100 per cent in 8 patients, amounting to 110 per cent in 2, and to 108 per cent in one. The blood sugar level was elevated in 7 (125 to 140 mg%). At the time of discharge those parameters had returned to normal.

SUMMARY

Environmental and climatic treatment in reconditioning centers on the Southern coast of the Crimean Peninsula was applied to patients with atherosclerotic ischemic heart disease. It was followed in the majority of instances by an improvement of the functional state of the heart muscle, as manifested by favorable changes in the electrocardiogram and ballistocardiogram.

A tendency toward a reduction of the serum cholesterol and an augmentation of the serum lecithin level caused in the majority of instances an increase in the ratio lecithin:cholesterol.

In patients with chronic coronary insufficiency, the signs of amelioration were less marked.

Chapter LIV

ASPECTS OF THE INFLUENCE OF A HOT AND HUMID ENVIRONMENT ON THE CARDIOVASCULAR SYSTEM OF MAN*

GEORGE E. BURCH and NICHOLAS P. DePASQUALE

(New Orleans, Louisiana, U.S.A.)

THE influence of climatic stress on the cardiovascular system of man has not been studied adequately, particularly for diseased man. Experimental data obtained from laboratory animals have been useful in the understanding of many important aspects of human cardiovascular function. However, translation of bioclimatologic data from laboratory animals to man is not always valid because man's thermoregulatory apparatus differs in many ways from that of other animals. For example, the eccrine sweat glands are more highly developed in man than in any other species of animal. In man, as in other mammals, heat is lost from the respiratory tract, but unlike most other animals the primary avenue of heat loss in man under conditions of extreme thermal stress is the evaporation of sweat from the surface of the body. It has not been sufficiently emphasized that valid data on the influence of climate on man can be obtained best from studies on man. Furthermore, psychic factors peculiar to man often play a significant part in the overall physiologic responses to thermal stress.

General Thermoregulatory Responses to a Hot and Humid Environment

Man, like all other homeothermic animals, maintains a relatively constant body temperature by balancing heat production with heat loss. In a comfortable or neutral environment, thermal equilibrium is maintained primarily through vasomotor regulation. Under such circumstances the amount of heat lost from the surface of the body by radiation and convection is regulated according to heat production by varying the dermal blood flow (1). When the environmental temperature and humidity increase so that body temperature can no longer be maintained by radiation and convection, man sweats and heat is lost from the surface of the body by evaporation (essentially 0.58 calorie/g of H_2O).

Vasomotor thermal regulation, per se, does not place an unusual load on the cardiovascular system; but when evaporative cooling is necessary to maintain thermal equilibrium, a burden is placed on the cardiovascular system, the magnitude of which is directly related to the degree of thermal stress (1, 2, 3). Following exposure to a hot and humid environ-

*Supported by grants from the U.S. Public Health Service.

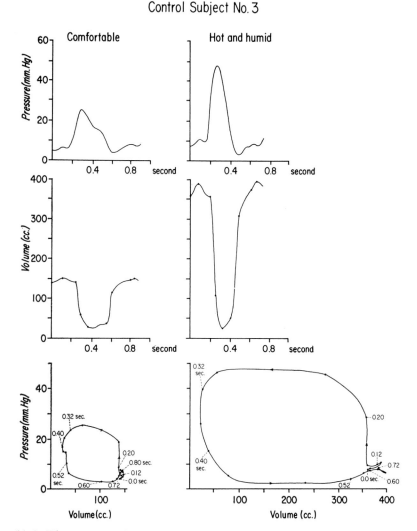

Figure 54–1. Time courses of pressure and volume of the right ventricle of a subject without cardiovascular disease, studied in comfortable and hot and humid environments. Exposure to a hot and humid environment was associated with a greater increase in stroke output than in stroke pressure.

ment, the dermal blood vessels dilate. The associated decrease in peripheral vascular resistance results in an increase in cardiac output and dermal blood flow. In fact, the dermal vasculature behaves like a large A-V fistula. Tachycardia and tachypnea develop (4). Eventually, total circulating blood volume increases. There is also an increase in systemic venous tone (5) which produces an elevation in the ventricular filling pressure to support the high cardiac output.

It is obvious from the above that exposure to a hot and humid environment is associated with profound circulatory

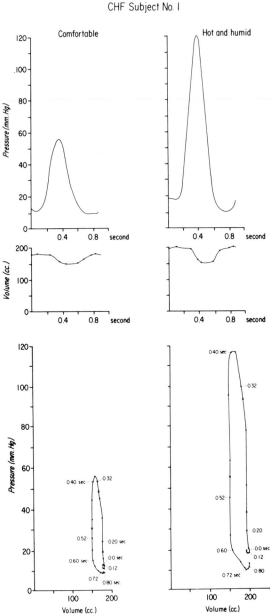

Figure 54–2. Time courses of pressure and volume of the right ventricle of a patient with chronic congestive heart failure and dilated heart, studied in comfortable and hot and humid environments. Exposure to a hot and humid environment was associated with a greater increase in stroke pressure than in stroke volume.

adjustments. The influence of a hot and humid environment on the normal and diseased cardiovascular system has been studied in the cardiovascular laboratories of the Tulane University School of Medicine for more than twenty years (1). The results of some of these studies are summarized briefly below.

Influence of a Hot and Humid Environment on Cardiac Performance in Normal and Diseased Man

There are no methods available by which it is possible to measure directly the work, power, and tension of the human heart. However, using certain assumptions, it is possible to calculate cardiac work, power and tension from the cardiac output and intraventricular pressure (6). These calculations and assumptions have been described in detail elsewhere (6, 7). In the present discussion only the performance of the right ventricle is considered. However, the same arguments and conclusions apply to the left ventricle.

The time courses of pressure and volume of the right ventricle of a normal male before and after exposure to a hot and humid environment are shown in Figure 54–1. It can be seen from this figure that exposure of a normal subject to a hot and humid environment was associated with a much greater increase in stroke output than in stroke pressure, resulting in a characteristic pressure-volume diagram which is of greater width than height (Fig. 54–1).

In contrast to the findings for the normal subject, exposure of a patient with chronic congestive heart failure and a dilated heart to a hot and humid environment was associated with a relatively greater increase in stroke pressure

Control Subject No. 3

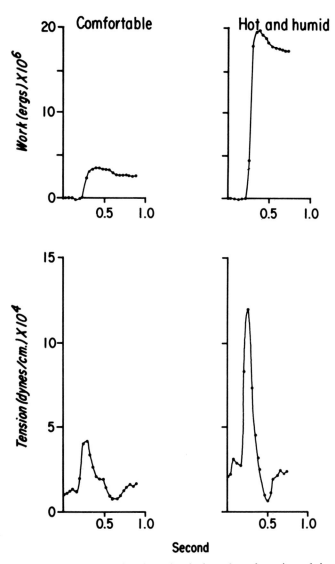

Figure 54–3. Time courses of calculated mechanical work and tension of the right ventricle of the same subject discussed in Figure 54–1.

than in stroke output, resulting in a characteristic pressure-volume diagram of greater height than width (Fig. 54–2).

Mechanical work (W) of the right ventricle may be expressed as

$$W = \int PdV$$

where P is the intraventricular pressure in dynes/cm² and V is the stroke output. It can be seen from Figures 54–3 and 4 that in the comfortable environment right ventricular work of the normal subject was essentially equal to that of the

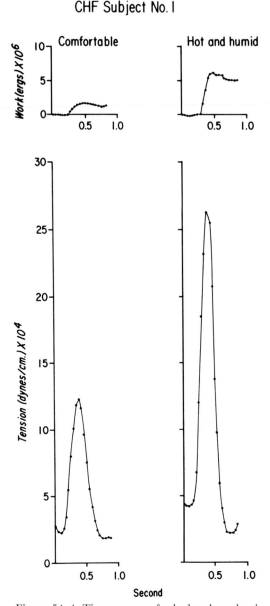

CHF Subject No. I

Figure 54–4. Time courses of calculated mechanical work and tension of the right ventricle of the patient with congestive heart failure discussed in Figure 54–3.

ject than for the patient with congestive heart failure (Fig. 54–3, 4). In other words, the myocardium of the patient with congestive heart failure was not capable of responding to a thermal stimulus with a significant increase in useful ventricular work. It should be emphasized that physiologic work must have increased markedly in the dilated heart.

If the ventricles are considered to be spherical, the tension (T) in a unit thickness of right ventricular wall during a cardiac cycle can be calculated from the following equation

$$T = \frac{RP}{2}$$

where R is equal to the radius of the ventricle and P is the ventricular pressure. More sophisticated mathematical approximations of ventricular contour, such as those obtained by considering the ventricle to be a hemi-ellipsoid of rotation as well as considering the variations in wall thickness, do not appreciably influence the interpretations of results obtained using the simple formula indicated above.

The increase in stroke output developed by the right ventricle of the normal subject following thermal stimulation was associated with an increase in wall tension (Fig. 54–3). Although the relative increase in myocardial tension in the hot and humid environment was greater for the normal than for the diseased heart, the absolute levels of tension were much higher for the diseased heart than for the normal heart (Figs. 54–3, 4). In other words, the dilated heart of the patient with congestive heart failure had to develop a greater tension to eject a smaller volume of blood than the normal-sized heart. In order to eject a stroke output comparable to the normal-sized heart,

patient with congestive heart failure. However, following exposure to a hot and humid environment there was a much greater increase in mechanical work (useful work) for the normal sub-

the myocardium of the dilated heart would have had to develop still greater increments of tension than those shown in Figure 54–4. When the limit of tension which the myocardium is capable of developing is reached, the ventricle can no longer increase stroke output upon demand.

Relation Between Cardiac Performance and Thermal Regulation

In order to understand all the implications of the findings described above on the influence of a hot and humid environment on cardiac performance, it is necessary to relate these findings to the general cardiovascular responses concerned with thermal regulation.

When a normal man is subjected to an environment which is becoming increasingly hot and humid, a point is reached at which radiation and convection can no longer maintain thermal balance. Indeed, heat may actually be absorbed from the environment. As a result, core temperature increases and initiates reflexes mediated through the hypothalamus, which result in sweating. For sweating to be effective the sweat must vaporize from the skin, and heat from the core must be conducted to the skin. In order to transport heat from the core to the skin, cardiac output and dermal blood flow must increase. In normal subjects there is no difficulty in meeting the demand for increased cardiac output associated with thermal stress. However, in patients with congestive heart failure and a dilated heart myocardial tension increases during systole rather than decreases as it does in the normal-sized heart. Thus, when it is necessary for the dilated heart to increase cardiac output, the muscle fibers of the

dilated heart must contract with even greater tension. The diseased, dilated heart may not be capable of developing enough tension to produce a sufficient increase in cardiac output to maintain thermal equilibrium. Under such circumstances heat storage occurs and core temperature increases. The increase in core temperature results in a still further demand for an augmented cardiac output. Thus, a vicious cycle is created which may result in death. In this regard, experiments in which normal subjects and patients with congestive heart failure and dilated hearts were exposed to a thermal stimulus are of interest (1, 4).

In normal subjects, exposure to a hot and humid environment was associated with an increase in skin temperature followed shortly by a rise in rectal temperature. Tachycardia, tachypnea, and, in some instances, hyperventilation developed after a variable period of time. Depending upon the duration of exposure, some subjects developed headache, restlessness, muscle tremor and visual disturbances. Similar effects were observed in patients with congestive heart failure. However, symptoms of worsening of their failure, such as dyspnea, orthopnea and even pulmonary edema, appeared after relatively short periods of exposure. In addition, gallop rhythm, pulsus paradoxus, arrhythmia, syncope and pulsus alternans were frequent findings. Signs of heat intolerance developed much sooner in patients with congestive heart failure than in normal subjects. In patients with chronic congestive heart failure, elimination of body heat is difficult even in a neutral environment. However, in a hot and humid environment the failure to eliminate heat is exaggerated and heat may actually be absorbed from the environment. The final result is cardiovascular collapse and death. These facts are illustrated by a recent study of heat disorders in 67 patients in New Orleans in which an overwhelming majority of patients had underlying cardiovascular disease.

CONCLUSIONS

It has been pointed out that a hot and humid environment evokes cardiovascular responses designed to maintain thermal balance. Whereas these responses offer little difficulty for the normal myocardium, the diseased heart may not be capable of responding to the thermal stress with an adequate increase in cardiac output and work to maintain thermal balance. Heat storage results and further demands are placed upon the myocardium. Thus, a vicious cycle begins which is maintained by multiple factors including intense sympathetic stimulation, excessive catecholamine production and venous hypertension, all of which drive the heart until cardiovascular collapse occurs.

It is important that patients with cardiovascular disease avoid excessive thermal stimulation. It is also important for the physician to realize that as long as a patient with a diseased, dilated heart has difficulty in eliminating body heat his heart is not at rest even if he is lying quietly in bed. Under such circumstances complete cardiac rest is not assured until the "load" placed upon the heart by the need of thermal balance is removed. This "load" can only be removed by placing the patient in a cool, air-conditioned environment and decreasing body heat production by restricting activity. On many occasions we have observed that during the summer

months a patient with a dilated heart failed to respond to therapy in a non-air-conditioned hospital ward even while at complete bed rest. However, placing the same patient in a cool, comfortable, air-conditioned ward with no change in therapy resulted in dramatic clinical improvement.

Although many of the observations presented above may seem obvious, it is surprising how often the deleterious effects of a hot and humid environment on patients with cardiovascular disease are ignored by physicians. Physicians will often put forth great effort to provide optimum therapy for patients with cardiovascular disease but will fail to consider problems related to difficulties with heat elimination. The elevated body temperature sometimes observed in patients with chronic congestive heart failure, which is associated with thermal imbalance (i.e., accumulation of heat), is even treated with antibiotics while a vigorous search is made for sources of infection. The failure to recognize the true cause of the hyperpyrexia as well as other problems due to defective heat elimination is a seriously neglected problem related to human bioclimatology. If such problems are given little attention in the laboratory, they are virtually ignored at the bedside. There is a need to emphasize human bioclimatology in medical teaching.

SUMMARY

A hot and humid environment increases the work and power output of the normal heart in an effort to meet the demands placed upon the circulation for thermal adjustments. Under these conditions which are characterized by intense cardiac stimulation, the increase in work and power output varies directly with the stress of the environment.

Patients with myocardial insufficiency are unable to increase their cardiac output of work and power, but in being driven to do so, fail further and, in turn, manifest acute congestive heart failure.

The importance of providing a comfortable environment to avoid the influences of heat and humidity must be kept in mind in the planning of programs for the prevention, treatment and rehabilitation of patients with heart disease.

REFERENCES

1. BURCH, G. E., and DEPASQUALE, N. P.: *Hot Climates, Man and His Heart.* Springfield, Thomas, 1962.

2. BURCH, G. E., and HYMAN, A.: Influence of a hot and humid environment upon cardiac output and work in normal man and in patients with chronic congestive heart failure at rest. *Amer Heart J, 53:*665, 1957.

3. BURCH, G. E., and HYMAN, A.: A study of the influence of tropical weather on output of volume, work and power by the right and left ventricles of man at rest in bed. *Amer Heart J, 57:*247, 1959.

4. BERENSON, G. S., and BURCH, G. E.: The response of patients with congestive heart failure to a rapid elevation in atmospheric temperature and humidity. *Amer J Med Sci, 223;*45, 1952.

5. THREEFOOT, H. K.: The response of the venous pressure of man to a hot and humid environment. *Amer J Med Sci, 224;*643, 1952.

6. BURCH, G. E., RAY, C. T., and CRONVICH, J. A.: The George Fahr Lecture; certain mechanical peculiarities of the human cardiac pump in normal and diseases states. *Circulation, 5;*504, 1952.

7. BURCH, G. E.: Theoretic considerations of the time course of pressure developed and volume ejected by the normal and dilated left ventricle during systole. *Amer Heart J, 50;*352, 1955.

SECTION IV

EDUCATIONAL ASPECTS

THE ROLE OF AN INTERNATIONAL ORGANIZATION IN THE PREVENTION OF CHRONIC CARDIOVASCULAR DISEASES WITH PARTICULAR REFERENCE TO RECONDITIONING

AUBREY R. KAGAN and ZDENĚK FEJFAR

(World Health Organization, Geneva, Switzerland)

THE World Health Organization seeks to apply knowledge available from all sources for the promotion of health and prevention of disease. Ischemic heart disease is an important cause of death in adults of well-to-do societies and is found in other communities. Whilst there may be speculation on whether it is increasing or not, it is certainly of great public health concern now in many countries. There is no reason to believe that it will not be of greater concern in other countries when immediate problems of malnutrition and infectious disease are controlled.

That infarction is connected with narrowed or blocked coronary arteries is demonstrated every day. That myocardial metabolism can be impaired by neurohumoral factors is harder to demonstrate in man. Thought through the centuries, and experiments in more recent years (though not conclusive), have pointed to the importance of physical, mental and metabolic harmony as important factors for long active life.

Dietary excess of animal fat or "saturated" fat, or carbohydrates, sedentary life, mental stress, particularly of a kind that evokes hemodynamic and metabolic "flight" or "fight" responses in a situation where the natural outlet is denied, and excess cigarette smoking have all been postulated as causative factors separately or in combination. Evidence implicating all these factors has thus far been incomplete. A W.H.O. Expert Committee on Arterial Hypertension and Ischemic Heart Disease (1) said in 1962:

"The possibility of applying preventive measures in ischemic heart disease is at present limited by the incompleteness of our understanding of etiology, and difficulties in early diagnosis. Recent evidence has suggested strong associations between ischemic heart disease and certain factors such as high blood cholesterol and hypertension, but at almost all points further information is needed before these relationships can be given practical application."

That committee expressed the view that "there are no effective means of preventing the occurrence of ischemic heart disease." Application of preventive measures, such as radical change in the diet on a nation-wide scale in people without apparent ischemic heart disease, was considered premature until the results of experimental trials in smaller population groups were known, for example, as described in the national dietary heart study in the USA. On the other hand, evidence has been presented by another WHO Expert Committee on Rehabilitation of Patients with Cardiovascular Diseases, 1963 (2) that many subjects with clinically apparent ischemic heart disease have been returned to former work activities and are enjoying optimum physical and mental function.

The same committee found that data are not yet available comparing the longevity of cardiacs who have been reconditioned for a prolonged period with those who have not been reconditioned (Technical Reports Series 270, p. 32).

The position has changed but little in the last year and all will agree that procedures designed to prevent the occurrence of ischemic heart disease in susceptibles who have not suffered from it, or deterioration in those who have, require further research.

Is the present evidence sufficient to take preventive action? Most would agree that there is sufficient reason for a personal physician with continuing intimate day to day knowledge and control of his patient to direct him into a way of life that would be advantageous. Some might consider the expenditure of private funds on a limited objective would be worthwhile or that there is sufficient evidence to justify the expenditure of public funds on a pilot public health project. This would be particularly so if such projects would contribute to better understanding and evaluation of these procedures. The evidence is insufficient to advocate a mass campaign on a national or international scale.

We are continually reminded that Snow took away a pump handle and stopped an epidemic of cholera long before the cause of cholera was known. Public health authorities today are ready to take effective measures without detailed knowledge of etiology, but in ischemic heart disease we have a galaxy of pump handles and most of them are firmly fixed.

Where then can an international organization help? Many questions need to be answered. Can reversal of the effect by drugs or simple rapid measures decrease the chance of ischemic heart disease?

Research is needed to clarify etiology, to test hypotheses in groups of people living in different environmental conditions, to establish early diagnosis of those with so-called latent ischemic heart disease, to prove or disprove empirical knowledge on how to promote better health.

The need is to clarify the role of neuro-humoral factors and mechanisms.

Can conditioning decrease the chance of getting ischemic heart disease? Controlled trials are also needed.

All the foregoing implies statement of objective, definition of terms and factors to be measured and their criteria, devising methods to assess these factors and testing these methods for comparability, planning a method for attacking these objectives with statistical advice so as to ensure that there is a good chance of answering the questions asked, finding the best places and the best personnel for carrying out these studies. Such studies are difficult, but we may take heart from the report on the feasibility of the national dietary heart study in the USA. Many "impossible" things turn out to be possible when a scientifically planned and rational approach is made.

WHO can and does help with this sort of study by bringing together material and people to obtain agreement on objectives and definitions, and by finding the most efficient ways of utilizing world resources—men, material, conditions, places—for carrying out such studies.

Already a number of WHO-inspired or adopted definitions in the cardio-pulmonary vascular field have met with wide approval and use (2–5).

The Cardiovascular Diseases Unit is helping to develop or encourage development of "comparable" methodology. Scientists and places have been found where what many have considered "impossible" can be achieved (e.g., autopsy of 90 per cent of all deaths in a demographic area, obtaining autopsies from home deaths, measuring stenosis of coronary arteries in longitudinally opened arteries). Studies of the living in the same areas are planned with the objective of improving early diagnosis.

In the field of neurohumoral mechanisms and ischemic heart disease, a report of a small group convened by the Organization, published in 1963 (6), indicates the importance of studying physiological variables over a prolonged period of time in "normals" and "abnormals" under habitual conditions.

WHO may help in other ways, such as obtaining and reporting comparable data, by pointing out the main trends in research, by helping workers in different areas to work in cooperation, and by stimulating and conducting studies in special and suitable places and situations. An important role is also the training of young research workers in these areas. Basic circulatory parameters should be measured during habitual life activities, and suitable techniques which will not influence those under investigation need to be developed. Some of these problems can be studied best by individuals, while others require cooperative effort.

It seems, however, that the problems of preventing ischemic heart disease has to be looked upon as the promotion of better health rather than the prevention of disease in the usual sense of the word. This requires deeper knowledge of the health of the human species throughout the life span. Knowledge of adequate nutrition during the development of the young organism and in adult life, the effort of work and the effect of lack of work on the healthy organism in all ages, and study of environmental stress fall into this category. The deeper studies of the functions of the healthy organism require stimulation and support, and it is hoped that by gradually increasing knowledge we shall be able to introduce step by step preventive measures for ischemic heart disease.

SUMMARY

Although it has been thought through the centuries that physical, mental and metabolic harmony are important factors for a prolonged active life, it is only in recent years that science has begun to produce supporting evidence. This evidence, however, is circumstantial and far from conclusive.

Before governments or communities can be advised to manipulate these factors to prevent ischemic heart disease, controlled trials are necessary to show what chances such action will have of preventing those without ischemic heart disease from developing it or those who have recovered from an acute attack of ischemic heart disease from a recurrence, or what improvement accrues from the specific action.

This type of trial is difficult to obtain but might be feasible if world resources of manpower, materials and experimental conditions were utilized and collaboration between scientists in different disciplines and different communities were increased.

This paper gives instances of how WHO has played a part in such endeavors.

REFERENCES

1. WHO Expert Committee on Arterial Hypertension and Ischemic Heart Disease, 1961 Technical Reports Series, 231, 1962.
2. WHO Expert Committee on Rehabilitation of Patients with Cardiovascular Diseases, 1963, Technical Reports Series, 270, 1964.
3. WHO Expert Committee on Prevention of Rheumatic Heart Disease, 1956. Technical Reports Series 126, 1957.
4. WHO Expert Committee on Chronic Cor Pulmonale, 1960. Technical Reports Series, 213, 1961.
5. WHO Expert Committee on Arterial Hypertension and Ischemic Heart Disease, 1961. Technical Reports Series, 231, 1962.
6. CHARVAT, J., DELL, P., and FOLKOW, B.: Mental Factors and Cardiovascular Diseases. *Cardiologia,* 44;124, 1964.

Chapter LVI

SOCIAL AND PREVENTIVE MEDICINE IN THE MEDICAL CURRICULUM

HANS SCHAEFER

(Heidelberg, Germany)

INTRODUCTION of a new topic into the medical curriculum invariably arouses the opposition of those who represent the traditional concepts of medical education. The new subject of "Social Medicine" is no exception in this respect. To a large measure, this may be due to misunderstandings concerning the nature and aims of that emerging branch of the medical sciences.

It appears necessary, therefore, to emphasize that Social Medicine has nothing whatever to do with "socialized" medicine (i.e., with the socialization of medical practice), which is strongly rejected in many countries.

The word "social," deriving from the Latin *socius* (companion), has a plain meaning and cannot be readily replaced by another term. Man is a social being, living in and creating societies and establishing inseparable relations between those societies and himself as an individual.

THE BASIC PROBLEMS

The basic problems of Social Medicine originate from the fact that conventional Medicine, although having succeeded remarkably well in controlling death i.e., in prolonging the span of our life, has failed in reducing the sum total of illness as expressed, for example, in the percentage of absentees from work.

In countries which operate systems of sickness insurance, the term "disease" has assumed a legally official character. This situation entails rather difficult financial implications in that no possibility exists to define the words "disease" or "illness" in a clearly circumscribed manner (1).

While the pattern of diseases, represented by the distribution of diagnoses in the general practice of recent years, has not undergone any major modifications (2), there has occurred a significant change in the behavior of various groups of people who are insured against illness. In Germany the absentee rate has recently increased from roughly 4 per cent to 6 per cent. In only about one-third of the population under investigation was this increase observed, and here it was due to a prolonged duration of illness (3). Thus, only a relatively small number of individuals accounted for it. The exact causes of this rise of morbidity are not clear but it cannot be interpreted simply as being due to fraud.

The problem of increasing morbidity is complicated by the fact that we do

TABLE 56–I

MORTALITY DIAGNOSES IN PER CENT
OF 1961 DEATHS

Diagnosis	Age Groups 24–35 years %	Age Groups 65–75 years %
Cancer	12.6	22.8
Arteriosclerosis	9.3	22.1
Cerebral vascular disease	1.9	18.8
Tuberculosis	5.7	1.7

TABLE 56–II

Diagnoses	Morbidity per 1000 of All Patients
1. Trauma	97
2. Pyogenic infections	93
3. Neuralgias, myalgias	79
4. Febrile conditions	68
5. Upper respiratory infections	35
6. Dermatitis, eczema	32
7. Abdominal pathology	31

not know the etiology of most of the common diseases. The problems of etiology require investigation by means of epidemiologic statistical methods. Accordingly, most types of therapy are, at present, limited to a merely symptomatic character.

The number of disease categories responsible for the highest mortality rates is comparatively small. A statistical survey from Germany (4) is shown in Table 56–I. Diagnoses other than those listed are far below the 5 per cent level. This means that approximately two-thirds of all people die from only 3 leading diseases. If strokes and arteriosclerosis are pooled in one group, 41 per cent of all persons between 65 and 75 years dies from diseases of the cardiovascular system. The etiology of these diseases is largely influenced by the "behavior" of man in the broadest sense of the term (i.e., by overeating, lack of physical activity, abuses, socioeconomic and other stress factors).

If we surmise that diseases occurring at such a high frequency have a common etiological background, common measures for their prevention (3) should become a possibility.

The practical implication of preventive principles faces some peculiar difficulties. The pattern of diagnoses made in general practice reveals that those diseases which

eventually become the causes of death play only a minor role among the various morbid entities which are diagnosed and treated during the patients' lifetime (5) (Table 56–II).

Obviously, the majority of diseases which provoke most of the subjective complaints are not those which ultimately lead to death. This does not necessarily mean that physicians and patients are unaware of the existence and the dangers of those insidious diseases, but, in general, they are not the object of medical care. In the statistics of the German Federal Republic, they constitute only about 6.5 per cent of all cases of illness reported and paid for by insurance companies (6).

It is common knowledge that tumors and arteriosclerosis remain undetected up to a certain stage of progression. To prevent these most fatal diseases it is, therefore, indispensable to complement the conventional techniques of diagnosis by a systematic search for predisposing risk factors and, accordingly, to introduce measures of mass prevention.

Procedures of preventive group therapy have been organized in many places but information on their mode of action and actual effectiveness is still inadequate. Psychosomatic factors are largely involved and must be taken into account in future pertinent investigations.

The more we envisage the total cost

of all matters connected with illness and medical care, the more the need for preventive action becomes obvious. In calculating these costs for West Germany and for the year 1963 (7), we included the expenditures for sickness insurance, invalidism, medical care, hospitals, medical schools (which constitute the smallest expense item of all), and the reduction of the total social product resulting from illness and early retirement. The sum mounted to about 30 billion dollars (i.e., more than one-quarter of the counry's entire social product). There can hardly be any question that a considerable portion of this sum could be saved by appropriate preventive measures.

SOCIAL AND PREVENTIVE MEDICINE IN MEDICAL EDUCATION

Classical, traditional medicine has no access to the above-mentioned vital problems. We believe, therefore, that a new form of medical scientific endeavor is needed. No detailed discussion of the definition and methods of such a new science will be attempted here. It should be pointed out, however, that, in essence, the science of Social Medicine has to deal with specific mutual relations between society and disease. This correlation includes all medical procedures in which not the individual but large groups of present, as well as prospective patients constitute the objects of research, diagnosis and treatment. In this respect, our new topic pertains to a collective, non-individualistic, and for the most part, noncurative field of medicine. It promotes a primarily theoretical endeavor largely concerned with research, but assuming the task of delivering rational concepts for preventive action and treat-

ment to those who are in immediate contact with prepatients and patients. In Anglo-American countries such ideas have long been put into effect in various fields of medicine.

The future physician receives almost no instruction concerning these problems, and it must be admitted that, under present conditions, it is difficult to organize an appropriate pertinent educational program because no single teacher's brain is capable of mastering all the disciplines involved. Physiology, evidently, must form the basis of the envisioned scientific building. Many influences, exerted by society on the individual, have to be described and analyzed as psychosomatic events, elicited through mediation of the forebrain, the limbic system, the hypothalamus and pituitary, and ultimately the autonomic nervous and endocrine systems. The spectrum of these multiple, both pathogenic and protective, effects may well be designated as "sociosomatic."

It is, of course, impossible to have physiologists working on such complex questions in every organized institute of Social and Preventive Medicine. The conventional departments such as physiology and psychology must take care of that. Moreover, epidemiologic studies are extremely expensive and it would be uneconomical to scatter such investigative efforts over a large number of medical schools. Most probably, a maximum of efficiency will be guaranteed by establishment of one or two central institutions per country, having at their disposal the staff, equipment and computers necessary to do concentrated research of the highest order.

Social Medicine Research Institutes at individual universities, staffed with only a few specialists each, would have to cover comparatively narrow problem areas in a way not much differing from the usual medical school set-up, but with a more distinct separation of research from teaching activities.

Due to the complexity and prevailing underdevelopment of the fields of Social Medicine and of Preventive Medicine with respect to the degenerative and chronic diseases, investigation must be planned and carried out on a very much larger scale than actual teaching.

It is important to keep in mind that the practically significant and useful results of extensive epidemiologic and related studies can be expected to be quite simple so that the actual teaching program for medical students will not need to occupy more than a comparatively small fraction of their time. Competent visiting guest lecturers could be entrusted with part of the formal educational obligations, spread out over a number of medical schools.

Even though we are still ignorant of the last fundamental causes of most pathological processes, we do know that epidemic diseases, such as atherosclerosis and ischemic heart disease, develop from a multifactorial background. For this reason, and because these fatal diseases are only rarely recognized at an early stage during the patient's lifetime, it appears evident that prevention (i.e., the timely elimination of risk factors), possesses a far greater importance for society than any other form of medical activity, including conventional medical research.

Apart from physiology and pathophysiology, the main subjects to be integrated into the field of Social and Preventive Medicine must be statistics, epidemiology, sociology and psychology.

The average university professor cannot possibly include all these disciplines in his own specialized teaching program. He is neither sufficiently familiar with the problems and facts in question nor is he willing, as a rule, to acquire an appropriate knowledge. He is bound to neglect matters which do not fit into his traditional concept and which are largely remote from his professional horizon. In the clinical field he is only infrequently confronted with the sociological problems of his patients and he himself has more often than not been raised in an environment untouched by serious social disorder. Thus, he rarely had or has an opportunity to develop a profound understanding of analogies, based on his own experience, and the world of many of his patients remains strange and incomprehensible to him. Hence, the need exists for a new type of academic teacher whose evolution will require the establishment of a new form of training.

The future of medicine with its increasingly important noncurative and nonindividual aspects will depend decisively on a change in the educational concepts of universities and medical colleges. Such a change will foreseeably help to save billions of dollars. What is more, it must be considered as one of the most urgent and most momentous developments in the adaptation of traditional medicine to the unfulfilled demands of our modern world and to the rapid changes of its technical, social and political structure.

SUMMARY

Conventional medicine and medical education in our modern world are characterized by paradoxical and disturbing inadequacies: (a) in spite of delayed mortality, morbidities are increasing, even though the general pattern of disease distribution has remained rather constant in recent years; (b) the etiology of most chronic diseases remains unknown, which limits their management to a merely symptomatic type of therapy, and (c) the overall morbidity spectrum, dealt with by medical practice, is dominated by nonfatal diseases. Preventive measures against the most fatal among them are nearly nonexistent.

In Germany the costs of all matters connected with illness amount to more than one-quarter of the total social product.

Traditional medicine does not meet these problems.

The social and preventive aspects of medicine, because of their "cross-sectional" character, demand the close cooperation of specialists from various disciplines.

Since the traditional university professor ignores and neglects the needs of social and preventive medicine, a new type of academic training is needed to keep teachers and students effectively in touch with sociological problems and with the practical requirements of early prevention.

Prevention of the degenerative and chronic diseases is the most urgently needed and the most promising obligation of modern medicine.

REFERENCES

1. SCHAEFER, H.: *Die Medizin heute*. Munich, R. Piper and Co. Verlag, 1963, p. 88.
2. BRAUN, R. N.: Die gezielte Diagnostik in der Praxis, Stuttgart, 1957, Tab. 2.
3. POTT, R.: Unpublished data.
4. Statistisches Jahrbuch für die Bundesrepublik Deutschland. Stuttgart and Mainz, 1961, p. 86.
5. BRAUN, R. N.: *Op cit.*
6. Statistisches Jahrbuch für die Bundesrepublik Deutschland. Stuttgart and Mainz, 1961, p. 82.
7. JAHN, H., and SCHAEFER, H.: Die volkswirtschaftliche Belastung durch das Phänomen "Krankheit" im weitesten Sinn, Mensch und Medizin, No. 5–6, 1965.

Chapter LVII

OBLIGATIONS OF MEDICAL EDUCATION IN THE MAINTENANCE OF NATIONAL HEALTH

ROBERT J. SLATER

(Burlington, Vermont, U.S.A.)

THE almost entirely curative attitude of our medical profession is reflected in a paucity of teaching programs which will educate future generations of physicians toward their obligation to protect public health against the widespread degenerative diseases of civilization, notably ischemic heart disease, the most fatal of all.

Modern developments in the pathophysiology of myocardial damage by a variety of factors constituted a major part of the agenda of the First International Conference on Preventive Cardiology, which was held at the University of Vermont in 1964. They strongly suggest that it is no longer necessary to face the problem of degenerative heart disease with discouragement and inaction. Some of the basic elements of pathogenesis and corresponding preventability can readily be incorporated into the teaching material of our current medical curricula since they are directly deducible from the present knowledge covered in cardiac physiology, biochemistry, pharmacology and pathology. Properly integrated instruction, cutting across the arbitrarily drawn borderlines of the above-named disciplines, should greatly improve the students' theoretical understanding of what approaches are necessary to reduce premature cardiac disease.

Even more important, however, is a systematic cultivation in every student of a philosophy of prevention-mindedness as an integral and prominent part of his professional conscience and initiative. In this respect we have a great deal to learn from the educational programs of other nations, and we would welcome a lively international exchange of teachers, as well as of students in this growing and vital field of medical education.

Chapter LVIII

TO PRACTICE WHAT WE PREACH

PAUL DUDLEY WHITE

(Boston, Massachusetts, U.S.A.)

ALL of us assembled here at this important International Conference on Preventive Cardiology are, I am quite sure, agreed on certain items of positive health. These are now wisely recommended to the public at large, which includes our patients, and should also include the families of our patients. It is also quite natural, therefore, that the public at large and our patients and their families look to us physicians and others interested in health to set the example. And I would like to outline the image of ourselves that we should present to these people to whom we are giving advice, after adding a word about the candidate for cardiovascular disease, that is, about heredity versus environment.

In the past it has been customary to deal mostly with possible environmental factors behind cardiovascular disease, such as diet, physical lethargy, stress, and tobacco, and to say little or nothing about heredity and the candidate for cardiovascular disease, partly because little or nothing seems to be possible in the way of correction of such an inherited background and partly because very few physicians pay any attention to the family history from the standpoint of protecting the young members of their families before they get sick. Actually it is quite easy to pick out many of the candidates for such a cardiovascular illness as coronary heart disease, and I shall give an example of men that I see every year, and apparently increasingly.

A young man 25-years-old has a father or a mother, or both, and a brother or two affected clinically by evident coronary heart disease in middle age. The young man himself and some of his family, especially those affected, have an elevated serum cholesterol much of the time, that is, over 300 mg% when not under treatment. The young man also has an elevated serum uric acid. He is of athletic build but has already cut down greatly his physical activity since starting his business career and a recent marriage. He is rapidly gaining weight and he smokes 2 or 3 packs of cigarettes a day. Here is the candidate who needs to make a change in his ways of life at once, to avoid, or at least to try to avoid, what has happened to his predecessors, that is, his father or mother, or older brother.

To return to environmental factors, it is quite obvious from statistical evidence and practical experience that obesity is, in the long run, harmful. Obese people are more likely to have hypertension and diabetes and cardiovascular disease than are those of optimal weight, or underweight. There is some question as to how the obesity develops—whether simply from calories *per se*, or from calories with a high percentage of saturated fats. But at any rate, we ourselves should not be obese. And if in addition we are, as noted above, candidates for cardiovascular disease early in life or in middle age, we should be unusually careful in the kind of food we eat. This is a well-recognized fact today.

The second simple rule of health is that of the need to utilize our muscles, especially those of our legs, for here, too, there is growing evidence that physical exercise which involves the use of the legs is not only physiologically and psychologically desirable, but now is also protective against the early development of serious atherosclerosic heart disease.

Thirdly, the use of tobacco has long been recognized by many of us, years before the recent report of the Surgeon General of the Public Health Service, to be a toxic substance to which men, and women too, can become addicted, and such addiction or habit is frequently very difficult to break. The harm from tobacco is now correctly stated to be more of a hazard to the lungs and the function of respiration than simply a cause of cancer and cardiovascular disease. The lungs function primarily for the exchange of gases, namely oxygen and carbon dioxide, and such an exchange is distinctly interfered with both physiologically and pathologically by the use of tobacco.

Other possibly harmful substances depend largely on the degree of exposure. This would include alcohol, which, in small amounts, is relatively harmless; an atmosphere that is contaminated with smoke other than that of tobacco; toxic fumes; and the excessive use of beverages such as coffee and tea, which for many people interfere with their sleep and nervous state.

If we physicians ourselves are willing to disregard these obvious factors of optimal health, we should at least try to persuade our junior colleagues and the medical students of today to start their careers in a healthier way than many of us have carried on.

Probably this advice to the members of this conference may be more important than all the advice that we pass out to the rest of the inhabitants of this globe. We are likely to persuade others by example much more than by recept to do what we think necessary in the prevention of cardiovascular disease, and even those individuals who are candidates, as indicated by studies of family health, can almost certainly be protected by these environmental factors if they begin in their youth to do so.

As a final note to this paper, may I quote from an article that I have written for the *Grade Teacher Magazine* as follows:

But can we expect our young children to rebel on their own against the bad habits of their parents and teachers? Of course not. We must set the example! We must make it possible for our youngsters in some way or another to walk or cycle at least part way to school again—and safely! We must not over-feed them from infancy onward as we have been doing! There is no advantage in having over-robust teenagers who are to die of heart attacks in their prime—in their forties and fifties—which is going on today. Also, the optimal use of our brains is dependent on a good circulation of blood thereto with strong heart and leg muscles and unobstructed arteries.

The answer is clear. The parent-teacher associations of the country must rise to the occasion and set the example in their own lives, which, incidentally, will probably save them too, since it is rarely too late to mend. This word to the wise should be sufficient.

GENERAL SUMMARY

Transdisciplinary and transcontinental integration of experimental, clinical and epidemiologic data concerning the origin of hypoxic (so-called "coronary" or "ischemic") and degenerative heart disease, even though still fragmentary, warrants the following schematic concept of fundamentally and jointly contributing pathogenic factors:

The causal factors listed under (B), on which this book is primarily focused, share the common denominator of myocardial oxygen-wasting adrenosympathetic overactivity.

Effective prevention can be expected from combined (a) limitation of dietary saturated, and supplementation of polyunsaturated fats; (b) environmental, emotional and sensory relaxation; (c) regular vigorous physical activity, and (d) abstinence from smoking.

In Western countries some of these principles are beginning to be implemented by a few local dietary and

PATHOGENESIS OF HYPOXIC HEART DISEASE

Basic Characteristics	(A) **Stable** (Predisposing)	(B) **Fluctuant** (Conditioning)
Categories of derangement	**Vascular structural**	**Myocardial metabolic**
Pathogenic features	Coronary atherosclerosis	Increased myocardial vulnerability to coronary atherosclerosis
Pathogenic mechanisms	Mechanical interference in **O_2 supply**	Neurogenic and hormonal biochemical interference in **O_2 consumption** and electrolyte balance
Causal backgrounds	(a) Heredity (b) Diet (c) Hypertension	(a) Socioeconomic and environmental stress (b) Lack of exercise (c) Nicotine

445

physical training programs and by governmental antismoking efforts. Vast government-, industry- and insurance-sponsored preventive reconditioning systems have been operated for many years in Eastern and Central Europe. They are based on temporary changes of environment, physical training, and indoctrination of lifelong health habits in thousands of rural reconditioning centers; promotion of large-scale active participation in sports, exercise breaks in industrial plants, instruction in creative, relaxing hobbies, and massive campaigns of public health education.

Conclusive statistical data on the morbidity and mortality effects of reconditioning and other programs are still missing but are now being assembled over extended periods. In the meantime, objective evidence of a favorable influence on predisposing autonomic nervous cardiovascular mechanisms and on general fitness has been obtained abroad in specially established institutes for research in social medicine and preventive reconditioning.

The uncontrolled mass mortality from degenerative heart disease, particularly in the prosperous nations of the West, demands a reorientation of medical school curricula, as well as a radical shift in professional and lay education toward the general comprehension and organized practical application of reasonably established principles of preventability.

The present book is being offered as a preliminary blueprint for organized action wherever such action is still underdeveloped.

W. Raab, M.D.
Editor

APPENDIX

SOME MOOT QUESTIONS REQUIRING FURTHER STUDY

1. What kind of mechanism is responsible for the muscular training-induced, sustained augmentation of cardiac vagal, and reduction of cardiac sympathetic tone and reactivity? Reflexes from muscular tissue or vessels? Changes in primary central nervous stimulus formation? (See Chapters 14, 15, 16, 37, 38, 50.)

2. Can beta-receptor blockers or other antiadrenergic drugs replace the cardioprotective effect of muscular training? (See Chapters 14, 15, 16, 37, 38, 50.)

3. How is the cardioprotective phenomenon of direct and "cross" resistance to cardiotoxic stresses (Selye) related to the cardioprotective effect of muscular training? Is the augmentation of myocardial potassium stores by subcardiotoxic stresses* involved in both? (See Chapter 18.)

4. How does the actual oxygen consumption and utilization of trained hearts compare with that of untrained or "detrained" ones under equal hemodynamic conditions? (See Chapters 14, 16, 37.)

5. Why is the intensive sympathetic stimulation and myocardial O_2 consumption during exercising relatively innocuous? Favorable intramyocardial microcirculatory dynamics and pressure gradients? Limited duration? Nonparticipation of potentially cardiotoxic corticoids? Availability of extra potassium, mobilized from the active skeletal muscles, for replenishment of myocardial potassium stores?† (See Chapters 40, 41, 42, 43.)

6. Which training patterns produce maximal cardioprotective effects with a minimum risk, sacrifice of time and of convenience, and how can motivation for lifelong exercise habits be best induced? (See Chapters 37, 39, 40.)

7. Does the emotion-induced simultaneous increase of catecholamine liberation and adrenal corticoid secretion‡ imply an aggravation of potential catecholamine cardiotoxicity under emotional stress? (See Chapters 18, 23, 24, 27.)

8. Which types of acute and chronic emotional stress cause maximally cardiotoxic sympathetic and adrenocortical stimulation? (See Chapters 23, 24, 27.)

9. Can the emotional augmentations of the blood corticoid level‡ and the

---

*Bajusz, E.: An ionic shift through which nonspecific stimuli can increase the resistance of the heart muscle. *Cardiologia, 45*:288, 1964.

†Rose, K. D., *et al.*: Serum electrolyte relationship to electrocardiographic change in exercising athletes. *J.A.M.A. 195*:111, 1966.

‡Mason, J. W., *et al.*: Concurrent plasma epinephrine, norepinephrine and 17-hydroxycorticosteroid levels during conditioned emotional disturbances in monkeys. *Psychosom. Med 23*:344, 1961.

corticoid-induced losses of body potassium be modified or prevented by muscular training?

10. Are the angiographically demonstrated coronary spasms equivalents of spontaneous events, or artifacts, provoked by contrast media?* (See Chapters 11, 12.)

11. Are the blood lipid and blood sugar elevations observed in cases of "coronary-proneness" and hypoxic heart disease caused by primary metabolic derangements or are they, at least in part, manifestations of the autonomic-nervous characteristics (adrenergic preponderance and over-reactivity) of such individuals? (See Chapters 9, 21, 24, 25, 31, 38, 39, 41.)

12. Can the early, premorbid risk evaluation concerning the predisposition to hypoxic heart disease be improved by the direct measurement of myo-

cardial, nerve-controlled functions (such as heart rate, isometric period) under standard sensory and mental stresses? (See Chapter 14.)

13. Is the psychological impact of sojourns in rural reconditioning centers superior to city gymnastics, in motivating trainees for continued adherence to healthful living habits? (See Chapters 39, 40, 41, 47, 48, 49.)

14. Is the incidence of hypoxic heart disease and of recurrences of myocardial infarctions demonstrably influenced by organized systematic mass reconditioning programs? (See Chapters 38, 39, 40, 41, 42, 43, 46, 47, 48, 49, 55.)

15. Should the fact that question 14 has not yet been answered conclusively, be considered a legitimate excuse for postponing any reasonably promising preventive action until "all the facts are known," and until all our "coronary-prone" contemporaries are dead?

W. RAAB

---

*Friesinger, G. C., *et al.*: Hemodynamic consequences of the injection of radiopaque material. *Circulation, 31:*730, 1965.

ADDITIONAL PERTINENT BOOKS AND REVIEWS

1. BECKMANN, P., WALINSKI, W., and DEWERTH, CHR.: *Internistische Uebungsbehandlung.* Stuttgart, Hippokrates-Verlag, 1961.
2. Conference on Prevention and Control of Cardiovascular Diseases, Bucharest, March 10–18, 1965, (WHO Reports).
3. DELIUS, L., *et al.*: *Studien zur Rehabilitation von Arbeitern mit Herzinfarkt. Deutsch Med Wschr, 89;*474, 519, 1964.
4. FELTON, J. S., and COLE, R.: The high cost of heart disease. *Circulation, 27;*957, 1963.
5. *Fizeecheskaya kul'tura—istotchnik dolgoletiya (Physical Culture—Source of Longevity).* Ed.: Moscow, Fizkul'tura y Sport, 1965.
6. FOX, S. M., and SKINNER, J. C.: Physical activity and cardiovascular health. *Amer J Cardiol, 14;* 731, 1964.
7. HELLERSTEIN, H. K.: Reconditioning and the prevention of heart disease. *Mod Med,* May 11, 1964, pp. 266–296.
8. HOLLMANN, W.: Körperliches Training als Prävention von Herz-Kreislaufkrankheiton, Hippokrates-Verlag, Stuttgart, 1965.
9. International Society of Cardiology: Meeting on Physical Activity and the Heart, Helsinki, 1964.
10. JOKL, E.: *Heart and Sport.* Springfield, Thomas, 1964.
11. KRAUS, H., and RAAB, W.: *Hypokinetic Disease—Diseases Produced by Lack of Exercise.* Springfield, Thomas, 1961.
12. KURASHOV, S. V.: Organizatsiya bor'by s syerdetchno-sosudistymi zabolyevaniyami. Moscow, 1960. (Organization of the control of cardiovascular diseases. Translated by Office of Technical Services, U.S. Dept. of Commerce, Washington, D. C.)
13. MELLEROWICZ, H.: *Präventive Cardiologie.* Berlin-Steglitz, Medicus Verlag, 1961.
14. MENSEN, H.: Frühprophylaxe des Herzinfarktes. *Allgemeine Therapeutik,* No. 4, 1965.
15. MYASNIKOV, A. L.: Myocardial necroses of coronary and non-coronary genesis. *Amer J Cardiol, 13;*435, 1964.
16. RAAB, W.: (a) The nonvascular metabolic myocardial vulnerability factor in "coronary heart disease." *Amer Heart J, 66:*685, 1963. (b) Emotional and sensory stress factors in myocardial pathology (in press).
17. RAHN, H.: Information explosion and communication crisis. *Physiologist, 7;*334, 1964.
18. RAYSKINA, M. E.: *Biokhimiya nyervnoy regulyatsii syerdtsa (Biochemistry of the nervous regulation of the heart).* Moscow, Medgiz, 1962.
19. REINDELL, H., *et al.*: Herz-Kreislaufkrankheiten und Sport. Munich, Johann Ambrosius Barth, 1960.
20. ROSENBAUM, F. F., and BELKNAP, E. L.: *Work and the Heart.* New York, Paul B. Hoeber, 1959.
21. SCHAEFER, H.: *Die Medizin heute.* Munich, Piper Verlag, 1963.
22. SELYE, H.: *The Pluricausal Cardiopathies.* Springfield, Thomas, 1961.
23. Smoking and Health. U.S. Department of Health, Education and Welfare, Office of the Surgeon General, Washington, D.C., U.S. Government Printing Office, 1964.
24. SPORT and LEIZURE: Internat'l. Council of Sport and Physical Education. Schorndorf bei Stuttgart, Verlag Karl Hofmann, 1964.
25. STAMLER, J., *et al.*: Approaches to the prevention of coronary heart disease. *J Amer Diet Ass, 40;* 415, 1962.
26. Symposium on Insurance Aspects of Cardiovascular Disease; Gubner, R. S., Guest Editor. *Amer J Cardiol, 13;*670–682, 1964.
27. TEICHMANN, W. (Ed.): Forschungs-methoden in der allgemainen Therapie. Sanitas Verlag i Bad Wörishofen, 1965.
28. World Health Organization: Report of Expert Committee on Ischemic Heart Disease, Technical Reports Series No. 231, Geneva, 1962.

APPEAL

TO HEALTH AUTHORITIES AND PRIVATE AGENCIES FOR INTERNATIONALLY COORDINATED PREVENTIVE ACTION AGAINST

ISCHEMIC HEART DISEASE

By

Participants in and Contributors to the FIRST INTERNATIONAL CONFERENCE ON PREVENTIVE CARDIOLOGY, University of Vermont, August 24 to 28, 1964, Burlington, Vermont, U. S. A.

Ischemic heart disease is one of the most common causes of premature invalidism and death in highly industrialized, prosperous countries. Despite much verbal emphasis on the need for early, pre-morbid prevention, systematically guided preventive action has been conspicuously lacking in some of the most afflicted areas of the world, while governments, insurance organizations, industries, and various private agencies in other countries have developed large-scale preventive reconditioning and public education programs over many years.

It is true that statistical data which would give unequivocal proof of the long-range preventive success of these programs concerning cardiac morbidity and mortality have not yet been assembled. However, our present-day knowledge concerning the pathophysiological fundamentals of ischemic heart disease and concerning the possibilities of effective counteraction is far more advanced and consolidated than generally realized by a large part of the medical profession and the lay public.

The first International Conference on PREVENTIVE CARDIOLOGY has made an effort to gather and to integrate pertinent but previously very poorly coordinated and utilized basic and clinical information from many lands into a scientifically sound pattern of preventive reasoning as the understructure for rational and determined preventive action.

Further postponement of such action with the excuse that complete scientific proof of its value must first be awaited for indefinite periods of time is unjustifiable in view of the gravity of the situation and in the light of the facts presented at the Conference.

Contemporary research has provided ample evidence that two main factors contribute jointly to the origin of ischemic heart disease, namely, (A) coronary atherosclerosis which limits the oxygen **supply** to the heart muscle, and (B) a disproportionate over-activity of the catecholamine-liberating adreno-sympathetic system which augments myocardial oxygen **consumption** beyond the "coronary reserve," thus inducing detrimental hypoxia.

Factor A is already being extensively investigated. It may possibly be reduced by dietary measures (low cholesterol, low fat) and by medicinal normalization of the blood pressure level. The equally important factor B is caused chiefly by emotional and sensory stresses, lack of physical exercise, and nicotine. Due to its functional nature, factor B is relatively easily amenable to such protective anti-adrenergic measures as environmental-emotional relaxation, habitual physical activity, and abstinence from smoking. These practices and rules are being put into effect and taught for life-long application in thousands of rural preventive reconditioning centers in several European countries. They are also effectively propagated there by vigorous public educational campaigns. Still fragmentary, but highly encouraging objective observations concerning the functionally favorable effects of reconditioning measures have been reported at the Conference.

In view of the urgency of the situation, the herewith undersigned are directing an earnest appeal to responsible health authorities and private agencies, especially in countries with a high incidence of ischemic heart disease but with under-developed reconditioning programs, to take the following active steps toward early prevention of uncontrolled premature cardiac mass mortality:

1. Improvement of **information on the pathogenesis and preventability of ischemic heart disease** by closely coordinating intercontinental experimental and clinical research programs and teams in consultation with the World Health Organization. Particular attention should be paid to the preventable neurogenic and hormonal metabolic features of myocardial ischemia and degeneration.

2. Internationally coordinated **investigation of the objective results of organized preventive reconditioning programs** (a) by the large-scale application of suitable screening tests for the selection of cardiac ischemia-prone reconditioning candidates; (b) by the study of immediate and long-range effects of supervised emotional and physical reconditioning and health indoctrination periods upon the parameters of those tests; (c) by the epidemiologic comparative long-range follow-up of suspected cardiac ischemia-prone individuals without and with exposure to reconditioning and health indoctrination periods, regarding cardiac morbidity and mortality.

3. **Establishment of scientifically conducted rural cardiac reconditioning centers,** partly equipped with research facilities and staffs, especially in severely afflicted, prosperous countries which do not yet have any reconditioning programs.

4. **Intercontinental exchange of reconditioning experts,** and training of young physicians, physical and health educators, and psychologists, in reconditioning techniques.

5. Incorporation into the official **medical school curricula** of brief courses, dealing with (a) the elementary features of cardio-vascular functional and

structural pathogenesis and their preventability; (b) principles of active prevention by appropriate living habits, and (c) the new physician's professional and moral obligation to propagate such habits both by counselling and by his personal example.

6. Initiation of systematic and incessant **public educational campaigns** via press, radio, TV, and special propaganda events, concerning: daily home exercising (calisthenics); avoidance of the unnecessary use of elevators and cars; out-door sports; hiking; fat-poor diet; non-smoking; cultivation of satisfying hobbies and, wherever possible, a positive, serene outlook on life.

In old age, cardiac death is not the worst of alternatives but it must no longer be permitted by responsible health agencies to destroy countless creative, useful lives without being faced by energetically guided attempts at rational preventive counter-action. Belated therapy and rehabilitation, no matter how ingeniously devised and carried out, are no adequate solution of the problem.

LIST OF SIGNATORIES

ABRAMS, H. K., M.D.; Med. Dir. Union Health Service, Chicago, Illinois (U. S. A.).

AIKEN, R. B., M.D.; Vermont State Health Commissioner, Burlington, Vermont (U. S. A.).

ALLARD, C., Ph.D.; Chief, Epidemiol. & Biochem. Depts., Institute of Cardiology, Montreal, Quebec (Canada).

ANDREWS, R. J., M.D.; Dir. Cardiol. Dept., Cape Hospital, Wilmington, North Carolina (U. S. A.).

BADAL, J., M.D., Docent; Dir. Harvey Heart Institute, Františkovy Lázne (Czechoslovakia).

BAHNSON, C., Ph.D.; Assoc. Prof. Psych., Jefferson Med. College, Philadelphia, Pennsylvania (U. S. A.).

BAJUSZ, E., M.D., Ph.D.; Assoc. Prof., Dept. of Path., Univ. of Montreal, Montreal, Quebec (Canada).

BECKMANN, P., M.D.; Med. Dir. Cardiovascular Reconditioning Center, Distr. Ins. Organization, Ohlstadt (West Germany).

BELLET, S., M.D.; Prof. and Dir. Div. of Cardiology, Univ. of Pennsylvania, Philadelphia, Pennsylvania (U. S. A.).

BENNETT, B. L.; Prof. Phys. Educ., Ohio State Univ., Columbus, Ohio (U. S. A.).

BISHOP, W. R., M.D.; Vice-Pres. and Med. Dir. Provident Life and Accident Ins. Co., Chattanooga, Tennessee (U. S. A.).

BLANKENSHIP, C., M.D.; Prof. and Chairman, Dept. of Community Health, Univ. of Louisville, Kentucky (U. S. A.).

BLOHMKE, M., M.D.; Inst. f. Work Medicine, Univ. Heidelberg (West Germany).

BLOOMFIELD, S. T., M.D.; Med. Res. Dept., Burroughs Wellcome & Co., Tuckahoe, New York (U. S. A.).

BLUMENFELD, A.; Med. Science Writer, New York City, N. Y. (U. S. A.).

BOUCHARD, R., M.D.; Asst. Prof. Med., Univ. of Vermont, Burlington, Vermont (U. S. A.).

BROWN, R. A., M.D.; Sr. Asst. Resident, Montreal General Hospital, Montreal, Quebec (Canada).

BRUNNER, D., M.D.; Prof. Physiol. Hygiene, Head Dept. of Medicine, Univ. of Tel-Aviv (Israel).

CANTIN, M., M.D., Ph.D.; Dept. Path., Univ. of Chicago, School of Medicine, Chicago, Illinois (U. S. A.).

CARDILLO, T. E., M.D.; Cardiologist, Eastman-Kodak Co., Rochester, New York (U. S. A.).

CHARLES, M. L., M.D.; Cardiologist, Pan-Am World Airways, Patrick Air Force Base, Florida (U. S. A.).

CHRISTIAN, P., M.D.; Prof., Dir. Inst. of Gen. Clin. Med., Univ. of Heidelberg, Heidelberg (West Germany).

COLMERS, R. A., M.D.; Cardiologist, FACC., Stamford, Conn. (U. S. A.).

COOPER, K. H., M.D.; Physician, U. S. Air Force, Brooks AFB, Texas (U. S. A.) (signature affixed with statement that it expresses only personal opinion and does not in any way reflect that of the U. S. Air Force).

COOPER, R. W., M.D.; Research Physician, Schering Corp., Bloomfield, New Jersey (U. S. A.)

CRESENZO, V. M., M.D.; Internist, Reidsville, North Carolina (U. S. A.).

CURETON, T. K., Ph.D.; Prof. Phys. Educ., Univ. of Illinois, Urbana, Illinois (U. S. A.).

DYER, N. A., M.D.; Dir. Bureau of Heart Dis. Control, West Virginia State Dept. of Health, Charleston, West Virginia (U. S. A.).

ERMAN, J. M., M.D.; Detroit, Michigan (U. S. A.).

EYRES, M. D., M.D.; Prof. of Prevent. Med., Univ. of S. Dakota, Vermillion, South Dakota (U. S. A.).

FARINA, A.; Instr. Phys. Educ., Boston Univ., Sargent Coll., Boston, Massachusetts (U. S. A.).

FEJER, I., M.D.; Cardiologist, Riverdale Hospital, Toronto, Ontario (Canada).

FRANKEL, L. J.; Dir. L. Frankel Foundation, Charlestown, West Virginia (U. S. A.).

GIALLORETO, O., M.D.; Asst. Prof. Med., Univ. of Montreal, Montreal, Quebec (Canada).

GRIFFIN, R. J., M.D.; Instr. Clin. Med., Wayne Univ., Detroit, Michigan (U. S. A.).

GRIFFITH, G. C., M.D.; Prof. Med., Univ. Southern California, Los Angeles, California (U. S. A.).

GROOVER, M. E., JR., M.D.; Assoc. Prof. Med., Univ. Oklahoma, Oklahoma City, Oklahoma (U. S. A.).

GRUBER, J. J., Ph.D.; Assoc. Prof. Phys. Educ., West Lafayette, Indiana (U. S. A.).

HAGAN, C. T., M.D.: Dir. Heart Station, St. Francis Hospital, Wichita, Kansas (U. S. A.).

HALHUBER, M. J., M.D.; Prof. Med., Univ. of Innsbruck, Innsbruck (Austria).

HARUMI, K., M.D., D.M.S.; Cardiologist, Univ. of Tokyo, Tokyo (Japan).

HAUCK, R. O., Ph.D.; Exec. Vice-Pres. and Dir. of Research, Knoll Pharmaceutical Co., Orange, New Jersey (U. S. A.).

HERRLICH, H. C., Ph.D.; Res. Assoc., Univ. of Vermont, Burlington, Vermont (U. S. A.).

HYDE, E. R., M.D.; Green Mountain Clinic, Northfield, Vermont (U. S. A.).

ISMAIL, A. H., M.D.; Assoc. Prof. of Research, Purdue Univ., West Lafayette, Indiana (U. S. A.).

JOKL, E., M.D.; Prof. and Dir. Phys. Educ. Res. Lab., Univ. of Kentucky, Lexington, Kentucky (U. S. A.).

JUSTER, I. R., M.D.; Cardiologist, Glens Falls Hosp., Glens Falls, New York (U. S. A.).

KASCH, F. W., Ed.D.; Prof. Phys. Educ., Dir. Adult Rehabil., San Diego State College, San Diego, California (U. S. A.).

KING, D. D., M.D.; Physician, Reidsville, North Carolina (U. S. A.).

KIPSHIDZE, N. N., M.D., D.M.S.; Dir. Inst. of Therapy, Tbilisi (Soviet Union).

KIRCHHOFF, H. W., M.D., Ph.D.; Med. Dir. Inst. of Aviation Med., Fürstenfeldbruck (West Germany).

KLOUDA, M. A., Ph.D.; Res. Assoc., Dept. Physiol., Loyola Univ., Stritch School of Med., Chicago, Illinois (U. S. A.).

KRAUS, H., M.D.; Assoc. Prof. Phys. Med. and Rehabil., New York Univ., New York City, New York (U. S. A.).

KREMER, H. U., M.D.; Asst. Prof. Clin. Med., Univ. of Pennsylvania, Philadelphia, Pennsylvania (U. S. A.).

KRZYWANEK, H. J., M.D.; Res. Assoc., Univ. of Vermont, Burlington, Vermont (U. S. A.).

LADUE, W. L., M.D.; Physician (Gen. Practice), Plattsburgh, New York (U. S. A.).

LAPICCIRELLA, V., M.D.; Prof., Lecturer in Med. Pathology, Univ. of Florence; Dir. Cardiol. Center, Montecatini (Italy).

LEACH, C. C., M.D.; Physician, Gen. Practice, Burlington, Vermont (U. S. A.).

LENEHAN, J. R., M.D.; Cardiologist, Hartford, Connecticut (U. S. A.).

LEPESCHKIN, E., M.D.; Prof. Exp. Med., Univ. of Vermont, Burlington, Vermont (U. S. A.).

LEVI, L., M.D.; Dir. Lab. Clin. Stress Research, Dept. Med. Karolinska Hospital, Stockholm (Sweden).

LIEBERMANN, B., M.D.; Chief Med. Consultant Calif. Dept. of Rehabil., Oakland, California (U. S. A.).

LINDBERG, H. A., M.D.; Assoc. Prof. Med., Northwestern Univ. Med. School, Chicago, Illinois (U. S. A.).

MARCHET, H., M.D.; Cardiologist, Inst. for Res. of Dis. of Civilization, Univ. of Innsbruck, St. Radegund (Austria).

MARTIN, C. G., M.D.; Med. Dir. Wesso Foundation, Oak Park, Illinois (U. S. A.).

MAUET, R. B., M.D.; Physician, Schenectady, New York (U. S. A.).

MAYER, G. A., M.D.; Lecturer in Med., Queen's Univ., Kingston, Ontario (Canada).

McCLUNG, L., M.D.; Physician, Gen. Practice, New Kensington, Pennsylvania (U. S. A.).

McCOY, H. I., M.D.; Chief, Dept. Med., Scripps Mem. Hospital, La Jolla, California (U. S. A.).

MELLEROWICZ, H., M.D.; Prof., Univ. of West Berlin, Dir. Inst. of Work Med., West Berlin (Germany).

MELVILLE, K. I., M.D.; Prof., Chairman Dept. Pharmacol., McGill Univ., Montreal, Quebec (Canada).

MINC, S., M.D.; Staff Member, Cardiol. Investig. Unit, Royal Perth Hospital, Perth (Australia).

MOISAN, C. E., M.D.; Physician, Richmond, Vermont (U. S. A.).

MYASNIKOV, A. L., M.D.; Dir. Inst. of Therapy of Soviet Acad. Med. Sciences, Member of Academy, Moscow (U. S. S. R.).

NAWATA, Y., M.D.; Res. Assoc., Univ. of Vermont, Burlington, Vermont (U. S. A.).

O'BRIEN, R. E., M.D.; Assoc. Prof. Med., Univ. of Vermont, Burlington, Vermont (U. S. A.).

PEISSNER, T.; Phys. Educ. Instructor, Bellows Free Academy, St. Albans, Vermont (U. S. A.).

PLUMMER, A. J., M.D.; Dir. of Macrobiology, CIBA Pharm. Co., Summit, New Jersey (U. S. A.).

POLLAK, J. J., M.D.; Fellow in Cardiol., Mary Hitchcock Hospital, Hanover, New Hampshire (U. S. A.).

PURSHOTTAM, N., M.D.; Asst. Prof. Prevent. Med., Univ. of California, School of Med., San Francisco, California (U. S. A.).

PUSHKIN, W., M.D.; Chief of Med., Charleston Gen. Hospital, Charleston, West Virginia (U. S. A.).

RAAB, W., M.D.; Em. Prof. Exp. Med., Univ. of Vermont, Burlington, Vermont (U. S. A.).

RANDALL, W. C., Ph.D.; Prof. and Chairman, Dept. Physiol., Loyola Univ., Stritch School of Med., Chicago, Illinois (U. S. A.).

REEVES, E. L., M.D.; Physician, Lewiston, Maine (U. S. A.).

REGAN, T. J., M.D.; Assoc. Prof. Medicine, Seaton Hall College of Med., Jersey City, New Jersey (U. S. A.).

RICHARDSON, J. A., Ph.D.; Prof. Pharmacol., Med. Coll. of South Carolina, Charleston, South Carolina (U. S. A.).

RITOTA, M. C., M.D.; Dir. of Research, Columbus Hospital, Newark, New Jersey (U. S. A.).

ROSENMAN, R. H., M.D.; Asst. Dir. Harold Brunn Institute, Mount Zion Hospital, Med. Center, San Francisco, California (U. S. A.).

RUSSEK, H. I., M.D.; Consultant on Cardiovas. Dis., U. S. Publ. Health Service Hospital, Staten Island, New York (U. S. A.).

RUTHERFORD, K., M.D.; Staff Physician, Oak Ridge National Lab., Oak Ridge, Tennessee (U. S. A.).

SAGER, R., M.D.; Assoc. Med. Dir., Health Ins. Phys., New York City, New York (U. S. A.).

SAWYER, W. A., M.D.; Med. Consultant, Internat. Assoc. of Machinists, Washington, D. C. (U. S. A.).

SCHAEFER, H., M.D.; Prof. and Dir. Physiolog. Inst., Univ. of Heidelberg, Heidelberg (West Germany).

SCHIMERT, G. E., M.D.; Prof. of Medicine, Dir. Inst. Preventive Cardiol., Univ. of Munich, Munich (West Germany).

SCHMIDT-DINCKLAGE, D.; Physiotherapist, Sonthofen (West Germany).

SELYE, H., M.D.; Prof. and Dir. Inst. Experim. Med. & Surg., Univ. of Montreal, Montreal, Quebec (Canada).

SHARNOFF, T. G., M.D.; Pathologist, Mt. Vernon Hospital, Mt. Vernon, New York (U. S. A.).

SIGLER, L. H., M.D.; Consulting Cardiologist, Adelphi Hospital, Brooklyn, New York (U. S. A.).

SLATER, R. J., M.D.; Dean, Univ. of Vermont Coll. of Med., Burlington, Vermont (U. S. A.).

SMITH, D. W., M.D.; Med. Dir., Greater New York Conf. of Seventh Day Adventists, New York City, New York (U. S. A.).

SMITH, R. H., M.D.; Regional Dir., Internat. Telephone & Telegraph Corp., Nutley, New Jersey (U. S. A.).

SMODLAKA, V., M.D., D.Sc.; Inst. of Phys. Med. and Rehabil., New York Univ. Med. School, New York City, New York (U. S. A.).

STANTON, H. C., Ph.D.; Cardiovasc. Group Leader, Dept. Pharmacol., Mead Johnson & Co., Evansville, Indiana (U. S. A.).

STARCICH, R., M.D.; Prof. Clin. Med., Univ. of Parma, Parma (Italy).

STEINBERG, H. H., M.D.; Asst. Med. Dir., Internat. Harvester Co., Chicago, Illinois (U. S. A.).

STOLBERG, D. C.; Asst. Prof. Univ. Toledo, Div. Health, Phys. Educ. and Recr., Toledo, Ohio (U. S. A.).

STULTZ, A. W., Ph.D.; Prof. Anatomy, Univ. of Vermont, Burlington, Vermont (U. S. A.).

TAUBER, J. B., M.D., Ph.D.; Works Physician, J. and L. Steel Corp., Aliquippa, Pennsylvania (U. S. A.).

TERRIEN, C. M., M.D.; Assoc. Prof. Med., Univ. of Vermont, Pres. Vermont Heart Assoc., Burlington, Vermont (U. S. A.).

TOMB, E. M.; Treasurer, Independent Citizens Research Foundation for Study of Degenerative Dis., New York City, New York (U. S. A.).

TOOR, M., M.D.; Prof., Head of Med. Dept. and Cardiopulm. Lab., Beilinson Hospital, Petach Tikva (Israel).

UPTON, L., M.D.; The Pentagon, Washington, D. C. (U. S. A.).

VAN HUSS, W. D.; Prof. Human Energy Lab., Michigan State Univ., East Lansing, Michigan (U. S. A.).

WARDWELL, W. J.; Assoc. Prof. Sociology, Univ. of Connecticut, Storrs, Connecticut (U. S. A.).

WASSERMIL, H., M.D.; Dir., Dept. Cardiovas. Rehabil., Beilinson Hospital, Petach Tikva (Israel).

WEAR, C. L.; Assoc. Prof. Phys. Educ. for Men, Univ. of Nebraska, Lincoln, Nebraska (U. S. A.).

WENZEL, D. G.; Prof. of Pharmacol., Dean, School of Pharmacy, Univ. of Kansas, Lawrence, Kansas (U. S. A.).

WHITE, P. D., M.D., Sc.D., LL.D.; Em. Clin, Prof. Med., Harvard Medical School, Boston, Massachusetts (U. S. A.).

WINTER, H. W. J., M.D.; Physician, Ohlstadt (West Germany).

WOLFFE, J. B., M.D.; Valley Forge Heart Hospital, Norristown, Pennsylvania (U. S. A.).

INDEX

(NOTE: Page numbers in **boldface** type indicate that the respective items either constitute the main subject on the thus marked page (s) or that they are discussed there with more details or emphasis than on the other pages listed under the same item.)